FOUNDATIONS OF
CLINICAL RESEARCH
APPLICATIONS TO PRACTICE

2nd Edition

Leslie Gross Portney, PhD, PT
Associate Professor
MGH Institute of Health Professions
Graduate Programs in Physical Therapy
Research Associate
Massachusetts General Hospital
Boston, Massachusetts

Mary P. Watkins, MS, PT
Clinical Associate Professor
MGH Institute of Health Professions
Graduate Programs in Physical Therapy
Clinical Associate
Massachusetts General Hospital
Boston, Massachusetts

Prentice Hall Health
Upper Saddle River, New Jersey 07458

Library of Congress Cataloging-in-Publication Data
Portney, Leslie Gross.
    Foundations of clinical research : applications to practice / Leslie Gross Portney, Mary
P. Watkins.—2nd ed.
        p. cm.
    Includes bibliographical references and index.
    ISBN 0-8385-2695-0
    1. Medicine—Research—Methodology.   I. Watkins, Mary P.   II. Title.
    R850.P56 2000
610'.72.—dc21
                                                                            99-055198

Publisher: *Julie Alexander*
Editor-in-Chief: *Cheryl Mehalik*
Acquisitions Editor: *Mark Cohen*
Editorial Assistant: *Melissa Kerian*
Director of Marketing: *Leslie Cavaliere*
Marketing Manager: *Kristin Walton*
Marketing Coordinator: *Cindy Frederick*
Director of Production and Manufacturing: *Bruce Johnson*
Managing Production Editor: *Patrick Walsh*
Production Liaison: *Cathy O'Connell*
Production Editor: *Michael Jennings, Carlisle Communications, Ltd.*
Senior Production Manager: *Ilene Sanford*
Creative Director: *Marianne Frasco*
Cover Design: *Maria Guglielmo*
Cover Director: *Jayne Conte*
Composition: *Carlisle Communications, Ltd.*
Presswork/Binding: *RR Donnelley and Sons, Harrisonburg*

ISBN 0-8385-2695-0

Prentice-Hall International (UK) Limited, *London*
Prentice-Hall of Australia Pty. Limited, *Sydney*
Prentice-Hall Canada Inc., *Toronto*
Prentice-Hall Hispanoamericana, S.A., *Mexico*
Prentice-Hall of India Private Limited, *New Delhi*
Prentice-Hall of Japan, Inc., *Tokyo*
Prentice-Hall (Singapore) Pte. Ltd.
Editora Prentice-Hall do Brasil, Ltda., *Rio de Janeiro*

ISBN 0-8385-2695-0

90000

9 780838 526958

To our families

Skip, Devon, Lindsay
Mom and Dad

John, Sarah, Leah
and the Friendship Trust

whose love and support
make all things possible

and

to all of our students

Thank you for the inspiration

Contents

APPENDICES

Preface

The second edition of this book will continue to serve as a comprehensive reference for a variety of research situations. As before, it is written for students and practitioners in the health professions as they become critical consumers of published research, and for those who are actively engaged in clinical research activities.

The framework of this text continues to reflect the process of research as a dynamic activity. The book is divided into five parts, each focusing on a different phase of the research process. Part I introduces the concept of research, and how theory and ethics impact our choices. Part II includes a complete discussion of measurement issues that affect research and clinical practice. In Part III, we consider the broad scope of experimental, exploratory and descriptive research designs. Part IV focuses on the application of statistical procedures, ranging from descriptive to multivariate methods. We continue to take a conceptual approach to statistics, although calculations are included for those who need to go through the steps of analysis to improve their understanding. Part V addresses communication issues, from the inception of a research project to the dissemination of results. Appendix A provides tables for statistical analysis. Appendix B is a handy guide for choosing statistical procedures based on design specifications. Appendix C is devoted to explanations of power analysis. Appendix D describes methods of data transformation. And Appendix E is a sample informed consent form, illustrating the required ethical elements.

We hope this text will always be a work in progress, as the directions and priorities of clinical research continue to evolve with the ever changing health care environment. When we started the revision, many people asked how much change there could be—after all, statistics and research design really haven't changed, have they? Our first inclination was to agree, until we began to consider how the concern for health care outcomes has changed the face of clinical research. Over the past decade we have seen a dramatic shift in research philosophies and paradigms that guide the conduct of research, the types of questions that are deemed important, the comprehensive nature of the measurement of outcomes, and the sophisticated use of data analysis procedures.

Changes in this edition were made to reflect popular approaches to analysis and design, and to address the focus of health care-related research through the 1990s and into the 21st Century. We have added or expanded several topics, including discussion of outcomes research and the disablement model, validity and diagnostic screening, meta-analysis, scales used in survey and outcomes research, logistic regression, measures of reliability, and data management to prepare for computer analysis. Examples throughout the text have been updated to reflect the contemporary concern for outcomes research and the need to adapt designs and measurement tools to address these issues. Appendix C now includes concepts of power analysis for correlation, regression, and chi-square as well as the *t*-test and analysis of variance. In the statistics chapters, we have provided simulated output from computer analysis in shaded boxes, assuming that most of us are using computer packages for this purpose, and will need to understand the information provided in such output. We have used SPSS as our model, although we have tried to describe this output in a generic format as much as possible.

Adding to an already large book meant leaving some things out or abbreviating their coverage. This we have also done, with careful consideration of the types of analysis that we have seen most often in the medical and health literature. We hope those who use the book will not find important information missing.

We have continually received feedback that one of the major strengths of the first edition was the use of examples from the clinical research literature. We have expanded the scope of these examples to reflect current trends in health care across multiple disciplines. Where examples are taken from published research, they have been chosen to illustrate specific designs or concepts. These studies were not necessarily selected on the basis of their validity or accuracy. We urge our readers to use their critical skills in evaluating research reports.

There can be no greater pleasure than the realization that one's efforts have been appreciated. We have been privileged to hear from people all over the globe who have found this book a useful text for classroom use as well as a comprehensive reference for clinical research. When the book was first published, we had hoped that it would serve a variety of purposes, and that it would find a variety of audiences. It has done that. Faculty, students and clinicians have realized that the scope of the book allows it to fulfill different needs at different times. We encourage faculty to use components of the book to fit the level of their students and their course objectives.

We have heard from colleagues and students in physical therapy, occupational therapy, speech therapy, nursing, exercise physiology, medicine, and public health—at the undergraduate, master's, and doctoral levels—and all have found an important use for the book. We have heard from people as far away as Taiwan, Thailand, Canada, Sweden, Australia, England, and Hong Kong. Thank you to everyone who has taken the time to come up to us at meetings or to call or write. We hope that our revisions will continue to provide this broadly applicable foundation for critical analysis of literature and implementation of clinical research studies.

As ever, we share our triumphs and disappointments with our families. The girls are older now—so are we. And Skip and John are still doing the dishes. We cannot find meaning in all of this without them.

Leslie G. Portney
Mary P. Watkins
Boston, 1999

Acknowledgments

We would like to acknowledge the special contributions of many individuals who gave of their time and wisdom to make this book a reality. Jack Echternach, EdD, PT, Old Dominion University; Susan Roush, PhD, PT, University of Rhode Island; Virgil Mathiowetz, PhD, OTR/L, University of Minnesota; and Marlene Aitken, PhD, Creighton University provided thorough reviews that were invaluable as we prepared the second edition. We are indebted to Diane Jette, DSc, PT, for her expertise in epidemiology and revision of Chapter 15. We are especially grateful to faculty and students at the MGH Institute of Health Professions whose ideas and insights helped to shape the book and improve the content, most notably Marianne Beninato, PhD, PT, Joan Fitzmaurice, RN, PhD, Kathy Gill-Body, MS, PT, NCS, Bette Ann Harris, MS, PT, Aimee Klein, MS, PT, OCS, Mary Knab, MS, PT, David Krebs, PhD, PT, Chris McGibbon, PhD, Susan Mercik Davis, MS, PT, and Patricia Sullivan, PhD, PT. We extend a hearty thanks to Carolyn Baum, PhD, OTR/L, and the faculty and students at Washington University School of Medicine, Programs in Occupational Therapy, who through the use of the book, have provided important feedback. Jay Piccarillo, MD, Jan Duchek, PhD, and Dorothy Edwards, PhD, shared the perspectives of medicine and psychology, which helped to define the applicability of the book across disciplines.

We are grateful to everyone at Appleton & Lange and Prentice Hall who have kept us on track over the years, especially our editors, Cheryl Mehalik and Mark Cohen. We thank them both for their advice, guidance, encouragement, and most of all their patience.

PART I

Foundations of Clinical Research

CHAPTER

1

A Concept of Research

The ultimate purpose of a profession is to develop a knowledge base that will maximize the effectiveness of practice. To that end, health professionals have recognized the necessity for documenting and testing elements of clinical practice through rigorous and objective analysis and scientific inquiry. The concept of **evidence-based practice** represents the fundamental principle that the provision of quality care will depend on our ability to make choices that have been confirmed by sound scientific data, and that our decisions are based on the best evidence currently available. If we look at the foundations of clinical practice, however, we are faced with the reality that often compels practitioners to make intelligent, logical, best-guess decisions when scientific evidence is not available.

This situation is even more of an issue because of the economic challenges confronting health care today. Clinical research has therefore become an imperative, driving clinical judgments, the organization of practice, and reimbursement. The task of addressing the needs of the present and future is one that falls on the shoulders of all clinicians—whether we function as consumers of professional literature or scientific investigators—to collect meaningful data, to analyze outcomes, and to critically apply research findings to promote changes that will foster effective and efficient methods of providing health care services. The purpose of this text is to provide a frame of reference that will bring together the comprehensive skills needed to promote critical inquiry as part of the clinical decision-making process.

In this chapter we develop a concept of research that can be applied to clinical practice, as a method of generating new knowledge and justifying intervention. Our exploration of this concept will build on an historic perspective of clinical research, an appreciation for the different ways one can acquire knowledge, identification of the different types of research that can be applied to clinical questions, and an understanding of the process of clinical research.

A DEFINITION OF CLINICAL RESEARCH

The concept of research in health professions has evolved with the development of techniques of practice and changes in the health care system. Traditionally, research has connoted controlled laboratory experiments, run by scientists in white lab coats using complex instrumentation; however, the maturation of a clinical profession brings with it the realization that research has a broader meaning as it is applied to the patients and situations encountered in practice. *Clinical research* is a structured process of investigating facts and theories and exploring connections. It proceeds in a systematic way to examine clinical conditions and outcomes, to establish relationships among clinical phenomena, to generate evidence for decision making, and to provide the impetus for improving methods of practice.

Clinical research must be *empirical* and *critical;* that is, results must be observable, documented, and examined for their validity.[1] This objective process is, however, also a dynamic and creative activity, performed in many different settings, using a variety of quantitative and qualitative measurement tools, and focusing on the application of clinical theory and interventions. It is a way of satisfying one's curiosity about clinical phenomena, of stimulating the intellectual pursuit of truth to understand or explain clinical events, and of generating new or different ways of viewing clinical problems.

Stressing the importance of objective documentation as an essential element in clinical research does not mean that practice can be reduced to a finite science. There is no pure "scientific method" that can account for the influence of intuition and creativity in clinical judgment. Making clinical decisions in the face of uncertainty and variability is part of the "art" of clinical practice. We cannot, however, dissociate the art from the science that supports it. The concept of the *scientist practitioner* has been proposed as a useful model to address the need for direct involvement of practitioners in establishing and testing the scientific and theoretical bases for therapeutic interventions.[2] This model implies that science and practice are two facets of the same fundamental entity. This is indeed a position we take as we explore the ways in which research supports and is driven by clinical decision-making processes and practice issues. Many approaches to scientific inquiry have been developed that provide a greater opportunity for clinicians to integrate research concepts into their practice. We address these various approaches in some detail as we explore the role of research in clinical professions.

CONTEMPORARY PERSPECTIVES

We can appreciate current standards and priorities in research as part of the historical shifts in rehabilitation and medicine in the United States through the latter half of the 20th century. Three major issues emerge as important elements in this process.

Changes in the Health Care System

The first issue concerns the noteworthy changes that have taken place in the structure and economics of health care delivery systems since the end of World War II. Early years in this period were characterized by a marked increase in the number of hospitals and physicians, striking development of new technology, and expanded insurance coverage through Medicare and Medicaid. These changes dramatically increased availability of technology and health care services, but also resulted in soaring costs that were seemingly unchecked.[3]

Through the 1970s and 1980s expenditures continued to rise, and those who provided reimbursement began to set cost-saving policies, leading to the prospective payment system and the onset of managed care. The federal government and regulatory agencies mandated documentation of the quality and cost of care. Suddenly, many of the decisions regarding evaluation and treatment were being dictated by the payers, who established tighter controls on prices. This dilemma was compounded by the lack of systematic data on outcomes of medical services to justify costs.[3, 4]

As we enter the 21st century, a new health care agenda has emerged, wherein consumers, payers, and providers of health services need to know more about the relative costs, safety, and effectiveness of all procedures used for diagnosis, treatment, and prevention. It is the strong emphasis on *effectiveness* at *reasonable cost* that has truly reshaped the research agenda, requiring that clinicians demonstrate how the outcomes of care reflect its quality.

Measurement of Outcomes

The second issue that has changed the focus of clinical research concerns the importance of documenting **outcomes.** The concept of looking at outcomes as the validation of quality care is not new. Historically, the triad of *structure, process,* and *outcomes* has been used as the barometer of quality.[5] Structure was assessed through organizational standards, and process by quality assurance programs looking at details such as charges and record keeping. Outcomes of care were typically assessed in terms of morbidity, mortality, length of stay, and readmissions. Today, the concept of outcomes has been expanded to fit with the World Health Organization's definition of health, which includes physical, social, and psychological well-being.[6] Looking at the effects of treatment now includes consideration of patient satisfaction, patient preferences, self-assessment of functional capacity, and quality of life. Clinicians and especially patients have always looked at functional outcome as the ultimate measure of the success of intervention. At this time, however, the state of health care has forced us to defend how outcomes are defined and documented, and how they are used to substantiate the efficiency and effectiveness of treatment.

To be meaningful the outcomes agenda must influence public policy, routine monitoring of medical care, and standardized assessment of patient outcomes.[7] Clinical practice databases must be developed to include functional outcome measures and other relevant information to contribute to the evaluation of outcomes.[8] Clinical managers now look at these data as a means of supporting practice and organizational structure. The objective of *outcomes management* has generated a renewed understanding of the link between clinical management decisions, treatment decisions, and measured documentation of effectiveness.[9, 10] The development of valid instruments to measure function and health status, in general and in disease-specific terms, has become a major thrust of health research and has provided a mechanism for understanding how functional outcomes relate to specific elements of health care.

The Disablement Model

The third issue in understanding the evolution of research is related to the overriding framework for the delivery of health care. This has historically been the *biomedical model,* which focuses on a linear relationship between pathology and resulting impairments

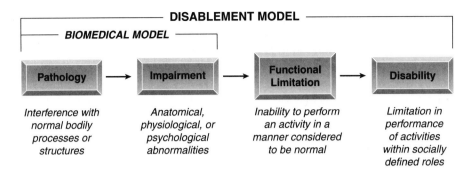

FIGURE 1.1   The disablement model, showing the relationship among pathology, impairments, functional limitations, and disability (using the terminology of Nagi[14]). The biomedical model is illustrated at one end of this hierarchy, focusing solely on the direct relationship between pathology and impairments.

(see Figure 1.1). Within this model, health is viewed as the absence of disease and the assumption is made that disease and injury can be treated and cured. The model confines attention to physical aspects of health, without consideration of how the patient is affected by illness.[11] The primary outcomes of interest under this model are the traditional endpoints of disease or death.[12, 13] However, as health care advances and people live longer, practitioners appreciate the inadequacies of the biomedical model for dealing with the common problems of aging, chronic disease, and disability, which do not fall within the rubric of "treat and cure," and the consequent need to look differently at the assessment of "successful" interventions.

The **disablement model** has been introduced as an alternative (see Figure 1.1), providing a framework for assessing the effect of acute and chronic conditions by expanding the biomedical model to emphasize functional consequences and social role. This model demonstrates the multidirectional relationships among pathology, impairments, functional limitations, and disability.[14, 15] Although variants of this model have been proposed with different terminology,[14, 16] they all include the basic elements of pathology, organ system dysfunction, restrictions in ADL, and limitations of role performance as a member of society.[17] Accordingly, this model provides a conceptual basis for looking at outcomes within the broader context of health, including psychological and social domains, general health status, well-being, and quality of life.[12, 18–20] It also provides a framework for research by suggesting theoretical relationships between impairments and functional outcomes, and behavioral or environmental risk factors that will influence those relationships.[18, 21]

Within the disablement model we must begin to identify which outcome measures are relevant. Health status and functional questionnaires provide one approach. We must also continue to look at changes in impairments and basic functional activities, such as gait or the performance of a particular functional or occupational task, to provide a complete picture of improvement. As we become more involved in the documentation of outcomes it is imperative that we understand the measurement properties of the tools we use so they can be applied and interpreted properly. We can then begin to ask questions that will verify how changes at the impairment level will directly or indirectly impact performance at the functional level. These questions will guide research on the efficacy of individual interventions and on different models of treatment selection, application, and management.[22] The assumption, of course, is that by describing and measuring the outcomes of care in a comprehensive way, we can more appropriately evaluate the success of treatment, make more informed clinical decisions, and change practice for the better.

SOURCES OF KNOWLEDGE

The information that is used to make clinical decisions and to support clinical research can be acquired in many different ways. As one participates in the pursuit of knowledge, it is interesting to reflect on the sources of information that guide our thinking and decision making. How do we decide which test to perform, which intervention should be most successful, which patients have the best chance of responding positively to a given treatment? Oftentimes clinical problems can be solved on the basis of scientific evidence, but in many situations such evidence does not exist. It is important, then, to consider how we come to "know" things, and how we can appropriately use what we know as we are faced with clinical problems.

Tradition

As members of an organized culture, we accept certain truths as givens. Something is thought to be true simply because people have always known it to be true. Within such a belief system, we inherit knowledge and accept precedent, without need for external validation. Rehabilitation science is steeped in tradition as a guide to practice and as a foundation for treatment. We have all been faced with clinical, administrative, or educational practices that are continued just because "that is the way they have always been done."

Tradition is useful in that it offers a common foundation for communication and interaction within a society or profession. Therefore, each generation is not responsible for reformulating an understanding of the world through the development of new concepts. Nevertheless, tradition as a source of knowledge poses a serious problem in clinical science, because many traditions have neither been evaluated for their validity nor been tested against potentially better alternatives. Sole reliance on precedent as a reason for making clinical choices generally stifles the search for new information, and may perpetuate an idea even when contrary evidence is available.

Authority

We frequently find ourselves turning to specialized sources of **authority** for answers to questions. If we have a problem with finances, we seek the services of an accountant. If we need legal advice for purchasing a home, we hire a real estate lawyer. In the medical profession we regularly pursue the expertise of specialists for specific medical problems. Given the rapid accumulation of knowledge and technical advances and the need to make decisions in situations when we are not expert, it is most reasonable and natural to place our trust in those who are authoritative on an issue by virtue of specialized training or experience.

Authorities often become known as expert sources of information based on their success, experience, or reputation. When an authority states that something is true, we accept it. As new techniques are developed, we often jump to use them without demanding evidence of their scientific merit, ignoring potential limitations, even when the underlying theoretical rationale is unclear.[23, 24] Too often we find ourselves committed to one approach over others, perhaps based on what we were taught, because the technique is empirically useful. This approach is necessary in situations when scientific evidence is unavailable; however, we jeopardize our professional responsibility if these techniques are not critically analyzed and if their effects are not scientifically documented.

The danger of uncritical reliance on authoritative canon is well illustrated by the unyielding belief in the medical tenets of Galen (A.D. 138–201), whose teachings were accepted without challenge in the Western world for 16 centuries. When physicians in the 16th and 17th centuries began dissecting human organs, they were not always able to validate Galen's statements. His defenders, in strict loyalty and unwillingness to doubt the authority, wrote that if the new findings did not agree with Galen's teachings, the discrepancy should be attributed to the fact that nature had changed![25]

Trial and Error

The **trial and error** method of data gathering was probably the earliest approach to solving a problem. The individual faced with a problem attempts one solution and evaluates its effects. If the effects are reasonably satisfactory, the solution is generally adopted. If not, another solution is tried. We use this method when we have no other basis for making a decision. We have all used trial and error at one time or another in our personal lives and in professional practice. Trial and error incorporates the use of intuition and creativity in selecting alternatives when one approach does not work.

The major disadvantage of trial and error is its haphazard and unsystematic nature and the fact that knowledge obtained in this way is usually not shared, making it inaccessible to others facing similar problems. In situations when a good response is not obtained, a continuous stream of different solutions may be tried, with no basis for sorting out why they are not working.

Trial and error is by nature extremely time consuming and limiting in scope, for although several possible solutions may be proposed for a single problem, the process generally ends once a "satisfactory" response is obtained. Experience is often based on these solutions, and when similar situations arise, a better solution, as yet untried, may never be tested. Therefore, a clinician using this method should never conclude that the "best" solution has been found.

Logical Reasoning

Many clinical problems are solved through the use of logical thought processes. Logical reasoning as a method of knowing combines personal experience, intellectual faculties, and formal systems of thought. It is a systematic process that has been used throughout history as a way of answering questions and acquiring new knowledge. Two distinctive types of reasoning are used as a means of understanding and organizing phenomena.

Deductive Reasoning

Deductive reasoning is characterized by the acceptance of a general proposition, or premise, and the subsequent inferences that can be drawn in specific cases. The ancient Greek philosophers introduced this systematic method for drawing conclusions by using a series of three interrelated statements, called a **syllogism,** containing (1) a major premise, (2) a minor premise, and (3) a conclusion. A classic syllogism will serve as an example:

1. All living things must die.   [major premise]
2. Man is a living thing.   [minor premise]
3. Therefore, all men must die.   [conclusion]

In deductive reasoning, if the premises are true, then it follows that the conclusion must be true. Scientists use deductive logic by beginning with known scientific principles or generalizations, and deducing specific assertions that are relevant to a specific question. The observed facts will cause the scientist either to confirm, to reject, or to modify the conclusion. The greater the accuracy of the premise, the greater the accuracy of the conclusion.

For example, we might reason that exercise will be an effective intervention to prevent falls in the elderly in the following ways:

1. Exercise improves postural stability.
2. People who fall have impaired postural stability.
3. Therefore, exercise will decrease the incidence of falls.

This system of deductive reasoning produces a testable hypothesis: If we develop an exercise program for individuals who have impaired stability, we should see a decrease in the number of falls. This has been the basis for several studies. For example, Wolf and colleagues used this logic as the theoretical premise for their study comparing balance training and tai chi exercise to improve postural stability in a sample of older, inactive adults.[26] Tinetti and coworkers designed a multiple-risk-factor intervention strategy, including exercise, aimed at modifying risk factors for falls in community-dwelling elderly persons.[27] Both studies found that the exercise groups either had a lower incidence of falls or delayed onset of falls, supporting the premise from which the treatment was deduced.

Of course, deductive reasoning does have limitations. Its usefulness is totally dependent on the truth of its premises. In many situations, the theoretical assumptions on which a study is based may be faulty or unsubstantiated, so that the study and its conclusions have questionable validity. In addition, we must recognize that deductive conclusions are only elaborations on previously existing knowledge. Deductive reasoning can organize what is already known and can suggest new relationships, but it cannot be a source of new knowledge. Scientific inquiry cannot be conducted on the basis of deductive reasoning alone because of the difficulty involved in establishing the universal truth of many statements dealing with scientific phenomena.

Inductive Reasoning

Inductive reasoning reflects the reverse type of logic, developing generalizations from specific observations. It begins with experience and results in conclusions or generalizations that are probably true. This approach to knowing was advanced in the late 16th century by Francis Bacon, who called for an end to reliance on authority as absolute truth. He proposed that the discovery of new knowledge required direct observation of nature, without prejudice or preconceived notions. Facts gathered on a sample of events could lead to inferences about the whole. This reasoning gave birth to the scientific approach to problem solving, and often acts as the basis for common sense. For example, we might observe that those patients who exercise do not fall, and that those who do not exercise fall more often. We might then conclude, through induction, that exercise will improve postural stability.

Inductive reasoning has its limitations as well. The quality of the knowledge derived from inductive reasoning is dependent on the representativeness of the specific observations used as the basis for generalizations. To be absolutely certain of an inductive conclusion, the researcher would have to observe all possible examples of the event, which is feasible only in the rare situations when the set of events in question is quite small. We therefore find ourselves relying mostly on imperfect induction based on incomplete observations. In the preceding example, if we observe the effects of exercise on a sample of elderly persons, and if balance and exercise responses are related to aging, our conclusion may not be valid for younger individuals.

Even with these limitations, the process of logical reasoning, both deductive and inductive, is an essential component of scientific inquiry and clinical problem solving. Both forms of reasoning are used to design research studies and interpret research data. Introductory statements in research articles often illustrate deductive logic, as the author explains how a research hypothesis was developed from an existing theory of the general body of knowledge. Inductive reasoning is used in the discussion section of a research report, where generalizations or conclusions are proposed from the data obtained in the study. Even though imperfect induction does not allow us to reach infallible conclusions, it is the clinical scientist's responsibility to critically evaluate the validity of the information and to draw reasonable conclusions. These conclusions must then be verified through further empirical testing.

The following statement, attributed to Galen, illustrates the potential for the abuse of logic:

> All who drink of this remedy recover in a short time, except those whom it
> does not help, who all die. Therefore, it is obvious that it fails only in incurable
> cases.[25]

The Scientific Method

The **scientific method** is the most rigorous process for acquiring new knowledge, incorporating elements of deduction and induction in a systematic and controlled analysis of phenomena. The scientific approach to inquiry is based on two assumptions related to the nature of reality. One is that nature is orderly and regular and that events are, to some extent, consistent and predictable. Second, we assume that events or conditions are not random or accidental and, therefore, have one or more causes that can be discovered. These assumptions allow us to direct clinical thinking toward establishing cause-and-effect relationships so that we can develop rational solutions to clinical problems.

The scientific approach has been defined as a *systematic, empirical, controlled, and critical examination of hypothetical propositions about the associations among natural phenomena.*[1] The *systematic* nature of research implies a sense of order and discipline that will ensure an acceptable level of reliability. It suggests a logical sequence that leads from identification of a problem, through the organized collection and objective analysis of data, to the interpretation of findings. The *empirical* component of scientific research refers to the necessity for documenting objective data through direct observation. Findings are thereby grounded in reality rather than in personal bias or subjective belief of the researcher.

The element of *control*, however, is the most important characteristic that sets the scientific method apart from the other sources of knowledge. To understand how one phenomenon relates to another, the scientist practitioner must attempt to control factors that are not directly related to the variables in question. Clinical problems such as pain, functional disability, cognitive dysfunction, deformity, cardiopulmonary insufficiency, or motor control concern highly complex phenomena and often involve the effects of many interacting factors. Investigators must be able to control extraneous influences to have critical confidence in research outcomes. This important concept is explored in greater detail in Chapter 9.

A commitment to *critical examination* means that the researcher must subject findings to empirical testing and to the scrutiny of other scientists. Scientific investigation is thereby characterized by a capacity for self-correction based on objective validation of data from primary sources of information. This characterization minimizes the influence of bias, and makes the researcher responsible for logical and defensible interpretation of outcomes.

Limitations of the Scientific Method

Although scientific research is considered the highest form of acquiring knowledge, it is by no means perfect, especially when it is applied to the study of human behavior and performance. The complexity and variability within nature and the environment and the unique psychosocial and physiological capacities of individuals will always introduce some uncertainty into the interpretation and generalization of data. These issues differentiate clinical research from laboratory research in physical and biological sciences, where environment and even heredity are often under complete control. This does not mean that the scientific method cannot be applied to human studies, but it does mean that clinical researchers must be acutely aware of extraneous influences to interpret findings in a meaningful way. Some clinical findings may actually be strengthened by the knowledge that patients generally improve with certain treatments despite physiological and environmental differences.

TYPES OF RESEARCH

The research process delineates a general strategy for gathering, analyzing, and interpreting data to answer a question. A variety of schema have been used to classify research strategies according to their purpose and objectives.

Basic Versus Applied Research

One system of classification is based on the objective of the research, or the degree of utility of the findings. **Basic research** is done to obtain empirical data that can be used to develop, refine, or test theory. Basic research is directed toward the acquisition of new knowledge for its own sake, motivated by intellectual curiosity, without reference to the potential practical use of results. Researchers who study how blood cells function or who examine the structure and function of parts of the brain are doing basic research. Of course, basic studies may eventually lead to numerous practical applications, such as developing a treatment for leukemia or grafting brain cells to treat Parkinsonism, but these are not the direct goals of the basic scientist.

In contrast, **applied research** is directed toward solving immediate practical problems with functional applications and testing the theories that direct practice. It is usually carried out under actual practice conditions on subjects who represent the group to which the results will be applied. Most clinical research falls into this category. When therapists study the effect of electrical stimulation for reducing muscle spasm or compare the effectiveness of eccentric and concentric exercises for increasing strength, they are doing applied research.

Although the distinction between basic and applied research appears to create a dichotomy, in reality a continuum exists between the two extremes. We recognize that rehabilitation and health care are applied sciences, but that many of the theories that guide practice are founded on basic science principles. Today, clinical research is often a hybrid, combining elements of both basic and applied science. Many studies provide clinical application and new knowledge that contributes to a theoretical understanding of behavior.

Experimental and Nonexperimental Research

Another common classification defines research as either experimental or nonexperimental. **Experimental research** refers to investigations in which the researcher manipulates and controls one or more variables and observes the resultant variation in other variables. The major purpose of an experiment is to compare conditions or intervention groups, to suggest cause-and-effect relationships. **Nonexperimental research** refers to investigations that are generally more descriptive or exploratory in nature and that do not exhibit direct control over the studied variables. This latter type of research is often referred to as *observational research,* to reflect the idea that phenomena are observed rather than manipulated.

A Continuum of Research

In a more practical schema, research can be viewed along a continuum that reflects the type of question the research is intended to answer. Within this continuum, illustrated in Figure

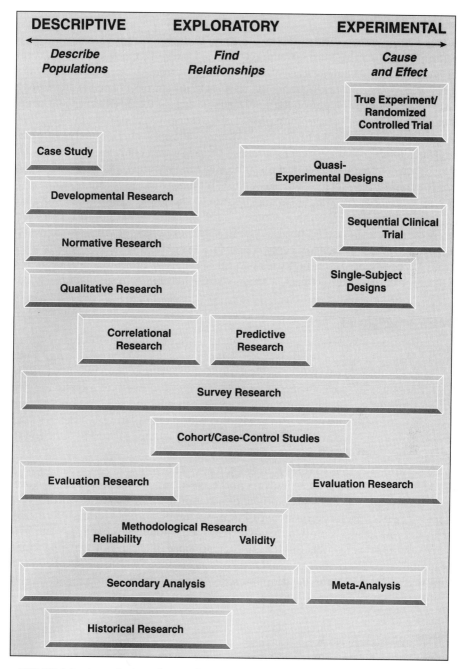

FIGURE 1.2 A continuum of research.

1.2, research methods are classified as descriptive, exploratory, or experimental. These classifications reflect different purposes of research, and within each one various types of research can be used. As a continuum suggests, however, different types of research can overlap in their purpose and may incorporate elements of more than one classification.

Descriptive Research

In **descriptive research** the researcher attempts to describe a group of individuals on a set of variables, to document their characteristics. Descriptive research may involve the use of questionnaires, interviews, or direct observation. Descriptive data allow researchers to classify and understand the scope of clinical phenomena, often providing the basis for further investigation. Several designs can be used within this approach.

A **case study,** or case series, may consist of a description of one or several patients, to document unusual conditions or the effect of innovative interventions. **Developmental research** is intended to investigate patterns of growth and change over time within selected segments of a population, or it may chronicle the natural history of a disease or disability. **Normative research** focuses on establishing normal values for specific variables, to serve as guidelines for diagnosis and treatment planning. **Qualitative research** involves collection of data through interview and observation, in an effort to characterize human experience as it occurs naturally, and to generate hypotheses about human behavior. In descriptive **evaluation research,** the investigator attempts to objectively assess a program or policy by describing the need for services or programs. **Surveys** or **questionnaires** are often used to collect descriptive information from small and large groups.

Exploratory Research

In **exploratory research** a researcher examines a phenomenon of interest and explores its dimensions, including how it relates to other factors. Using **correlational methods,** the researcher is able to search for these relationships and may generate predictions that these relationships suggest. *Predictive models* can then be used as a basis for decision making, setting expectations, and prognosis. By establishing associations, researchers can also test or model theoretical propositions. Many efforts in outcomes research use this approach to study relationships among pathologies, impairments, functional limitations, and disability.

In **epidemiology** health researchers examine associations to describe and predict risks for certain conditions using **cohort** and **case-control studies. Methodological studies** will use correlational methods to demonstrate reliability and validity of measuring instruments. As large databases begin to develop, researchers often use **secondary analysis** as a mechanism for exploring relationships. This approach involves the use of data that were collected for another purpose, but provide an opportunity for ongoing analysis. **Historical research** reconstructs the past, on the basis of archives or other records, to generate questions or suggest relationships of historical interest to a discipline.

Experimental Research

Experimental designs provide a basis for comparing two or more conditions. They control or account for the effects of extraneous factors, providing the greatest degree of confidence in the validity of outcomes and allowing the researcher to draw meaningful conclusions about observed differences. The **randomized clinical trial (RCT)** is considered the "gold standard" of experimental designs, typically involving the controlled comparison of an experimental intervention and a placebo. There are, however, many alternative models, some simple and others more complex, that provide opportunities to examine the cause of outcomes, including the systematic study of one or several individuals within the clinical environment. These include **single-subject designs** and **sequential clinical trials.** Experimental **evaluation research** is an objective assessment of the success of a program or policy, proving a method for documenting quality of care, and the efficacy or efficiency of therapeutic programs.

In **quasi-experimental research** the degree of control is limited by a variety of factors, but interpretable results can still be obtained. When true experimental conditions cannot be achieved, these designs permit comparisons, but they also acknowledge the limitations placed on conclusions. **Meta-analysis** is a process of statistically combining the findings from several studies to obtain a summary analysis.

Quantitative and Qualitative Research

In categorizing clinical research, scientists often describe studies by distinguishing between quantitative and qualitative methods. Quantitative methods may be used all along the continuum of research approaches, whereas qualitative data are generally applied to descriptive or exploratory research. **Quantitative research** involves measurement of outcomes using numerical data under standardized conditions. The advantage of the quantitative approach is the ability to summarize scales and to subject data to statistical analysis. Quantitative information may be obtained using formal instruments which address physical or physiological parameters, or by putting subjective information into an objective numerical scale.

Qualitative research is more concerned with subjective, narrative information, which typically is obtained under less structured conditions. In qualitative methodology, "measurement" is based on open-ended questions, interviews, and observations, as the researcher attempts to capture the context of the data, to better understand how phenomena are experienced by individuals. The purpose of the research may be to simply describe the state of conditions, or it may be to explore associations, formulate theory, or generate hypotheses.

THE RESEARCH PROCESS

Clinical research involves a systematic process of sequential steps that guide thinking, planning, and analysis. Whether one is collecting quantitative or qualitative data, using the research process ensures that there is a reasonable and logical framework for a study's design and conclusions. We conceptualize research as a series of nine sequential steps shown in Figure 1.3, recognizing that the order may vary and the steps may overlap in different research models. These steps can be subdivided into five general phases.

Phase I: Identify the Research Question

The first phase of the research process involves delimiting the area of research and formulating a specific research question that provides an opportunity for scientific testing (see Chapter 7). During this stage, the researcher must define the type of individual to whom the results will be generalized. Through a review of scientific literature, the

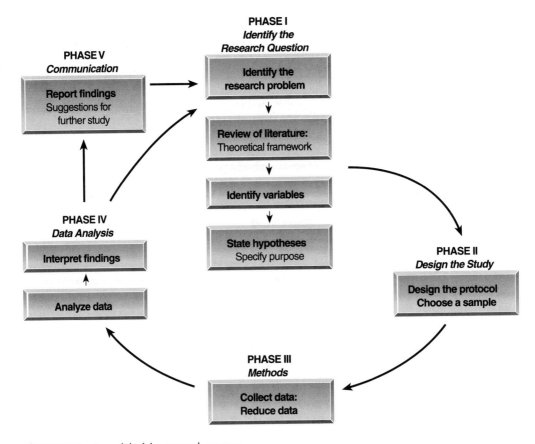

FIGURE 1.3   A model of the research process.

researcher should be able to provide a rationale for the study, a justification of the need to investigate the problem, and a theoretical framework for interpreting results. Research hypotheses are proposed to predict how response variables and treatment variables will be related and to predict clinically relevant outcomes. In descriptive or qualitative studies, guiding questions may be proposed that form the framework for the study.

Phase II: Design the Study

In phase II, the researcher designs the study and plans methods of subject selection, testing, and measurement so that all procedures are clearly mapped out (see Chapters 8 through 16). The choice of research method reflects how the researcher conceptualizes the research question. Many alternative approaches are available, depending on the nature of the data and the type of subjects. The researcher must carefully define all measurements and interventions so that the methods for data analysis are clear. The completion of the first two phases of planning results in the formulation of a *research proposal* (see Chapter 29).

Phase III: Methods

During the third phase of the research process, the researcher implements the plans designed in phases I and II. *Data collection* is typically the most time-consuming part of the research process. After data are collected and recorded, the researcher must reduce and collate the information into a useful form for analysis. Forms or tables are created for compiling the "raw data." Just as much attention to precision must be given during data reduction as during data collection.

Phase IV: Data Analysis

The fourth phase of the research process involves analyzing, interpreting, and drawing valid *conclusions* about the obtained data. It is the pulling together of all the materials relevant to the study, to apply them to a generalized or theoretical framework. Statistical procedures are applied to summarize quantitative information in a meaningful way, usually with the assistance of a computer (see Chapters 17 through 28). It is at this stage that the research hypothesis will be either supported or rejected. In qualitative studies, the researcher will look for themes that characterize the data. Through the analysis of results, the study should also lead to new questions that will stimulate further study.

Phase V: Communication

Research done in a vacuum is of little use to anyone. Researchers have a responsibility to share their findings with the appropriate audience so that others can apply the information either to clinical practice or to further research. Research reports can take many forms including journal articles, abstracts, oral presentations, and poster presentations. Students may be required to report their work in the lengthier form of a thesis or dissertation (see Chapter 30).

Finally, no research project is a dead end. Results of one study always lead to new questions. Researchers contribute to the advancement of their own work by offering suggestions for further study and recommending what kinds of additional studies would be useful for contributing to the theoretical foundations addressed in the current study.

UNDERSTANDING METHOD, CONTENT, AND PHILOSOPHY

The focus of a text such as this one is naturally on the methods and procedures of conducting research—on the mechanisms of how research is done: how phenomena are observed and measured; how different types of research fit varied research questions; how to design conditions so that relationships can be examined; and how to control and manipulate variables to demonstrate cause-and-effect relationships. By understanding the processes, definitions, and analytic procedures of research, the clinician has the building blocks to structure an investigation or interpret the work of others.

Methodology is only part of research, however. Research designs and statistical techniques cannot lead us to a research question, nor can they specify the technical procedures needed for studying that question. Designs cannot tell us what to investigate, nor do they assign meaning to the way clinical phenomena behave. Two other aspects are equally important to the concept of research: a knowledge of the subject matter that will be studied and the research philosophy of the clinical discipline.

A thorough knowledge of content related to a research question is necessary to determine relevant applications of the methods for answering the question. The researcher must be able both to determine which instruments are appropriate for measuring different variables and to apply measurement tools properly. The scientific bases for observed responses must be thoroughly understood to design a study and interpret results. Without a complete background in the relevant content, the researcher may make serious errors in data collection and analysis.

The philosophy of a discipline concerns itself with the way the subject matter is conceptualized, the overall significance of the knowledge generated by research, and what scientific approaches will contribute to an understanding of practice. How one conceives of a discipline's objectives and the scope of practice will influence the kinds of questions one will ask. We must recognize the influence of professional values on these applications. These values reflect the researcher's inclinations to consider treatment alternatives, to search for new knowledge to substantiate certain types of clinical decisions, or to investigate particular types of questions with particular methods. For instance, different paradigms will direct some clinical investigators to study behavior at the level of impairments versus outcomes, or to use qualitative versus quantitative methods.

There is no right or wrong in these contrasts. As we explore the variety of research approaches, we urge the readers to continually use their own framework for applying these methods. Our emphasis on clinical examples throughout the book is a limited attempt to demonstrate these connections. It is also relevant to consider the interdisciplinary clinical associations inherent in health care, the team approach to patient care, and the shared research agendas that might emerge from such associations. The framework that supports a research question might be broader than any one discipline's objectives and might be well served by a team of professionals.

COMMENTARY

Research and Clinical Problem Solving

As we discuss the clinical research process, it is also useful to recognize the analogy that can be drawn between research and clinical problem solving. Clinical problem solving begins with the definition of specific clinical problems, which are understood within the context of a theoretical framework. The clinician then generates a list of alternative solutions and selects one reasonable course of action. The process continues with the design of a plan of care, implementation of that plan, and the evaluation of change. It is easy to see the commonalities of this process to the design and analysis of a research question, as presented in Figure 1.3.

Two major differences distinguish clinical problem solving from clinical research, however. One difference is the purpose for which each process is used. Problem solving is used to determine solutions to particular clinical problems. Research concerns broader questions about recurrent phenomena, and is used to obtain knowledge that is generalizable beyond individual situations. In problem solving, the process usually ends with a solution. In research, outcomes generate more questions. The outcomes of clinical decisions may be shared with colleagues, but as a rule, the decisions are not intended to contribute to an overall understanding of the clinical problem beyond the immediate situation. In contrast, the goal of clinical research is to contribute to a scientific understanding of clinical phenomena, to predict outcomes and strengthen the theoretical foundations of treatment and evaluation.

The other difference between these processes concerns the degree of control that is required. Problem solving is used within the clinical environment, and deals with events and variations within that environment as they occur naturally. In contrast, the researcher attempts to control or at least account for the environment, to have confidence that observed differences are due to the imposed intervention and not due to extraneous environmental influences.

The experienced clinician will also recognize that information is not always available to justify clinical decisions. Therefore, research questions often develop out of clinical practice. In this way, problem solving and clinical research become interdependent. Research provides information on which to base clinical decisions, and problem solving contributes to the development of research questions. Both processes involve the application of orderly and systematic procedures to guide the interpretation of outcomes.

As the various approaches to clinical research and the development of clinical theory are explored further in this text, we will continue to focus on the idea that research and practice are inseparable components of clinical science and that clinicians are uniquely qualified to study and analyze their intervention techniques in a clinical environment.

KEY TERMS

evidence-based practice
outcomes
disablement model
tradition
authority
trial and error
deductive reasoning
syllogism
inductive reasoning
scientific method
basic research
applied research
experimental research
nonexperimental research

observational research
descriptive research
case study (series)
developmental research
normative research
qualitative research
evaluation research
surveys
questionnaires
exploratory research
correlational methods
predictive models
epidemiology
cohort studies

case-control studies
methodological studies
secondary analysis
historical research
experimental designs
randomized clinical trials
  (RCT)
single-subject designs
sequential clinical trials
quasi-experimental
  research
meta-analysis
quantitative research

REFERENCES

1. Kerlinger FN. *Foundations of Behavioral Research.* New York: Holt, Rinehart & Winston, 1973.
2. Barlow DH, Hayes SC, Nelson RO. *The Scientist Practitioner: Research and Accountability in Clinical and Educational Settings.* New York: Pergamon Press, 1984.
3. Relman AS. Assessment and accountability: the third revolution in medical care. *N Engl J Med* 1988;319:1220–2.

4. Wennberg JE, Freeman JL, Culp WJ. Are hospital services rationed in New Haven or over-utilised in Boston? *Lancet* 1987;1:1185–9.

5. Donabedian A. *Explorations in Quality Assessment and Monitoring.* Ann Arbor, MI: Health Administration Press, 1980.

6. World Health Organization. Constitution. *WHO Chronicle* 1947;1:29.

7. Ware JE. Conceptualizing and measuring generic health outcomes. *Cancer* 1991;67:774–9.

8. Shields RK, Leo KC, Miller B, Dostal WF, Barr R. An acute care physical therapy clinical practice data base for outcomes research. *Phys Ther* 1994;74:463–70.

9. Ellwood PM. Outcomes management: a technology of patient experience. *N Engl J Med* 1988;318:1549–1556.

10. Hart DL, Geril AC, Pfohl RL. Outcomes process in daily practice. *PT Magazine* 1997; 5(9):68–77.

11. Minaire P. Disease, illness and health: theoretical models of the disablement process. *Bull World Health Org* 1992;70:373–9.

12. Bergner M. Quality of life, health status and clinical research. *Med Care* 1989;27:S148–S156.

13. Wilkins EG, Lowery JC, Smith Jr DJ. Outcomes research: a primer for plastic surgeons. *Ann Plast Surg* 1996;37:1–11.

14. Nagi SZ. Disability concepts revisited: implications for prevention. In: Pope AM, Tarlov AR, eds. *Disability in America: Toward a National Agenda for Prevention.* Washington, DC: Division of Health Promotion and Disease Prevention, Institute of Medicine, National Academy Press, 1991.

15. Verbrugge LM, Jette AM. The disablement process. *Soc Sci Med* 1994;38:1–14.

16. World Health Organization. International Classification of Impairments, Disabilities and Handicaps. Geneva: WHO, 1980.

17. Whiteneck GG, Fongeyrollas P, Gerhart KA. Elaborating the model of disablement. In: Fuhrer MJ, ed. *Assessing Medical Rehabilitation Practices: The Promise of Outcomes Research.* Baltimore: Brookes Publishing, 1997.

18. Jette AM. Physical disablement concepts for physical therapy research and practice. *Phys Ther* 1994;74:380–6.

19. Patrick DL, Bergner M. Measurement of health status in the 1990s. *Ann Rev Public Health* 1990;11:165–83.

20. Pope AM, Tarlov AR. *Disability in America: Toward a National Agenda for Prevention.* Washington, DC: Division of Health Promotion and Disease Prevention, Institute of Medicine, National Academy Press, 1991.

21. Jette AM. Outcomes research: shifting the dominant research paradigm in physical therapy. *Phys Ther* 1995;75:865–970.

22. Whyte J. Toward a methodology for rehabilitation research. *Am J Phys Med Rehabil* 1994;73:428–35.

23. Harris SR. How should treatments be critiqued for scientific merit? *Phys Ther* 1996;76:175–81.

24. Rothstein JM. Editors note: Say it ain't so. *Phys Ther* 1994;74:175–81.

25. Silverman WA. *Human Experimentation: A Guided Step into the Unknown.* New York: Oxford University Press, 1985.

26. Wolf SL, Barnhart HX, Ellison GL, Coogler CE. The effect of Tai Chi Quan and computerized balance training on postural stability in older subjects. *Phys Ther* 1997;77:371–81.

27. Tinetti ME, Baker DI, McAvay G, et al. A multifactorial intervention to reduce the risk of falling among elderly people living in the community. *N Engl J Med* 1994;331:821–7.

CHAPTER

2

The Role of Theory in Clinical Research

Clinical research is a systematic method for evaluating the effectiveness of treatment and for establishing a basis for inductive generalizations about intervention. The ultimate goal is to further the intellectual progress of the profession by contributing to its scientific base through the development of **theory.** Theories are created out of a need to organize and give meaning to a complex collection of individual facts and observations. Methods are the means by which we conduct investigations in a reliable and valid way so that we can understand clinical phenomena. But it is theory that lets us speculate on the questions of why and how treatment works, accounting for what we observe. Theories provide the explanations for findings within the context of what is already known from the successes and failures of previous investigations. As we continue to examine observations, we try to create theoretical generalizations to form a basis for predicting future outcomes. Without such explanations we risk having to reinvent the wheel each time we are faced with a clinical problem.

A theory is a set of interrelated concepts, definitions, or propositions that specifies relationships among variables and represents a systematic view of specific phenomena.[1] Theories have always been a part of human cultures, although not all theories have been scientific. Philosophy and religion have historically played a significant part in the acceptance of theory. The medieval view that the world was flat was born out of the theory that angels held up the four corners of the earth. Naturally, the men of the day were justified in believing that if one sailed toward the horizon, eventually one would fall off the edge of the earth. Such theories went untested because of a lack of instrumentation and because it was not considered necessary to test that which was already known to be true.

In contrast, scientific theory deals with the empirical world of observation and experience, and requires constant verification. We use theory to generalize beyond a specific situation and to make predictions about what *should* happen in other similar situations. The validity of these predictions can be tested through research. The purpose of this chapter is to define the elements of theory and to describe mechanisms for developing and testing clinical theories.

PURPOSES OF THEORIES

Theories can serve several purposes in science and clinical practice, depending on how we choose to use them. Theories *summarize* existing knowledge, giving meaning to isolated empirical findings. They provide a framework for interpretation of observations. For example, theories of motor learning bring together the results of many separate studies that have examined schedules of practice, types of skills, psychomotor components of performance, and other elements of the learning process. Theories are also used to *explain* observable events by showing how variables are related. For instance, a theory of motor learning would explain the relationship between feedback and feedforward mechanisms in the learning, performance, and refinement of a motor skill.

Theories allow us to *predict* what should occur, given a set of specific circumstances. For example, one theory of motor learning states that greater changes take place during stages of initial learning than during later stages, as illustrated by a decelerating learning curve. On the basis of this theory, we could anticipate that a patient using an exercise device for the first time will experience a spurt of improvement in force output during early trials as a result of practice that will not necessarily be related to strength increases.[2] Theories can also provide a basis for predicting phenomena that cannot be empirically verified. For instance, through deductions from mathematical theories, Newton was able to predict the motion of planets around the sun long before technology was available to confirm their orbits. The element of prediction also affords us a measure of control. This concept is illustrated by analysis of the germ theory of disease, which explains how organisms in the environment cause disease states. The theory allows us to predict how changes in the environment will affect the incidence of disease. This, in turn, suggests mechanisms to control disease, such as the use of drugs, vaccines, or attention to hygiene.

Theories also help to stimulate the *development of new knowledge* by providing motivation and guidance for asking significant clinical questions. On the basis of a theoretical premise, a clinician can use the process of deduction to formulate a hypothesis which can then be tested, providing evidence to support, reject, or modify the theory. For instance, based on the theory that reinforcement will facilitate learning, a clinician might deduce that verbal encouragement will decrease the time required for a patient to learn a home program. This hypothesis can be tested by comparing patients who do and do not receive reinforcement, and, if supported, the hypothesis will lend credence to the original theory. A wide variety of hypotheses can be deduced from this same theory. For instance, a clinician may hypothesize that reinforcement will improve learning for spinal cord–injured patients working to master the use of a hand splint. The results of testing each hypothesis will provide additional affirmation of the theory or demonstrate specific situations when the theory is not substantiated.

Theory provides the basis for asking a question in applied research. Sometimes there will be sufficient background in the literature to build this framework; other times the researcher must build an argument based on what is known from basic science. In descriptive or exploratory research, the study's findings may contribute to the development of theory. The researcher uses a theoretical premise to project how the variables being studied should be related and what outcomes are expected. The theoretical framework is usually discussed within the introduction or discussion section of a paper.

Without a theoretical framework a researcher will be unable to understand the implications of his findings, and observations will not have a context.

COMPONENTS OF THEORIES

Concepts and Constructs

The role that theory plays in clinical practice and research is best described by examining the structure of a theory. Figure 2.1 shows the basic organization of scientific thought, building from observation of facts to laws of nature.

The essential building blocks of a theory are **concepts.** Concepts are abstractions that allow us to classify natural phenomena and empirical observations. From birth we begin to structure empirical impressions of the world around us in the form of concepts, such as "mother," "father," "play," or "food," each of which implies a complex set of recognitions and expectations. We develop these concepts within the context of experience and feelings, so that they meet with our perception of reality. We supply labels to sets of behaviors, objects, or processes that allow us to identify them and discuss them.

We use concepts in professional communication in the same way. Even something as basic as a "wheelchair" is a concept from which we distinguish chairs of different types, styles, and functions. Almost every term we incorporate into our understanding of human and environmental characteristics and behaviors is a conceptual entity. When concepts can be assigned values, they can be manipulated as variables, so that their relationships can be examined. In this context, variables become the concepts used for building theories and planning research. Variables must be operationally defined; that is, the methods for measuring or evaluating them must be clearly delineated.

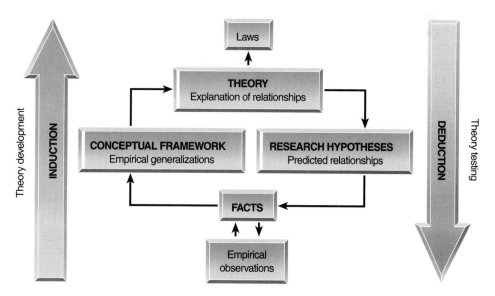

FIGURE 2.1 A model of scientific thought, showing the circular relationship between facts and theory and the integration of inductive and deductive reasoning.

Some concepts are observable and easily distinguishable from others. For instance, a wheelchair will not be confused with an office chair. Other concepts, however, are less tangible and can be defined only by inference. Concepts that represent nonobservable behaviors or events are called **constructs.** Constructs are invented names for abstract variables that cannot be seen directly, but are inferred by measuring relevant or correlated behaviors that are observable. The construct of intelligence, for example, is one that we cannot see, and yet we give it very clear meaning. We evaluate a person's intelligence by observing his behavior, the things he says, what he "knows." We can also measure a person's intelligence using standardized tests and use a number to signify intelligence. An IQ score of 125 tells us something about that individual, but the number by itself has no empirical value. We cannot observe 125 intelligence "points" like we can 125 degrees of motion. Constructs are often manipulated as variables in psychosocial and behavioral research.

Propositions

Once the concepts that relate to a theory are delineated, they are formed into a generalization, or **proposition.** Propositions state the relationship between variables, which can be described in several ways. For example, a *hierarchical* proposition shows a vertical relationship, establishing ordered levels of concepts. Maslow's theory of the relationship of human needs to motivation demonstrates this principle.[3] He described five levels, beginning at the bottom with basic physiological needs, moving up to safety, social needs, esteem, and finally ending at the top with self-actualization, or the fulfillment of one's self. A *temporal* proposition orders concepts in time and states a sequence of events. For instance, one theory of motor development proposes that mobility must precede stability in the development of motor skill.[4] Similarly, developmental theory states that the appearance of postural reactions and motor milestones in infants progresses sequentially with age.[5] A *quantitative* proposition is based on the frequency or duration of a specific behavior. For example, theories of fatigue are partly based on the concept of repetitions of exercise and how that relates to muscular endurance.[6]

Models

Many of the concepts we deal with in professional practice are so infinitely complex that we cannot truly comprehend their real nature. In an effort to understand them we try to simplify them within the context of a **model** that serves as an analogy for the real phenomenon. To understand the concept of an "atom," for example, it was helpful for scientists to delineate a conceptual model that is likened to a solar system. The intricacies of genetic processes were clarified by the development of a helical model of DNA. Function of the neuromuscular system is often taught using a model of the muscle spindle. These models are considered simplified approximations of reality. The model leaves out much of the detail, but describes the conceptual structure closely enough to give us a better understanding of the phenomenon. Models are symbolic representations of the elements within a system. Whereas a theory is an explanation of phenomena, a model is a structural representation of the concepts that comprise the theory.

Some physical models are used to demonstrate how the real behavior might occur. For example, engineers study models of bridges to examine the stresses on cables and the effects of different loading conditions. The benefit of such models is that they obey the same laws as the original, but can be controlled and manipulated to examine the effects of various conditions in ways that would not otherwise be possible. Rehabilitation engineers develop prototypes of prostheses or motor-driven wheelchairs to evaluate their performance and to perfect their design. Scientists also use animal models to mimic specific anatomical or physiological deficits in the human to examine the effects of pathology, trauma, and intervention.

Sometimes a model is a schematic representation, such as an architect's plans or a map. Therapists might use this type of model when evaluating a client's home for architectural barriers, by drawing a diagram of rooms and doorways and plotting out the spatial requirements for use of a wheelchair. Such a model provides opportunities for considering the implications of different approaches without physically carrying them out, and facilitates making appropriate changes when necessary. Computer simulations are the most recent contributions to the development of physical models. Scientists can experiment with an infinite number of variations in design and can analyze the implications of each without risk or major expense.

A model can also represent a process rather than a real object. For example, decision-making models can be used to define the progression of physical dysfunction or to show how examination and treatment should proceed for the development of effective intervention.[7,8] A model of motor learning suggests the stages one goes through in the course of learning and perfecting a motor skill. The disablement model (shown in Figure 1.1) creates a structure to understand the theoretical relationship between impairments and functional abilities, and can be used to offer explanations as to why specific impairments might lead to certain types of disability.[9]

Statistical models are used to describe the quantitative relationship among variables by using symbols to represent them. Statistical models in physical science allow for accurate prediction of quantities, such as the summary of the relationship between force, mass, and acceleration ($F = m \times a$). In the behavioral sciences, however, statistical models are less precise, usually containing some degree of error resulting from the variability of human behavior and physical characteristics. For instance, a clinician might want to determine the level of strength a patient could be expected to achieve following a period of training. A model that demonstrates the influence of a person's height, weight, and age on muscle strength would be useful in making this determination.[10] This type of quantitative model can serve as a guide for setting long-term goals and for predicting functional outcomes. Research studies provide the basis for testing these models and estimating their degree of accuracy for making such predictions (see Chapter 27).

TYPES OF THEORIES

Historically, theories have been developed in two ways. **Inductive theories** are data based and evolve through a process of inductive reasoning, beginning with empirically verifiable observations. Through multiple investigations and observations, researchers determine those variables that are related to a specific phenomenon and those that are not. The patterns that emerge from these studies are developed into a systematic conceptual framework, which forms the basis for generalizations. For instance, this process was used by Skinner in the formulation of his theories of learning and behavior, based on previous work and his own observations of human behavior.[11] Through the examination and clarification of the interrelationships between stimuli and responses, he formulated a systematic explanation for the observed behaviors. Glaser and Strauss used the term "grounded theory" to describe the development of theory by reflecting on experience.[12]

The alternative approach to theory building is the intuitive approach, whereby a theory is developed on the basis of great insight and intuitive understanding of an event and the variables most likely to impact on that event. This type of theory, called a **hypothetical-deductive theory,** is developed with few or no prior observations, and often requires the generation of new concepts to provide adequate explanation. Freud's theory of personality fits this definition.[13] It required that he create concepts such as "id," "ego," and "superego" to explain psychological interactions and motivations. Because they are not developed from existing facts, hypothetical-deductive theories must be continually tested in the real world to develop a database that will support them. Einstein's theory of relativity is an excellent example of this type of theory; it was first advanced in 1905 and is still being tested and refined through research.

Most theories are formulated using a combination of both inductive and hypothetical-deductive processes. Observations initiate the theoretical premise, and then hypotheses derived from the theory are tested. As researchers go back and forth in the process of building and testing the theory, concepts are redefined and restructured. This process occurs along a circular continuum between fact and theory, whereby a theory can be built on facts, but must also be tested by them (Fig 2.1).

CHARACTERISTICS OF THEORIES

As we explore the many uses of theories in clinical research, we should also consider criteria that can be used to evaluate the utility of a theory. First and foremost, a theory should provide a thorough and *rational explanation* of observed facts. It should provide a basis for classifying relevant variables and predicting their relationships. A theory should also provide a means for its own verification; that is, it should be sufficiently developed and clear enough to permit deductions that form testable hypotheses.

A good theory is *economical*. It should be the most efficient explanation of the phenomenon, using only those concepts that are truly relevant and necessary to the explanation offered by the theory. Complex theories are difficult to interpret and less likely to provide meaningful direction to practice or research. Theories are also most useful when they apply to a broad range of situations, not one specific segment of a discipline.

A theory should also be *important*. It should reflect that which is judged significant by those who will use it. In this sense, theories become the mirror of a profession's values and identity. When we examine the theories that are adopted by clinicians in the course of their practice, their intellectual investments become clear. For example, many therapists rely on neurophysiological theory as a basis for choosing therapeutic exercise techniques that use diagonal and rotational patterns of motion, as opposed to the traditional use of anatomical theory as a basis for exercises in straight planes. This suggests that research is needed to test hypotheses that predict the superiority of multiple-plane movement over single-plane exercise for given purposes.

Lastly, a theory is fluid. It must be *consistent with observed facts* and the already established body of knowledge, but it must also be able to shift and grow as knowledge progresses. Theories reflect the present state of knowledge and must adapt to changes in that knowledge as technology and scientific evidence improve. Therefore, a theory is only a tentative explanation of phenomena. It should be reasonable according to what has been observed, but may not be the only explanation. Many theories that are accepted today will be discarded tomorrow. Some will be "disproved" by new evidence, and others may be superseded by new theories that integrate the older ones. For instance, the *disengagement theory of aging* was originally proposed to account for observations of age-related decreases in social interaction.[14] The explanation this theory offered was that older individuals withdrew from social involvements in anticipation of death. As sociological theory progressed, however, new perspectives emerged, such as *exchange theory,* which suggested that interactions in old age become limited because the old have fewer resources to offer, therefore bringing less to a relationship.[15] In a further generation of exchange theory, *socioemotional selectivity theory* tries to explain reduced social exchange of older persons as a function of increasing selectivity in interactions.[16] This theory suggests that older persons decide to reduce emotional closeness with some people while they increase closeness with others; that is, interactions reflect the rewards of specific emotional support with a selective group of individuals. This evolution of theory illustrates how the explanations of an observed psychosocial phenomenon have continued to change as our understanding and perceptions of social interaction have grown.

THEORY AND RESEARCH

Every theory serves, in part, as a research directive. The empirical outcomes of research can be organized and ordered to build theories using inductive reasoning. Conversely, theories must be tested by subjecting deductive hypotheses to scientific scrutiny. The processes of theory development and theory testing are represented in the model shown in Figure 2.1. It integrates the concepts of inductive and deductive reasoning as they relate to the elements of theory design.

Theory Development

As the previous examples illustrate, theories are not discovered, they are created. A set of observable facts may exist, but they do not become a theory unless someone has the insight to understand the relevance of the observed information and pulls the facts together to make sense of them. Certainly, many people observed apples falling from trees before Newton was stimulated to consider the force of gravity.

The basic process of theory development is induction. It begins with multiple observations that lead to a collection of facts within a specific area of interest. These facts may be derived from the results of research studies or from empirical observations, but they are not mere speculations. Facts must then be conceptualized into a framework that allows for generalization of concepts. This process involves a degree of abstraction and imagination, as ideas are manipulated and concepts reorganized, until some structural pattern is evident in their relationship.

Theory Testing

When we speak of testing a theory, we should realize that a theory itself is not testable. The validity of a theory is derived through the empirical testing of hypotheses that are deduced from it and from observation of the phenomenon the theory describes. The hypotheses predict the relationships of variables included in the theory. The results of research will demonstrate certain facts, which will either support or not support the hypothesis. If the hypothesis is supported, then the theory from which it was deduced is also supported.

When we compare the outcomes of individual research studies with predicted outcomes, we are always aware of the potential for disconfirmation of the underlying theory. In essence, the more that research does *not* disconfirm a theory, the more the theory is supported. This may sound backward, but in actuality we can never "prove" or confirm a theory. We can only demonstrate that a theoretical premise does not hold true in a specific situation. When a research hypothesis is tested and it is *not rejected*—that is, the study turns out the way we expected—we cannot state that the underlying theory is definitely true. To make such a statement, we would have to verify every possible application of the theory and demonstrate that the outcomes were absolutely consistent. As this is not feasible, we can only interpret individual hypotheses and conclude that a theory has not been disproved.

Utilization of Theory in Research and Practice

Clinicians are actually engaged in theory testing on a regular basis in practice. Specific therapeutic modalities are chosen for treatment because of expected outcomes that are based on theoretical assumptions. Therefore, the theory is tested each time the clinician evaluates treatment outcomes. When a theory is used as the basis for a treatment, the clinician is, in effect, hypothesizing that the treatment will be successful. If results are as expected, the theory has been supported. When evidence is obtained that does not support a theory, or that cannot be explained by the theory, alternative explanations must be considered. There may be reason to question how measurements were taken and how concepts were defined, to determine if these were truly consistent with the theory's intent. The validity of the theory may be questioned, or the application of the theory to the specific problem being studied may need to be reevaluated. It may also be necessary to reexamine the theory and modify it, so that it does explain the observed outcome. If this is not practical, a new theory may need to be considered that will encompass this and all previous observations.

Continuous research is needed to contribute to the foundations of practice. Understanding clinical phenomena cannot be achieved in a single study. It is a process within a community of researchers involving discussion, criticism, and intellectual exchange to analyze the connection between new and previous findings and explanations. This type of exchange allows the inconsistencies to surface, to identify findings that cannot be explained by current theories. This process can serve as a catalyst for a *paradigm shift*, or a change in the basic framework that governs the way knowledge is pursued.[17] For example, the focus on outcomes in research represents a paradigm shift in rehabilitation science, as constructs such as disability and quality of life become a major focus, rather than the traditional emphasis on changes in physical impairments.[18] By looking at outcomes in this way, researchers recognize that questions and their underlying theories will take a different direction than in the past.

The importance of theory for understanding research findings is often misunderstood. Whenever a research question is formulated, there is an implicit theory base that suggests how the variables of interest are related. Unfortunately, many authors do not make this foundation explicit.[19] Empirical results are often described with only a general explanation, or an admission that the author can find no explanation. It is the author's responsibility, however, to consider what is known, to examine potential relationships, and to help the reader understand the context within which the results can be understood. It is incumbent upon all researchers to project their expectations into the realm of theory, to offer an interpretation of findings, and thereby to contribute to the growth of knowledge.[20]

THEORY AND LAW

When a theory reaches the level of absolute consistency in outcomes, it is called a **law.** Laws generally have a wider scope than theories, and allow precise predictions. For example, Newton made many mathematical observations that were used to describe the motion of the planets around the sun. These motions can be described with great precision, allowing great accuracy of prediction. What started as a theoretical observation eventually came to be accepted as a universal law. Generally, laws are not established in the applied sciences, as they are in the physical sciences. The nature of human beings and their interactions with the environment does not allow our theories to become so precise in their prediction. We are left, therefore, with the necessity of continuing the quest for affirmation of our theories.

COMMENTARY

Applying Theory

History documents many dramatic changes in society's acceptance of theories, such as the belief that the world was round, not flat, and that the sun was the center of the solar system. In medicine we are aware of significant modifications to our understanding of the human body, as evidenced in the shift from Galen's view of "pores" in the heart to Harvey's theory of circulation. We have also witnessed major changes in cultural values that have influenced the acceptance of some theories, such as the effect of the feminist movement on theories of social interaction and management.

The fact that scientists are constantly adapting or developing theories to accommodate new information is, of course, healthy and of critical importance to clinical science if we expect our treatments to reflect the most up-to-date scientific information available. We cannot ignore the possibility that any theory will need to be modified or discarded. At any given time a particular theory will be accepted by some scientists for some purposes, and not by others. Theories need to be tested in different ways in a variety of contexts. Research is, therefore, essential to the continued refinement of the theoretical basis for treatment.

How one views theory in the interpretation of behavior has a direct impact on how research questions will be formulated. For instance, if we observe a child balancing atop a large ball, we would expect to see the child lift his head and search for the horizon with his eyes. Depending on the underlying theoretical premise we assign to this behavior, we might interpret the response as a reflexive righting reaction or as a biomechanical adjustment of balance. In an effort to document the effects of treatment to improve the child's performance, each of these explanations would suggest very different research questions and different approaches to treatment.

We should also be careful not to assign the rank of theory to an individual's teachings or an "approach" to treatment. For example, neurophysiological treatment approaches, often given imposing names such as neurodevelopmental treatment (NDT) or proprioceptive neuromuscular facilitation (PNF), are not theories, but are developed from theories of motor control and neurophysiology. Many of these theories are derived from animal studies, and we must be equally careful not to automatically project these explanations onto the human animal. We use these theories as a basis for our treatments because they are all we have to go on given the limits of our knowledge and technology.

Much of clinical practice is based on empirical successes which clinicians have attempted to explain using theories that are currently accepted. As new knowledge is advanced, these theories may be dismissed or changed. This does not mean that the treatment does not work. It only suggests that the theory was incorrectly applied to that situation and that we do not yet fully understand why the treatment is successful. We must continue to test theories in an effort to refine them in the context of human behavior, and eventually reformulate them to reflect more precisely what we actually observe in practice.

KEY TERMS

theory
concepts
variables
constructs

propositions
model
inductive theories

hypothetical-deductive
theories
law

REFERENCES

1. Kerlinger FN. *Foundations of Behavioral Research.* New York: Holt, Rinehart & Winston, 1973.
2. Mawdsley RH, Knapik JJ. Comparison of isokinetic measurements with test repetitions. *Phys Ther* 1982;62:169–72.
3. Maslow AH. *Motivation and Personality.* 2d ed. New York: Harper & Row, 1970.
4. Stockmeyer SA. An interpretation of the approach of Rood to the treatment of neuromuscular dysfunction. *Am J Phys Med* 1967;46:900–61.
5. Bobath B. *Abnormal Postural Reflex Activity Caused by Brain Lesions.* 2d ed. London: Heineman Medical Books, 1971.

6. Maughan RJ, Harmon M, Leiper JB, Sale D, Delman A. Endurance capacity of untrained males and females in isometric and dynamic muscular contractions. *Eur J Appl Physiol* 1986;55:395–400.
7. Harris BA, Dyrek DA. A model of orthopaedic dysfunction for clinical decision making in physical therapy practice. *Phys Ther* 1989;69:548–53.
8. Schenkman M, Butler RB. A model for multisystem evaluation, interpretation, and treatment of individuals with neurologic dysfunction. *Phys Ther* 1989;69:538–47.
9. Verbrugge LM, Jette AM. The disablement process. *Soc Sci Med* 1994;38:1–14.
10. Falkel J. Plantar flexor strength testing using the cybex isokinetic dynamometer. *Phys Ther* 1978;58:847–50.
11. Gewirtz JL, Pelaez-Nogueras M. B. F. Skinner's legacy to human infant behavior and development. *Am Psychol* 1992;47:1411–22.
12. Glaser B, Strauss A. *The Discovery of Grounded Theory.* Chicago: Aldine Publishing, 1967.
13. Keutz PV. The character concept of Sigmund Freud. *Schweiz Arch Neurol Neurochir Psychiatr* 1971;109:343–65.
14. Cummings E, Henry WE. *Growing Old: The Process of Disengagement.* New York: Basic Books, 1961.
15. Bengtson VL, Dowd JJ. Sociological functionalism, exchange theory and life-cycle analysis: a call for more explicit theoretical bridges. *Int J Aging Hum Develop* 1981;12:55–73.
16. Carstensen LL. Social and emotional patterns in adulthood: support for socioemotional selectivity theory. *Psychol Aging* 1992;7:331–8.
17. Kuhn T. *The Structure of Scientific Revolutions.* New York: Norton, 1962.
18. Jette AM. Outcomes research: shifting the dominant research paradigm in physical therapy. *Phys Ther* 1995;75:865–970.
19. Bengtson VL, Burgess EO, Parrott TM. Theory, explanation, and a third generation of theoretical development in social gerontology. *J Gerontol* 1997;52B:S72–S88.
20. Royce JR. Pebble picking versus boulder building. *Psychol Rep* 1965;16:447–50.

3

Ethical Issues in Clinical Research

The purpose of this chapter is to complete our conceptual framework by discussing the ethical issues that have an impact on clinical research. We will describe the principles and practices that have become standards in the planning and implementation of research involving human subjects. These principles elucidate the ethical obligation of researchers to engage in meaningful research and to acknowledge the participation of not only the subjects under study but also professional colleagues who contribute substantially to a research project. We will cite the major documents that define public policy. For the ethical practice of research, the evolution of our standards has occurred within the last half of the twentieth century in response to prior conduct that was antithetical to the dignity and respect of all persons. Now a clear system is in place that is intended to protect everyone who is asked to participate in clinical studies.

INTEGRITY OF THE RESEARCHER

Researchers have a responsibility for honesty and integrity in all phases of the research process, beginning with their choice of a research question. Researchers who are health professionals have an obligation to set priorities and to pursue questions that are relevant to important health care issues. Today, for example, we see an emphasis on research to examine the outcomes of emerging health care strategies for the twenty-first century. Changes in the population profile and public health problems have stimulated research in specific areas such as geriatrics and acquired immune deficiency syndrome (AIDS). The research direction of most clinical scientists is affected by external forces such as the priorities of funding agencies. These complex factors influence the selection of ongoing research efforts.

Researchers also have an ethical responsibility to do clinical research that is meaningful.[1] We should be able to justify a project based on the potential scientific value of its results. This implies an obligation to base our research on rational, theoretical principles and to carry it out according to a sound research design with an appropriate sample. It also suggests that research should be conducted by competent investigators who have the expertise to do reliable and valid work. It is not ethical to involve patients in a study, with potential risks to them, when the study has little chance of making a scientific contribution.

During data collection researchers must be careful to minimize the effect of personal bias in measurement. Rosenthal has described several types of experimenter bias that can have significant effects on experimental outcomes.[2] These include unconscious or purposeful inaccuracies in measurement that will tend to support the research hypothesis and the influential interactions between researcher and subject that alter the subject's behavior. Bias cannot be eliminated entirely simply because of human nature, but it should be recognized and controlled as much as possible.

Statistical procedures should be appropriate, and should not be used to manipulate data for the sole purpose of obtaining a significant result. All data should be included in an analysis, and true differences or the lack of true differences should be reported. Unfortunately, there have been many instances of fraudulent reports in the medical research community. These serve only to hinder the pursuit of truth and progress. Researchers should be aware of potential conflicts of interest. It is not unusual today to find research funded by government or private agencies or equipment manufacturers. The researcher should know who will control the dissemination of information. Technically, research data belong to the agent providing the funds.[3] That agent may want to suppress results that do not conform to expectations. The researcher should be clear on who owns the data and who has access to it once the project is completed.

A researcher has an obligation to publish findings and to be thorough and honest in the reporting of results. Credit of authorship is an issue for research publications. Authors should have made major contributions to a project,[4] although many research directors are routinely listed as a formality. The order in which authors are listed in the byline is usually determined according to each individual's contribution. Agreements about authorship should be made early in the course of a project to avoid later conflicts. Most research involves the input of many contributors, and researchers should not hesitate to give authorship credit where it is due. Authors should also give credit to those who helped during the project, but who might not merit authorship, through an acknowledgment.

PROTECTION OF HUMAN RIGHTS IN CLINICAL RESEARCH

Our primary professional purpose in conducting clinical research is to document the effectiveness and efficiency of treatment intervention. Our patients or normal subjects are therefore the *sine qua non* of our research activities. Commitment to the protection of their rights and dignity must be inherent in the design of any clinical research project.

Guiding Principles

Research with human subjects requires adherence to three basic principles: autonomy of each individual, beneficence, and justice.[5] Personal **autonomy** refers to self-determination and the capacity of individuals to make decisions affecting their lives and to act on those decisions. Beauchamp and Childress describe autonomous action as intentional, carried out with understanding and without controlling influence.[6] It is essential that researchers demonstrate all due respect for the elements of autonomy. Some individuals who may be appropriate subjects for research, such as children or patients with cognitive problems, may be unable to understand adequately. In these cases, the researcher is obliged to ensure that a surrogate decision maker is available, has the ability to make a reasoned decision, and is committed to the well-being of the compromised individual.

Beneficence refers to the obligation to attend to the well-being of individuals. All who engage in clinical research are bound by two rules associated with this mandate: (1) "Do no harm," which is a cornerstone of medical ethics asserted in the Hippocratic oath; and (2) "Maximize possible benefits and minimize possible harm."[7] The balance between risks and benefits must be weighed as a part of the decision to go forward with a specific project. Risks may be physical, economic, social, or psychological. Potential benefits may include new knowledge that can be applied to future subjects or patients, or that may have a direct impact on study participants, such as improved health status. The point is that the "risks to the subjects [must be] reasonable in relation to anticipated benefits."[8] The analysis of the *risk-benefit* relationship measures the probability and magnitude of benefit against the probability of anticipated harm or discomfort.[6] For example, if a new, powerful chemotherapeutic agent with known serious side effects requires testing, the selection of normal subjects would be unacceptable; whereas testing on subjects who are terminally ill, and for whom the drug has the potential to effect a positive change, might be acceptable.

Justice refers to fairness in the research process, or the equitable distribution of the benefits and burdens.[5] This principle speaks to the fair selection of subjects who are appropriate for a given study, drawn from a defined population that is most likely to benefit from the research findings. The selection of subjects should not be discriminatory on some irrelevant criterion, but based on reasons directly related to the problem being studied.[7] The principle of justice also has meaning in multigroup studies when subjects have an equal chance of being assigned to an experimental or control or alternative group. Current practices are followed to ensure consideration of and adherence to these three basic principles.

Use of Control Groups

An historical dilemma for medical researchers has been the need for a **control group,** or placebo group, as a basis for experimental comparison. Randomized clinical trials (RCTs) have become an accepted way to determine whether an intervention has a significant effect on subjects who receive the treatment compared with those who receive no treatment or a sham treatment. The RCT is preferred for this purpose over observation or retrospective analysis of data. Through the process of random assignment of subjects to the treatment or control group, researchers are best able to control confounding variables that could affect the outcome of the study.[6] A dilemma arises, however, especially when the researchers are also the clinicians responsible for the care of the patients who might be potential research subjects. Rothman and Michels reported several examples of this problem in drug studies where a placebo condition was employed, when, in fact, effective therapeutic methods existed.[9] An alternative used in many studies is a comparison of two or more treatments, with no placebo control. In this case, the research goal is to determine which of the alternative treatments is more effective. This allows us to say that one treatment is different from another, but it does not establish if treatment conditions are more effective than no intervention at all (see Chapter 10).

The researcher can support the concept of a control group from several perspectives. First, there may be some clinical conditions for which no treatments have been effective. In that case, it is necessary to compare a new treatment with a no-treatment condition. It is also necessary to make such a comparison when the purpose of the research is to determine whether a particular treatment approach is not effective. In situations when the efficacy of a treatment is being questioned because current knowledge is inadequate, it may actually be more ethical to take the time to make appropriate controlled comparisons than to continue clinical practice using potentially ineffective techniques. As a form of compensation, a researcher may offer the experimental treatment to control group patients after data collection is complete, if results indicate that treatment is beneficial. When a study is planned that includes a control group, the researcher is obliged to inform the potential participants of this fact. Subjects should know that there is an equal chance that they will either receive or not receive the experimental treatment. As clinician-researchers, we are obliged to discuss alternative treatments that would be appropriate for each patient-subject if such alternatives are employed in clinical practice. This is an important element of the informed consent process that will be discussed later in this chapter.

Evolution of Regulations for the Conduct of Research Involving Human Subjects

Establishment of formal guidelines delineating rights of research subjects and obligations of professional investigators became a societal necessity as clear abuses of experimentation came to light. In the United States, many unconscionable studies have been identified over the years.[10] In one case, elderly patients were injected with live malignant cancer cells without their knowledge.[11] Another much publicized study, begun in the 1930s, withheld treatment from men with syphilis to observe the natural course of the disease.[12] This study continued until the early 1970s, long after penicillin had been identified as an effective cure. The first formal guidelines document written in this century was the *Nuremberg Code of 1947*. This document was developed in response to the criminal experimentation on captive victims by Nazi physicians during World War II. It clearly emphasized that the human subject should voluntarily consent to participate as a research subject. Consent should be given only after the subject has sufficient knowledge of the purposes, procedures, inconveniences, and potential hazards of the experiment. This principle underlies the current practice of obtaining informed consent prior to initiation of clinical research or therapeutic intervention. The *Nuremberg Code* also addresses the competence of the investigator, that research "should be conducted only by scientifically qualified persons."

The *Declaration of Helsinki* was adopted by the World Medical Association in 1964, and was revised in 1975, 1983, and again in 1989 (Table 3.1).[13] This document addressed for the first time the concept of independent review of research protocols by a committee of individuals who are not associated with the proposed project (principle 2). These and

TABLE 3.1. DECLARATION OF HELSINKI[13]

The International Code of Ethics for Biomedical Research

Basic Principles

1. Biomedical research involving human subjects must conform to generally accepted scientific principles and should be based on adequately performed laboratory and animal experimentation and with a thorough knowledge of the scientific literature.

2. The design and performance of each experimental procedure involving human subjects should be clearly formulated in an experimental protocol which should be transmitted to a specially appointed independent committee for consideration, comment, and guidance.

3. Biomedical research involving human subjects should be conducted only by scientifically qualified persons and under the supervision of a clinically competent medical person. The responsibility for the human subject must always rest with a medically qualified person and never rest on the subject of the research even though the subject has given his or her consent.

4. Biomedical research involving human subjects cannot legitimately be carried out unless the importance of the objective is in proportion to the inherent risk to the subject.

5. Every biomedical research project involving human subjects should be preceded by careful assessment of predictable risks in comparison with foreseeable benefits to the subject or to others. Concern for the interest of the subject must always prevail over the interests of science and society.

6. The right of the research subject to safeguard his or her integrity must always be respected. Every precaution should be taken to respect the privacy of the subject and to minimize the impact of the study on the subject's physical and mental integrity and on the personality of the subject.

7. Physicians should abstain from engaging in research projects involving human subjects unless they are satisfied that the hazards involved are believed to be predictable. Physicians should cease any investigation if the hazards are found to outweigh the potential benefits.

8. In the publication of the results of his or her research, the physician is obliged to preserve the accuracy of the results. Reports on experimentation not in accordance with the principles laid down in this Declaration should not be accepted for publication.

9. In any research on human beings, each potential subject must be adequately informed of the aims, methods, anticipated benefits, and potential hazards of the study and the discomfort it may entail. He or she should be informed that he or she is at liberty to abstain from participation in the study and that he or she is free to withdraw his or her consent to participation at any time. The doctor should then obtain the subject's freely given informed consent, preferably in writing.

10. When obtaining informed consent for the research project the physician should be particularly cautious if the subject is in a dependent relationship to him or her or may consent under duress. In that case the informed consent should be obtained by a physician who is not engaged in the investigation and who is completely independent of this official relationship.

11. In the case of legal incompetence, informed consent should be obtained from the legal guardian in accordance with national legislation. Where physical or mental incapacity makes it impossible to obtain informed consent, or when the subject is a minor, permission from the responsible relative replaces that of the subject in accordance with national legislation.

12. The research protocol should always contain a statement of the ethical considerations involved and should indicate that the principles enunciated in the present Declaration are complied with.

Medical Research Combined with Professional Care (Clinical Research)

1. In the treatment of the sick person, the physician must be free to use a new diagnostic and therapeutic measure, if in his or her judgment it offers hope of saving life, reestablishing health or alleviating suffering.

Continued

TABLE 3.1 *Continued*

2. The potential benefits, hazards and discomfort of a new method should be weighed against the advantages of the best current diagnostic and therapeutic methods.

3. In any medical study, every patient—including those of a control group, if any—should be assured of the best proven diagnostic and therapeutic method.

4. The refusal of the patient to participate in a study must never interfere with the physician-patient relationship.

5. If the physician considers it essential not to obtain informed consent, the specific reasons for this proposal should be stated in the experimental protocol for transmission to the independent committee.

6. The physician can combine medical research with professional care, the objective being the acquisition of new medical knowledge, only to the extent that medical research is justified by its potential diagnostic or therapeutic value for the patient.

Non-Therapeutic Biomedical Research Involving Human Subjects (Non-clinical Biomedical Research)

1. In the purely scientific application of medical research carried out on a human being, it is the duty of the physician to remain the protector of the life and health of that person on whom biomedical research is being conducted.

2. The subjects should be volunteers—either healthy persons or patients for whom the experimental design is not related to the patient's illness.

3. The investigator of the investigating team should discontinue the research if in his/her judgment it may, if continued, be harmful to the individual.

4. In research on man, the interest of science and society should never take precedence over consideration related to the well-being of the subject.

other essential principles set forth in this document have been incorporated into the U.S. Department of Health and Human Services (DHHS) Rules and Regulations.[8] The *Declaration of Helsinki* also states that reports of research that have not been conducted according to stated principles should not be accepted for publication (principle 8). This principle has led to an editorial challenge to professional journals to obtain assurance that submitted reports of human studies do indeed reflect proper attention to ethical conduct. DeBakey suggests that all reports should contain information on the procedures used for obtaining informed consent and ethical review.[14] Many journals now require acknowledgment that informed consent was obtained from subjects used in any research project.

Based on the ethical principles guiding biomedical research and the rules and regulations promulgated pursuant to the 1974 National Research Act (PL-93-348), procedures to ensure protection of human subjects in research have been delineated and are now considered "standard" throughout the United States. There must be a fully developed research proposal that identifies the problem or question to be studied and provides the rationale of, need for, and importance of the study. The research design must be clearly stated and deemed appropriate to answer the question. Informed consent must be obtained from individuals or their legally authorized representatives. This is usually accomplished by a signature affixed to a written informed consent document. Both the written proposal and the informed consent form are submitted to an Institutional Review Board for approval.

The National Research Act established the National Commission for the Protection of Human Subjects of Biomedical and Behavioral Research. The deliberations and recommendations of this commission resulted in *The Belmont Report* that delineates the guiding principles discussed previously in this chapter and the manner in which these principles apply to human research studies.[7] Based on that report, both the DHHS and the Food and Drug Administration (FDA) established the rules and regulations that govern the conduct of research in the United States today. The Office for Protection from Research Risks (OPRR) is the administrative arm of the DHHS that is responsible for implementing the regulations and providing guidance to those who conduct human studies.

THE INSTITUTIONAL REVIEW BOARD

According to federal regulations, projects funded through federal agencies must be reviewed by an institutional committee prior to implementation to ensure that the rights of research subjects are protected.[8] As a rule, most institutions require that all projects involving human subjects must be submitted for review, regardless of funding considerations. According to federal regulations, an **Institutional Review Board (IRB)** must be composed of at least five members. It may not consist of all males, or all females, or all members of one professional group, although the IRB must be able to competently review the scientific details of proposed research. At least one member must be concerned primarily with nonscientific issues and may be a lawyer, clergyman, or ethicist. One member must not be otherwise affiliated with the institution where the research is to be conducted. One of the responsibilities of the OPRR is to approve IRB documents that ensure compliance with the ethical principles and regulations.

Review of Proposals

The responsibility of the IRB is to review research proposals at convened meetings. The decision to approve, require modifications in, or disapprove a proposal must be that of a majority. In arriving at a decision, the IRB considers the scientific merit of the project, the competence of the investigators, the risk to subjects, and the feasibility based on identified resources. If the project is not scientifically sound or practical, there can be no benefit; therefore, no risk to subjects is justified. Reviewers will consider the evidence that the risks and discomforts to the subject have been minimized and are sufficiently outweighed by the potential benefits of the proposed study. This is the **risk-benefit ratio.** The board also studies the procedures for selecting subjects, ensuring voluntary informed consent based on complete and understandable descriptions and confidentiality. The majority of proposals submitted to an IRB are reviewed in this detailed manner.

Expedited or Exempt Review

Some categories of research activity, however, may qualify for an expedited review or may be exempted from the review process. A project may qualify for **expedited review** in circumstances such as "recording data from subjects 18 years of age or older using noninvasive procedures routinely employed in clinical practice" and "moderate exercise by healthy volunteers."[8] In the case of an expedited review, the chairman and at least one designated member of the IRB conduct the review. The advantage of expedited review is that it is usually completed in less time than that required for a full board review.

Certain projects may be **exempted** from committee review if they are surveys, interviews, or studies of existing records, provided that the data are collected in such a way that subjects cannot be identified. Surveys or interviews will only be given exempt status if they do not deal with sensitive issues such as drug abuse, sexual behavior, or criminal activity. Secondary analysis of existing data from databases where subject information is coded to avoid any personal identifiers may be exempt. On the other hand, when actual patient clinic records are used, IRB approval is required.[15] Researchers must describe methods of coding data to ensure patient confidentiality. All proposals for human subject projects must be submitted to the IRB, which then determines whether a project qualifies for full review, expedited review, or is exempt.

Institutional Guidelines

Each institution establishes its own guidelines for review in accordance with federal and state regulations. Clinicians should therefore become familiar with the requirements in their own institutions. Clinicians should also be aware that the process can take several weeks, depending on the IRB's schedule and whether the proposal needs revision. This review process should be included in the timetable for any research project. No research on human subjects should be done without prior review and approval of a designated review committee.

ELEMENTS OF INFORMED CONSENT

Perhaps the most important ethical tenet in human studies is the individuals' ability to agree to participate with full understanding of what will happen to them. The **informed consent** process and all of its elements address the basic principles of autonomy, beneficence, and justice. The components of the process consist of **information elements,** including disclosure of information and the subjects' comprehension of that information, and **consent elements,** ensuring the voluntary nature of participation and the subjects' competence to consent.[6]

Information Elements
Subjects Must Be Fully Informed

The informed consent process begins with an invitation to participate. A statement of the purpose of the study permits potential subjects to decide whether they believe in or agree with the worth and importance of the research. The process then requires that the researcher provide, in writing, a fair explanation of the procedures to be used and how they will be applied. This explanation must be complete, with no deception by virtue of commission or omission. Subjects should know what will be done to them, how long it will take, what they will feel, what side effects can be expected, and what types of questions they may be asked. If subjects cannot read the informed consent document, it should be read to them. Children should be informed to whatever extent is reasonable for their age. Subjects should also know why they have been selected to participate in terms of inclusion criteria for the study, such as clinical condition or age. If the subjects are patients, they should understand the distinction between procedures that are experimental and procedures, if any, that are proposed to serve their personal needs.

An ethical dilemma occurs when complete disclosure of procedures might hinder the outcomes of a study by biasing the subjects so that they do not respond in a typical way. When the risks are not great, review boards may allow researchers to pursue a deceptive course, but subjects must be told that information is being withheld and that they will be informed of all procedures after completion of data collection. For example, when the research design includes a control or placebo group, subjects will not know what treatment they are receiving. They should know that they will be told their group assignment at the completion of the study.

An important aspect of informed consent is the description of all reasonable foreseeable risks or discomforts to which the patient will be subjected, directly or indirectly, as part of the study. **Risk** refers to physical, psychological, or social harm that goes beyond expected experiences in daily life. The researcher should detail the steps that will be taken to protect against these risks and the treatments that are available for potential side effects. For example, if a patient is likely to become fatigued as a result of performing maximal physical exercise, the researcher may include rest periods during the experimental trial. If a patient is receiving electrical stimulation, the researcher would explain the risk of shock and how that risk is minimized by proper grounding and by regular inspection of the equipment. The subject should be advised against such behaviors as taking certain medications or driving a car, which could be hazardous during or after the experimental period. A statement should be included whereby subjects agree to exercise appropriate caution. They are not bound by this, but they should understand the potential harm of not honoring the agreement. If the research involves more than a minimal risk, a statement should be included concerning the availability of medical care and whether compensation will be provided. Subjects should also be informed of new information, such as the identification of previously unknown risks, that becomes available during the course of the study. This may affect their willingness to continue participation. The researcher also delineates the potential **benefits** of participation. Some studies may result in a beneficial reduction of symptoms. For example, subjects who participate in a study to test the effectiveness of treatment for migraine headaches may find their pain relieved by the experimental treatment. The subject should be advised that such a benefit is possible but is not guaranteed. Studies that are geared more toward theory testing may provide no direct benefits. The researcher should explain the potential application of theoretical findings and how the findings will contribute to future research or future patient care.

When a study involves a form of therapeutic intervention, subjects must be informed that alternative treatments are available and that they have the right to choose among them instead of accepting the experimental intervention. Patients must also be told if "standard" treatments to which they are entitled are being withheld as part of the study. This information is essential if a patient is to make an informed decision about accepting the experimental conditions.

Subject Information Should Be Confidential and Anonymous

Research subjects should be told what steps are being taken to ensure confidentiality of all information, including descriptive and experimental data. When possible, a subject's anonymity should be protected. This issue becomes important with surveys, for example, when respondents wish to remain unidentified. In experimental situations anonymity is often not feasible, but the researcher can code the data without using names. Identifying codes can be kept separate from the rest of the data. Researchers should also be aware of this responsibility when disseminating results.

If the subject is to be videotaped or photographed during the study, this fact should be disclosed in the consent form. The subject should know who will have access to tapes or photographs, who will keep them, and how they will be used. Subjects retain the right to review such material and to withdraw permission for its use at any time. Subjects should also be informed if one-way windows will be used and who will be the observers.

The Informed Consent Form Must Be Written in Lay Language

Informed consent is more than telling subjects about the research; the process implies that they understand what they are being told and what they are reading. The language must be clear and basic so that the average reasonable individual can follow it. Professional jargon is unacceptable. Instead of "perform a maximal isometric contraction," the subject should be told to "pull up as hard as you can without moving." This is the language that clinicians use routinely in patient education. As a rule of thumb, language should be written for the lowest educational level that would be expected for subjects.

The Researcher Must Offer to Answer Questions at Any Time

The researcher is responsible for ensuring that the subject understands all relevant information. A verbal description is almost always a part of the process, so that the researcher can "personalize" the information for each subject. The subjects should have sufficient time to assimilate the details of the proposed project, prior to making their decision to participate. They should feel free to question the procedures at any time during the course of the study, and should be provided with the name and telephone number of an appropriate contact person.

Consent Elements

Consent Must Be Voluntary

Subjects should participate in a research project of their own free will. Patients are usually quite motivated to help, but they must be informed that there is no penalty to them if they refuse. Some studies may involve monetary compensation for participation. It should be clear if such compensation will be received whether or not the subject completes the study.

Special Consideration Must Be Given to Subjects Who Are Particularly "Vulnerable"

Some individuals cannot give informed consent because they may not be able to understand the information. In cases of mental illness, developmental disability, or diminished mental capacity, the ability of the subject to consent must be evaluated by the researcher and others who know the subject well. If the subject is not competent, consent must be provided by a legal guardian or advocate.[5, 6]

The regulations regarding children as research subjects require that parents or guardians give permission for participation. Furthermore, if children are considered competent to understand, regardless of age, their assent—that is, their affirmative agreement to participate—must be obtained and documented. Researchers should be particularly cautious about influencing subjects who are considered "captive."[16] For example, there are specific regulations regarding research involving prisoners.[8] More subtle circumstances exist with the use of students or nursing home residents. In both cases, the sense of pleasing those in authority may affect the subjects' decisions.

Subjects Must Be Free to Withdraw Consent at Any Time

The informed consent document must indicate that the subjects are free to discontinue participation for any reason at any time without prejudice; that is, the subjects must be assured that no steps will be taken against them, and, if they are patients, that the quality of their care will not diminish. This can occur before or during an experiment, or even after data collection when subjects might request that their data be discarded. It should also be clear that the researcher will discontinue the experiment at any time if necessary for the subjects' safety or comfort.

The Informed Consent Form

All subjects must give informed consent prior to participating in a project. This is done by providing a written informed consent form that is signed and dated by the subject, researcher, and a witness. Subjects should receive a copy of this form and the researcher must retain a signed copy. Although it is a general contractual agreement, the informed consent form is not binding on subjects.[17] Subjects never waive their rights to redress if their participation should cause them harm. The form should not contain language that appears to release the researcher from liability. The required elements of an informed consent form are listed in Table 3.2. A sample informed consent form can be found in Appendix E. The format of this sample informed consent form is used in many institutions. It specifically identifies and acknowledges all the elements of informed consent. Of special note, the signature page should not stand alone, but must contain some of the text of the document to show that the signatures are applied in the context of the larger document.

Although written consent is preferable, some agencies allow oral consent in selected circumstances. In this case, a written "short form" can be used that describes the information presented orally to the subject or the subject's legally authorized representative.[5] This short form is submitted to the review committee for approval.

TABLE 3.2.   ELEMENTS OF INFORMED CONSENT

1. **Purpose of the research project**
   - A clear explanation of the reason for doing the study and why it is important
   - Reason for selecting this particular individual

2. **Procedures**
   - A clear, detailed explanation of what will be done to or by the individual

3. **Risks and discomforts**
   - Truthful and inclusive statements of risks that may result, and discomforts that can be expected

4. **Benefits**
   - A description of potential benefits to the individual participant, to the general knowledge, or to future administration of health care

5. **Alternatives to participation**
   - A description of reasonable alternative procedures that might be used in the treatment of this individual when a treatment intervention is being studied

6. **Confidentiality**
   - Statements of the procedures used to ensure the anonymity of the individual in collecting, storing, and reporting information and who (persons or agencies) will have access to the information

7. **Request for more information**
   - A statement that the individual may ask questions about or discuss participation in the study at any time, naming an individual to contact

8. **Refusal or withdrawal**
   - A statement that the individual may refuse to participate or discontinue participation at any time without prejudice

9. **Injury statement**
   - A description of measures to be taken if injury occurs as a direct result of the research activity

10. **Consent statement**
    - A confirmation that the individual consents to participate in the research project

11. **Signatures**
    - Participant
    - Parent or guardian (for the care of minors)
    - Assent of minors over age 7 years
    - Witness

Informed Consent and Usual Care

Clinical research projects are often designed to test specific treatment protocols that are accepted as standard care, and subjects are recruited from those who would receive such treatments. Clinicians often ask if informed consent is necessary for a research project when the procedures would have been used anyway. The answer is yes! Even when treatment is viewed as usual care, patients are entitled to understand alternatives that are available to them. Patients must always be informed of the use of the data that are collected during their treatments, and they should have sufficient information to decide to participate, regardless of whether treatment is viewed as experimental or accepted clinical practice.

This situation is somewhat different, however, when analysis of patient responses is based on use of medical records, that is, when the study is a retrospective analysis of data. It is not necessary to obtain the consent of individual patients under these circumstances. It is necessary to obtain approval from an IRB, however, to ensure confidentiality and ethical use of the data.

COMMENTARY

A Patient Care Perspective

The concepts of informed consent for human research have also been applied to medical practice in widespread state legislation.[18] Patients entering hospitals are asked to sign standard consent forms that indicate agreement to routine medical care and tests. Additional forms are signed for surgery or special tests. This practice has not been applied as readily to clinical situations in allied health, although the concepts of disclosure and voluntary participation are becoming more important to the protection of patients' rights.[19] Although the idea of explaining treatments to patients is by no means unusual, the structure and formal requirements of informed consent have important implications for the patient-provider relationship. The clinician can give the patient a description of the planned treatment and available alternatives and explain inherent risks, consequences, advantages, and disadvantages. Clinicians recognize the possibilities of inflicting harm on patients through thermal modalities, resistive exercise, or mobilization and should identify these potential effects prior to treatment. It is not necessary for the average patient to understand the physiological rationale for treatment, but clinicians should be able to explain things in reasonable detail and within the scope of the patient's understanding.[17] With sufficient information, patients can participate in the setting of treatment goals, consider whether they want to be treated, and express their preference for particular types of treatment. In this manner, patients, like research subjects, can assume an appropriate role in making decisions about the activities that affect their lives.

KEY TERMS

autonomy
beneficence
justice
control group
Institutional Review Board
    (IRB)

risk-benefit ratio
expedited review
exempt review
informed consent
information elements
consent elements

risk
benefits

REFERENCES

1. Weijer C, Dickens B, Meslin EM. Bioethics for clinicians: 10. Research ethics. *Can Med Assoc J* 1997;156:1153–7.

2. Rosenthal R. *Experimenter Effects in Behavioral Research.* New York: Appleton-Century-Crofts, 1966.

3. Fox DJ. *Fundamentals of Research in Nursing.* Norwalk, CT: Appleton-Century-Crofts, 1982.

4. International Committee of Medical Journal Editors. Uniform requirements for manuscripts submitted to biomedical journals. *JAMA* 1997;277:927–34.

5. Levine RJ. *Ethics and Regulation of Clinical Research.* 2d ed. Baltimore: Urban & Schwarzenberg, 1986.

6. Beauchamp TL, Childress JF. *Principles of Biomedical Ethics.* New York: Oxford University Press, 1994.

7. The National Commission for the Protection of Human Subjects of Biomedical and Behavioral Research. *The Belmont Report: Ethical Principles and Guidelines for the Protection of Human Subjects of Research.* Washington, DC: DHEW, 1979.

8. Title 45 Code of Federal Regulations. Part 46: *Protection of Human Subjects* (HHS). Washington, DC: US Government Printing Office, 1994.

9. Rothman KJ, Michels KB. The continuing unethical use of placebo controls. *N Engl J Med* 1994;331:394–8.

10. Beecher HK. Ethics and clinical research. *N Engl J Med* 1966;274:1354–60.

11. Langer E. Human experimentation: New York verdict affirms human rights. *Science* 1966;151:663.

12. *Final Report of the Tuskegee Syphilis Study Ad Hoc Advisory Panel.* Washington, DC: United States Public Health Service, 1973.

13. World Medical Association. Declaration of Helsinki. Recommendations guiding physicians in biomedical research involving human subjects. *JAMA* 1997;277:925–6.

14. DeBakey L. *The Scientific Journal: Editorial Policies and Practices.* St. Louis: CV Mosby, 1976.

15. Huston P, Naylor CD. Health services research: reporting on studies using secondary data sources [editorial]. *Can Med Assoc J* 1996;155:1697–1709.

16. Hayter J. Issues related to human subjects. In: Down F, Fleming J, eds. *Issues in Nursing Research.* New York: Appleton-Century-Crofts, 1979, 107–47.

17. Michels E. Research and human rights. Part 1. *Phys Ther* 1976;56:407–12.

18. Ozzi WM. Survey of the law of informed consent in physician-patient relationships. *Leg Med* 1982;117–36.

19. Purtilo RB. Applying the principles of informed consent to patient care. Legal and ethical considerations for physical therapy. *Phys Ther* 1984;64:934–7.

CHAPTER

4

Principles of Measurement

Scientists and clinicians use measurement as a way of understanding, evaluating, and differentiating characteristics of people and objects. **Measurement** provides a mechanism for achieving a degree of precision in this understanding, so that we can describe physical or behavioral characteristics according to their quantity, degree, capacity, or quality.[1] We can document that a patient's shoulder can flex to 75 degrees, rather than say motion is "limited," or indicate that the air temperature is 95°F, rather than just "hot." This facility helps us communicate information in objective terms, giving us a common sense of "how much" or "how little" without ambiguous interpretation. Principles of measurement, therefore, are basic to our ability to describe phenomena, demonstrate change or relationship, and communicate this information to others.

Measurement is used as a basis for making decisions or drawing conclusions in several ways. At its most basic level, measurement is used to describe the quality or quantity of an existing variable, such as the measurement of intelligence, attitude, range of motion, or muscle strength. We can also use measurement to make absolute decisions based on a criterion or standard of performance, such as the requirement that a student achieve at least a grade of C to pass a course or that a certain degree of spinal curvature be present to indicate a diagnosis of scoliosis. We use measurement as a basis for choosing between two courses of action. In this sense a clinician might decide to implement one treatment approach over another based on the results of a comparative research study. Clinicians use measurement as a means of evaluating a patient's condition and response to treatment—that is, we measure change or progress. We also use measurements to compare and discriminate between individuals or groups. For instance, a test can be used to distinguish between children who do and do not have learning disabilities or between different types of learning disabilities. Finally, measurement allows us to draw conclusions about the predictive relationship between variables. We might use grades on a college entrance examination to predict a student's ability to succeed in an academic program. We can measure the functional status of an elderly patient to determine the level of assistance that will be required when the patient returns home. There are virtually no decisions or clinical actions that are independent of some type of measurement.

Measurement has been defined as the *process of assigning numerals to variables to represent quantities of characteristics according to certain rules.*[2] The purpose of this chapter is to explore this definition as it is applied to clinical research. In doing so, we consider several aspects of measurement theory and discuss how these relate to measurement, analysis, and interpretation of clinical variables.

QUANTIFICATION AND MEASUREMENT

The first part of the definition of measurement emphasizes the process of *assigning numerals to variables.* A numeral is a symbol or label in the form of a number. A variable is a property that can differentiate individuals or objects. It represents an attribute that can have more than one value. Value can denote quantity, such as age or blood pressure, or quality, such as sex or geographic region. Numerals are used to represent qualitative values, with no quantitative meaning. Therefore, we can assign numerals to football players, or code data on a questionnaire using a "0" to represent Male and a "1" to represent Female. A numeral becomes a mathematical number only when it represents a known quantity.

A number reflects how much of an attribute or variable is present. A **continuous variable** can theoretically take on any value along a continuum within a defined range. Between any two values an indefinitely large number of fractional values can occur. In reality, continuous values can never be measured exactly, but are limited by the precision of the measuring instrument. For instance, joint range could be measured as 50 degrees, 50.5 degrees, or even 50.3 degrees, depending on the gradations on the goniometer and skill of the measurer. Strength, distance, weight, and chronological time are other examples of continuous variables.

Other variables can be described only in whole units, and are considered **discrete variables.** Heart rate, for example, is measured in beats per minute, not in fractions of a beat. Variables such as the number of trials needed to learn a motor task or the number of children in a family are also examples of discrete variables. Qualitative variables represent discrete categories, such as male/female. When qualitative variables, such as gender, can take on only two values, they are called **dichotomous variables.**

Precision refers to the exactness of a measure. For statistical purposes, this term is used to indicate the number of decimal places to which a number is taken. Therefore, 1.473826 is a number of greater precision than 1.47. The degree of precision in a measurement is a function of the sensitivity of the measuring instrument and data analysis system as well as the variable itself. It is not useful, for example, to record blood pressure in anything less than integer units (whole numbers with no decimal places). It may, however, be meaningful to record strength to a tenth or hundredth of a kilogram.

THE INDIRECT NATURE OF MEASUREMENT

The definition of measurement also indicates that measured values *represent quantities of characteristics.* Most measurements are a form of abstraction or conceptualization; that is, very few variables are measured directly. Range of motion and length are among the few examples of measures that involve direct observation of a physical property. We can actually see how far a limb rotates or how tall a person is, and we can compare angles and heights between people. Most characteristics are not directly observable, however, and we can measure only a correlate of the actual property. Therefore, most behavioral variables are actually indirect measures of these characteristics. For example, we do not observe temperature, but only the height of a column of mercury in a thermometer; we are not capable of visualizing the electrical activity of a heartbeat or muscle contraction, although we can evaluate the associated recording of an electrocardiogram (EKG) or electromyogram (EMG); force is observable only as the reading on a dynamometer, not as movement of the contractile elements of muscle. For most variables, then, we use some form of direct observation to *infer* a value for a phenomenon.

Constructs

The ability to measure a variable, no matter how indirectly, is dependent on one's ability to define it. Unless we know what a term means we cannot show that it exists. This is not difficult for variables such as temperature, weight, and heart rate, which can be defined by direct physical or physiological methods, but is much harder for abstract terms such as intelligence, health, strength, or pain. Any explanation of what these variables mean will undoubtedly involve descriptions of behaviors or outcomes that indicate if someone is "intelligent," "healthy," "strong," or "in pain"; however, there is no logical, unidimensional definition that will satisfy these terms. For instance, intelligence cannot be assessed as a single estimate of verbal performance, memory, or quantitative skill, but is conceptualized as a complex, combined measure of IQ. Different aspects of strength may be assessed by dynamometry, strain gauges, lifting weights, or manual resistance, with specific reference to type of contraction, joint position, speed of movement, and type of resistance. No single measurement can be interpreted as an absolute measure of a person's "strength."

These types of abstract variables are called **constructs** (see Chapter 2). Measurement of a construct is based on expectations of how a person who possesses the specified trait would behave, look, or feel in certain situations. Therefore, a construct is associated with some value or values that are assumed to represent the original variable. Some constructs are derived from one or more quantities of other variables.[3] For instance, velocity is calculated by first determining values for distance and time. Work is derived from the product of force and distance. These constructs have no inherent meaning except as a function of other constructs.

Most constructs must be defined as a function of many interrelated concepts or multiple dimensions. For example, we each have a conceptual understanding of the clinical term "disability," but researchers still struggle to develop meaningful ways to measure it. How might a physical therapist look at disability as compared with an occupational therapist, nurse, psychologist, neurologist, orthopedist, or social worker? Can we devise a scale so that one sum or average number is indicative of a patient's level of disability? Many such scales exist. But can we make the inferential leap from this number to an assessment of the psychological, social, physical, and physiological manifestations of disability? To do so we must be able to define the construct of disability in terms of specific and limited properties of behavior that are relevant to our own frame of reference. It is important to appreciate this difficulty in operationally defining construct measures as a basis for interpretation of clinical variables.

RULES OF MEASUREMENT

The last element of the definition of measurement concerns the need for establishing purposeful and precise *rules* for assigning values to objects. These rules designate how numbers are to be assigned, reflecting both amount and units of measurement. In some cases the rules are obvious and easily learned, as in the use of a yardstick (inches), scale (pounds), goniometer (degrees), or dynamometer (pounds of force). This is not the case for many clinical variables, for which the rules of measurement must be invented. Concepts such as sensation, quality of life, muscle tone, manual resistance, gait, function, and developmental age have been operationally defined by researchers who have developed instruments with complex rules of measurement that are by no means intuitive or obvious. Often these rules require rigorous training and practice for the instruments to be applied effectively.

The criteria for assigning values and units to these types of variables must be systematically defined so that levels of the behavior can be objectively differentiated; that is, rules of assignment stipulate certain relationships among numbers or numerals. For example, we assume that relationships are consistent within a specific measurement system, so that objects or attributes can be equated or differentiated. For instance, we assume that either *a* equals *b*, or *a* does not equal *b*, but both cannot be true. We also assume that if *a* equals *b*, and *b* equals *c*, then *a* should also equal *c*.

Numbers are also used to denote relative order among variables. If *a* is greater than *b*, and *b* is greater than *c*, it should also be true that *a* is greater than *c*. We can readily see how this rule can be applied to a direct variable such as height. Similarly, we might assume that if A is stronger than B, and B is stronger than C, then A is also stronger than C. As logical as this may seem, however, there are measurement scales that do not fit within this structure. For example, if patient A receives a Good+ grade on a manual muscle test, and patient B receives a Good grade, we cannot assume that patient A is stronger than patient B. The "rules" for manual muscle testing define a system of order that is valid *within* an individual, but not *across* individuals. A similar system is employed with a visual analogue scale for evaluating pain. Two patients may mark a point at 6.5 cm, but there is no way to establish that their levels of pain are equal. If, after a period of treatment, each patient marks a point at 2.0 cm, we know that their pain has decreased, but we still do not know if one patient has more pain than the other. Therefore, a researcher must understand the conceptual basis of a particular measurement to appreciate how the rules for that measurement can logically be applied and interpreted.

Rules of measurement also apply to the acceptable operations with which numerals can be manipulated. For instance, not all types of data can be subjected to arithmetic operations such as division and multiplication. Some values are more appropriately analyzed using proportions or frequency counts. The nature of the attribute being measured will determine the rules that can be applied to its measurement. To clarify this process, four **scales** or **levels of measurement** have been identified—nominal, ordinal, interval,

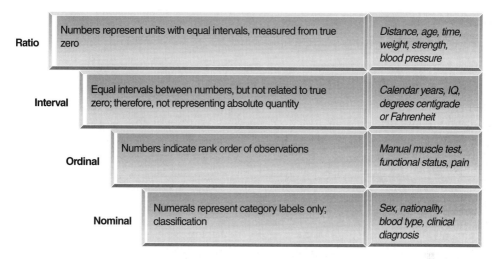

FIGURE 4.1   Summary of characteristics of scales of measurement.

and ratio—each with a special set of rules for manipulating and interpreting numerical data.[4] The characteristics of these four scales are summarized in Figure 4.1.

Nominal Scale

The lowest level of measurement is the **nominal scale,** also referred to as the *classificatory scale.* Objects or people are assigned to categories according to some criterion. Categories may be coded by name, number, letter, or symbol, although none of these have any quantitative value. They are used purely as labels for identification. Blood type, handedness, type of mental illness, side of hemiplegic involvement, and area code are examples of nominal variables. Questionnaires often code nominal data as numerals for responses such as (0) no and (1) yes, (0) male and (1) female, or (0) disagree and (1) agree.

Based on the assumption that relationships are consistent within a measurement system, nominal categories are *mutually exclusive,* so that no object or person can logically be assigned to more than one category. This means that the members within a category must be equivalent on the property being scaled, but different from those in other categories. We also assume that the rules for classifying a set of attributes are *exhaustive;* that is, every subject can be accurately assigned to one category. Classifying sex as male–female would follow these rules. Classifying hair color as only blonde or brunette would not.

The numbers or symbols used to designate groups on a nominal scale can be altered without changing the values or characteristics they identify. The categories cannot, therefore, be ordered on the basis of their assigned numerals. The only permissible mathematical operation is *counting* the number of subjects within each category, such as 35 males and 65 females. Statements can then be made concerning the frequency of occurrence of a particular characteristic or the proportions of a total group that fall within each category.

Ordinal Scale

Measurement on an **ordinal scale** requires that categories be rank-ordered on the basis of an operationally defined characteristic or property. Data are organized into adjacent categories exhibiting a "greater than–less than" relationship. Many clinical measurements are based on this scale, such as sensation (normal > impaired > absent), spasticity (none < minimal < moderate < severe), and balance (good > fair > poor). Most clinical tests of constructs such as function, strength, and development are also based on ranked scores. Surveys often create ordinal scales to describe attitudes or preferences (strongly agree > agree).

The intervals between ranks on an ordinal scale may not be consistent and, indeed, may not be known. This means that although the objects assigned to one rank are considered equivalent on the rank criterion, they may not actually be of equal value along the continuum that underlies the scale. Therefore, ordinal scales often record ties even when true values are unequal. For example, manual muscle test grades are defined according to ranks of Normal > Good > Fair > Poor > Trace > Zero.[5] Although Good is always stronger than Fair, this scale is not sensitive enough to tell us what this difference is. Therefore, the interval between grades Good and Fair on one subject will not necessarily be the same as on another subject, and one Good muscle may not be equal in strength to another Good muscle.

Ordinal scales can be distinguished on the basis of whether they contain a natural origin, or true zero point. For instance, military rank is ordinal, but has no zero rank. Manual muscle testing grades have a true zero, which represents no palpable muscle contraction. In some cases, an ordinal scale can incorporate a natural origin within the series of categories, so that ranked scores can occur in either direction away from the origin (+ and −). This type of scale is often constructed to assess attitude or opinion, such as agree/neutral/disagree. For construct variables, it may be impossible to locate a true zero. For example, what is zero function? A category labeled "zero" may simply refer to performance below a certain criterion or at a theoretical level of dependence.

Limitations for interpretation are evident when using an ordinal scale. Perhaps most important is the lack of arithmetic properties for ordinal "numbers." Because ranks are assigned according to discrete categories, ordinal scores are essentially labels, similar to nominal values; that is, an ordinal value does not represent quantity, but only relative *position* within a distribution. Manual muscle test grades can be written as 5, 4, 3, 2, 1, 0, rather than using word categories, but these numbers have no more arithmetic meaning than Good, Fair, and Poor. No matter how one chooses to label categories, the ranks do not change. Any scheme can be used to assign values, as long as the numbers get bigger with successive categories. Therefore, we know a manual muscle test grade of 4 is greater than 2, but it does not mean twice as much strength. We know that the distance from 2 to 3 is not equal to the distance from 3 to 4, even within one individual. Thus, the difference between two ordinal scores will be difficult to interpret.

This concern is relevant to the use of ordinal scales in clinical evaluation, especially those that incorporate a sum. For instance, the Functional Independence Measure (FIM) uses the sum of 18 items, each scored 1–7, to reflect the degree of assistance needed in functional tasks.[6] The Oswestry Low Back Pain Disability Questionnaire is scored as the total of 10 items, each scored on a 0–5 scale, with higher scores representing greater disability.[7] The sums are used to describe a patient's functional level, but their interpretation for research purposes must acknowledge that these numbers are not true quantities, and therefore, have no coherent meaning.[8] Therefore, ordinal scores are generally considered appropriate for descriptive analysis only. Although ordinal numbers can be subjected to arithmetic operations, such as calculating an average rank for a group of subjects or subtracting to document change over time, such scores are not meaningful as true quantities. Issues related to interpreting ordinal scores are discussed further in Chapter 6.

Interval Scale

An **interval scale** possesses the rank-order characteristics of an ordinal scale, but also demonstrates known and equal distances or intervals between the units of measurement. Therefore, relative difference and equivalence within a scale can be determined. What is not supplied by an interval scale is the absolute magnitude of an attribute, because interval measures are not related to a true zero (similar to an ordinal scale without a natural origin). This means that negative values may represent lesser amounts of an attribute. Thus, the standard numbering of calendar years (B.C. and A.D.) is an interval scale. The year 1 was an arbitrary historical designation, not the beginning of time. Measures of temperature using Fahrenheit and Celsius scales are also at the interval level. Both have artificial zero points that do not represent a total absence of heat and can indicate temperature in negative degrees. Within each temperature scale we can identify that the numerical difference between 10° and 20° is equal to the numerical difference between 70° and 80° (in each case 10°); however, these differences are based on the numerical values on the scale, not on the true nature of the variable itself. Therefore, the actual difference in amount of heat or molecular motion generated between 10° and 20° is not necessarily the same as the difference between 70° and 80°.

Because of the nature of the interval scale, we must consider the practical implications for interpreting measured differences. Interval values can be added and subtracted, but these operations cannot be used to interpret actual quantities. For example, we could use an interval scale, such as that shown in the lower scale of Figure 4.2, to calculate the sum $6 + 2 = 8$; however, if we arbitrarily reset zero at a point five units higher, as in the upper scale, maintaining the integrity of the intervals, measurement of the same quantities will now yield the sum $1 + 2 = 3$. Although the relative position of each quantity is the same, the actual values of each measurement are quite different. Therefore, it is not reasonable to develop a ratio based on interval data because the numbers cannot be logically measured against true zero.

Because the actual values within any two interval scales are not equivalent, one interval scale cannot be directly transformed to another. For instance, the designation of

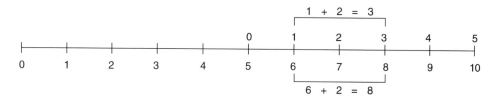

FIGURE 4.2 An interval scale, showing quantities expressed with two different zero points.

100°C cannot be compared with 100°F; however, because the actual values are irrelevant, it is the ordinal positions of points or the equality of intervals that must be maintained in any mathematical operation. Therefore, we can transform scales by multiplying or adding a constant, which will not change the relative position of any single value within the scale. After the transformation is made, intervals separating units will be in the same proportion as they were in the original scale. This is classically illustrated by the transformation of Fahrenheit to Celsius by subtracting 32 and multiplying by 5/9.

Ratio Scale

The highest level of measurement is achieved by the **ratio scale,** which is an interval scale with an absolute zero point that has empirical, rather than arbitrary, meaning. A score of zero at the ratio level represents a total absence of whatever property is being measured. Therefore, negative values are not possible. Range of motion, height, weight, and force are all examples of ratio scales. Although a zero on such scales is actually theoretical (it could not be measured), it is nonetheless unambiguous. Numbers on this scale reflect actual amounts of the variable being measured. It makes sense, then, to say that one person is twice as heavy as another, or that one person is half as tall as another. Ratio data can also be directly transformed from one scale to another, so that 1 in. = 2.54 cm, and 1 lb = 2.2 kg. All mathematical and statistical operations are permissible with ratio level data.

Identifying Measurement Scales

As shown in Figure 4.1, the four scales of measurement constitute a hierarchy based on the relative precision of assigned values, with nominal measurement at the bottom and ratio measurement at the top. Although most variables will be optimally measured at one level of measurement, it is always possible to operationally define a variable at lower levels. Suppose we were interested in measuring step length in a sample of four children. We could use a tape measure with graduated centimeter markings to measure the distance from heelstrike to heelstrike. This would constitute a ratio scale because we have a true zero point on a centimeter scale and clearly equal intervals. Our measurements would allow us to determine the actual length of each child's step, as well as which children took longer steps than others. Hypothetical data for such measures are presented in Table 4.1.

We could convert these ratio measures to an interval scale by arbitrarily assigning a score of zero to the lowest value and adjusting the intervals accordingly. We would still

TABLE 4.1. HYPOTHETICAL DATA FOR STEP LENGTH MEASURED ON DIFFERENT SCALES

Subject	Ratio Measure	Interval Measure	Ordinal Measure	Nominal Measure
A	23	4	2	Long
B	24	5	3	Long
C	19	0	1	Short
D	28	9	4	Long

know which children took longer steps, and we would have a relative idea of how much longer they were, but we would no longer know what the actual step length was. We would also no longer be able to determine that Subject D takes a step 1.5 times as great as Subject C. In fact, using interval data, it erroneously appears as if Subject D takes a step 9 times the length of Subject C.

An ordinal measure can be achieved by simply ranking the childrens' step lengths. With this scale we no longer have any indication of the magnitude of the differences. On the basis of ordinal data we could not establish that Subjects A and B were more alike than any others. We can eventually reduce our measurement to a nominal scale by setting criteria for "long" versus "short" steps and classifying each child accordingly. With this measurement we have no way of distinguishing any differences in performance between Subjects A, B, and D.

Clearly, we have lost significant amounts of information with each successive reduction in scale. It will always be to the researcher's advantage, therefore, to achieve the highest possible level of measurement. Data can always be manipulated to use a lower scale, but not vice versa. In reality, clinical researchers usually have access to a limited variety of measurement tools, and the choice is often dictated by the instrumentation available and the clinician's preference or skill. Therefore, we must distinguish between the level of measurement it is theoretically possible to achieve for a given variable and the level that is actually achieved.

COMMENTARY

When Is an Ordinal Measure Not an Ordinal Measure?

Identifying the level of measurement for a particular variable is not always as simple as it seems. The underlying properties of many behavioral variables do not fit neatly into one scale or another. For example, behavioral scientists continue to question the classification of IQ scores as either ordinal or interval measures.[9] Can we assume that intervals are equal, so that the difference between scores of 50 and 100 is the same as the difference between 100 and 150, or are these scores only reflective of relative order? Is everyone with a score of 100 equally intelligent? Most likely the true scale is somewhere between ordinal and interval. Consider the use of a visual analog scale to evaluate the intensity of pain. A patient makes a mark along a 10-cm line to indicate his level of pain, on a continuum from "no pain" to "pain as bad as it could be." The mark can be measured in precise millimeters from the left anchor. When the patient makes a second mark, however, to show a change in pain level, can we interpret the distance on a ratio scale, or does it actually represent a ranked or ordinal measurement? Is the patient able to equate the exact difference in millimeters with his change in pain? How different is this from asking the patient to rate his level of pain on an ordinal scale of 1–10? Researchers have shown that these questions are not simple, and can be affected by many factors such as instructions given to subjects, the length of the line, and the words used at the anchors.[10–12] These considerations bear out the multidimensional influences on measurement properties.

An understanding of the scales of measurement is more than an academic exercise. The importance of determining the measurement scale for a variable lies in the determination of which mathematical and statistical operations are appropriate and which interpretations are meaningful for the data. In the classical view, nominal and ordinal data can be described by frequency counts; interval data can be added or subtracted; and only ratio data can be subjected to multiplication and division.[4] According to these guidelines, tests of statistical inference that require arithmetic manipulation of data (as opposed to just ranking scores) should be applied only to variables on the interval or ratio scale; however, we find innumerable instances throughout the clinical and behavioral science literature where these statistical operations are used with ordinal data. The question is how serious are the consequences of misassumptions about scale properties to the interpretation of statistical research results? Some say quite serious,[8] while a number of other respected references indicate that the answer is "not very."[2, 13] Many researchers are comfortable constructing ordinal scales using categories that are assumed to logically represent equal intervals of the test variable and treating the scores as interval data,[14–16] especially when the scale incorporates some type of natural origin. Velleman and Wilkinson propose that the four measurement scales may not be sufficient for categorizing all forms of measurement, and that the level of measurement must be determined within the context of the instrument and the questions asked of the data.[17] They suggest that statistical procedures should be applied according to what is meaningful in the data, not strictly by the scale used. Transformations of data may change the measurement attributes, or new information about a measure may help to interpret the data differently. They suggest, for instance, that values such as percents and fractions may need to be handled differently, depending on how they are derived and how they will be used.

Because ordinal measures occur frequently in the behavioral and social sciences, this issue is of significant importance to the reasonable interpretation of clinical data. Kerlinger suggests that most psychological and educational scales approximate equal intervals fairly well, and that the results of statistical analyses using these measures provide satisfactory and useful information.[13] Many scales used in clinical practice have not, however, been subjected to sufficient validation for us to be totally comfortable with this assumption. It is by no means clear how we can interpret intervals between manual muscle testing grades. Could we say that the interval between Good and Fair is the same as the interval between Fair and Poor? How can we judge intervals within functional status measures? Is the difference in disability level between independent function and minimal assistance the same as the difference between minimal assistance and moderate assistance? Are we able to distinguish small amounts of change, or is there a threshold of change that must occur before we see a change in grade?[18]

We will not attempt to settle this ongoing statistical debate. This issue will take on varied importance depending on the nature of the variables being measured and the precision needed for meaningful interpretation. For the most part, it would seem appropriate to continue treating ordinal measurements as ranked rather than interval data; however, if the interval approach is defensible, the degree of error associated with this practice may be quite tolerable in the long run.[19] Clinical researchers must scrutinize the underlying theoretical construct that defines a scale to determine if it can reasonably support the idea of equal intervals. A technique called Rasch analysis has been used to examine the structure of ordinal scales, and to statistically convert an ordinal scale to one with equal intervals. See Chapter 14 for further discussion of this concept.

It may also be useful to examine the number of categories the scale comprises. For example, a pain scale with 10 points can be conceptualized as more continuous than one with 5 points, thereby allowing for a different interpretation of intervals and perhaps more precise measures of change. The researcher has to recognize that any mathematical manipulation can be performed on any set of numbers, but those manipulations may not contribute to an understanding of the data. It is the researcher's responsibility to propose and test meaningful hypotheses.[20, 21]

Perhaps it is also prudent to caution against judging the worthiness of a measurement based on its scale. Although ratio and interval data provide greater precision, they may not provide the best measurement under given clinical conditions. Moreover, clinicians will often utilize ratio measures to make ordinal judgments about a patient's condition;[22] that is, the exact value of range of motion (ratio) may not be as important as the determination that the patient has improved in functional level (ordinal), or simply that he is ready to return to work (nominal). No matter how data are analyzed, researchers are always responsible for justifying the application of statistical procedures and the subsequent interpretations of the data.

KEY TERMS

measurement
continuous variable
discrete variable
dichotomous variable
precision

constructs
scales
levels of measurement
nominal scale
   (classificatory scale)

ordinal scale
interval scale
ratio scale

REFERENCES

1. Michels E. Evaluation and research in physical therapy. *Phys Ther* 1982;62:828–34.
2. Nunally JC. *Psychometric Theory.* 2d ed. New York: McGraw-Hill, 1978.
3. Michels E. Measurement in physical therapy. On the rules for assigning numerals to observations. *Phys Ther* 1983;63:209–15.
4. Stevens SS. Mathematics, measurement and psychophysics. In: Stevens SS, ed. *Handbook of Experimental Psychology.* New York: Wiley, 1951.
5. Hislop HJ, Montgomery J. *Daniels and Worthingham's Muscle Testing: Techniques of Manual Examination.* 6th ed. Philadelphia: WB Saunders, 1995.
6. Linacre JM, Heinemann AW, Wright BD, Granger CV, Hamilton BB. The structure and stability of the Functional Independence Measure. *Arch Phys Med Rehabil* 1994;75:127–32.

7. Fairbank JC, Couper J, Davies JB, O'Brien JP. The Oswestry low back pain disability questionnaire. *Physiotherapy* 1980;66:271–3.
8. Merbitz C, Morris J, Grip JC. Ordinal scales and foundations of misinference. *Arch Phys Med Rehabil* 1989;70:308–12.
9. Glass GV, Hopkins KD. *Statistical Methods in Education and Psychology.* 2d ed. Englewood Cliffs, NJ: Prentice-Hall, 1984.
10. Jensen MP, Karoly P. Self-report scales and procedures for assessing pain in adults. In: Turk DC, Melzack R, eds. *Handbook of Pain Assessment.* New York: Guilford Press, 1992.
11. Price DD, Bush FM, Long S, Harkins SW. A comparison of pain measurement characteristics of mechanical visual analogue and simple numerical rating scales. *Pain* 1994;56:217–26.
12. Price DD, Harkins SW, Baker C. Sensory-affective relationships among different types of clinical and experimental pain. *Pain* 1987;28:291–9.
13. Kerlinger FN. *Foundations of Behavioral Research.* New York: Holt, Rinehart & Winston, 1973.
14. Gaito J. Measurement scales and statistics: resurgence of an old misconception. *Psychol Bull* 1980;87:564.
15. Hasselkus BR, Safrit MJ. Measurement in occupational therapy. *Am J Occup Ther* 1976;30:429–36.
16. Anderson NH. Scales and statistics: parametric and nonparametric. *Psychol Bull* 1961;58:305.
17. Velleman PF, Wilkinson L. Nominal, ordinal, interval and ratio typologies are misleading. *Am Statistician* 1993;47:65–72.
18. Andres PL, Skerry LM, Thornell B, Portney LG, Finison LJ, Munsat TL. A comparison of three measures of disease progression in ALS. *J Neurol Sci* 1996;139 (Suppl):64–70.
19. Guilford J. *Psychometric Methods.* 2d ed. New York: McGraw-Hill, 1954.
20. Marcus-Roberts HM, Roberts FS. Meaningless statistics. *J Educ Stat* 1987;12:383.
21. Johnston MV, Keith RA, Hinderer SR. Measurement standards for interdisciplinary medical rehabilitation. *Arch Phys Med Rehabil* 1992;73:S3–S23.
22. Rothstein JM, Echternach JL. *Primer on Measurement: An Introductory Guide to Measurement Issues.* Alexandria, VA: American Physical Therapy Association, 1993.

CHAPTER

5

Reliability

The usefulness of measurement in clinical research and decision making depends on the extent to which clinicians can rely on data as accurate and meaningful indicators of a behavior or attribute. The first prerequisite, at the heart of measurement, is **reliability,** or the extent to which a measurement is consistent and free from error. Reliability can be conceptualized as reproducibility or dependability. If a patient's behavior is reliable, we can expect consistent responses under given conditions. A reliable examiner is one who will be able to measure repeated outcomes with consistent scores. Similarly, a reliable instrument is one that will perform with predictable consistency under set conditions. Reliability is fundamental to all aspects of measurement, because without it we cannot have confidence in the data we collect, nor can we draw rational conclusions from those data.

The second prerequisite is **validity,** which ensures that a test is measuring what it is intended to measure. Validity is necessary for drawing inferences from data, and determining how the results of a test can be used. Both reliability and validity are essential considerations as we explore ways in which measurement is used in both clinical practice and research. We will address issues of validity in depth in the next chapter.

The purpose of this chapter is to present the conceptual basis of reliability and to describe different approaches for testing the reliability of clinical measurements. Statistical techniques for reliability testing are presented in Chapter 26.

MEASUREMENT ERROR

The nature of reality is such that measurements are rarely perfectly reliable. All instruments are fallible to some extent, and all humans respond with some inconsistency. Consider the simple process of measuring an individual's height with a tape measure. If measurements are taken on three separate occasions, either by one tester or three different testers, we can expect to find some differences in results from trial to trial, even when the individual's true height has not changed. If we assume all the measurements were made using the same exact procedures and with equal concern for accuracy, then we cannot determine which, if any, of these three values is a true representation of the subject's height; that is, we do not know how much error is included in these measurements.

Theoretically, then, it is reasonable to look at any *observed score (X)* as a function of two components: a *true score (T)* and an *error component (E)*. This relationship is summarized by the equation

$$X = T \pm E \tag{5.1}$$

This expression suggests that for any given measurement (X), a hypothetically true or fixed value exists (T), from which the observed score will differ by some unknown amount (E). The true component is the score the subject would have gotten had the measurement been taken by a perfect measuring instrument under ideal conditions. The difference between the true value and the observed value is **measurement error,** or "noise" that gets in the way of our finding the true score. For example, if we measure a height of 65 in., when the true height is 65.5 in., our assessment will be too short; that is, our measurement error is −0.5 in. On a second assessment, if we measure 66 in., our measurement error will be +0.5 in. In reality, we cannot calculate these error components because we do not know the true score. Therefore, we must find a way of *estimating* how much of our measurement is attributable to error and how much represents an accurate reading. That estimate is reliability.

To understand reliability, we must distinguish between two types of measurement errors: systematic and random. **Systematic errors** are predictable errors of measurement. They occur in one direction, consistently overestimating or underestimating the true score. Such error is constant and biased. Therefore, if a systematic error is detected, it is usually a simple matter to either correct it by recalibrating the system or adjust for it by adding or subtracting the appropriate constant. For example, if the end of a tape measure is incorrectly marked, so that markings actually begin 0.25 in. from the end, measurements of height will consistently record values that are too long by 0.25 in. We can correct this error by cutting off the extra length at the end of the tape or by subtracting 0.25 in. from all measurements. By definition, systematic errors are constant and, therefore, do not present a problem for reliability. Systematic errors are primarily a concern of validity, because, although they are consistent, test values are not true representations of the quantity being measured.

Random errors of measurement are due to chance and can affect a subject's score in an unpredictable way from trial to trial. They are as likely to increase the observed score as to decrease it. Random errors occur from unpredictable factors such as fatigue, inattention, mechanical inaccuracy, or simple mistakes. If the patient moves slightly while her height is being measured or does not stand fully erect each time measurements are taken, scores will be inconsistent. The tester might observe markings at an angle and read them incorrectly, or the tape measure might be stretched out more on one occasion than another. Reliability focuses on the degree of random error that is present within a measurement system. As random errors diminish, the observed score moves closer to the true score, and the measurement is more reliable. The assumption is made that random error is not related to the magnitude of the true score, and that if enough measurements were taken, random errors would eventually cancel each other out, making the average score a good estimate of the true score.

Sources of Measurement Error

The development or testing of a measuring instrument typically involves specification of a protocol that maximizes the reliability of the instrument; that is, procedures are detailed to ensure consistent application and scoring. In developing such a protocol, researchers have to address known or expected sources of error that could limit the reliability of the test. Once these errors are identified, they can often be controlled or eliminated to some extent. Generally, measurement errors can be attributed to three components of the measurement system: (1) the individual taking the measurements (often called the tester or *rater*), (2) the measuring instrument, and (3) the variability of the characteristic being measured. Many sources of error can be minimized through careful planning, training, clear operational definitions, and inspection of equipment. Therefore, a testing protocol should thoroughly describe the method of measurement, which must be uniformly performed across trials. Isolating and defining each element of the measure reduces the potential for error, thereby improving reliability.

Even when the anticipated sources of error are controlled, a researcher is still faced with the unpredictability of the environment and the human response as a normal and inevitable part of measurement. Many instruments, especially mechanical ones, will always be subject to some level of background noise and random fluctuation of performance. Responses of raters and subjects will be influenced by variable personal characteristics, such as motivation, cooperation, or fatigue, and environmental factors such as noise and temperature. These contributions to error may not be controllable. We assume that these factors are random and, therefore, their effect will be canceled out in the long run.

The most difficult challenge to reliability testing occurs when the response being measured is inherently unstable. For instance, if we measure blood pressure, we might expect a natural fluctuation from session to session. When a response is very unstable, no one measurement can be considered an accurate representation of it, and it is virtually impossible to estimate the reliability of the instrument used to measure it. It is important, therefore, for researchers to understand the theoretical and practical nature of response variables, so that sources of error in reliability testing can be interpreted properly.

Regression toward the Mean

When we examine the effect of measurement error on reliability, we must also consider the extremeness of observed scores; that is, very high scores may reflect substantial positive error and very low scores may reflect substantial negative error. Cook and Campbell used the example of students taking academic exams to illustrate this concept.[1] Everyone has, at one time or another, done worse than they expected on a test, with any number of possible "excuses," such as getting a poor night's sleep, being distracted, or accidentally marking the wrong space on the answer sheet. If we think of these factors as random sources of error, then the low grade is not an accurate assessment of the student's knowledge or ability; that is, the student's true score is confounded by negative error. On a subsequent test this student's grade is likely to be higher because, all things being equal, these negative "errors" would probably not be operating to the same extent. Conversely, if a student obtained an unusually high score on the first test, we might suspect that favorable conditions were operating (positive error), such as several good guesses on questions for which the student did not really know the answer. On a second test, this student is just as likely to score lower, because these favorable conditions would not necessarily exist.

This phenomenon is called **regression toward the mean.** It suggests that extreme scores on a pretest are expected to move closer, or regress, toward the group average (the mean) on a second test; that is, the error component of an extreme pretest score is likely to be less extreme on a posttest. Therefore, using our student example, higher test scores will decrease and lower test scores will increase, moving closer to the class average. The reliability of the test will have an impact on the extent to which this effect will be present. As a more reliable score contains less error, a reliable test should produce a score close to the true score. Thus, there is less chance for regression to occur. If the tests are not reliable, the error component within each test will be large, and therefore, the chances of observing a regression effect are considerably higher.

Regression toward the mean is potentially most serious in situations when subjects are specifically assigned to groups on the basis of their extreme scores. For instance, we might be interested in the differential effect of a particular teaching technique on different levels of students. Suppose we give a class a pretest to determine their initial ability and find that the average score is 80. Then we distinguish two experimental groups on the basis of these pretest scores, one composed of those scoring above 90 and the other of those scoring below 70. According to regression theory, we would expect to see both groups respond with scores closer to 80 (the total group mean) on a second test, even if the teaching technique had no effect. The effect can be minimized, however, if we can improve the reliability of the test as a measure of student ability.

RELIABILITY COEFFICIENTS

Reliability can be conceptually defined as an estimate of the extent to which a test score is free from error, that is, to what extent observed scores vary from true scores. As it is not possible to know the true score, the true reliability of a test can never be calculated; however, we can estimate reliability based on the statistical concept of **variance,** which is a measure of the variability or differences among scores within a sample. The larger the variance, the greater the dispersion of scores; the smaller the variance, the more homogeneous the scores. If we were to measure a patient's blood pressure 10 times, we do not expect the scores to be identical—they will exhibit a certain amount of variance. Some of this total variance in observed scores will be the result of true differences among the scores (the patient's blood pressure actually changed), and some can be attributed to random sources of error, such as position of the arm or skill of the tester. Reliability is a measure of how much of this total variance is attributable to true differences between scores. Therefore, reliability can be expressed as a ratio of the true score variance to the total variance, or

$$\frac{\text{true score variance}}{\text{true score variance} + \text{error variance}} = \frac{T}{T + E} \qquad (5.2)$$

This ratio yields a value called the **reliability coefficient.** From this ratio, we can see that reliability increases as the observed score approaches the true score ($T + E \rightarrow T$). With maximum reliability (zero error), this ratio will produce a coefficient of 1.00; that is, the observed score *is* the true score. As error increases $(T + E \rightarrow E)$, the ratio approaches zero. The reliability coefficient can range between 0.00 and 1.00, with 0.00 indicating no reliability and 1.00 indicating perfect reliability. There are actually many reliability coefficients, each applied under different design conditions and with different types of data.

Magnitude of the Reliability Coefficient

Because reliability is hardly ever perfect, reliability coefficients of 1.00 are rare. Therefore, reliability cannot be interpreted as an all-or-none condition. It is a property of a measurement system that is attained to varying degrees. Most researchers establish limits that define "acceptable" levels of reliability. Although such limits are essentially arbitrary, as a general guideline coefficients below .50 represent poor reliability, coefficients from .50 to .75 suggest moderate reliability, and values above .75 indicate good reliability. We hasten to add, however, that these limits must be based on the precision of the measured variable and how the results of the reliability test will be applied. For instance, researchers may be able to tolerate lower reliability for measurements that are used for description of groups, whereas those used for decision making or diagnosis of individuals need to be higher, perhaps at least .90 to ensure valid interpretations of findings. When only one form of measurement exists for a particular variable, researchers are often faced with the choice of using a less reliable test or no test at all. For some purposes, even a test with moderate reliability can add sufficient information to justify its use, especially when used in conjunction with other tests.[2] "Acceptable reliability" is a judgment call by the researcher or clinician who understands the nature of the measured variable and whether the measurements are precise enough to be used meaningfully.

Correlation and Agreement

Many reliability coefficients are based on measures of correlation. Although we discuss the concept of correlation in detail in Chapter 23, it is necessary to provide a brief introduction here to understand how reliability coefficients can be interpreted. **Correlation** reflects the degree of association between two sets of data, or the consistency of position within the two distributions. For example, if we were to measure height and shoe size on a sample of adult men, we would probably find a correlation between the two variables; that is, those with big feet tend to be tall and those with small feet tend to be short.

Reliability can be interpreted in a similar way. For instance, if we measured height on two separate occasions, we would expect that the tallest man on test 1 would also be the tallest on test 2; the shortest man on test 1 would also be measured as the shortest on test 2. If the relative position of each subject remains the same from test to test, we would obtain a high measure of correlation. We assume that any variations in observed measurements are due to random error. If systematic errors occur, the correlation would be unaffected because each subject's relative position will not change, meaning that systematic errors of measurement will not have any effect on the size of the reliability coefficient.

Consider the two sets of scores shown in Figure 5.1. In both sets the scores are *directly proportional* for X and Y; hence, their relationship is depicted on a straight line. The relative positions of the scores are also consistent; that is, the highest score in X is paired

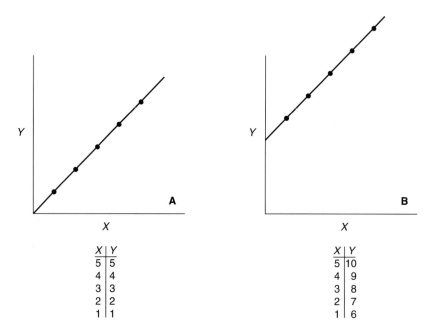

X	Y
5	5
4	4
3	3
2	2
1	1

X	Y
5	10
4	9
3	8
2	7
1	6

FIGURE 5.1   Examples of the association between X and Y in two sets of scores. In (A) the graph shows a *line of identity,* where each measure on X and Y is equal, resulting in perfect correlation as well as agreement, indicating excellent reliability. In (B) there is still perfect correlation, but no agreement, illustrating poor reliability.

with the highest score in Y, and so on. The scores in graph A also show direct **agreement** for each pair of scores. This is not the case in graph B, where all pairs disagree. But both graphs show perfect correlation! Therefore, while correlation tells us how the scores vary together, it cannot tell us the extent of agreement between the two sets of measurements. For most research and clinical applications, however, the essence of reliability is agreement between the two tests; that is, we want to know that the actual values obtained by two measurements are the same, not just proportional to each other. For example, range of motion measurements are used to evaluate joint dysfunction on the basis of actual, not relative, limitations. We need to know the true value of the limitation, not just that one patient is more limited than another. It would not be enough to know that repeated measurements were proportionally consistent; it would be necessary to establish that repeated tests resulted in the same angular measurements. Therefore, the correlation coefficient is not effective as a measure of reliability. Statistical approaches to reliability testing should include estimates of agreement that can be used in conjunction with correlation.

TYPES OF RELIABILITY

Estimates of reliability vary depending on the type of reliability being analyzed. We discuss four general approaches to reliability testing: test–retest reliability, rater reliability, alternate forms reliability, and internal consistency. For each approach we identify the most commonly used reliability coefficients. These statistical indices are detailed in Chapter 26.

Test–Retest Reliability

One basic premise of reliability is the stability of the measuring instrument; that is, a reliable instrument will obtain the same results with repeated administrations of the test. **Test–retest reliability** assessment is used to establish that an instrument is capable of measuring a variable with consistency. In a test–retest study, one sample of individuals is subjected to the identical test on two separate occasions, keeping all testing conditions as constant as possible. The coefficient derived from this type of analysis is called a *test–retest reliability coefficient.* This estimate can be obtained for a variety of testing tools, and is generally indicative of reliability in situations when raters are not involved, such as self-report survey instruments and physical and physiological measures with mechanical or digital readouts. If the test is reliable, the subject's score should be similar on multiple trials. In terms of reliability theory, the extent to which the scores vary is interpreted as measurement error.

Because variation in measurement must be considered within the context of the total measurement system, errors may actually be attributed to many sources. Therefore, to assess the reliability of an instrument, the researcher must be able to assume stability in the response variable. Unfortunately, many variables change over time. For example, a patient's self-assessment of pain may change between two testing sessions. We must also consider the inconsistency with which many clinical variables naturally respond over time. When responses are labile, test–retest reliability may be impossible to assess.

Test–Retest Intervals

Because the stability of a response variable is such a significant factor, the time interval between tests must be considered carefully. Intervals should be far enough apart to avoid fatigue, learning, or memory effects, but close enough to avoid genuine changes in the measured variable. The primary criteria for choosing an appropriate interval are the stability of the response variable and the test's intended purpose. For example, if we were interested in the reproducibility of electromyographic measurements, it might be reasonable to test the patient on two occasions within a week. Range of motion measurements can often be repeated within a day or even within a single session. Measures of infant development might need to be taken over a short period, to avoid the natural changes that rapidly occur at early ages. If, however, we are interested in establishing the ability of an IQ test to provide a stable assessment of intelligence over time, it might be more meaningful to test a child using an interval of one year. The researcher must be able to justify the stability of the response variable to interpret test–retest comparisons.

Carryover and Testing Effects

With two or more measures, reliability can be influenced by the effect of the first test on the outcome of the second test. For example, practice or carryover effects can occur with repeated measurements, changing performance on subsequent trials. A test of dexterity may improve because of motor learning. Strength measurements can improve following warm-up trials. Sometimes subjects are given a series of pretest trials to neutralize this effect, and data are collected only after performance has stabilized. A retest score can also be influenced by a subject's effort to improve on the first score. This is especially relevant for variables such as strength, where motivation plays an important role. Many researchers will not let subjects know their first score to control for this effect.

It is also possible for the characteristic being measured to be changed by the first test. A strength test might cause pain in the involved joint and alter responses on the second trial. Range of motion testing can stretch soft tissue structures around a joint, increasing the arc of motion on subsequent testing. When the test itself is responsible for observed changes in a measured variable, the change is considered a **testing effect.** Oftentimes, such effects will be manifested as systematic error, creating consistent changes across all subjects. Such an effect will not necessarily affect reliability coefficients, for reasons we have already discussed.

Reliability Coefficients

Test–retest reliability has traditionally been analyzed using the Pearson product-moment coefficient of correlation (for interval-ratio data) or the Spearman rho (for ordinal data). As correlation coefficients, however, they are limited as estimates of reliability. The **intraclass correlation coefficient (ICC)** has become the preferred index, as it reflects both correlation and agreement. The ICC actually has several forms. Model 3 is appropriate for test-retest reliability (see Chapter 26). With nominal data, **percent agreement** can be determined and the **kappa** statistic applied.

Rater Reliability

Many clinical measurements require that a human observer, or *rater,* is part of the measurement system. In some cases, the rater is the actual measuring instrument, such as in a manual muscle test or joint mobility assessment. In other situations, the rater must observe performance and apply operational criteria to subjective observations, as in a gait analysis or functional assessment. Sometimes a test necessitates the physical application of a tool, and the rater becomes part of the instrument, as in the use of a goniometer or the taking of blood pressure. Raters may also be required simply to read or interpret the output from another instrument, such as an electromyograph, or force recordings on a dynamometer. However the measurements are taken, the individual performing the ratings must be consistent in the application of criteria for scoring responses.

This aspect of reliability is of major importance to the validity of any research study involving testers, whether one individual does all the testing or several testers are involved. Data cannot be interpreted with confidence unless those who collect, record, and reduce the data are reliable. In many studies, raters undergo a period of training, so that techniques are standardized. This is especially important when the measuring devices are new or unfamiliar or when subjective observations are used. Even when raters are experienced, however, rater reliability should be documented as part of the research protocol.

To establish rater reliability the instrument and the response variable are considered stable, so that any differences between scores are attributed to rater error. In many situations, this may be a large assumption, and the researcher must understand the nature of the test variables and the instrumentation to establish that the rater is the true source of observed error.

Intrarater Reliability

Intrarater reliability refers to the stability of data recorded by one individual across two or more trials. When carryover or practice effects are not an issue, intrarater reliability is usually assessed using trials that follow each other with short intervals. Reliability is best established with multiple trials (more than two), although the number of trials needed is dependent on the expected variability in the response. In a test–retest situation, when a rater's skill is relevant to the accuracy of the test, intrarater reliability and test–retest reliability are essentially the same estimate. The effects of rater and the test cannot be separated out.

Many researchers automatically assume that intrarater reliability is achieved simply by having one experienced individual perform all measurements; however, the objective nature of scientific inquiry demands that even under expert conditions, rater reliability should be evaluated. Expertise by clinical standards may not always match the level of precision needed for research documentation. By establishing statistical reliability, those who critique research cannot question the measurement accuracy of data, and research conclusions will be strengthened.

Rater Bias.   We must also consider the possibility for bias when one rater takes two measurements. Raters can be influenced by their memory of the first score. This is most relevant in cases when human observers use subjective criteria to rate responses, but can operate in any situation when a tester must read a score from an instrument. The most effective way to control for this type of error is to blind the tester in some way, so that the first score remains unknown until after the second trial is completed; however, as most clinical measurements are observational, such a technique is often unreasonable. For instance, we could not blind a clinician to measures of balance, function, muscle testing, or gait, when the tester is an integral part of the measurement system. The major protections against tester bias are to develop grading criteria that are as objective as possible, to train the testers in the use of the instrument, and to document reliability across raters.

Interrater Reliability

Interrater reliability concerns variation between two or more raters who measure the same group of subjects. Even with detailed operational definitions and equal skill, different raters are not always in agreement about the quality or quantity of the variable being assessed. Intrarater reliability should be established for each individual rater before comparing raters with each other.

Interrater reliability is best assessed when all raters are able to measure a response during a single trial, where they can observe a subject simultaneously and independently, and thus eliminate true differences in scores as a source of measurement error when comparing raters' scores. Videotapes of patients performing activities have proved useful for allowing multiple raters to observe the exact same performance.[3, 4]

Simultaneous scoring is not possible, however, for many variables that require interaction of the tester and subject. For example, range of motion and manual muscle testing could not be tested simultaneously by two clinicians. With these types of measures, rater reliability may be affected if the true response changes from trial to trial. For instance, actual range of motion may change if the joint tissues are stretched from the first trial. Muscle force can decrease if the muscle is fatigued from the first trial.

Researchers will often decide to use one rater in a study, to avoid the necessity of establishing interrater reliability. Although this is useful for attempting consistency within the study, it does not strengthen the generalizability of the research outcomes. If interrater reliability of measurement has not been established, we cannot assume that other raters would have obtained similar results. This, in turn, limits the application of the findings to other people and situations. Interrater reliability allows the researcher to assume that the measurements obtained by one rater are likely to be representative of the subject's true score, and therefore, the results can be interpreted and applied with greater confidence.

Reliability Coefficients

The intraclass correlation coefficient (ICC) should be used to evaluate rater reliability. For interrater reliability, ICC model 2 or 3 can be used, depending on whether the raters are representative of other similar raters (model 2) or no generalization is intended (model 3). For intrarater reliability, model 3 should be used (see Chapter 26).

Alternate Forms

Many measuring instruments exist in two or more versions, called equivalent, parallel, or alternate forms. Interchange of these alternate forms can be supported only by establishing their parallel reliability. **Alternate forms reliability** testing is often used as an alternative to test–retest reliability with paper-and-pencil tests, when the nature of the test is such that subjects are likely to recall their responses to test items. For example, we are all familiar with standardized tests such as the Scholastic Aptitude Test (SAT) and the Graduate Record Examination (GRE), professional licensing exams, or intelligence tests, which are given several times a year, each time in a different form. These different versions of the tests are considered reliable alternatives based on their statistical equivalence. This type of reliability is established by administering two alternate forms of a test to the same group, usually in one sitting, and correlating paired observations. Because the tests are ostensibly different, they can be given at relatively the same time without fear of bias from one to the other. Although the idea of alternate forms has been applied mostly to educational and psychological testing, there are many examples in clinical practice. For example, clinicians use parallel forms of gait evaluations, tests of motor development, strength tests, functional evaluations, and range of motion tests. Many of these have not been tested for alternate forms reliability.

The importance of testing alternate forms reliability was illustrated in a study of hand dynamometers. One popular brand is available in several models, each with slightly different design features. Flood-Joy and Mathiowetz compared three of these models on a sample of normal adults.[5] To control for extraneous sources of error, they calibrated the dynamometers before and after each use and standardized instructions and positions of testing. The investigators found significant differences between strength scores using the three instruments. Therefore, test–retest strength measurements using these devices would have to be made with the same instrument, or patients might appear to be stronger or weaker simply because of the error between instruments. Establishing this method comparison is necessary if absolute values are to be compared or equated across tests, and to generalize findings from one study to another or from research to practice.

Reliability Coefficients

Correlation coefficients have been used most often to examine alternative forms reliability. The determination of *limits of agreement* has been proposed as a useful estimate of the range of error expected when using two different versions of an instrument. This estimate is based on the standard deviation of difference scores between the two instruments (see Chapter 26).

Internal Consistency

Software instruments such as questionnaires, written examinations, and interviews are ideally composed of a set of questions or items designed to measure particular knowledge or attributes. **Internal consistency,** or **homogeneity,** reflects the extent to which items measure various aspects of the same characteristic and nothing else. For example, if a professor gives an exam to assess students' knowledge of research design, the items should reflect a summary of that knowledge; the test should not include items on anthropology or health policy. If we assess a patient's ability to perform daily tasks using a physical function scale, then the items on the scale should relate to aspects of physical function only. If some items evaluated psychological or social characteristics, then the items would not be considered homogeneous. The scale should, therefore, be grounded in theory that defines the dimension of physical function, thereby distinguishing it from other dimensions of function.

The most common approach to testing internal consistency involves looking at the correlation among all items in a scale. For most instruments, it is desirable to see some relationship among items, to reflect measurement of the same attribute, especially if the scale score is summed. Therefore, for inventories that are intended to be multidimensional, researchers generally establish subscales that are homogenous on a particular trait (even though items are often mixed when the test is administered). For example, the Medical Outcomes Trust Short Form-36 (SF-36) health status measure is composed of eight subscales: physical function, limitations in physical role, pain, social function, mental health, limitations in emotional role, vitality, and general health perception.[6] Each of these subscales has been evaluated separately for internal consistency.[7]

Split-half Reliability

If we wanted to establish the reliability of a questionnaire, it would be necessary to administer the instrument on two separate occasions, essentially a test–retest situation. Oftentimes the interval between testing is relatively brief, to avoid the possibility for true change. Recall of responses, then, becomes a potential threat, as it might influence the second score, making it impossible to get a true assessment of reliability. One solution to this problem is the use of parallel forms, but this shifts the measure of reliability to a comparison of instruments, rather than reliability of a single instrument.

A simpler approach combines the two sets of items into one longer instrument, with half the items being redundant of the other half. One group of subjects takes the test at a single session. The items are then divided into two comparable halves for scoring, creating two separate scores for each subject. Typically, questions are divided according to odd and even items. This is considered preferable to comparing the first half of the test with the second half, as motivation, fatigue, and other psychological elements can influence performance over time, especially with a long test. Reliability is then assessed by correlating results of two halves of the test. If each subject's half-test scores are highly correlated, the whole test is considered reliable. This is called **split-half reliability.** This value will generally be an underestimate of the true reliability of the scale, since the reliability is proportional to the total number of items in the scale. Therefore, because the subscales are each half the length of the full test, the reliability coefficient is too low.

The obvious problem with the split-half approach is the need to determine that the two halves of the test are actually measuring the same thing. In essence, the two halves can be considered alternate forms of the same test; however, the split-half method is considered superior to test–retest and alternate forms procedures, because there is no time lag between tests and the same physical, mental, and environmental influences will affect the subjects as they take both sections of the test.

Reliability Coefficients

The statistic most often used for internal consistency is **Cronbach's coefficient alpha (α).**[8] This statistic can be used with items that are dichotomous or that have multiple choices.* Conceptually, coefficient α is the average of all possible split-half reliabilities for the scale. This statistic evaluates the items in a scale to determine if they are measuring the same construct or if they are redundant, suggesting which items could be discarded to improve the homogeneity of the scale. Cronbach's α will be affected by the number of items in a scale. The longer the scale, the more homogeneous it will appear, simply because there are more items.

For split-half reliability, the **Spearman-Brown prophecy statistic** is used as an estimate of the correlation of the two halves of the test. A fuller discussion of internal consistency statistics can be found in Chapter 26.

We can also assess internal consistency by conducting an **item-to-total correlation;** that is, we can examine how each item on the test relates to the instrument as a whole. To perform an item-to-total correlation, each individual item is correlated with the total score, omitting that item from the total. If an instrument is homogeneous, we would expect these correlations to be high. With this approach it is not necessary to create a doubly long test. If items are dichotomous, the point-biserial correlation coefficient should be

---

*When items are dichotomous, Cronbach's alpha is identical to a statistic called KR-20 (Kuder-Richardson formula 20).

used (see Chapter 23); if there are more than two response alternatives, the Pearson product-moment correlation coefficient is appropriate (see Chapter 23).[9]

GENERALIZABILITY

Measurement in clinical research or practice is never used as an end unto itself. Measurements are used as information for decision making, evaluation, or prediction. The score we obtain from a test is given a meaning beyond the specific situation in which it was taken; that is, we make generalizations about performance or behavior based on measurements. In many ways, reliability provides the foundation for making such generalizations, as we must have confidence in the dependability of measurements if they are to be applied in different situations or used to make decisions for future action. On this basis, Cronbach and his colleagues introduced the idea that reliability theory should be more accurately conceptualized in terms of **generalizability theory.**[10] They suggested that every individual score can be thought of as a sample from a universe of possible scores that might have been obtained under the same testing conditions. These specific testing conditions define the universe to which measures of reliability can be generalized. For example, we can test the grip strength of a patient with rheumatoid arthritis using a hand dynamometer. A single measured score of 15 pounds would be one of a universe of possible scores that might have been obtained under the same testing conditions, using the same dynamometer, at the same time of day, and by the same examiner. Because most research involves taking small samples of measurements, we assume that our observations are representative of this infinite distribution of possible scores. A single measurement then becomes the *best estimate* of a true score under those testing conditions. Reliability is essentially a measure of how good an estimate that measurement is.

According to classical reliability theory, an individual's observed score can be partitioned into a true component and an error component. The true score is assumed to be a fixed value that exists independently of any other conditions of measurement. Therefore, any differences between the observed score and the true score are due to random error. This theory also assumes that the error component is undifferentiated; that is, it comes from many different sources in an unbiased form. If we accept this premise, then we should be comfortable applying a given reliability estimate to any other situation when the same measurement is taken, because the error in each situation should be equally random. In generalizability theory, however, the conditions of testing are not considered independent factors; that is, the true score is a function of an underlying theoretical component *only as it exists under specific conditions.*[11] This means that not all variations from trial to trial should be attributed solely to random error. If we can identify relevant testing conditions that influence test scores, then we should be able to explain and predict more of the variance in a set of scores, effectively leaving less variance unexplained as error.

The concept of generalizability, therefore, forces us to interpret reliability within a multidimensional context, that is, in relation to a set of specific testing conditions. Each condition that defines this context is called a **facet.**[10] A particular combination of facets characterizes the universe to which reliability can be generalized. The researcher determines which facets are relevant to the measurement of a particular variable. By specifying those facets of greatest relevance, it is possible to statistically determine how much of the variance in observed scores can be attributed to each facet.

For instance, we could set up a test–retest situation and obtain two sets of ratings for a sample of 10 patients. By comparing these two sets of scores, we can establish the reliability of data across two occasions. Therefore, "occasion" becomes a facet of reliability. These occasions may be trials within one session or over two separate days. How these occasions are defined determines how the results can be generalized. Similarly, if we collect data from four clinicians' ratings within a single session, we can establish the reliability of data across four raters. Therefore, "rater" becomes a facet of reliability. In this case, we would have to establish the criteria that would characterize these raters, such as their years of experience or special training. Then results can be generalized to other raters with similar training.

The concept of generalizability is a clinically useful one, especially in terms of the development and standardization of measurement tools, because it provides a frame of reference for interpretation of reliability coefficients. Because we cannot expect to verify the reliability of every instrument on every patient for every rater, we must be able to document those characteristics that are relevant to generalizing measurement consistency. Generalizability theory also emphasizes that reliability is not an inherent quality of an instrument, but exists only within the context in which it was tested. Accordingly, we cannot automatically assume that estimates of reliability from one study can be applied to other raters, environments, testing conditions, or types of patients, unless we specifically address these factors in our analysis. Most reliability studies look at rater as the most important single facet. The essence of generalizability theory suggests, however, that other facets must be examined before an instrument's reliability can be fully understood.

In effect, then, there is no one coefficient that provides a complete estimate of reliability for a given test or measurement. Separate coefficients that address different facets can be obtained and applied to relevant situations. Without such documentation, it is not possible to make reasonable claims of general reliability for any instrument. Statistical and design considerations that are appropriate for generalizability studies are discussed further in Chapter 26.

Population-Specific Reliability

The concept of generalizability also emphasizes the need to consider characteristics of those involved in establishing reliability, including the patients or subjects being tested and the raters who do the testing. Reliability that is established on subjects from one population cannot automatically be attributed to other populations. This has been termed **population-specific reliability.** Clearly, factors such as pain, deformity, weakness, anxiety, and spasticity can alter the way a patient responds to a measurement and the consistency with which a clinician can take those measurements. Doing a manual muscle test on a patient with shoulder pain may be a different experience from doing the test on someone with limited range of motion. Range of motion measurements may be difficult to standardize among patients with joint deformities, joint pain or tenderness, or severe limitations of movement. Similarly, rater reliability must take into account the skill, experience, and training of the individual performing the test. Therefore, reliability of measurement must be documented according to the characteristics of a specific group of individuals who will be part of the measurement.

PILOT TESTING

When choosing an instrument for clinical or research measurement, it would certainly make sense to use a tool for which reliability has already been demonstrated. Even then, however, there is no guarantee that the same degree of reliability will be achieved in every situation. Therefore, researchers often perform pilot studies to establish reliability prior to the start of actual data collection. This study should be a routine part of the research process, especially when observational measurements are used. It allows the researcher to determine if raters are adequately trained to obtain valid measurements. It may be important to consider, however, that specific characteristics of the pilot test situation may be quite different from those that will be encountered during data collection. At the least, raters are often much more careful when they know the scores will be examined for reliability. Some studies have shown that raters' responses are less reliable during data collection than during sessions specifically designed for testing reliability.[12–14] Mitchell suggests that actual data collection should include multiple trials of each measurement, and that these trials should be assessed for reliability as part of the study's data analysis.[11] Although training and testing prior to data collection are essential for developing measurement accuracy, the validity of an experiment will be well served by documenting the error rate of measurement within the actual data used for analysis. For generalization of findings, it is probably more meaningful to report the reliability of these data than those obtained during pilot testing.

COMMENTARY

What Is the True Score?

It is hard to imagine any measurement system that is free from error. The concept of reliability is based on the premise that we can expect some deviation from the "true score" in every measurement we take. This presents an interesting dilemma when quantitative performance data are collected. If we take measures of range of motion or strength, for example, how do we determine which scores are useful for analysis? What strategies can we apply in data collection procedures to ensure the most reliable outcome? In addition to test–retest and rater reliability studies, most researchers recognize the need for taking more than one measurement of a behavior or characteristic whenever possible. But then we must ask: Out of these several trials, which value best represents the individual's true score?

Most investigators will not use the first score alone as the test value. The initial trial is often confounded by a warm-up or learning effect that will be evident as performance improves on subsequent trials. Some researchers use the final score in a series. They rationalize that the last repetition in a set of trials will be stabilized following warm-up or practice effects; however, depending on the number of trials, the final score may also be influenced by fatigue and, therefore, will not necessarily represent the subject's true effort.

A more common approach is to take the "best" score. Many researchers prefer using the subject's best effort as a reflection of what the subject is maximally capable of doing. If we consider reliability theory, however, then this is not necessarily the most accurate representation, because random error can contribute both positive and negative components to an observed score. Therefore, any observed score may be an overestimate or an underestimate of the true score. It is possible that the subject's maximal score in a set of two or three trials may actually be a function of positive error. Using the maximal score for data analysis may lend a positive bias to the outcome that would not be seen if the study were repeated on another sample.

Theoretically, then, the most representational score should be achieved through the mean or average score, because the sum of the error components over an infinite number of trials would be zero. Thus, the true score can be thought of as the average of the observed scores for a large number of trials, with the error components canceled out. Of course, there is room for argument in this rationale, because this theory operates in the "long run"; that is, we can expect a canceling of error components over an infinite number of trials. With only a few trials, this may be an unrealistic assumption; however, studies have shown that taking a mean value provides a more reliable measurement than any single value in a series of trials.[15, 16]

Which score should be used? There is no ready answer to this question. Researchers grapple with this decision for every study, based on the types of variables being measured and the precision those measurements achieve. It is often useful to take a series of measurements and estimate reliability using both single scores and average scores, to determine which approach provides the most reliable basis for data analysis. Generally, reliability of measurements that are less stable can be improved if averages are used. Reliability is also an important issue in statistical inference, as greater error (low reliability) will reduce the chances of finding statistically significant differences between groups. Therefore, the researcher always tries to make measurements as reliable as possible. This issue does reinforce, however, the constant need to confirm reliability.

KEY TERMS

reliability
validity
measurement error
systematic errors
random errors
regression toward the mean
variance
reliability coefficient
correlation
agreement

test–retest reliability
testing effect
intraclass correlation coefficient (ICC)
percent agreement
kappa
intrarater reliability
interrater reliability
alternate forms reliability
internal consistency
homogeneity

split-half reliability
Cronbach's coefficient alpha
Spearman-Brown prophesy formula
item-to-total correlation
generalizability theory
facet
population-specific reliability

REFERENCES

1. Cook TD, Campbell DT. *Quasi-experimentation: Design and Analysis Issues for Field Settings.* Boston: Houghton Mifflin, 1979.
2. Guilford J. *Psychometric Methods.* 2d ed. New York: McGraw-Hill, 1954.
3. Krebs DE, Edelstein JE, Fishman S. Reliability of observational kinematic gait analysis. *Phys Ther* 1985;65:1027–33.
4. Stuberg WA, White PJ, Miedaner JA, Dehne PR. Item reliability of the Milani-Comparetti Motor Development Screening Test. *Phys Ther* 1989;69:328–35.
5. Flood-Joy M, Mathiowetz V. Grip strength measurement: a comparison of three Jamar dynamometers. *Occup Ther J Res* 1987;7:235.
6. Ware JE, Sherbourne CD. The MOS 36-item Short-Form Health Survey (SF-36): I. Conceptual framework and item selection. *Med Care* 1992;30:473–83.
7. McHorney CA, Ware Jr JE, Lu JF, Sherbourne CD. The MOS 36-item Short-Form Health Survey (SF-36): III. Tests of data quality, scaling assumptions, and reliability across diverse patient groups. *Med Care* 1994;32:40–66.
8. Cronbach LJ. *Essentials of Psychological Testing.* 5th ed. New York: Harper & Row, 1990.
9. Nunally JC. *Psychometric Theory.* 2d ed. New York: McGraw-Hill, 1978.
10. Cronbach LJ, Gleser GC, Nanda H, Rajaratnam N. *The Dependability of Behavioral Measurements: Theory of Generalizability for Scores and Profiles.* New York: Wiley, 1972.
11. Mitchell SK. Interobserver agreement, reliability, and generalizability of data collected in observational studies. *Psychol Bull* 1979;36:376.
12. Reid JB. Reliability assessment of observational data: a possible methodological problem. *Child Dev* 1970;41:1143.
13. Taplin PS, Reid JB. Effects of instructional set and experimenter influence on observer reliability. *Child Dev* 1973;44:547.
14. Romanczyk RG, Kent RN, Diament C, et al. Measuring the reliability of observational data: a reactive process. *J Appl Behav Anal* 1973;6:175.
15. Beattie P, Isaacson K, Riddle DL, Rothstein JM. Validity of derived measurements of leg-length differences obtained by use of a tape measure. *Phys Ther* 1990;70:150–7.
16. Mathiowetz V, Weber K, Volland G, Kashman N. Reliability and validity of grip and pinch strength evaluations. *J Hand Surg [AM]* 1984;9:222–6.

6

Validity of Measurements

Measurement validity concerns the extent to which an instrument measures what it is intended to measure. Validity places an emphasis on the objectives of a test and the ability to make inferences from test scores or measurements. For instance, a goniometer is considered a valid instrument for testing range of motion (ROM), because we can assess joint range from angular measurements. A ruler is considered a valid instrument for calibrating length, because we can judge how long an object is by measuring inches or centimeters. We would, however, question the validity of assessing low back pain by measuring leg length because we cannot make reasonable inferences about back pain based on that measurement.

Therefore, validity addresses what we are able to do with test results. Tests are usually devised for purposes of discrimination, evaluation, or prediction. For instance, we may ask the following questions: Is the test capable of *discriminating* among individuals with and without certain traits? Can it *evaluate* change in the magnitude or quality of a variable from one time to another? Can we make useful and accurate *predictions* or diagnoses about a patient's potential function based on the outcome of the test? These are all questions of test validity.

The determination of validity for any test instrument can be made in a variety of contexts, depending on how the instrument will be used, the type of data it will generate, and the precision of the response variables. The purpose of this chapter is to define different types of validity and to describe the application of validity testing for clinical measurements.

VALIDITY AND RELIABILITY

Validity implies that a measurement is relatively free from error; that is, a valid test is also reliable (Fig. 6.1). An instrument that is inconsistent cannot produce meaningful measurements. If we use a goniometer with a loose axis that alters alignment, our results will no longer be valid indicators of joint range. Random measurement error will make it difficult to determine a true reading.

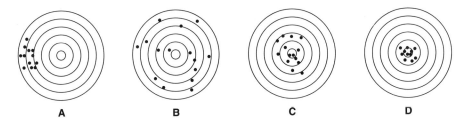

FIGURE 6.1 Representation of targets to illustrate the relationship between reliability and validity. (A) Scores are highly reliable, but not valid, demonstrating systematic error. (B) Scores are neither reliable nor valid, demonstrating random error. (C) Reliability has improved but is still low; scores are somewhat valid. (D) Scores are both reliable and valid.

An invalid test can be reliable, however (Fig. 6.1). For instance, we could obtain reliable measures of leg length time after time, but those measurements would still not tell us anything about back pain. Similarly, we might be able to establish that the reliability of leg length measurements is greater than the reliability of scores on a less objective test, such as a graphic pain scale, but this fact could not be used to support the validity of leg length as a measure of back pain. In addition we must consider the effect of systematic error or bias in the recording of data. If a tape measure is incorrectly marked, so that readings are consistently one inch more than the actual length, we may see strong reliability, but we will not have a valid measure of length.

These examples illustrate the importance of separating out issues of reliability and validity when evaluating a test. Although reliability is a prerequisite to validity, this relationship is unidirectional; that is, reliability sets the limits of validity, but it is no guarantee of it. Low reliability is automatic evidence of low validity, whereas strong reliability does not automatically suggest strong validity.

VALIDITY OF INFERENCES

In Chapter 4 we discussed the indirect nature of clinical measurement. We explained that most clinical variables are assessed by taking a correlate of the actual property being measured; that is, we make inferences about the magnitude of a particular variable based on a relevant observable behavior or response. Validity is basic to establishing these inferences. We must be able to document that the instrument's output is related and proportional to the actual variable of interest, and that the values assigned to a variable are representative of that response. We can verify that a thermometer is a valid instrument for measuring temperature, because mercury expands and contracts in proportion to changes in heat. A dynamometer is valid for measuring strength, because the transducer responds with a signal proportional to the exerted force. Similarly, it is logical to assess the level of serum creatinine in the body as an indicator of renal disease, since the kidneys regulate the level of creatinine in the body. Unfortunately, for the measurement of more abstract variables, such as intelligence, function, and perception, measurement scales are not so obviously related to the variable of interest, and validity is harder to verify.

We also draw inferences from tests that go beyond the simple values assigned to a variable. When we measure a patient's muscle strength or range of motion, it is not the muscle grade or joint angle that is of interest for its own sake, but what those values mean in terms of the integrity of the patient's musculoskeletal system. We use those values to infer something about the cause of that person's symptoms, the degree of disability, or the level of improvement following treatment. If we were told that the scores were not related to any other characteristics or future performance, we would wonder why anyone bothered to measure them.

Measurements are important, therefore, insofar as they allow us to make generalizations beyond a specific score. For example, clinical trials in Duchenne muscular dystrophy have examined the effects of various drug interventions by documenting changes in manual muscle test grades, range of motion, pulmonary function, and functional status.[1] These assessments can be considered valid for the measurement of the effectiveness of drug intervention only if we can make inferences about the state of the disease or disease progression based on their values.

At issue here is the *specificity of validity.* Just like reliability, validity is not inherent to an instrument, but must be evaluated within the context of the test's intended use and a specific population. The question of validity should not be, "Is an instrument valid?" It is more accurately, "How valid is it for a given purpose?" For instance, manual muscle testing, which was first developed to evaluate patterns of denervation in patients with poliomyelitis,[2] may not be valid for use on patients who exhibit upper motor neuron involvement because grading criteria do not account for the interference of abnormal muscle tone or reflexes. Similarly, an instrument designed to assess function in patients who have had a stroke may not be valid for patients with Alzheimer's disease. In another context, an instrument designed to describe the health status of a specific population may not be appropriate for assessing change in an individual's function. Therefore, validity is not a universal characteristic of an instrument. The researcher is always responsible for presenting evidence to support the validity of a measurement method for the specific question being investigated.

Because measurement inferences are difficult to verify, establishing validity is not as straightforward as establishing reliability. For many variables there are no obvious rules or formulas for judging that a test is indeed measuring the critical property of interest. Like reliability, we do not think of validity in an all-or-none sense, but rather as a characteristic that an instrument has to a varying degree. It is often a source of frustration to clinical scientists that, when dealing with abstract constructs, the documentation of test validity may never be complete.

Validation procedures are based on the types of evidence that can be offered in support of a test's validity. We can think of validation as a process of hypothesis testing, determining if scores on a test are related to specific behaviors, characteristics, or levels of performance. Evidence to support hypotheses is generally defined according to four types of validity: face validity, content validity, criterion-related validity, and construct validity (Table 6.1). These categorizations are helpful for differentiating approaches to validity testing, but it is important to remember that all types of validity address the degree of confidence we have in the inferences we draw from test scores.[3]

TABLE 6.1. TYPES OF MEASUREMENT VALIDITY

Face validity: Indicates that an instrument appears to test what it is supposed to test. The weakest form of measurement validity.

Content validity: Indicates that the items that make up an instrument adequately sample the universe of content that defines the variable being measured. Most useful with questionnaires and inventories.

Criterion-related validity: Indicates that the outcomes of one instrument, the target test, can be used as a substitute measure for an established gold standard criterion test. Can be tested as concurrent or predictive validity.

    Concurrent validity: Establishes validity when two measures are taken at relatively the same time. Most often used when the target test is considered more efficient than the gold standard and, therefore, can be used instead of the gold standard.

    Predictive validity: Establishes that the outcome of the target test can be used to predict a future criterion score or outcome.

        Prescriptive validity: Establishes that the interpretation of a measurement is appropriate for determining effective intervention.

Construct validity: Establishes the ability of an instrument to measure an abstract construct and the degree to which the instrument reflects the theoretical components of the construct.

FACE VALIDITY

The least rigorous method for documenting a test's validity is face validation. **Face validity** indicates that an instrument *appears* to test what it is supposed to and that it is a plausible method for doing so. To establish face validity, one must be clear about the definition of the concept that is being measured. For some instruments, face validity is easily established because the instrument measures the property of interest through some form of direct observation. Therefore, face validity is generally attributed to tests of range of motion, length, strength, tactile discrimination, sensation, gait, and balance. The separate items on a functional status scale, such as eating, dressing, and transferring, would have face validity. Some instruments do not have obvious face validity, and must be validated in some other way to document their usefulness. For instance, the measurement of temperature using a mercury thermometer does not have face validity; however, physicists can show how mercury reacts to changes in molecular motion and heat to provide validation.

For scientific purposes, face validity should not be considered sufficient documentation of a test's validity because there is no standard for judging it or determining "how much" of it an instrument has.[4] Essentially, face validity is assessed as all or none. Therefore, assessments of face validity are considered subjective and scientifically weak. Whenever possible, a more stringent validation criterion should be applied that is capable of evaluating the degree of validity present in an instrument. There will be times, however, when no other form of validation is possible, when an instrument is one of a kind, and no other instrument or test can be used for comparison. In that case, the investigator may be forced to rely on face validity to justify an instrument's use. The disadvantage of relying on face validation as the only justification for a test is that it provides no clout against potential challenges because it is based solely on the opinion of the investigator. Goldsmith suggests that one way to evaluate face validity is to determine who the stakeholders are, such as patients, physicians, physical therapists, occupational therapists, or social workers, and then to describe a simple percentage of how many consider the test credible.[5]

Face validity serves an important purpose, however, in that an instrument lacking in face validity may not be acceptable to those who administer it, those who are tested by it, or those who will use the results. For example, respondents on a questionnaire may not answer questions with honesty or motivation if they do not see the relevance of the questions. Patients may not be compliant with repeated testing if they do not understand how a test relates to their difficulty. Consumers of research reports may not accept results if they feel the test is irrelevant. Therefore, although face validity should not be considered sufficient, it is a useful property of a test.

CONTENT VALIDITY

Most behavioral and educational variables have a theoretical domain or universe of content that consists of all the behaviors, characteristics, or information that could possibly be observed about that variable. **Content validity** refers to the adequacy with which this universe is sampled by a test. Because the content universe is only theoretical, it must be defined by representative parts of the whole. An instrument is said to have content validity if it covers all parts of the universe of content and reflects the relative importance of each part. Content validity is an especially important characteristic of questionnaires, examinations, inventories, and interviews that attempt to evaluate a range of information by selected test items or questions.

Content validity demands that a test is free from the influence of factors that are irrelevant to the purpose of the measurement. For instance, a test of gross motor skills should not contain items that assess fine motor skills, nor should it be influenced by the patient's anxiety level or ability to read. If these factors influence the patient's score, the test would be measuring something other than what it was intended to measure and would not be a valid reflection of gross motor skill. Perhaps more importantly, content validity means that the test contains all the elements that reflect the variable being studied. For example, an evaluation of pain using a visual analogue scale (VAS) that assesses the intensity of an individual's pain reflects only one element of the experience of pain. A tool such as the McGill Pain Questionnaire may have greater content validity because it includes a comprehensive assessment of many elements of pain such as location, quality, time, and intensity.[6]

The determination of content validity is essentially a subjective process. There are no statistical indices that can assess content validity. Claims for content validation are made by a panel of "experts" who review the instrument and determine if the questions satisfy the content domain. This process often requires several revisions of the test. When all agree that the content domain has been sampled adequately, content validity is supported.

In some ways, content validation and face validation are similar concepts, in that both are based on subjective judgments, and both indicate that the test *appears* to be serving its intended purpose. There is, however, an important distinction between these two procedures. Face validity is a post hoc form of validation; that is, it is a judgment made after an instrument is constructed. Conversely, content validity evolves out of the planning and construction of a test. It is derived through a complete and rational evaluation of a test's objectives and how its component parts reflect the theoretical basis for the test. Therefore, face validity can be considered a component of content validity.

Content validity is specific to the content universe as it is defined by the researcher. For some content areas this will be fairly obvious. For instance, an instructor preparing a final examination can determine if the questions address each unit covered during the semester and if the requested information was included in course materials. Other content universes are less obvious. Consider the following: What range of activities are representative of "function"? Should a functional status questionnaire include questions related to physical, cognitive, social, and emotional function? How important are each of these domains to the assessment of function of a patient with a stroke, a patient with spinal cord injury, or a well elderly person? If we are interested in dressing skills, how many different tasks must be sampled to make a valid judgment? Will physical therapists define this universe differently from occupational therapists or nurses?

These types of questions must be answered by the researcher before the validity of the test can be determined. The answers will depend on the rationale for the test, the operational definitions of the test variable, and the specific objectives of the test instrument. The content universe should be described in sufficient detail so that the domain of interest is clearly identified for all who use the instrument.

CRITERION-RELATED VALIDITY

Criterion-related validity is the most practical approach to validity testing and the most objective. It is based on the ability of one test to predict results obtained on another test. The test to be validated, called the *target test,* is compared with a **gold standard,** or criterion measure that is already established or assumed to be valid. When both tests are administered to one group of subjects, the scores on the target test are correlated with those achieved by the criterion measure. If the correlation is high (the correlation coefficient is close to 1.00), the target test is considered a valid predictor of the criterion score. For instance, we can investigate the validity of heart rate (the target test) as an indicator of energy cost during exercise by correlating it with values obtained in standardized oxygen consumption studies (the criterion measure). We could establish the validity of observational gait analysis (the target test) by comparing results with those obtained with computerized motion analysis systems (the criterion measure). In each case, the criterion measure is known or assumed to be a valid indicator of the variable of interest, and therefore, comparable results achieved with the target test are supportive of that test's validity.

Validity of the Criterion

The most crucial element of criterion validation is the ability to demonstrate validity of the criterion measure. If the criterion is not valid, it is plainly useless as a standard. Several characteristics can be used to judge the utility of a criterion measure. First, it is necessary to demonstrate its reliability in a test–retest situation, so that the instrument's stability is confirmed. Second, the criterion and target ratings should be *independent* and *free from bias.* For instance, if we use a supervisor's ratings as the criterion to validate a new scale of clinical competence for evaluating staff performance, we want to be sure that the supervisor's relationship with the staff does not influence the rating. We also want to blind the supervisor to the staff person's scores on the clinical scale to avoid the temptation of giving higher ratings to those who achieved higher clinical scores. It is often helpful to have different raters perform the target and criterion tests.

A third, and probably the most important, characteristic of a good criterion is its relevance to the behavior being measured by the target test. We must be able to establish that the criterion is a valid measure of the variable being addressed by the target test; that is, the *criterion and the target test must be measuring the same thing.* For instance, some studies have used measures of range of motion to document changes in joint pain. One might believe that active movement in a joint will be proportional to the amount of pain experienced during movement. Others might argue, however, that ROM measures do not assess pain and would be inappropriate as a criterion for validation of other pain scales. This issue is of obvious importance to the interpretation of correlations between tests.

In many areas of physical and physiological science, standard criteria are readily available for validating clinical tools. For example, to validate methods of measuring physical activity levels, we can use oxygen consumption data;[7] to validate a new method of measuring range of motion, we can refer to the standard universal goniometer.[8] Unfortunately, choosing a gold standard for more abstract constructs is not always as obvious a task. If we want to establish the validity of a functional status questionnaire, with what referent should it be compared? What standard can be used to validate a scale designed to assess perceptions of quality of life in a nursing home population? How can we establish an external criterion to judge a person's degree of pain? Sometimes the best a clinician can do is use another instrument that has already achieved a degree of validation or acceptance. For abstract variables such as these, criterion validation is not always feasible, and a more complex approach—construct validation—is necessary. This process is discussed in the next section.

Criterion-related validity is often separated into two components: concurrent validity and predictive validity. These approaches are differentiated on the basis of the time frame within which predictions are made.

Concurrent Validity

Concurrent validity is studied when the measurement to be validated and the criterion measure are taken at relatively the same time (concurrently), so that they both reflect the same incident of behavior. This approach to validation is useful in situations when a new or untested tool is potentially more efficient, easier to administer, more practical, or safer than another more established method, and is being proposed as an alternative instrument. For instance, clinicians interested in measuring leg length differences have used a variety of clinical methods, such as a tape measure and palpation of both iliac crests, most of which are accepted on the basis of their face validity. Taking measurements from radiographs is generally considered the most accurate approach,[9] but this method is costly and involves some risk to the patient. Therefore, one group of investigators used radiographic data as the gold standard to establish the validity of a tape measure for determining leg length differences.[10] These investigators found a high correlation between these two methods, suggesting that the measurements taken with the tape measure were valid indicators of leg length inequality; that is, measurements obtained with the tape measure were useful predictors of measurements that would have been obtained using the radiographic technique. Of course, the validity of these conclusions is limited to the extent that radiographs are an accurate gold standard for calculating leg lengths.

Predictive Validity

Predictive validity attempts to establish that a measure will be a valid predictor of some future criterion score. A test with good predictive validity helps an investigator make successful decisions by providing a basis for predicting outcomes or future behaviors. To assess predictive validity, a target test is given at one session and is followed by a period of time after which the criterion score is obtained. The interval between these two tests is dependent on the time needed to achieve the criterion, and may be as long as several years. The relationship between the target and criterion scores is examined to determine if the target test score is a valid predictor of the outcome on the criterion measure.

A classic example is the use of college admissions criteria, such as the Scholastic Aptitude Test (SAT) or grade point average (GPA), based on their presumed ability to predict future academic success. In health care, predictive validity is an essential concept in screening procedures, prognosis, and setting of long-term goals. We engage in prediction when we examine the relationship between impairments and functional limitations or disability. For example, Jette et al. were able to show that musculoskeletal impairments, particularly decrements in hand function, are important indicators in the progression of physical disability in the elderly.[11] Magaziner et al. studied 536 patients aged 65 or older who had a hip fracture, and followed them for one year following hospital discharge.[12] They demonstrated that affective status, cognitive function, and social contact were important predictors of recovery, as measured by walking ability and ability to perform activities of daily living (ADL), suggesting areas where discharge planning efforts should focus.

We also estimate the potential for rehabilitation or change on the basis of a patient's initial status. For instance, Katz and coworkers studied a sample of 105 patients who underwent arthroscopic partial meniscectomy, to identify factors that were predictive of poor outcomes.[13] They examined demographic factors, medical history, preoperative impairments and functional status, and operative variables to determine their relationship to postoperative function, as measured by the SF-36 Physical Activity Scale. Through multivariate statistical analyses, they found that the extent of cartilage damage, workers' compensation, and preoperative functional status were most predictive of a poor outcome. The authors suggested that these findings should be routinely measured and incorporated into prognostic data, to provide a basis for discussing the advantages and disadvantages of the procedure with patients.

A practical limitation exists, however, when trying to assess the predictive validity of screening procedures. One must be able to follow subjects who *do* and *do not* have positive initial findings, so that follow-up measures can distinguish between them. For instance, in setting admissions criteria, presumably we only choose the most qualified students. Therefore, when examining the outcome of academic success we are not able to determine if those with lesser scores would have also succeeded. They were never given the chance. This makes it difficult to truly determine if the admissions criteria have predictive validity.

Prescriptive Validity

In most clinical situations, pre-treatment data are used as criteria for deciding on a course of treatment. Our decisions are based on the assumption that the inferences we draw from these measurements have validity for this purpose. The term **prescriptive validity** has been used to distinguish the situation in which predictor variables are used as the basis for choosing an appropriate intervention.[14] For example, we often assess a patient's balance to determine what type of assistive device they should use to maximize safety during walking. If we use a specific measure of balance as a target test, and prescribe a particular assistive device based on this score, we would then want to determine if the patient did, indeed, maintain safe ambulation while using the device. Over time, if we used this same balance test on many patients, perhaps we could evaluate the outcome by collecting data on the number of times patients fell or lost their balance while walking with the device. If the outcome showed that patients did not fall, then we would have evidence of the prescriptive validity of the balance test. It helped us choose an appropriate ambulation device. If we find out in the end that the device did not effectively improve safety, then our balance test, although valid and reliable as a measure of impairment, was not valid for selecting treatment; that is, the data were not able to lead us to a correct *prescriptive* decision. To truly establish this validity, however, we would have to compare the results when we assigned an assistive device using some other test criterion, to determine if there was a lower incidence of falls using the balance score.

Prescriptive validity can be compromised if outcome measurements are not chosen carefully. For instance, if we evaluated the outcome of safe ambulation by measuring gait speed, we might not see much of a change over time. Perhaps patients continue to walk slowly, but maintain their balance. In this case we would not be able to accurately assess the prescriptive validity of the balance score. Therefore, judgment about the prescriptive validity of an initial evaluation must be taken within the context of the desired outcome.

CONSTRUCT VALIDITY

Construct validity reflects the ability of an instrument to measure an abstract concept, or construct. The process of construct validation presents a considerable challenge to the researcher because constructs are not "real"; that is, they are not directly observable and exist only as concepts that are constructed to represent an abstract trait. Because constructs are typically multidimensional, it is not easy to determine if an instrument is actually measuring the variable of interest.

For example, everyone agrees that "health" is an important clinical construct, but because of its complexity, clinicians are generally unable to agree on how it should be defined or measured. Therefore, the definition of such a construct as "health status" can be determined only by the instrument used to measure it. A test that focuses only on physical activity will suggest a very different definition than a more global test that also incorporates cognitive, social, and psychological elements. Similarly, a scale that looks at activities of daily living according to categories of self-care, transfers, and dressing will provide a different perception of function than one that also evaluates locomotion, housekeeping, and recreation skills. An instrument that evaluates ADL according to an individual's perception of the *difficulty* performing given tasks will produce a measurement that is interpreted differently than one which focuses on the *time* needed to perform, the *assistance* required, or another that assesses the level of *pain* associated with specific tasks. Each of these provide a different theoretical foundation for defining the construct of function.

Part of construct validity, therefore, is based on content validity; that is, one must be able to define the content universe that represents that construct to develop a test to measure it. Beyond content, however, constructs must also be defined according to their underlying *theoretical context*. Thus, the "meaning" of a construct is based on assumptions about how an individual with that trait would behave under given conditions and how the various dimensions that form the construct interrelate. One can generate hypotheses regarding the overt behaviors of individuals with high and low scores on the test. An instrument is said to be a valid measure of a construct when its measurements support these theoretical assumptions.

For example, pain is a difficult construct to define, as it represents a subjective phenomenon rather than a performance behavior. However, we may also question whether pain is a stimulus, a perception, a response, or a behavior. Looking at the construct of pain, then, requires that we conceptualize what is actually being evaluated. For instance, Sim and Waterfield discuss the "experience of pain" as a subjective outcome that varies from individual to individual.[15] They describe the pain experience as having sensory, affective, evaluative, cognitive, and behavioral dimensions, with sensory, emotional, and physiological outcomes (Fig. 6.2). Further analysis suggests the need to look at memory, cultural factors, social networks, sex and age, personality, and other elements that contribute to the individual perception of pain. The differentiation between chronic and acute pain is more than just the time over which the pain occurs. Then there are characteristics of pain such as intensity, quality, location, and duration.

How one chooses to measure pain, therefore, will affect greatly how the outcome will be interpreted. For instance, a VAS using the anchors of "no pain" to "pain as bad as it could be" would be focusing solely on intensity, and could not distinguish a pin prick from a headache or a burn. The Oswestry Low Back Pain Disability Questionnaire looks at back pain with reference to disabling effects, rather than the subjective nature of the pain.[16] The Pain and Distress Scale evaluates mood and behavior changes associated with acute pain, but not the severity of the pain itself.[17] The construct is defined, therefore, by the instrument used to measure it. Different elements may be important, depending on the clinical or research situation.

Because of the abstract and complex nature of constructs, construct validation is never quite fully realized. Each attempt to validate an instrument provides evidence to support or refute the theoretical framework behind the construct. Construct validation is an ongoing process, wherein we are continually learning more about the construct and testing its predictions. This evidence can be gathered by a variety of methods. Some of

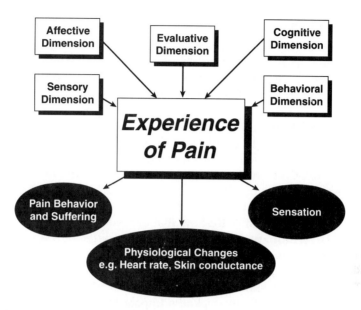

FIGURE 6.2   Theoretical model of the multidimensional nature of the experience of pain, illustrating how the construct of pain may be conceptualized. Several dimensions contribute to the individual nature of the experience, as well as how the outcomes of the pain experience are perceived. (Adapted from Sim J, Waterfield J. Validity, reliability and responsiveness in the assessment of pain. *Physiother Theory Pract* 1997; 13:23–37.)

the more commonly used procedures include the known groups method, convergence and discrimination, factor analysis, hypothesis testing, and criterion validation.

Known Groups Method

The most general type of evidence in support of construct validity is provided when a test can discriminate between individuals who are known to have the trait and those who do not. Using the **known groups method,** a criterion is chosen that can identify the presence or absence of a particular characteristic, and the theoretical context behind the construct is used to predict how different groups are expected to behave. Therefore, the validity of a particular test is supported if the test's results document these known differences.

For example, Gregory-Flock and Yerxa examined the construct validity of the prone extension postural test as a measurement of vestibular function in children.[18] They studied children from 4 to 8 years old who did and did not have learning disabilities. They based their study on the theory that the ability to maintain the prone extension posture is an indicator of vestibular function and that vestibular dysfunction is generally associated with learning disability. By analyzing the statistical difference between the two groups' performance on the test, they were able to show that the normal children and the children with learning disabilities had different ranges of scores, supporting the construct validity of the test as a measure of vestibular function.

Convergence and Discrimination

Campbell and Fiske have suggested that the construct validity of a test can be evaluated in terms of how its measures relate to other tests of the same and different constructs.[19] In other words, it is important to determine what a test measures as well as what it does not measure. This determination is based on the concepts of convergence and discrimination.

Convergent validity indicates that two measures believed to reflect the same underlying phenomenon will yield similar results or will correlate highly. For instance, if two health status scales are valid methods for measuring quality of life, they should produce correlated scores. Convergence also implies that the theoretical context behind the construct will be supported when the test is administered to different groups in different places at different times. Convergence is not a sufficient criterion for construct validity, however. It is also necessary to show that a construct can be differentiated from other constructs. **Discriminant validity** indicates that different results, or low correlations, are expected from measures that are believed to assess different characteristics. Therefore, the results of an intelligence test should not be expected to correlate with results of a test of gross motor skill.

To illustrate these concepts, the Sickness Impact Profile (SIP) has been compared with several other measures of function in an effort to establish its construct validity. The SIP is a health status measure that indicates the changes in a person's behavior due to sickness, scored on the total scale as well as on separate physical and psychosocial subscales.[20] Convergent validity has been supported by a high correlation between the physical dimension of the SIP scale and the Arthritis Impact Measurement Scale,[21] and a strong correlation between the psychosocial SIP scale and the Carroll Rating Scale for Depression.[22] Discriminant validity is illustrated by a lower correlation between the physical SIP scale and the depression score.[22] These types of studies are part of the ongoing nature of construct validity testing, continually examining how an instrument functions as a measure of a theoretical construct.

Campbell and Fiske also suggest that validity of a test should be evaluated in terms of both the characteristic being measured and the method used to measure it. They call this a *trait-method unit*[19]; that is, a trait cannot be assessed independently of some method. Therefore, the validity of the assessment must take both elements into account. On the basis of this concept, a validation process was proposed that incorporates an analysis of two or more traits measured by two or more methods. The intercorrelations of variables within and between methods are arranged in a matrix called a *multitrait–multimethod matrix*. By arranging scores in this way, we can verify that tests measuring the same trait produce high correlations, demonstrating convergent validity; and those that measure different traits produce low correlations, demonstrating discriminant validity. For example, Shields and Cicchetti studied emotion regulation among school-age children.[23] They explored the construct validity of the Emotion Regulation Q-Scale using a sample of 223 maltreated or impoverished children, aged 6 to 12 years. Using a multitrait–multimethod matrix they were able to demonstrate excellent convergence among the Emotion Regulation Q-Scale and other established measures of affect regulation. The new scale also had low correlations with measures of related constructs, such as assessments of ego resiliency. Therefore, they concluded that the scale was able to distinguish between maltreated and comparison children and between groups of well-regulated versus dysregulated children. The advantage of including more than one construct in this analysis is that the researcher can establish that the concepts are truly distinct, rather than simply different labels for the same underlying attribute.

Factor Analysis

Another common approach to construct validation is the use of a statistical procedure called **factor analysis.** The concept of factor analysis is based on the idea that a construct contains one or more underlying dimensions, or different theoretical components. For instance, intelligence has been analyzed in terms of perception, quantification, word fluency, verbal ability, spatial ability, memory, and reasoning.[24] Within each of these "dimensions" we can identify a variety of tasks or performance variables that together will provide an evaluation of that particular dimension. A valid test of intelligence should be able to measure and discriminate among these components. For example, the theoretical component of perception can be measured by facial perceptions and mirror reading. Quantification can be measured by the ability to identify numbers and to perform arithmetic tasks. If we were to measure a whole series of specific variables that relate to intelligence, and we were to correlate these measures, we would find that certain variables would be correlated with each other in distinct groupings. For example, facial perception and mirror reading should be correlated with each other; number identification and arithmetic tasks should be correlated with each other; but the perception variables should not be correlated with the quantification variables. These separate groupings of correlated variables are called *factors*. A factor represents a subset of test items or behaviors that are related to each other, but are not related to items in other factors; that is, each factor represents a unique combination of items that reflects a different theoretical component of the construct. The statistical basis for this process is quite complex and beyond our current discussion, but we will devote considerable attention to it in Chapter 27 when we discuss multivariate statistics.

Hypothesis Testing

Because constructs have a theoretical basis, an instrument's validity can also be assessed by using it to test specific hypotheses that support the theory. For instance, the construct validity of the Functional Independence Measure (FIM) was assessed by Dodds et al., based on the assumption that the instrument should be able to distinguish functional differences between people with varied clinical conditions.[25] The construct of function that forms the foundation for the FIM relates to the burden of care, or the degree of assistance needed for a patient to fulfill activities in ADL, mobility, and cognitive domains. Using this theoretical premise, the authors proposed three hypotheses: (1) FIM scores should decrease with increasing age and comorbidities; (2) the score should be related to a patient's discharge destination according to the level of care provided in that setting (such as home or skilled nursing facility); and (3) there should be a relationship between FIM scores and degree of severity for patients with amputations, spinal cord injury, and stroke. Using data collected on more than 11,000 patients, their results supported some hypotheses better than others, demonstrating a strong relationship between FIM scores and discharge destination, and severity of spinal cord injury and stroke. This type of analysis provides distinct evidence of construct validity for the instrument, but it leaves unanswered many theoretical questions regarding its use over the broad range of reha-bilitation situations. Therefore, it also points to the need for continued testing to deter-mine how the FIM score relates to various diagnoses and clinical findings.

Criterion Validation

Construct validity can also be supported by comparison of test results with those of rel-evant criterion tests. This approach is not used as often as other approaches, because it is typically difficult to find a suitable criterion. In most cases, when a new instrument is developed to measure a construct, it is because no other acceptable instruments are available. Therefore, no standard can be applied to test it; however, it is often possible to find criterion tests that can be applied to subparts of the overall instrument. For exam-ple, Podsiadlo and Richardson used the Berg Balance Scale, gait speed, and a measure of function as criterion values to establish the construct validity of the timed "Up & Go" test.[26] These individual criterion tests were assumed to represent components of the overall construct of mobility that the "Up & Go" test was intended to measure. Through a series of correlations the authors were able to demonstrate that each criterion test was related to the outcome variable, and although these were not perfect correlations, taken together they supported the overall concept that was being evaluated.

EVALUATING DIAGNOSTIC PROCEDURES

Many measuring instruments are specifically designed as *diagnostic* or *screening* tools. In a traditional medical framework, a diagnostic test is used to screen for the presence or absence of a disease or abnormal condition. Clinical researchers have expanded upon this concept to include tests that are intended to identify individuals with functional deficits, those who would benefit from specific intervention strategies, or those for whom treatment has produced clinically meaningful outcomes. In essence, then, we may consider the process of *diagnosis* in the same way that we view *prognosis*. As we dis-cuss the use of diagnostic procedures, we can easily substitute "outcome" for "disease" to apply these principles to prognostic tests as well. Because diagnostic procedures in-volve allocation of resources and potential risks to patients, and are used for clinical de-cision making, it is important to verify their validity.

Test Results

The results of a diagnostic procedure may be dichotomous, categorical, or continuous. The simplest tests will have only a dichotomous outcome: positive or negative. Tests that look for presence or absence of cancer will generate such an outcome. A categorical test would involve ratings on an ordinal scale such as $+++$, $++$, $+$, $-$ to reflect the level of involvement. A continuous scale provides the most information regarding the outcome, such as a test measuring degrees of range of motion or hearing decibel level.

The ideal diagnostic test, of course, would always be accurate in discriminating be-tween those with and without the disease or condition; it would always have a positive result for someone with the disease, whether a mild or severe case, and a negative result in everyone else. We determine the quality of a screening test by comparing the test result with known diagnostic findings obtained by a **gold standard.** The gold standard will reflect the true event—either the presence or absence of the condition. The assumption is made that the individual performing the test is blind to the true condition, eliminating possible bias. In some situations, the gold standard will be another concurrent test, such as an X ray or blood test. In other situations, it will be obtained at a future time, as with an autopsy or long-term outcome. Sometimes there is no clear gold standard, especially when using this approach for prognosis, and an outcome measure must be defined, such as need for further hospitalization or length of stay. One goal of outcomes research is to define measures that are appropriate standards for determining that a treatment has achieved an acceptable level of success.

Sensitivity and Specificity

The validity of a diagnostic test is evaluated in terms of its ability to accurately assess the presence and absence of the target condition. A diagnostic test can have four possible outcomes, summarized in the 2 × 2 arrangement shown in Table 6.2. Classification is assigned according to the true presence or absence of disease (Dx+ or Dx–) versus positive or negative test results. In Table 6.2 the cells labeled *a* and *d* represent **true positives** and **true negatives,** respectively, that is, individuals who are correctly classified as having or not having the target condition. Cell *b* reflects individuals who are incorrectly identified as having the condition (**false positives**), and cell *c* represents those who are incorrectly identified as not having the condition (**false negatives**).

TABLE 6.2   SUMMARY OF ANALYSIS FOR SCREENING TEST RESULTS

	Diagnosis (Dx) (presence or absence of target condition)		
Screening test results	**Dx+**	**Dx-**	**Total**
Positive	*a* (true positive)	*b* (false positive)	*a + b*
Negative	*c* (false negative)	*d* (true negative)	*c + d*
Total	*a + c*	*b + d*	

$$\text{Sensitivity} = \frac{a}{a + c}$$

$$\text{Specificity} = \frac{d}{b + d}$$

$$\text{Positive predictive value (PV+)} = \frac{a}{a + b}$$

$$\text{Negative predictive value (PV–)} = \frac{d}{c + d}$$

Sensitivity is the test's ability to obtain a positive test when the target condition is really present, or a true positive. Using the notation presented in Table 6.2, sensitivity is calculated as $a/(a + c)$. This value is the proportion of individuals who test positive for the condition out of all those who actually have it, or the probability of obtaining a positive test in patients who have the target condition. The sensitivity of a test increases as the number of persons with the condition who are correctly classified increases; that is, fewer persons with the disorder are missed.

Specificity is the test's ability to obtain a negative test when the condition is really absent, or a true negative. This value is given by $d/(b + d)$, which represents the proportion of individuals who test negative for the condition out of all those who are truly normal, or the probability of a negative test in those who do not have the target condition. A highly specific instrument will rarely test positive when a person does not have the disease.

To illustrate the application of these measures, Amendt and coworkers studied the validity of an instrument, called a Scoliometer, which was designed to assess axial trunk rotation.[27] The trunk angle measured by the Scoliometer was used to screen for the presence or absence of scoliosis. Screening results were compared with those obtained using radiographic data as the gold standard. For this example, we refer to a portion of their data using a trunk angle of 5 degrees as the criterion level to indicate the presence of scoliosis, as shown in Table 6.3. The sensitivity of this test was strong, at 94%. Of the 16 patients diagnosed as having scoliosis (according to the radiographic data), 15 tested pos-

TABLE 6.3 SENSITIVITY, SPECIFICITY, AND PREDICTIVE VALUES FOR A SCREENING TEST FOR SCOLIOSIS USING A CRITERION OF 5 DEGREES OF TRUNK ROTATION

Screening test results	Diagnosis of scoliosis		Total
	Dx+	Dx-	
Positive	15	13	28
Negative	1	5	6
Total	16	18	34

$$\text{Sensitivity} = \frac{a}{a + c} = \frac{15}{16} = 94\%$$

$$\text{Specificity} = \frac{d}{b + d} = \frac{5}{18} = 28\%$$

$$\text{PV+} = \frac{a}{a + b} = \frac{15}{28} = 54\%$$

$$\text{PV-} = \frac{d}{c + d} = \frac{5}{6} = 83\%$$

Source: Amendt LE, Ause-Ellias KL, Eybers JL, et al. Validity and reliability testing of the Scoliometer. *Phys Ther* 1990; 70:108.

itive using the Scoliometer. The specificity of the test, however, was only 28%. Only 5 of the 18 patients who did not have scoliosis tested negative. Therefore, although all those with scoliosis were identified, a large percentage of patients who did not have scoliosis tested positive.

Predictive Value

In addition to sensitivity and specificity, the usefulness of a clinical screening tool can be assessed by its feasibility. A test must demonstrate that it is an efficient use of time and resources and that it yields a sufficient number of accurate responses to be clinically useful. This characteristic is assessed by the test's predictive value. A **positive predictive value** (PV+) estimates the likelihood that a person who tests positive actually has the disease. With the notation given in Table 6.2, PV+ = $a/(a + b)$, which represents the proportion of those who tested positive who were true positives. Therefore, a test with a high positive predictive value will provide a strong estimate of the actual number of patients who have the target condition. Similarly, a **negative predictive value** (PV–) indicates the probability that a person who tests negative is actually disease free. Therefore, PV– = $d/(c + d)$, which is the proportion of all those who tested negative who were true negatives. A test with a high negative predictive value will provide a strong estimate of the number of people who do not have the target condition.

For the scoliosis study (Table 6.3), the positive predictive value of 54% tells us that about half of those who tested positive actually had scoliosis; that is, approximately one of every two patients who tested positive was actually normal. The negative predictive value was higher at 83%. Therefore, approximately four of five patients who tested negative were normal.

Predictive value may be of greatest importance in deciding whether to implement a screening program. When the positive predictive value is low, only a small portion of those who test positive actually have the target condition. Therefore, considerable resources will probably be needed to evaluate these people further to separate false positives, or unnecessary treatments will be applied. Policy decisions are often based on a balance between the use of available resources and the potential harmful effects resulting from not identifying those with the target condition.[28]

The predictive value of a test is related to its sensitivity and specificity. With a more sensitive test, positive cases are identified more readily; that is, we will not miss many true cases. Therefore, it is less likely that an individual with a negative test will have the disease, which leads to a high negative predictive value. With a more specific test, negative cases are identified more readily. Therefore, it is less likely that an individual with a positive test will actually be normal, which results in a high positive predictive value.

Prevalence

Sensitivity, specificity, and predictive value are also influenced by the prevalence of the target condition in the population.[29] **Prevalence** refers to the number of cases of a condition existing in a given population at any one time. For a test with a given sensitivity and specificity, the likelihood of identifying cases with the condition is increased when prevalence is high (the condition is common). Therefore, when prevalence is high, a test will tend to have a higher positive predictive value. When prevalence is low (the condition is rare), one can expect many more false positives, just by chance. A positive predictive value can be increased either by increasing the specificity of the test (changing the criterion) or by targeting the screening program to a subgroup of the population that is at high risk for the target condition.

Choosing a Cutoff Score

Although continuous scales are considered preferable for screening because they are more precise, they must generally be converted to a dichotomous outcome for diagnostic purposes; that is, a **cutoff score** must be established to demarcate a positive or negative test. For example, a specific level of blood pressure (a continuous scale) is used to determine if a patient should or should not be placed on a therapeutic regimen for hypertension (dichotomous). In the previous example, a score of 5 degrees was considered indicative of scoliosis. However, if a cutoff score of 10 degrees was used, the sensitivity and specificity would be different. The problem, then, is to determine what cutoff score should be used. This decision point must be based on the relative importance of sensitivity and specificity, or the cost of incorrect outcomes versus the benefits of correct outcomes. For instance, predicting a storm that does not occur (false positive) has little cost relative to the danger of failing to predict a storm that does occur (false negative).

Suppose that a balance test is used to predict if an elderly individual is at risk for falling, and the individual with a high score is referred to a balance exercise program. If the individual is not truly at risk (false positive), the outcome may be considered low cost, compared with the situation when an individual who is at risk is not correctly diagnosed (false negative), not referred for treatment, and injures herself in a fall. Therefore, it would be reasonable to set the cutoff score low to avoid false negatives, thereby increasing sensitivity. Conversely, consider a scenario in which a test is used to determine the presence of a condition that requires life-threatening surgery. A physician would want to avoid the procedure for a patient who does not truly have the disease. For this situation, the threshold might be set high to avoid false positives, increasing specificity. We would not want to perform this procedure unless we knew for certain that it was warranted.

Obviously it is desirable for a screening test to be both sensitive and specific. Unfortunately, there is usually a compromise between these two characteristics. One way to evaluate this decision point would be to look at several cutoff points to determine the sensitivity and specificity at each point. We could then look at the relative trade-off to determine the most appropriate cutoff score. Those who use a screening tool must decide what levels of sensitivity and specificity are acceptable, based on the consequences of false negatives versus false positives. It is often necessary to combine the results of several screening tests to minimize the trade-off between specificity and sensitivity.

Receiver Operating Characteristic (ROC) Curves

The balance between sensitivity and specificity can be examined using a graphic representation called a **receiver operating characteristic (ROC) curve.** This procedure actually evolved from radar and sonar detection strategies developed during World War II to improve **signal-to-noise ratios.** Suppose we were listening to a radio station that has a weak signal. As we increase the gain of this signal we not only pick up the desired signal, but also background noise. At lower settings, we will hear the signal more than the noise. There will come a point, however, as we increase the gain, that the noise will grow faster than the signal; that is, the signal has reached its full capacity, but the noise continues to increase. If we set the gain to its maximum, we may claim that the signal is strong, but the noise will be so great that the signal will be indecipherable. Therefore, the optimal setting will be where we detect the largest ratio of signal to noise. This is essentially what we are trying to do with a diagnostic test. We want to detect the "signal" (the presence or absence of the disease—the true positive and true negative) with the least amount of interference possible (incorrect diagnoses—false positive and false negative). The ROC curve diagrams this relationship. It allows us to answer the question: How well can a test discriminate between signal and noise—can it discriminate between the presence or absence of disease?[30]

Constructing the ROC Curve

The process of constructing an ROC curve involves setting several cutoff points for a test and calculating sensitivity and specificity at each one. The curve is then created by plotting a point for each cutoff score that represents the proportion of patients correctly identified as having the condition on the Y-axis (true positives) against the proportion of patients incorrectly identified as having the condition (false positives) on the X-axis. The Y-axis represents sensitivity, and the X-axis represents one minus specificity (1−specificity).*

To illustrate this process, consider the use of the timed "Up & Go" test to screen for risk for falls. The test requires that an individual rises from a standard arm chair, walks a distance of 3 meters, turns, walks back, and sits down.[26] Scores are recorded in seconds, documenting the time to complete the task. We have created a hypothetical dataset for a sample of 150 subjects who, based on their past year history of falls, have been identified as "at risk" (they have fallen at least once, $n = 70$) or "not at risk" (they have not fallen, $n = 80$). Table 6.4A shows the distribution of timed scores for the subjects in each group. These continuous scores have been converted to a 6-category ordinal scale.

Table 6.4B shows the distribution of scores at 5 cutoff points. It is generally recommended that at least 4 to 6 points should be used to plot an ROC curve. We calculate the sensitivity and specificity of the test at each cutoff point. For this example, lower scores indicate better balance, and therefore, less likelihood to fall. Higher scores will result in a "diagnosis" of "at risk" for falls. Table 6.4B shows the number of true positives and false positives for each cutoff point, and the corresponding values for sensitivity and 1– specificity. For example, if we use a cutoff score of 10 sec, then all those who obtained a score of 10 sec or less will be considered "not at risk." Those with a score greater than 10 sec will be diagnosed "at risk." With this cutoff score, 66 of the fallers have been correctly identified "at risk;" (true positives) and 46 of the non-fallers have been correctly diagnosed. This leads to a corresponding sensitivity of .94 and specificity of .58. Therefore, 34 of the non-fallers

---

*If we take all those who are diagnosed **negative** ([b + d] in Table 6.2), out of this total (100%) those who tested negative (true negatives) equal 1.00–d (specificity). Therefore, the remainder, or those who tested positive (false positives), would be 1.00–specificity.

TABLE 6.4   DATA FOR CREATING THE ROC CURVE IN FIGURE 6.3

A. Hypothetical Scores for the Timed "Up & Go" Test

	Time	Known Group	
		"At Risk" (Fallers) $n = 70$	"Not at Risk" (Non-Fallers) $n = 80$
	≤ 10 sec	4	46
	11–20 sec	2	10
	21–30 sec	7	12
	31–40 sec	3	8
	41–50 sec	6	2
	> 50 sec	48	2

B. True Positive and False Positive Rate, Plotted on ROC Curve

Cutoff Point	True Positives	False Positives	Sensitivity	Specificity	1–Specificity
10 sec	66	34	.94	.58	.42
20 sec	64	24	.91	.70	.30
30 sec	57	12	.81	.85	.15
40 sec	54	4	.77	.95	.05
50 sec	48	2	.69	.975	.025

have been incorrectly diagnosed "at risk" (false positives), which results in 1–specificity of .42. Similarly, with a cutoff score of 20 sec, all those who obtained a score of 20 sec or lower will be considered "not at risk." Those with scores above 20 sec will be diagnosed "at risk." When this cutoff score is used, 64 fallers are correctly diagnosed and 24 non-fallers are incorrectly diagnosed "at risk." This leads to a corresponding sensitivity of .91 and 1–specificity of .30. These values are then plotted to create the ROC curve (Fig. 6.3).[†]

Interpreting the ROC Curve

The ROC curve is plotted on a square with values of 1.0 for sensitivity and 1–specificity at the upper left and lower right corners, respectively. A perfect test instrument will have a true positive rate of 1.0 and a false positive rate of 0.0, resulting in a curve that essentially fills the square; that is, it will go from the origin to the upper left corner to the upper right corner (Fig. 6.4A). A noninformative curve occurs when the true positive and false positive rates are equal, which means that the test provides no better information

---

[†]The curve is completed at the origin and the upper right hand corners, reflecting cutoff points above and below the highest and lowest scores. For example, with a cutoff score at zero, *all subjects* will be diagnosed "at risk." Therefore, all those truly "at risk" are correctly diagnosed (true positive rate is 100%), and all those "not at risk" are incorrectly diagnosed (false positive rate is 100%). Similarly, with a cutoff score above 50 sec, *all subjects* will be diagnosed "not at risk." Therefore, all those truly "at risk" will be incorrectly diagnosed (true positive rate is zero), and all those "not at risk" will be correctly diagnosed (false positive rate is zero).

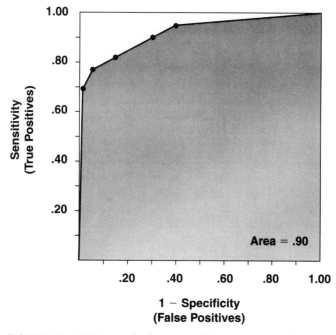

FIGURE 6.3   ROC curve for hypothetical data shown in Table 6.4. Curve shows the relationship between sensitivity and 1–specificity of the timed "Up & Go" test at five cutoff points.

than a 50:50 chance. This curve starts at the origin and moves diagonally to the upper right corner (Fig. 6.4B).

Area under the curve.   If we wanted to compare two tests to determine which was a better diagnostic tool, we would look to see which curve more closely approximates the perfect curve. This provides only a visual basis of comparison, however, and a quantitative standard is more definitive. The best index for this purpose is a measure of the area under the ROC curve.[‡] This value equals the probability of correctly choosing between normal and abnormal signals. This means that, given a test with an ROC curve area of .90 (as in Figure 6.3) and presented with a randomly chosen pair of patients (one with the disease and one without), the clinician would choose the correct diagnosis 90% of the time. Therefore, the area represents the ability of the test to discriminate between the diseased and nondiseased state. A perfect test has an area of 1.00; using such a test would allow the clinician to always identify the patient with disease.

[‡]Statistical procedures for calculating the area under the curve are cumbersome by hand, but are based on the nonparametric Wilcoxon rank sum statistic, W.[31-33] Computer programs can be written for these calculations.[34,35] Many statistical programs, such as SPSS and SAS, will construct ROC curves. In addition to the determination of area, the standard error of the area and confidence intervals can be obtained, which are most useful for comparing curves of different tests.

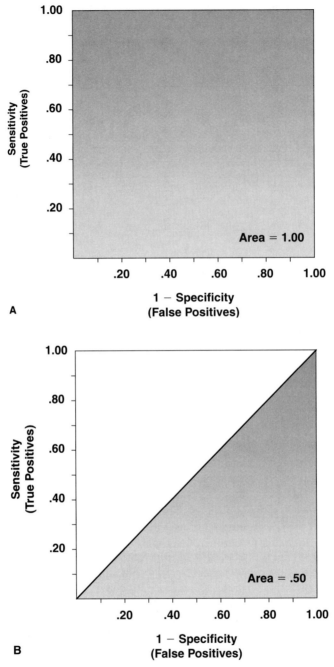

FIGURE 6.4 (**A**) ROC curve with 100% accuracy. Curve runs parallel to Y-axis and curves at the upper left corner. (**B**) Curve drawn at 45-degree angle represents diagnosis which is no better than chance.

Choosing a cutoff point. In addition to making comparisons, or describing the relative effectiveness of a test for identifying disease, one can also use the ROC curve to decide which cutoff point would be most useful. Most ROC curves have a steep initial section, which reflects a large increase in sensitivity with little change in the false positive rate. A relatively flat region across the top is also typical. Neither of these sections of the curve makes sense for choosing a cutoff point, as they represent little change in one component of the curve. Usually the best cutoff point will be at the point where the curve turns. In Figure 6.3, a marked turn occurs at the second cutoff point, suggesting that a cutoff point of 40 sec would provide the best balance between sensitivity and specificity for this test. At that point, we would miss diagnosing risk for 16 of the 70 individuals who have fallen, and we would incorrectly target 4 of the 80 nonfallers. The final choice, however, must be based on how the clinician and patient see the impact of an incorrect identification. The ROC curve should only act as a guide for that decision.

MEASURING CHANGE

As clinicians and researchers, we could reasonably argue that a primary goal of treatment is to effect a positive change in a patient's status. The difference between the outcome and the initial score is called a **change score,** or **gain score.** The use of change scores as the basis for analysis of treatment outcomes is pervasive throughout clinical research. This practice is actually quite complex, however, in terms of statistical interpretation. Perhaps the most important consideration is the purpose of measuring change. Consider four goals. The first is to measure change in an individual's performance or condition. Second, we measure differences between individuals in the amount of change, to distinguish those who changed a lot from those who changed a little. Third, we seek to identify factors that contribute to a good response. Fourth, we intend to draw inferences about treatment effects by looking at group differences.

Four major issues affect the validity of change scores:[36]

1. Level of measurement. The use of nominal, ordinal, interval, or ratio data is an important consideration in the calculation of change scores. Nominal scores, of course, cannot be subtracted, and therefore, cannot demonstrate change. At the other end of the continuum, true change can only be measured using ratio scores, because all measures have known quantities. Interval level data present a problem for evaluating change (refer to Figure 4.2), because although we can determine the *distance* of change, we do not know the true *amount* of change. The risk of misinference is greatest, however, with ordinal measures because the distance between intervals is not known and may not be equal.[37]

This situation becomes troublesome for clinical researchers, as so many tools used to measure impairments, function, and quality of life are based on ordinal scores. Assessment of change with such tools must take into account their limitations for interpretation. To illustrate, consider the Functional Independence Measure (FIM) which is used extensively within rehabilitation settings.[38] This instrument includes 18 items related to independence in physical and cognitive domains. Each item is scored on a 1–7 ordinal scale, with lower scores representing the need for more assistance. We would have to question an assumption, however, that would equate a 1-point improvement from 1 to 2 points with the same "amount" of improvement from 6 to 7 points. Similarly, a change from 1 to 2 points on a manual muscle test could not be validly equated with a change from 3 to 4 points. Therefore, efforts to show improvement in individual patients or groups through change scores can be ambiguous.

This measurement issue is a concern for interpretation of scores. For instance, most functional scales present a total score, derived by summing item scores. This process could be considered meaningless if the "numbers" that are used to create the sum have no inherent mathematical relationship; that is, an ordinal number is nothing more than a categorical label, and has no arithmetic properties. Therefore, the sum may be uninterpretable.[37] Taking this argument one step further, using a change score derived from these sums may be equally uninterpretable for research purposes.

Interestingly, experts do not agree on the seriousness of this issue.[36] Some believe that functional scales, for example, include approximately equal intervals in the sense that each point represents a clinically useful and measurable "step" in the continuum from dependence to independence. Specialized statistical applications, such as Rasch analysis (see Chapter 14), have been developed as a way of transforming an ordinal scale into equal intervals. Nonparametric statistics can also be used to appropriately analyze ordinal values.

2. Reliability.   A second important issue in evaluating the validity of change concerns the reliability of the factor being measured. This consideration refers back to the concept of error and measurement theory (Chapter 5). Let us assume that we take a pretest measurement, and that the true value does not change. On a subsequent posttest the score will probably be different because of random measurement error. Now we subtract the pretest from the posttest to obtain a change score. Assuming that the *true score* has not changed, measurement theory suggests that the difference will cancel out the true score, essentially leaving nothing but error in the change score. Therefore, even with true change, reliability is a necessary precondition for the application of change scores. Streiner and Norman suggest that one should only use change scores when the reliability of a measure exceeds 0.50,[3] although for many clinical variables reliability should probably be higher. It is important to remember, however, that being reliable does not automatically imply that a measure will be able to detect change.

3. Stability.   In addition to the reliability of the measurement system, we must also consider the stability of the variable being measured. If we are working with a variable that is labile, it may be difficult to determine if change is a function of improvement in a therapeutic element, or if it is a reflection of an unstable behavior. For instance, measurement of blood pressure may vary from trial to trial with no true change in physiological status, whereas measures of function should be fairly stable even though precise performance may vary from time to time. Establishing stability may require that several measurements be taken at both baseline and outcome to demonstrate that the performance is reliable.

4. Linearity.   A fourth concern in the interpretation of improvement is the linearity of change.[36] Sometimes the extent to which a variable changes will depend on its starting point. For instance, a patient who has had a total knee replacement may find it easier to improve from 70 degrees to 90 degrees than from 90 degrees to 110 degrees of knee flexion. For patients with a frozen shoulder, we may see substantial improvement in shoulder abduction ROM in one who starts out limited to 60 degrees, as compared with one who starts out at 90 degrees, simply because there is more range to gain.

Therefore, when describing the effectiveness of a therapeutic program, information should be included about gains as a function of initial scores. It would be useful to know if the likelihood of improvement is similar across all levels of pretest scores. Patterns may become evident when the starting point is examined. If some patients do not improve as much as others, it would be helpful to understand if their status upon admission was different: Those with greater impairments may need to be treated differently.

One solution to this problem is the use of the analysis of covariance (see Chapter 24) to create a standardized value, called the **residualized gain score.** This process uses a regression analysis, which is based on the correlation between pretest and posttest scores, to predict what a posttest score *would be* if everyone started at the same pretest level. Therefore, the residualized gain score removes the effect of initial differences to determine who changed more or less than was expected, accounting for where they started. This solution can also be used when bias is introduced as a function of extreme scores. Changes that are measured on a posttest can, under such conditions, reflect the phenomenon of *regression toward the mean* (see Chapter 5). The consequence of this effect is an overestimate of the difference between initial and outcome scores.

Linearity is also a factor if the increments within the measurement scale are not sufficient to detect small degrees of change that might occur at higher or lower levels (ceiling and floor effects). For instance, Andres and coworkers examined changes in strength in patients with amyotrophic lateral sclerosis using manual muscle test grades (ordinal scale) and isometric force measures with a strain gauge (ratio scale).[39] They found that early changes in strength were evident with the ratio scale measure, which were not evident using the ordinal measure. Significant changes in functional strength occurred within a single manual muscle test grade. During later stages, strength decrements were more dramatic and were clear with both measures. The choice of tool, therefore, could make a distinct difference in evaluative decisions early in the disease.

Responsiveness to Change

If we are interested in documenting change, one of the first choices we must make is which measuring instrument we will use. For some variables this decision is rather straightforward. When we want to measure ROM or strength, for instance, we have a fairly traditional set of tools to employ. For more abstract variables, however, such as function and quality of life, the outcomes movement has generated a vast set of questionnaires that can be applied in different situations. Much of the research in the development of these tools has focused on construct validity, determining if the instrument is able to reflect a person's status at a given point in time. However, if we intend to use an instrument for evaluation, we must extend our concern for validity beyond the construct itself to a discussion of the **responsiveness** of the instrument, or its ability to detect change over time.

The characteristic of responsiveness can be considered a component of test validity. It is an important quality if a test is to be used to assess the effectiveness of intervention; that is, the score must change in proportion to the patient's status change, and must remain stable when the patient is unchanged. This change must also be large enough to be statistically significant for research purposes, and precise enough to show increments of meaningful change for clinical purposes.

Analysis of Responsiveness

Change scores. Researchers have looked at responsiveness in two fundamental ways. One approach has been to use a pretest–posttest design, statistically analyzing differences in change scores over time using repeated measures *t*-tests or analyses of variance.[40–42] Measurements may be taken once before and after, or there may be multiple measures as the individual is followed over time.[43] This approach may involve only one group of subjects, or it may incorporate two or more groups. The groups would be formed according to different expectations of change; that is, a treatment group would be expected to show change but a nontreated group would be expected to stay the same. A significant difference, then, would demonstrate that the instrument was able to distinguish between the two groups.

Effect size. We might also be interested in comparing responsiveness across different instruments. As clinicians become more involved in assessing outcomes, we find that we have multiple choices of outcome measures, some generic and other condition-specific. Many of these instruments are intended for use across varied populations. It would be important, therefore, to determine which instruments will be most responsive under certain conditions, so we could choose the most efficient mechanism for demonstrating treatment effectiveness. For example, Jette and Jette measured changes in health status following physical therapy care in patients with spinal impairments.[44] They analyzed change in each of the eight subscales of the SF-36. Because these scales are based on distinct theoretical dimensions, however, change scores cannot be directly compared. A standardized score that is unit free is needed to make these comparisons.

A common solution to this problem involves the use of **effect size** as a comparative value. Effect size is a standardized measure of change, typically from initial to final measurement, that allows comparison across different units.[45] In their study of spinal impairments, Jette and Jette determined effect size by subtracting the initial score from the final score and dividing the result by the standard deviation for the initial score.[44] Therefore, an effect size of .5 indicates a change equal to one-half of the initial standard deviation.§ The degree of change, then, is viewed as a function of the distribution of scores at the start. The more variable the subjects are before treatment, the more difficult

---

§Using a somewhat different approach, Liang et al. looked at five established health status instruments to determine the optimal scale for evaluating orthopedic outcomes in patients with total joint arthroplasty.[40] They introduced the term *standardized response mean,* defined as the ratio of the mean change score divided by the standard deviation of the change scores. The estimate of change in this case will reflect the distribution of change scores, not initial scores, potentially resulting in a less variable standard. Further statistical comparisons can also be made using this value by calculating its standard error and confidence intervals. Clearly, the interpretation of effect size will depend on how the researcher chooses to conceptualize it.

it will be to demonstrate a strong effect following intervention. Many researchers use Cohen's suggested interpretation of effect size, whereby scores below .4 are considered small, .5 is considered moderate, and .8 is considered large (see Appendix C). These conventions are only guides, however, and must be further interpreted in terms of the clinical phenomenon being studied and the extent of change that is clinically meaningful. In many situations, a small change may be very important.

ROC curve. Another way to look at responsiveness is to consider it a way of discriminating between those who have changed and those who have not. Therefore, we can look at change as a "diagnosis," or the determination of whether a clinically important change has occurred.[46] For example, one could set a cutoff point to say that a change of at least 10 points is necessary to reflect meaningful change. The amount of change that would be considered meaningful would be a clinical decision, based on the maximum possible score, the precision of the variable being measured, and the increments that are reasonable to document differences with that instrument. Because there will be random error in the scale scores, as with any measurement, we can expect to see some scores change even when no true change has occurred (false positive), and no change for some patients who have really improved (false negative), depending on where we have set the cutoff point. We can, therefore, describe responsiveness in terms of sensitivity and specificity. By setting different cutoff points, we can plot an ROC curve to quantify this property. For example, Stratford et al. looked at four questionnaires for assessing pain and function in patients with low back pain.[47] They set different cutoff scores to represent change for each test and constructed four ROC curves. They then compared the area under the curves to determine which would be preferred for detecting change over time in this population (Fig. 6.5).

CRITERION REFERENCING AND NORM REFERENCING

The validity of a measurement is also related to how one makes judgments from the test results. Tests may be developed to assess performance based on an absolute criterion. The results of a **criterion-referenced test** are interpreted relative to a standard that represents an acceptable model or level of performance. If we know that a patient with a total knee replacement needs at least 90 degrees of knee flexion to negotiate stairs, then we will establish 90 degrees as an acceptable outcome. A functional test will establish how much assistance a patient needs to perform certain tasks using specific definitions of dependence and independence. In educational programs, clinical performance evaluations set a criterion that represents entry-level competence. Similarly, a grade of 70 on a test might be used to specify competence for the material being tested. This absolute standard will indicate passing, regardless of how the rest of the group performs. The validity of a criterion-referenced score, of course, depends on the validity of the criterion. So if we set a passing score on an exam, that score should represent competence, and should differentiate those who are competent from those who are not competent.

Many tests are specifically designed to determine if an individual is "normal," that is, if an individual performs within the average range of a reference group. Such a test is considered **norm-referenced.** The normal values are determined by testing a large

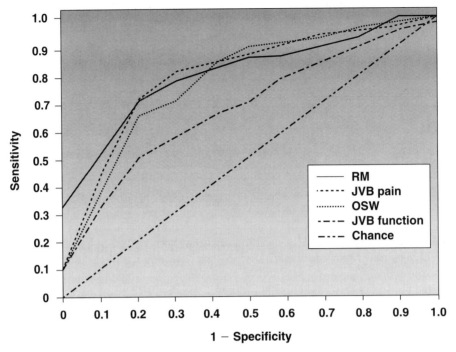

FIGURE 6.5 Receiver operating characteristic (ROC) curves for four low back pain questionnaires: Roland-Morris (RM), Jan van Breeman (JVB) pain scale and function scale, and the Oswestry (OSW). Areas under the curve were as follows: RM = 0.79; JVB pain = 0.79; JVB function = 0.66; and OSW = 0.78. A significant difference was found between the area for the JVB function questionnaire and the other three questionnaires. (From Stratford PW, Binkley J, Solomon P, et al. Assessing change over time in patients with low back pain. *Phys Ther* 1994; 74: 528–33, Figure p. 531. Reprinted with permission of the American Physical Therapy Association.)

group that meets a certain profile. The mean of the distribution of scores for the reference sample is used as the standard, and the variability (standard deviation) is used to determine how an individual performs relative to the sample. For example, standardized tests such as the SAT or GRE are scored relative to the group taking the test at that administration. When we assess a patient's pulmonary function or muscle strength based on normal values that have been determined according to age and sex, we are using a norm-referenced standard. If a professor decides to curve test scores so that the grades of the majority of the class are considered a C, regardless of the absolute score, then the test would be norm referenced. Several developmental tests, such as the Bayley Scales of Infant Development[48] or the Gesell development scales,[49] are based on data collected on children within specified age groups. These standardized tests allow the clinician to determine if a child's developmental status falls within the range of the majority of children in that age group. Therefore, the identification of problems is based on this reference group. The validity of a norm-referenced test will depend on the validity of the sample that was used to provide the normal values.

The distinction between criterion-referenced and norm-referenced scores is an important one, and should be understood by those who administer and interpret tests. The relative utility of these scores will depend on the purpose of the test and the action that will be taken based on the results. Norm-referenced tests are primarily used to establish placement or for diagnosis, as in standardized college board exams or developmental tests. A criterion-referenced test is used to examine the proficiency of performance along a continuum of skill, and does not depend on the performance of others. Criterion-based scores are generally more useful for establishing treatment goals and measuring change, as they tend to be based on an analysis of the tasks that are required for successful performance. Both types of tests should demonstrate reliability and validity.

CROSS-VALIDATION

The purpose of validation studies is to document that a test can be used effectively for a particular purpose. When we deal with predictive tests or screening procedures, we collect data on an experimental sample and use these data to create predictive equations or cutoff scores that will be applied to the larger population. For example, if we want to determine the appropriate criteria for screening scoliosis patients, we would look at results obtained on a particular sample and then apply the most effective cutoff score to other samples.

Unfortunately, the data obtained on an experimental sample are often different from those that would be obtained on a sample of different subjects. Therefore, the error components within predictive equations or cutoff scores will usually be greater for subsequent samples than they were for the original sample. This means that the test's accuracy will not necessarily be as great as it was on the original sample.

The predictive models or cutoff scores obtained from validation studies should, therefore, always be cross-validated on a second sample, to determine if the test criteria can be generalized across samples. **Cross-validation** is accomplished by trying out a previously developed test on a new group with characteristics as close as possible to those of the original. Of course, we assume that the original and test groups are both good representatives of the population for which the test will be used. It is also possible to cross-validate the test on a sample with different characteristics that may be appropriate for the test. For instance, certain perceptual tests may be used for different age groups and could be validated across groups of children and adults. If cross-validation is not documented, a substantial reduction in the validity of a test on subsequent applications can be anticipated.

COMMENTARY

The Ongoing Pursuit of Validity

The process of developing a measuring instrument involves several stages of planning, test construction, reliability testing, and validation.[55] In the planning stages, the purpose of the test must be stipulated, including specification of the relevant content universe or the theoretical construct and the target population for which the instrument will be used. A literature review is usually necessary, to determine that an appropriate instrument does not already exist and to formulate operational definitions of the construct to be measured. For educational or physical tests, these operational definitions will refer to specific content that the subject is expected to know or perform. For physiological or behavioral tests, operational definitions must specify how the construct theory will be manifested in a person's actions or responses. The literature will often help identify the types of test items that are likely to best evaluate the construct of interest.

Validation is almost never a complete process, nor is it ever accomplished with only one study. Numerous research efforts are required to substantiate a test's validity. Therefore, validation is an ongoing process. The choice of which type of evidence is required to document validity will depend on the test's purpose. For most instruments, more than one method will be used. In many instances, construct validity will subsume the other forms of evidence and require that multiple approaches to validation be used.

Concepts of validity are of vital importance in the contemporary health care environment, where outcomes and quality of life constructs are seen as relevant end points for evaluating the success of treatment and justifying continued intervention. As clinicians become more familiar with the vast number of generic and condition-specific health instruments that are being used, they must also be able to determine which instrument is appropriate for which patient, and they must be able to interpret scores with meaningful analyses. If an instrument is used to demonstrate change or improvement, but it is not sensitive enough to pick up small but clinically important changes, then the treatment will appear unsuccessful. As we attempt to use these tools to show effectiveness, we must understand the concepts of validity to make reasonable judgments and more informed choices. Given the large number of instruments that are presently available, we can contribute to our understanding of their capabilities by applying them in varied settings with different populations, to determine their useful measurement properties.

■■■■■   KEY TERMS   ■■■■■

measurement validity
face validity
content validity
criterion-related validity
gold standard
concurrent validity
predictive validity
prescriptive validity
construct validity
known groups method
convergent validity
discriminant validity
multitrait–multimethod
    matrix

factor analysis
true positives
true negatives
false positives
false negatives
sensitivity
specificity
positive predictive value
negative predictive value
prevalence
cutoff score
receiver operating
    characteristic (ROC)
    curve

signal-to-noise ratio
change score
gain score
residualized gain score
responsiveness
standardized response
    mean (SRM)
criterion-referenced test
norm-referenced test
cross-validation

REFERENCES

1. Florence JM, Pandya S, King WM, et al. Clinical trials in Duchenne dystrophy. Standardization and reliability of evaluation procedures. *Phys Ther* 1984;64:41–5.
2. Williams M. Manual muscle testing: development and current use. *Phys Ther Rev* 1956;36:797.
3. Streiner DL, Normal GR. *Health Measurement Scales: A Practical Guide to Their Development and Use*. 2d ed. New York: Oxford Press, 1995.
4. Sechrest L. Reliability and validity. In: Bellack AS, Hersen M, eds. *Research Methods in Clinical Psychology*. New York: Pergamon Press, 1984, 24–54.
5. Goldsmith CH. Commentary: Measurement validity in physical therapy research. *Phys Ther* 1993;73:113–4.
6. Melzack R, Katz J. The McGill Pain Questionnaire: appraisal and current status. In: Turk DC, Melzack R, eds. *Handbook of Pain Assessment*. New York: Guilford Press, 1992.
7. Balogun JA, Martin DA, Clendenin MA. Calorimetric validation of the Caltrac accelerometer during level walking. *Phys Ther* 1989;69:501–9.
8. Petherick M, Rheault W, Kimble S, Lechner C, Senear V. Concurrent validity and intertester reliability of universal and fluid-based goniometers for active elbow range of motion. *Phys Ther* 1988;68:966–9.
9. Fisk JW, Baigent ML. Clinical and radiological assessment of leg length. *N Z Med J* 1975;81:477–80.
10. Beattie P, Isaacson K, Riddle DL, Rothstein JM. Validity of derived measurements of leg-length differences obtained by use of a tape measure. *Phys Ther* 1990;70:150–7.
11. Jette AM, Branch LG, Berlin J. Musculoskeletal impairments and physical disablement among the aged. *J Gerontol* 1990;45:M203–M208.
12. Magaziner J, Simonsick EM, Kashner TM, Hebel JR, Kenzora JE. Predictors of functional recovery one year following hospital discharge for hip fracture: a prospective study. *J Gerontol* 1990;45:M101–M107.
13. Katz JN, Harris TM, Larson MG, et al. Predictors of functional outcomes after arthroscopic partial meniscectomy. *J Rheumatol* 1992;19:1938–42.
14. Rothstein JM, Echternach JL. *Primer on Measurement: An Introductory Guide to Measurement Issues*. Alexandria, VA: American Physical Therapy Association, 1993.
15. Sim J, Waterfield J. Validity, reliability and responsiveness in the assessment of pain. *Physiother Theory Pract* 1997;13:23–38.
16. Fairbank JC, Couper J, Davies JB, O'Brien JP. The Oswestry low back pain disability questionnaire. *Physiotherapy* 1980;66:271–3.
17. Zung WW. A self-rating pain and distress scale. *Psychosomatics* 1983;24:887–90, 892–4.
18. Gregory-Flock JL, Yerxa EJ. Standardization of the prone extension postural test on children ages 4 through 8. *Am J Occup Ther* 1984;38:187–94.
19. Campbell DT, Fiske DW. Convergent and discriminant validation by the multitrait-multimethod matrix. *Psychol Bull* 1959;56:81.
20. Bergner M, Bobbitt RA, Kressel S, Pollard WE, Gilson BS, Morris JR. The sickness impact profile: conceptual formulation and methodology for the development of a health status measure. *Int J Health Serv* 1976;6:393–415.
21. Hendricson WD, Russell IJ, Prihoda TJ, Jacobson JM, Rogan A, Bishop GD. An approach to developing a valid Spanish language translation of a health-status questionnaire. *Med Care* 1989;27:959–66.
22. Brooks WB, Jordan JS, Divine GW, Smith KS, Neelon FA. The impact of psychologic factors on measurement of functional status. Assessment of the sickness impact profile. *Med Care* 1990;28:793–804.

23. Shields A, Cicchetti D. Emotion regulation among school-age children: the development and validation of a new criterion Q-sort scale. *Dev Psychol* 1997;33:906–16.

24. Thurstone L, Thurstone T. *Factorial Studies of Intelligence.* Chicago: University of Chicago Press, 1941.

25. Dodds TA, Martin DP, Stolov WC, Deyo RA. A validation of the Functional Independence Measurement and its performance among rehabilitation inpatients. *Arch Phys Med Rehabil* 1993;74:531–6.

26. Podsiadlo D, Richardson S. The timed "Up & Go": a test of basic functional mobility for frail elderly persons. *J Am Geriatr Soc* 1991;39:142–8.

27. Amendt LE, Ause-Ellias KL, Eybers JL, Wadsworth CT, Nielsen DH, Weinstein SL. Validity and reliability testing of the Scoliometer. *Phys Ther* 1990;70:108–17.

28. Ibrahim MA. *Epidemiology and Health Policy.* Rockville, MD: Aspen, 1985.

29. Hennekens CH, Buring JE. *Epidemiology in Medicine.* Boston: Little Brown, 1987.

30. Centor RM. Signal detectability: the use of ROC curves and their analyses. *Med Decis Making* 1991;11:102–6.

31. Beck JR, Shultz EK. The use of relative operating characteristic (ROC) curves in test performance evaluation. *Arch Pathol Lab Med* 1986;110:13–20.

32. Centor RM, Schwartz JS. An evaluation of methods for estimating the area under the receiver operating characteristic (ROC) curve. *Med Decis Making* 1985;5:149–56.

33. Hanley JA, McNeil BJ. The meaning and use of the area under a receiver operating characteristic (ROC) curve. *Radiology* 1982;143:29–36.

34. Centor RM. A Visicalc program for estimating the area under a receiver operating characteristic (ROC) curve. *Med Decis Making* 1985;5:139–48.

35. Gorog G. An Excel program for calculating and plotting receiver-operator characteristic (ROC) curves, histograms and descriptive statistics. *Comput Biol Med* 1994;24:167–9.

36. Johnston MV, Keith RA, Hinderer SR. Measurement standards for interdisciplinary medical rehabilitation. *Arch Phys Med Rehabil* 1992;73:S3–S23.

37. Andres PL, Skerry LM, Thornell B, Portney LG, Finison LJ, Munsat TL. A comparison of three measures of disease progression in ALS. *J Neurol Sci* 1996;139 (Supp):64–70.

38. Liang MH, Fossel AH, Larson MG. Comparisons of five health status instruments for orthopedic evaluation. *Med Care* 1990;28:632–42.

39. Chambers LW, Haight M, Norman G, MacDonald L. Sensitivity to change and the effect of mode of administration on health status measurement. *Med Care* 1987;25:470–80.

40. MacKenzie CR, Charlson ME, DiGioia D, Kelley K. Can the Sickness Impact Profile measure change? An example of scale assessment. *J Chronic Dis* 1986;39:429–38.

41. Stratford PW, Binkley JM, Riddle DL. Health status measures: strategies and analytic methods for assessing change scores. *Phys Ther* 1996;76:1109–23.

42. Deyo RA, Centor RM. Assessing the responsiveness of functional scales to clinical change: an analogy to diagnostic test performance. *J Chronic Dis* 1986;39:897–906.

43. Stratford PW, Binkley J, Solomon P, Gill C, Finch E. Assessing change over time in patients with low back pain. *Phys Ther* 1994;74:528–33.

44. Bayley N. *The Bayley Scales of Infant Development.* New York: The Psychological Corporation, 1969.

45. Knobloch H, Stevens F, Malone AF. *Manual of Developmental Diagnosis: The Administration and Interpretation of the Revised Gesell and Amtruda Developmental and Neurological Examination.* Hagerstown, MD: Harper & Row, 1980.

III

Designing Clinical Research

CHAPTER

7

The Research Question

The first step in any research effort is to identify the specific question that will be investigated. This is the most important and often most difficult part of the research process, because it controls the direction of all subsequent planning and analysis. The delineation of a precise question is an analytic and evolutionary process, requiring a thorough search through the literature to determine what information is already available on the topic. Throughout the search the researcher reexamines and redefines the purpose of the research, honing it and clarifying it until, finally, a "researchable" question is asked.

The overall process for identifying a research question is illustrated in Figure 7.1. It starts with the selection of a research topic that sparks some interest, and the subsequent exploration of that topic by examining issues in clinical practice and theory, and reading the professional literature. This information leads to the identification of a research problem, a broad statement that begins to focus the direction of study. The problem is then refined to a research question, which is specific and defined. The question may actually be in the form of a statement or an interrogatory; in either case, it delimits the purpose of the study. Several components will shape the question, including an evaluation of its importance and feasibility, specification of the population to be studied, development of a research rationale to support the question, and a description of the specific variables to be studied. Throughout this process, the researcher relies on a comprehensive review of the literature to provide the background necessary for decision making. The research question is then translated into a statement that reflects the expected outcomes of the study, clarifying the research objectives in the form of hypotheses or a statement of purpose.

The purpose of this chapter is to clarify this framework for developing and refining a feasible research question, to define the different types of variables that form the basis for the question, to describe how research objectives guide a study, and to discuss how the review of literature contributes to this process.

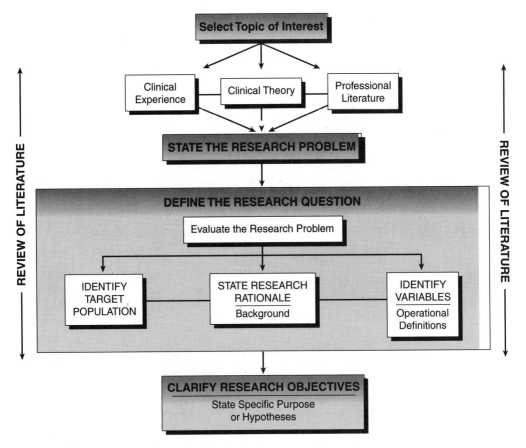

FIGURE 7.1   Illustration of the process for developing a research question.

SELECTING A TOPIC

The research process begins when a researcher identifies a specific **topic** of interest. Many beginning researchers approach the initial phase of the research process by "looking for a question." Students may be required to generate a question for a project to meet academic requirements. Certainly there is no paucity of clinical problems that need to be investigated; however, developing a research question should not be merely a fishing expedition. The intellectual and problem-solving processes that are part of all clinical or academic endeavors will generate questions of interest. Questions grow out of these experiences because the clinician or researcher feels a need to know something that is not already known, to resolve a conflict, or to clarify some piece of information that is not sufficiently documented. Even in situations when the research task is an academic exercise, the investigator's intellectual curiosity is bound to uncover some uncertainty or special interest that can be translated into a research question. Clinicians are usually able to identify that they are interested in studying a certain patient population, a specific type of intervention, a clinical theory, or a fundamental policy issue in the profession.

THE RESEARCH PROBLEM

Once a topic is identified, the process of clarifying a research problem begins by sorting through ideas, facts and theories based on clinical experience, and professional literature to determine what we know, what we do not know, and what we need to find out. The application of this information will lead to identification of a **research problem** that will provide the foundation for delineating a specific **research question** that can be answered within a single study. Typically, research problems start out broad, and concern general clinical problems or theoretical issues. They must be manipulated and modified several times before they become narrowed sufficiently to propose a specific question. Reading the literature and discussing ideas with colleagues are invaluable as one works toward crystallizing a research question. For instance, a researcher might be interested in exploring issues related to wound care. This topic may suggest a research problem such as, "How can we effectively treat pressure ulcers?" This problem could then be addressed in many ways, leading to several different types of studies. For example, one researcher might look at the effects of ultrasound for promoting healing. Another might use electrical stimulation. Many other approaches could be taken to address the same general problem. Each approach will contribute to the overall knowledge base that helps us understand the problem. Beginning researchers are often unprepared for the amount of time and thought required to formulate a question that is testable. It is sometimes frustrating to accept that only one small facet of a problem can be addressed in a single study.

Clinical Experience

Research problems often emerge from some aspect of practice that presents a dilemma. A clinician's knowledge, experience, and curiosity will influence the types of questions that are of interest. We often ask why a particular intervention is successful for some patients but not for others. Would a particular treatment be more or less effective if we changed the technique of application or combined it with other treatments? Are new treatments more effective than established ones? What outcomes can be expected following a particular intervention?

Often, through trial and error, clinicians find interesting solutions to clinical problems. These present a challenge to objectively document effects of treatment on specific patient populations. Treatments that are based in tradition or authority should also be examined, to test their underlying assumptions in the effort to support evidence-based practice. Can we substantiate the effects of craniosacral therapy?[1] Does the theory of therapeutic touch hold up under scientific scrutiny?[2] In many cases, our empirical observations suggest that a treatment works and we do not feel a need to pursue documentation further; however, evidence-based practice requires systematic study of traditional treatment biases and a critical analysis of treatment alternatives.

Research problems may reflect a need to describe patterns of normal behaviors or the natural history of clinical phenomena. What values can we use to judge the degree of dysfunction we find in our patients? Does one clinical problem consistently accompany others? What is the natural progression of physical disability following a specific injury or onset of disease? Questions about methodology are also of interest. How can we measure change? What tools are needed to document and evaluate patient problems? Many new instruments have been developed in recent years for measuring physical, physiological, and psychological performance. These need to be analyzed for reliability and validity under varied clinical conditions and on different patient groups.

Clinical Theory

Clinicians will often examine the theories that govern their practice as a source of research questions. Theories allow us to explain relationships and to predict outcomes based on given information (see Chapter 2); however, theories are applicable only to the extent that they can be empirically confirmed. For example, the validity and scope of theories that address motor control, motor learning, cognitive and physical development, neuromuscular function, language acquisition, personal interaction, or compliance can be tested in clinical situations. To formulate a specific research question, a clinician must first examine the principles behind a theory and then determine what clinical outcomes would support or not support the theory. The answers will be the basis for a research question. Consider the theoretical premise that stresses produced during hand activities contribute significantly to joint changes and deformity in patients with rheumatoid arthritis. Hasselkus and coworkers explored this theory by generating a deductive hypothesis that proposed that the dominant hand would be subjected to greater daily stresses than the nondominant hand.[3] If the theory is true, then the dominant hand would be expected to exhibit greater joint changes than the nondominant hand. The attempt to verify this theoretical premise led to a study of the relationship between hand dominance and joint mobility in arthritis.

Professional Literature

Reference to professional literature plays an essential role in the delineation of a research problem and ultimately in the derivation of the specific research question. In the initial phases, the literature will help the researcher determine the issues of importance. Using this information, an initially broad or vague problem can begin to take a more structured and concise form. This initial review of the literature is preliminary and not necessarily extensive. The researcher will explore a variety of references on a particular subject and examine a breadth of materials to become oriented to practical and theoretical issues, and the kinds of variables or clinical problems that others have addressed.

Professional literature provides the basis for developing a research problem in several ways. First, it will clarify holes in professional knowledge, areas where we do not have sufficient information for clinical decision making. For example, Kramer and coworkers were interested in studying functional loss following stroke and hip fracture.[4] The literature showed that the effectiveness of different rehabilitation options for restoring function for these patients had not been examined. This finding led them to a study of functional outcomes comparing rehabilitation hospitals and traditional and subacute nursing homes.

Another common source of ideas derives from conflicts in the literature, when studies present contradictory findings. For instance, many researchers have looked at the effect of electrical stimulation on strength changes in knee muscles following knee surgery; however, some studies have shown significant effects and others have not. Snyder-Mackler and colleagues investigated this question further by clarifying the type of stimulator and dosage of stimulation needed to enhance recovery of patients following anterior cruciate ligament (ACL) reconstruction.[5] Professional literature may also identify disagreements due to differences or flaws in study design or measurement methods. For example, Beurskens et al. were interested in the effect of lumbar traction for treating back pain, and found that many former studies lacked good baselines, did not use appropriate outcome measures, or did not incorporate blinding into the design.[6] Their approach was to develop a randomized trial that controlled these effects to compare high-dose and low-dose traction in patients with nonspecific low back pain.

In many instances, replication of a study is a useful strategy to correct for design limitations or to examine outcomes with different populations. A study may be repeated using the same variables and methods or slight variations of them. Replication is an extremely important process in research, because one study is never sufficient to confirm a theory or to verify the success or failure of a treatment. We are often unable to generalize findings of one study to a larger population because of the limitations of small sample size in clinical studies. Therefore, the more studies we find that support a particular outcome, the more confidence we can have in the validity of those findings. Another approach is to consider *suggestions for further study*, which are usually presented at the end of an article and offer ideas for pursuing that line of research. These sources of research questions are ideal for beginning researchers because they do not require that the research process begin from scratch.

Research questions may also arise out of data from descriptive studies, which document trends, patterns, or characteristics that can subsequently be examined more thoroughly using alternative research approaches. For example, many descriptive studies have documented characteristics of elderly patients who fall.[7] These findings provide a rich source of questions concerning how we might intervene to prevent falls.

IMPORTANCE AND FEASIBILITY OF THE RESEARCH QUESTION

Throughout the process of identifying and refining a research question, three general criteria should be considered to determine whether the question is worth pursuing: The question should be important, answerable, and feasible.

The Question Should Be Important

Clinical research should have potential impact on treatment, on theoretical foundations, or on policies related to practice. Basic research should address questions that contribute to scientific knowledge and theory. Because of the commitment of time and resources required for research, a researcher should believe that the effort is worthy of investigation; that is, it should generate new information that will further the profession's knowledge base. Although it is important to keep a project simple and direct, it should not be so trivial as to make no difference to anyone. Researchers should consider if the outcomes of the study will resolve inconsistencies in previous research, or if they will contribute to explanations of clinical theory. It may be relevant to ask how often this clinical problem occurs in practice. Will the findings provide useful information for clinical decision making or be generalizable to other clinical situations? Will others be interested in the results? Statements that support the importance of the research question are often considered the *justification* for a study. We often say that the research question must be able to pass the "so what?" test; that is, the results should be meaningful and useful. Researchers should look at trends in practice and health care to identify those problems that have clinical or professional significance for contributing to evidence-based practice.

The Question Should Be Answerable

Not all questions can be studied scientifically. For instance, questions involving judgments or philosophical issues are often difficult to study. We should not consider asking, "Are all patients entitled to treatment regardless of their ability to pay for services?" If this issue is of interest, however, related questions can be investigated: What is the extent of health insurance coverage for different age groups or socioeconomic groups? What types of treatments are being denied reimbursement by various insurers? These questions are not the same as the original question, but they would provide related information that can be used by clinicians in considering the ethical and moral consequences of the issue.

Questions that begin with "why" are also difficult to answer using clinical research methods. Why does one treatment approach work better than another for reducing spasticity? The answer to such a question goes beyond the capability of clinical tools. Rather than asking why a patient responds a certain way to a treatment, we can document that a treatment does or does not change the level of response and examine whether that response supports a particular theory. Similarly, it is not the function of science to judge if one or another treatment is "preferable." Such judgments reflect personal values but are not based on research evidence.

The research problem should also incorporate variables that can be defined and measured. Consider the question, "How can we improve a patient's motivation to exercise?" How can we define the term "motivation"? What criteria can be established to assess that a person is motivated? How will those who are motivated be distinguished from those who are not motivated? Motivation becomes a construct for which some relevant measure must be identified. If a variable cannot be adequately defined, it cannot be studied.

The Question Should Be Feasible

Many factors influence the feasibility of a research study. The researcher must have the necessary skill, background, and resources to be able to complete the project properly. In many cases, consultants and advisors will be needed for technical and statistical assistance. Can a realistic timetable be developed? Pilot studies are helpful for estimating the time requirements of a study. Are sufficient numbers of subjects available, and can they be counted on to participate? Problems often occur when patients are discharged or develop medical complications that prevent their participation. What type of space is needed to carry out the project, and when will it be available? Can the necessary equipment be obtained? Does the project have the necessary administrative support? What are the budgetary requirements of the project? Investigators will typically incur costs for a computerized literature search, photocopying articles, obtaining laboratory equipment and supplies, and so on. Lastly, are the rights of subjects being protected? The researcher must determine risks and benefits, and be able to justify the demands placed on the subject during data collection (see Chapter 3). These considerations must be addressed prior to continuing with plans for a study. Many research questions will be refocused by the practicalities of the process.

TARGET POPULATION

As we proceed with the development of a research question, we must identify *who* we want to study. The **target population** refers to the group of individuals to which the results of the study will apply. It represents the totality of all members of this group who conform to a designated set of specifications. For example, suppose we are interested in studying the effectiveness of electrical stimulation for increasing muscle strength. We could designate a healthy population of "normal" subjects as our population, or we could select patients with total knee replacements or ACL reconstruction; however, further restriction may be necessary to make this designation clear and appropriate, considering both practical and theoretical issues. Once again, the literature is a consistent source of information for decision making. Should the subjects be within a certain age range? Will we include males and females? Should we specify a time since onset of pain or surgery? Is the cause of the knee surgery a relevant factor? Does it matter if symptoms are unilateral or bilateral? Other considerations may be based on availability of patients. For instance, the age range of the population may be dictated by the age range of patients at the researcher's facility. We might specify a general target population of otherwise healthy males between 20 and 40 years of age with no prior history of orthopedic or neuromuscular dysfunction, who have had an ACL repair within the last 6 months. The definition of the target population should be sufficiently clear and complete that it will be obvious who will and who will not be considered a member (see Chapter 8).

THE RESEARCH RATIONALE

Once the research problem has been defined, a full review of literature will establish the background for the research question. This foundation will clarify the **research rationale** that will support the research question, guide decisions in designing the study, and most importantly, provide the basis for interpreting results. The rationale presents a logical argument that shows how the question was developed. It provides a **theoretical framework** by explaining the constructs and mechanisms behind the question. It helps us understand why the question makes sense. The research rationale includes references to previous research as well as logical assumptions that can be made from current theory. Without a strong rationale, the results of a study will be hard to interpret.

For example, many researchers have looked at the effectiveness of electrical stimulation for increasing muscle strength in healthy populations and in patient populations. Some studies have focused on the comparison of neuromuscular electrical stimulation (NMES) and voluntary exercise. The research rationale for these studies focuses on the suggested mechanisms for this effect.[8] Why should electrical stimulation be expected to produce strength gains? One explanation proposes that training with NMES is similar to strengthening with voluntary exercise in terms of muscle physiology. If this is true, then we should be able to observe comparable strength gains with each technique, and the protocol for strengthening with NMES should follow currently accepted guidelines for voluntary exercise, including frequency, number of repetitions and load. Another mechanism suggests that NMES selectively recruits high-force muscle fibers, thereby increasing muscle strength. Researchers have used this rationale as the basis for comparing the recruitment order of fast- and slow-twitch muscle fibers during NMES and voluntary exercise. The study rationale, therefore, demonstrates current knowledge of muscle physiology, theories related to how exercise increases functional strength, the physiological properties of neuromuscular electrical stimulation, and an understanding of what other studies have been able to demonstrate. These concepts form a logical foundation for the research question.

VARIABLES

Now we must specify *what* we want to test. **Variables** are the building blocks of the research question. A variable is a property that can differentiate members of a group or set. It represents a concept, or **factor,** that can have more than one *value.* By definition, variables are characteristics that can vary. A factor becomes a variable by virtue of how it is used in a study. For instance, if we want to compare levels of back pain between men and women, then pain and gender are the variables of interest. Pain can take on a range of values, depending on how we measure it, and gender can take on two "values" (male and female). If, however, in another study, we compare the effects of two different treatments for decreasing back pain in men, then gender is no longer a variable. It has only one "value" (male), and is therefore a constant. In this latter example, type of treatment and pain are the variables of interest.

Research is performed to examine the relationship among variables or describe how variables exist in nature. In descriptive and correlational studies, variables represent the phenomena being examined, and their measurement may take many forms. The investigator looks at these characteristics one at a time, and describes their values and their interrelationships. In predictive and experimental studies the investigator examines relationships among two or more variables to predict outcomes or to establish that one variable influences another. For these latter types of studies, research variables are generally classified as independent or dependent, according to how they are used.

Independent and Dependent Variables

A *predictor variable* is an **independent variable.** It is a condition, intervention or characteristic that will predict or cause a given outcome. The *outcome variable* is the **dependent variable,** which is a response or effect that is presumed to vary depending on the independent variable.

In a predictive study the researcher investigates how variables tend to go together, and tries to establish if the presence and the quantity of the independent variable are predictive of the dependent variable. For example, suppose we were interested in studying the relationship between low back pain and one's age and sex. The dependent variable (the outcome variable) would be back pain and the independent variables (predictor variables) are the characteristics of age and sex. These types of studies often involve several independent variables, as the researcher tries to establish how different factors interrelate to explain the outcome variable.

Comparative studies investigate causal relationships, in which the independent variable is controlled and the dependent variable is measured. For instance, researchers have compared the effect of a back class versus usual medical care to determine if the back class was an effective program for reducing low back pain.[9] Outcomes included changes in a disability score and a pain scale rating. In this example the independent variable is the back class (intervention), and the two dependent variables are the disability and pain scores (response). A change in the dependent variables is presumed to be caused by the "value" of the independent variable; that is, the dependent variable is a function of the independent variable.

In comparative studies, independent variables are given values called **levels.** The levels represent groups or conditions that will be compared. Every independent variable will have at least two levels. For example, in the study comparing a back class and usual care, the independent variable of "intervention" has two levels: back class and usual care. If the study had included additional interventions, such as physical therapy or bed rest, it would have changed the number of *levels* of the variable, not the number of variables.

Comparative studies can be designed with more than one independent variable. We could look at the patients' gender in addition to intervention, for instance, to determine if effectiveness of a back class is different for males and females. We would then have two independent variables: type of intervention and gender, each with two levels. A study can also have more than one dependent variable. In the previously mentioned study, researchers measured both disability rating and pain. Dependent variables are not described as having levels.

Sometimes an independent variable is based on a continuous scale, but categories are created that classify the levels of the variable. For instance, we could study the effect of varied dosages of ultrasound (independent variable) on changes in low back pain (dependent variable). We could describe the independent variable according to increments of 0.5, 1.0, and 1.5 watts/cm^2. In another study we could examine changes in pain during successive 2-minute intervals of a 10-minute ultrasound treatment. In this case the independent variable is the number of minutes of treatment application, with five intervals or levels. In both of these studies, we would be interested in establishing the pattern or *trend* of response changes. In some cases the intervals used for a quantitative variable are arbitrary; other times they are based on specific clinical parameters, previous research findings, or theoretical values. For instance, theory might suggest that results would fall in a staircase pattern or a linear function. Therefore, the range and number of levels chosen must be sufficient to describe these trends fully. To study dosage, we might want to determine if changes in pain are proportional to dosage level, or if there is a critical dosage below which changes will not occur. To study changes over time, we might be interested in observing the rate of decrease, to determine if it is a steady decline or if a plateau occurs at some point during the treatment.

Operational Definitions

Once the variables of interest have been identified, the researcher still faces some major decisions. Exactly what procedures will be used? What questions do we need to ask ourselves to refine the purpose of the study? If we are interested in studying the effects of different interventions on back pain, exactly what will be the interventions? How will they be applied? Do we want to look at a treatment against a control condition, compare two different treatment approaches, or look at two variations of the same technique? How will we measure a change in back pain? Are we interested in pain at the time that treatment session begins or when it ends? On the same day or later in the week? What aspect of pain should we measure? As the research question continues to be refined we continually refer to the literature and our clinical experience to make these judgments. How often will subjects be treated? In what position will the subjects be tested? How often will they be tested? These questions must be answered before adequate definitions of variables are developed.

Variables must be defined in terms that explain how they will be used in the study. For research purposes, we distinguish between conceptual definitions and operational definitions. A *conceptual definition* is the dictionary definition, one that describes the variable in general terms, without specific reference to its methodological use in a study. For instance, "back pain" can be defined as the degree of discomfort in the back. This definition is useless, however, for research purposes because it does not tell us what measure of discomfort is used or how we could interpret discomfort.

In contrast, an **operational definition** defines a variable according to its unique meaning within a study. The operational definition should be sufficiently detailed so that another researcher could replicate the procedure or condition. Independent variables are operationalized according to how they are manipulated by the investigator. For example, in the study comparing a back class and usual care, an operational definition for the independent variable "back class" should include the number of sessions, the type of training and materials, expectations of compliance, who will teach the class, and so on. The subjects' activities and other treatment specifications should be included. We also need to describe the control group's activities of usual care. Operational definitions for independent variables must differentiate the various levels of the variable.

Dependent variables are operationally defined by describing the method of measurement, including delineation of tools and procedures used to obtain measurements. A variable like "low back pain" could be defined operationally as the score on a visual analogue scale (VAS), reflecting the magnitude of pain at a particular time of day under specific activity conditions. An individual reading this definition should be able to know precisely how the variable "pain" could be interpreted in this study.

Some variables do not require substantial operational definitions. The application of the term "age", for example, is readily understood, as is the identification of male and female. It is usually sufficient to define variables such as height and weight simply by specifying units of measurement and the type of measuring instrument. Some variables can be defined according to standardized criteria, such as manual muscle tests and intelligence; however, many variables whose definitions appear self-evident still present sufficient possibilities for variation that they require explanation. Consider the concept of hand preference. We often take for granted the designation of right handed or left handed; but when used in a study that concerns laterality, this may not be sufficient. Some researchers might accept the hand used for writing as the preferred hand. Others may want to include mixed handedness, and use a standardized test for dominance.[10]

There are many examples of concepts for which multiple measurements may be acceptable. Researchers often find themselves faced with having to choose which method best represents the variable for purposes of a single study. For example, back pain can be measured using a VAS, the McGill Pain Questionnaire, or the Oswestry Disability Rating Scale. The results of studies using these different tools would be analyzed and interpreted quite differently because of the different information provided by each form. The measurement properties, feasibility of use, and sensitivity of an instrument should be considered in choosing the most appropriate dependent variable. A comparison of measurement methods can also become the basis for a research question.

There may be instances when the reader of a research report does not agree with the validity of an operational definition set forth by an investigator. For example, some researchers have examined changes in pain as a function of decreased usage of medication;[11] others have considered greater active joint range of motion a useful indicator.[12] These investigators have made certain assumptions about the relationship between pain and intake of medication or mobility. Some clinicians might argue, however, that these measures could be influenced by a subject's pain tolerance and that a more stoic individual might demonstrate changes in the measured variable that are not necessarily representative of changes in pain. The importance of the operational definition is that it communicates exactly how the term is being used so that the reader understands the researcher's conceptualization of the variable and the implications of the findings. Whatever measure is chosen will reflect only certain characteristics of the construct, and thereby influence our interpretation of changes. It is the researcher's responsibility to justify the operational definition in terms of the purpose of the research.

RESEARCH OBJECTIVES

The final step in delineating a researchable question is to clarify the objectives of the study. This step is the culmination of all the reasoning and reading that has gone before to determine the target population, describe the research rationale, and define the research variables. These objectives may also be presented as *hypotheses, specific aims,* or the *purposes* of the research. The terms used will vary among researchers, journals, and disciplines. Most importantly, however, this statement must specifically and concisely delineate what the study is expected to accomplish.

The four general types of research objectives are to evaluate measuring instruments, to describe populations or clinical phenomena, to explore relationships, and to make comparisons between groups. To illustrate, let us again assume that we are generally interested in studying low back pain. Through clinical experience and a review of literature we find that low back pain affects a significant number of individuals as a result of work-related injuries.[13] We could approach this topic in several ways. In choosing an approach, it may be helpful to be thinking about how the results of the study would be integrated back into clinical practice.

1. Many research problems stem from the lack of appropriate *measuring instruments* to document outcomes. Studies may involve the investigation of reliability and validity in measuring tools to determine how different instruments can be used meaningfully for clinical decision making. Sometimes the problem will address different uses of a known tool, and other times it will suggest the need for a new instrument. For instance, researchers have looked at use of the SF-36 as a measure of function for patients with low back pain.[14] Others have considered the need for a new tool to assess the extent of recovery and potential for return to work.[15]

2. The intent of the study may be *descriptive,* in an effort to characterize clinical phenomena or existing conditions in a particular population. As an example, researchers have interviewed patients with low back pain to describe reasons for repeated medical visits.[16] Di Fabio and Boissonnault studied changes in health-related quality of life for patients with common orthopedic disorders, including low back pain, to describe patient perceptions between initial assessment and discharge from physical therapy.[17] These studies provide data that form a foundation for generating additional questions. For instance, Di Fabio's data suggested the need to further examine diagnostic categories, types of treatments, and preinjury functional level to see if these factors differentially influence quality of life.

3. A third type of research objective is the *exploration of relationships* to determine how clinical phenomena interact. For instance, one research team followed Belgian steel workers to investigate the relationship between occurrence of low back pain and prior personal, anthropometric, or functional characteristics.[18] In another study, investigators evaluated leg length discrepancy, hip flexor tightness, and lower extremity acquired laxity or overuse as predictive factors for low back pain in college athletes.[19] By determining such relationships, these types of studies suggest risk factors that contribute to functional limitations and provide ideas for prevention and treatment options.

4. The study may be based on a *comparison,* in an attempt to define a cause-and-effect relationship using an experimental model. This type of study evaluates differences between groups or the effectiveness of interventions. For example, researchers have compared the effect of exercise and motivational programs on the compliance and degree of disability of patients with chronic back pain.[20] Loisel et al. compared four treatment models to determine which would be more effective for decreasing pain, reducing absence from work, and improving time to return to work.[21] The study previously described, looking at a back class and usual care, is a comparative study.[9]

The choice of one of these approaches will frame the research design, the types of data collection that will be appropriate, and the applicable data analysis procedures. Many studies incorporate more than one approach. For example, in a study of patients with low back pain who were receiving workers' compensation, the study was designed to describe levels of disability and return to work, and to explore the relationship of compliance and pain with disability and work status.[13]

Specific Aims

Descriptive studies will usually be based on *specific aims* or *guiding questions* that describe the study's purpose. For instance, researchers may specify that they want to describe attitudes about a particular issue, the demographic profile of a given patient group, or the natural progression of a disease. Survey researchers will design a set of questions to organize a questionnaire. Because descriptive studies have no fixed design, it is important to put structure into place. Setting specific aims or guiding questions allows the researcher to organize data and discuss findings in a meaningful way.

Hypotheses

For exploratory and experimental studies involving the investigation of relationships, the researcher must be more precise in setting expectations. This process requires that the researcher propose an educated guess about the outcome of the study. This guess is presented as a statement called a **hypothesis:** a declarative statement that predicts the relationship between the independent and dependent variables, specifying the population that will be studied. The purpose of the study is to test the hypothesis and, ultimately, to provide evidence so that the researcher can accept or reject it. The researcher generally formulates a **research hypothesis** following identification of the problem, a review of relevant literature, and final conceptualization of the research variables. A research question might ask, "Is knee range of motion improved by the addition of continuous passive motion (CPM) to a postoperative rehabilitation program following total knee replacement?"[22] The clinical researcher may then hypothesize that "Knee range of motion in flexion and extension at time of discharge will be greater for patients who receive CPM following total knee replacement than for those who do not receive CPM." Hypotheses are developed at the outset to provide a definitive structure for the investigation by assisting the researcher in planning the design and methods, and in determining the data analysis procedures. Hypotheses also provide the reader of a research report with an understanding of what the researcher was expecting to find.

Characteristics of Hypotheses

Useful hypotheses can be evaluated according to several criteria. Consider the statement, "Patients with total knee replacements who receive CPM following surgery will have fewer postoperative complications." This statement includes a reference to a target population, but is not complete because it contains only one variable—the number of postoperative complications. CPM treatment is not a variable in this statement because only one condition is presented. We can modify the statement to express a relationship and thereby make it a complete hypothesis: "Patients with total knee replacements who receive CPM following surgery will have fewer postoperative complications than patients who do not receive CPM." Now CPM is an independent variable, with two levels. We will be able to distinguish the responses of those patients who receive CPM from those who do not. Hypotheses usually incorporate phrases such as "greater than," "less than," "different from," or "related to" as a way of indicating the type of relationship that is being examined.

An acceptable hypothesis must be testable and should be based on a sound rationale. This implies that a body of knowledge exists that will support the hypothesis. A researcher does not propose a hypothesis purely on the basis of speculation. Hypotheses can be derived from theory or suggested from previous research, clinical experience, or observation. *Deductive hypotheses* are based on a theoretical premise, allowing the clinician to predict what outcomes would be expected under a given set of conditions. When contradictions exist in the literature, researchers must examine these variances to draw relevant parallels with their own research questions. *Inductive hypotheses* are based on trends, regularities, patterns, or relationships that are observed in clinical practice. Clinicians can also use other sources of knowledge such as authority, tradition, and trial and error as bases for formulating a hypothesis. When a new area is being addressed, the researcher's own experiences and logical reasoning may be the only foundation available.

Stating the Hypothesis

A **research hypothesis** states the researcher's true expectation of results, guiding the interpretation of outcomes and conclusions. Analysis of data is based on testing a statistical hypothesis, which differs from the research hypothesis in that it will always express no difference or no relationship between the independent and dependent variables. The statistical hypothesis is called the **null hypothesis** (see Chapter 18).

Researchers use a great deal of flexibility when phrasing research hypotheses. The same research problem can be translated into a hypothesis in different ways. Some research hypotheses predict *no difference* between variables:

1. There is no difference in the level of physical therapy use in acute care facilities for the treatment of inpatients and outpatients served by Medicare before and after the onset of the Medicare prospective payment system.[23]

More often, research hypotheses propose a relationship in terms of a difference. Some do not predict the direction of that difference:

2. There will be a difference in acute or chronic low back pain treated with either TENS [transcutaneous electrical nerve stimulation] or gentle mechanical massage, as measured by scores on the McGill Pain Questionnaire, and ROM [range of motion] of straight leg raise and back flexion.[24]

Hypotheses 1 and 2 are considered **nondirectional hypotheses** because they do not predict a direction of change. In other cases, a researcher will have a definite idea about the expected direction of outcomes. Consider the following hypotheses:

3. Women who receive physical therapy as part of their postmastectomy rehabilitation program will demonstrate a greater improvement in shoulder motion and level of performance of functional activities as compared to a group of patients who do not receive physical therapy.[25]

4. Change scores on the Gross Motor Function Measure will be higher than change scores on the Peabody Developmental Gross Motor Scale in a sample of children with cerebral palsy.[26]

These are examples of **directional hypotheses.** They not only describe the relationship between variables in terms of a difference, but they also assign a direction to that difference.

Hypotheses can also be phrased to predict a *relationship,* between variables, rather than a *difference,* as illustrated by the following:

5. There is a relationship between low scores on tests designed to measure constructional praxis and body scheme integration and failure to gain independence in upper extremity dressing at time of discharge.[27]

6. A significant relationship will be demonstrated between total risk scores on the Movement Assessment of Infants (MAI) at 4 months and scores on the Gross Motor Scale of the Peabody Developmental Motor Scales (PDMS) at 4.5 years.[28]

Hypothesis 5 is considered directional because the authors predict the presence of a relationship between two variables and the direction (direct or inverse) of that relationship. We can expect that the lower a patient's perceptual test score, the greater the incidence of failure to achieve functional independence. Hypothesis 6 does not tell us the expected direction of the proposed relationship.

Research hypotheses can be phrased in simple or complex forms. A **simple hypothesis** includes one independent variable and one dependent variable. For example, hypotheses 1, 4, and 6 are simple hypotheses. A **complex hypothesis** contains more than one independent or dependent variable. Hypotheses 2 and 3 contain two dependent variables. Hypothesis 5 specifies two independent variables. Complex hypotheses are often nondirectional because of the potential difficulty in clarifying multiple relationships. Complex hypotheses are efficient for expressing expected research outcomes in a research report, but they cannot be tested. Therefore, for analysis purposes, such statements must be broken down into several simple hypotheses. Several hypotheses can be addressed within a single study.

REVIEWING THE LITERATURE

Every research project can be considered an extension of all the thoughts and investigation that have gone before it. The results of each study contribute to that accumulated knowledge and thereby stimulate further research. For this process to work, researchers must be able to identify relevant research and theory, which is accomplished through the **review of literature.** The review of literature is actually conducted in two phases. The initial review is a preliminary one, intended to achieve a general understanding of the state of knowledge in the area of interest. Once the research problem has been clearly formulated, however, the researcher begins a full and extensive review that will provide a detailed and complete understanding of the relevant background.

Scope of the Review of Literature

Clinicians and students are often faced with a dilemma in starting a review of literature in terms of how extensive a review is necessary. How do researchers know when they have read a sufficient amount of material? There is no magic formula to determine that 20, 50, or 100 articles will provide the necessary background for a project. The number of references needed for a review depends first on the researcher's familiarity with the topic. A beginning researcher may have limited knowledge and experience, and might have to cover a wider range of materials to feel comfortable with the information. In addition, the scope of the review will depend on how much research has been done in the area, and how many relevant references are available. Obviously, when a topic is new and has been studied only minimally, fewer materials will exist. In that situation, it is necessary to look at studies that support the framework for a question. When a topic has been researched extensively, the researcher need only choose a representative sample of articles to provide sufficient background. The important consideration is the relevancy of the literature, not the quantity. Researchers will always read more than they will finally report in the written review of literature.

The review of literature should focus on several aspects of the study. As we have already discussed, the researcher tries to establish a theoretical framework for the study based on generalizations from other studies. It is often necessary to review material on the patient population, to understand the underlying pathology that is being studied. Researchers should also look for information on methods, including equipment used and operational definitions of variables. Often it is helpful to replicate procedures so that results have a basis for comparison with previous studies. It may be helpful to see what statistical techniques have been used by others for the same reason.

Literature also provides the basis for validating assumptions. **Assumptions** are concepts or principles that are assumed to be true, based on documented evidence or accepted theoretical premises. Assumptions allow us to continue our research without having to document every aspect of our procedures. For instance, if a study involves strength testing over several trials, the research protocol might call for a 2-minute rest between trials, based on the assumption that this time interval will be sufficient to avoid fatigue effects. This assumption can be validated by reviewing the literature on fatigue and recovery rates, rather than testing it on every subject.

The review of literature should be as current as possible, but should include some classical works as well. It is generally practical, however, to limit the review of older studies, so as not to review every historic document in the field. Experienced researchers know that, if not confined somehow, a review of literature can go on forever. As early as possible, the researcher should try to delimit the research question so that relevance of an article can be determined, and irrelevant articles can be ignored. The review should cover all relevant studies, even if findings are contradictory to the study's objectives. It is helpful to check the reference lists at the end of recent articles. The classical works will soon be evident, as they are usually referenced repeatedly. As more and more is read, the researcher will begin to find the same references cited again and again, and will have an indication that most relevant sources have been obtained. The review of literature should not be confined to published research studies. Subjective papers may be used as sources of information, and clinical reports may broaden an understanding of the clinical context of the problem.

Primary and Secondary Sources

It is important to differentiate the roles of primary and secondary sources in a review of literature. A **primary source** is a report or document provided directly by the person who authored it. Most research articles in professional journals are primary sources, as are oral presentations of direct research results, diaries, interviews, and eyewitness accounts. A **secondary source** is a description or review of one or more studies presented by someone other than the original author. Review articles and most textbooks are secondary sources, as are newspaper accounts and biographies.

Both primary and secondary references are important to the literature review. Reference lists in textbooks are often an excellent way to start the review, to identify references that are relevant to the topic; however, secondary references should not be considered substitutes for primary sources. They are most useful for providing bibliographical information on relevant primary sources. Beginning researchers should try to avoid the temptation to rely solely on secondary sources just because they conveniently summarize many studies. Secondary references often provide insufficient, inaccurate, or biased information about other studies. Researchers are often amazed when they go back to a primary source to discover how different their own interpretation of results can be from those provided in review articles.

As another consideration in choosing references, researchers should know whether a journal is refereed. This means that articles are reviewed by content experts before being accepted for publication, assuring a certain level of quality. Refereed journals generally require several levels of review and revision prior to publication. Papers in non-refereed journals do not undergo this scrutiny.

Organizing the Review of Literature

Because the review of literature can be extensive, researchers usually find it helpful to establish a process for organizing references as they read them. The first step is to identify the relevant information from each reference. The research question, key elements of the method, findings, and conclusions should be summarized. If a reference is being used for a specific purpose, such as a description of a particular outcome instrument, this should be indicated. The researcher should critique each article for validity of design and measurement, and record critical comments. The summary should include how data were analyzed and a description of the pertinent results. The researcher should indicate how each article is related to the research study and other articles. This information will be invaluable when writing a review of literature for an article or thesis. It will allow the researcher to look through reference summaries and find those studies that present similar or conflicting information (see Chapter 30). Some people keep these records on index cards for each article. More recently, researchers have begun to take advantage of computer programs that provide a structure for cataloging references by author, title, or keywords. Many of these reference manager programs allow the researcher to download the full reference, including abstracts, from the internet.

Locating Sources

Although most of us have had some experience obtaining references for term papers or assignments, many efficient strategies for locating research references are worth mentioning. The library, of course, is where this process begins. Most clinicians have access to a departmental or institutional library, but medical and university libraries will usually be more complete. Those who need assistance using the catalogs or reference materials should not hesitate to contact a reference librarian. Articles, books, or theses that are not available at a local facility can often be obtained through an *interlibrary loan*. Many facilities also provide access to full text downloads of articles, often for a fee. Some academic institutions provide a password for students and faculty to access online journals.

Many specialized library resources are available to assist the researcher in locating references on specific topics. We have summarized several of these sources in Table 7.1. A variety of **indexes** are available for health science literature, providing bibliographic listings of articles, books, and conference proceedings. **Abstract journals** provide short summaries of articles, allowing the researcher to judge quickly if the content is relevant. Most indexes can also be accessed by computer through online services, the internet, or CD-ROM. Some facilities charge a fee for the use of these services, and librarians are often able to help facilitate a successful search. However, many of these programs are interactive and menu driven, so that even researchers with little experience can use them easily. A computer search can save hours of the researcher's time. It allows the researcher to view the full citation and abstract of an article, to determine if it is relevant. The citation can then be printed or downloaded for future reference. Depending on the program used, the report generated may include only authors and titles, the full bibliographic reference, reference and abstract, or full text of the article (see Figure 7.2).

TABLE 7.1.   SOME COMMONLY USED INDEXES AND DATABASES FOR REFERENCES AND ABSTRACTS

Title	Database	Coverage*
Indexes		
Index Medicus	MEDLINE	1966
	AIDSLINE	1980
	BIOETHICSLINE	1973
Science Citation Index	SCISEARCH	1965
Cumulative Index to Nursing and Allied Health Literature	CINAHL	1983
Hospital and Health Administration Index	HealthSTAR	1975
Educational Resources Information Center	ERIC	1966
Books in print	BOOKS IN PRINT	Current
National Technical Information Service	NTIS	1964
Sport Bibliography	SPORT	1975
Current Contents	CCON	Current
Abstracts		
Excerpta Medica	EXCERPTA MEDICA	1975
Psychological Abstracts	PSYCH ABSTRACTS	1967
	MENTAL HEALTH ABSTRACTS	1969
	PSYCHLIT	
Biological Abstracts	BIOSIS PREVIEWS	1969
Sociological Abstracts	SOCIOLOGICAL ABSTRACTS	1963
Dissertation Abstracts International	DISSERTATION ABSTRACTS ONLINE	1861
Carcinogenesis Abstracts	CANCERLIT	1963

*Starting dates of coverage for databases only. Indexes may cover references for a longer period.

AU	- Underwood MR
AU	- Morgan J
TI	- The use of a back class teaching extension exercises in the treatment of acute low back pain in primary care.
LA	- Eng
MH	- Acute Disease
MH	- *Exercise Therapy
MH	- Low Back Pain/*therapy
MH	- Support, Non-U.S. Gov't
PT	- JOURNAL ARTICLE
PT	- RANDOMIZED CONTROLLED TRIAL
DP	- 1998 Jan
TA	- Fam Pract
PG	- 9-15
IP	- 1
VI	- 15
AB	- BACKGROUND: Back extension exercises are commonly recommended to treat acute low back pain. Evidence of their beneficial effect is, however, weak. OBJECTIVES: We aimed to demonstrate a benefit of teaching back extension exercises in addition to usual GP care for acute low back pain. METHODS: Patients with acute simple low back pain of less than 28 days duration, presenting to a GP, were randomized either to attend a back class or to receive conventional management. Outcome was measured using changes in the Oswestry disability score and visual analogue pain scale (VAS) on six occasions during 1 year and also a VAS and patient assessment of degree of disability during the previous 6 months at 1 year. RESULTS: Seventy-five patients were recruited. The principal outcome measures showed no difference between the two groups. The treatment group reported less chronic disability at 1 year (50% versus 14%, P < 0.007). CONCLUSIONS: A treatment effect has not been demonstrated, but some patients who would otherwise have reported mild pain were pain free after 1 year. This approach to treating back pain has not been shown to be effective. More much larger studies, with more intensive treatment, are required in order to decide whether physical therapy in primary care is beneficial as treatment for acute back pain.
SO	- Fam Pract 1998 Jan; 15(1): 9–15

(AU) Author, (TI) Title, (LA) Language, (MH) Medical subject heading, (PT) Publication type, (DP) Date of publication, (TA) journal title, (PG) pages, (IP) issue, (VI) volume, (AB) Abstract, (SO) complete source.

FIGURE 7.2 A sample MEDLINE report (abbreviated version).

Most indexes and databases in the medical field use **Medical Subject Headings (MeSH)** that have been adopted by the National Library of Medicine.* This listing provides a powerful reference system for performing a search.[29] When a desired topic is not found in the subject headings, the researcher must find synonyms or related terms that are listed. Many journals publish **key words** with an article that refer to these headings.

Boolean Logic

When performing a search, it is important to fine-tune the choice of key words or reference terms to narrow the search. Most databases and search engines use a system called **Boolean logic,** named for George Boole, a French mathematician who invented it in the mid 1800's. Boolean logic utilizes three primary operators, AND, OR and NOT, to refine or broaden a search. For example, suppose we are interested in finding references on back pain. We might enter the terms: back AND pain. Limiting results to the last 10 years, this search yields 8,692 citations! If our topic is actually focused on physical therapy intervention for back pain, we might limit the search further: back AND pain AND physical therapy. This brings the list down to 877 citations.

Sometimes the topic of interest can be identified by more than one term, and the researcher needs to provide both as options. For instance, we might look at both "back" and "spine" as terms for our current search. We could then enter: back OR spine AND pain AND physical therapy. This search yields 1,007 references. The term OR can be very useful when several synonyms exist for a concept, and they are used interchangeably in the literature.

We can also limit the search by indicating specific terms that we do not want included. In this example, we could specify: back OR spine AND pain AND physical therapy NOT massage. The term NOT allows us to eliminate references that include massage. Now only 962 references are listed. Obviously, we need to further delimit this search to make it manageable. We need to use terms that will be specific to our needs. For instance, including the words "AND acute" in our list leaves 146 citations. The search can be narrowed further by limiting articles to the last 5 years, to the English language, or even to a specific journal or author.

Databases

MEDLARS (*MEDical Literature Analysis and Retrieval System*) is the computerized system of databases offered through the National Library of Medicine (NLM).† Of these, the most commonly used database in health-related sciences is MEDLINE, corresponding to the *Index Medicus.* Other useful databases included in MEDLARS are AIDSLINE with information on AIDS and related topics, BIOETHICSLINE which covers ethics and related public policy issues, CANCERLIT which covers major cancer topics, and Health-

---

*The MeSH VOCABULARY FILE can be accessed through *Grateful Med.* It contains an online dictionary or thesaurus of current biomedical subject headings, subheadings, and other terms.

†The National Library of Medicine offers free access to several medically related databases. *PubMed* provides access to MEDLINE (*http://www.ncbi.nlm.nih.gov/PubMed/*). *Grateful Med* provides access to a fuller range of databases and allows the researcher to limit searches by language, publication type, etc. (*http://igm.nlm.nih.gov*).

STAR (*Health Services, Technology, Administration and Research*) which emphasizes evaluation of patient outcomes and administrative aspects of health care.

Several other important indexes are also available as databases. These include CINAHL (*Cumulative Index to Nursing and Allied Health Literature*), which provides access to citations from all nursing journals as well as primary journals in more than a dozen allied health disciplines, including occupational and physical therapy, cardiopulmonary technology, respiratory therapy, and social services; ERIC (*Educational Resources Information Center*), sponsored by the National Institute of Education, including citations in education and psychology; and PYSCHLIT, which covers topics in psychology and psychiatry. *Current Contents* can also be accessed online, providing a weekly publication of the tables of contents of several hundred journals, with emphasis on life sciences, but including physical and behavioral sciences, engineering, and education.

PILOT TESTING

The development of a research question is basic to the entire research effort. Typically, the process requires many revisions and reconsiderations of ideas and approaches before variables are defined and a research hypothesis is proposed. As ideas develop, researchers constantly go back to the literature to see what has already been done, to define variables, and to clarify theory. This process can be greatly facilitated by carrying out a **pilot study** to test the feasibility of a project and to help clarify decisions about operational definitions and procedures. The pilot study is a trial run of the actual methods, and may reveal limitations in the design that were not foreseen, allowing the researcher to make the necessary modifications. Sometimes the measuring instruments must be tested to determine their reliability or validity. If a survey questionnaire is used, a pilot study can reveal if questions or instructions are ambiguous. The researcher can get an idea of how long data collection will take and if adequate resources are available to complete the project. The pilot study should be carried out using the actual research procedures, so that conditions accurately represent what the researcher can expect during data collection. The number of subjects tested in a pilot will vary, depending on how efficient the procedures are and how the information will be used. When the pilot study is used only to verify that procedures work, two or three subjects may be sufficient. When the study is intended to provide a basis for reliability of instrumentation, a larger sample is necessary. When extensive revisions are needed, a second pilot study may be useful to evaluate the effectiveness of those changes. Pilot studies are well worth the time and effort, because errors and instrumentation failures are very costly when they occur after data collection has already begun.

COMMENTARY

Putting the Horse before the Cart

Albert Einstein once wrote that "the formation of a problem is far more often essential than its solution. . . . to raise new questions, new possibilities, to regard old problems from a new angle, requires creative imagination and marks real advance in science."[30] It is no exaggeration to speak of the extreme importance of the development of the right question. This process is often arduous and painstaking; however, it forms the foundation for all that will follow and crystallizes the researcher's expectations for results. The research question is developed in detail in a research proposal, which provides a specific and comprehensive outline of the entire research project, including the delineation of variables and a basis for hypotheses (see Chapter 30). A strong research study addresses questions that are clearly delineated and that lead to conclusions within the limits of the research design. If the question is too vague, it cannot guide the development of data collection or analytic methods. Beginning researchers often spin their wheels as they search for what to measure, rather than starting their search with the delineation of a specific and relevant question. It does not matter how complex or simple the design—it is not as important to know how to answer the question as it is to know how to ask the question.[31]

A clear research question also allows those who read about the study to understand its intent. It is easy to report data on any response, but those data will be totally irrelevant if they do not form the context of a specific question. Those who read the literature will find themselves lost in a sea of results if a question has not been clearly stated at the outset. The presentation of results and discussion in an article or oral paper should focus on those data that address the question, thereby delimiting the theoretical framework within which the results of the study will be interpreted.

In the process of doing research, novice researchers will often jump to a methodology and design, eager to collect and analyze data. It is an unfortunate situation, which has occurred all too often in our experience, when a researcher has invested hours of work and has obtained reams of data, and cannot figure out what to do with the information. There is nothing more frustrating than a statistical consultant trying to figure out what analysis to perform, and asking the researcher, "What is the question you are trying to answer?" The frustrating part is when the researcher realizes that the question cannot be answered with the data that were collected.

That said, we must consider a special circumstance that is common in the contemporary research environment. Many researchers today are faced with opportunities for research using databases that have been collected for other reasons, but that provide interesting information for answering questions of clinical significance. This situation requires a modification of the process we have outlined here, because the data are already in place before the question is developed. The researcher has no control over which variables were chosen, how subjects were selected, or what operational definitions were used. The challenge in this case is to know the database well, to understand the variables that are included, and to review the literature sufficiently so that the researcher can determine what questions are reasonable. The theoretical rationale for the question must be clear. Researchers often have definite questions in mind, but they find that the data will not support the question. With secondary data analysis, the question must be refined to fit the data, as obviously, the data cannot be manipulated. This will often limit the questions that can be asked. This form of research is a rich source of information in outcomes research. Researchers must be clearly aware of the limitations they face when using a preexisting set of data (see Chapter 16).

KEY TERMS

topic
research problem
research question
target population
research rationale
theoretical framework
variable
factor
independent variable
dependent variable

levels
operational definition
hypothesis
research hypothesis
null hypothesis
nondirectional hypothesis
directional hypothesis
simple hypothesis
complex hypothesis
review of literature

assumptions
primary source
secondary source
indexes
abstract journals
Medical Subject Headings
 (MeSH)
key words
Boolean logic
pilot study

REFERENCES

1. Hanten WP, Dawson DD, Iwata M, Seiden M, Whitten FG, Zink T. Craniosacral rhythm: reliability and relationships with cardiac and respiratory rates. *J Orthop Sports Phys Ther* 1998;27:213–8.
2. Rosa L, Rosa E, Sarner L, Barrett S. A close look at therapeutic touch. *JAMA* 1998;279:1005–10.
3. Hasselkus BR, Kshepakaran KK, Safrit MJ. Handedness and hand joint changes in rheumatoid arthritis. *Am J Occup Ther* 1981;35:705–10.
4. Kramer AM, Steiner JF, Schlenker RE, et al. Outcomes and costs after hip fracture and stroke: a comparison of rehabilitation settings. *JAMA* 1997;277:396–404.
5. Snyder-Mackler L, Delitto A, Stralka SW, Bailey SL. Use of electrical stimulation to enhance recovery of quadriceps femoris muscle force production in patients following anterior cruciate ligament reconstruction. *Phys Ther* 1994;74:901–7.
6. Beurskens AJ, de Vet HC, Koke AJ, et al. Efficacy of traction for non-specific low back pain: a randomised clinical trial. *Lancet* 1995;346:1596–600.
7. Whedon MB, Shedd P. Prediction and prevention of patient falls. *Image J Nurs Sch* 1989;21:108–14.
8. Lake DA. Neuromuscular electrical stimulation. An overview and its application in the treatment of sports injuries. *Sports Med* 1992;13:320–36.
9. Underwood MR, Morgan J. The use of a back class teaching extension exercises in the treatment of acute low back pain in primary care. *Fam Pract* 1998;15:9–15.
10. Crovitz HF, Zener KE. A group-test for assessing hand- and eye-dominance. *Am J Psychol* 1962;75:271.
11. Hollinger JL. Transcutaneous electrical nerve stimulation after cesarean birth. *Phys Ther* 1986;66:36–8.
12. Inaba MK, Piorkowski M. Ultrasound in treatment of painful shoulders in patients with hemiplegia. *Phys Ther* 1972;52:737–42.
13. Di Fabio RP, Mackey G, Holte JB. Disability and functional status in patients with low back pain receiving Worker's Compensation: A descriptive study with implications for the efficacy of physical therapy. *Phys Ther* 1995;75:180–193.
14. Ren XS, Kazis L, Lee A, et al. Comparing generic and disease-specific measures of physical and role functioning: results from the Veterans Health Study. *Med Care* 1998;36:155–66.
15. Williams RM, Myers AM. A new approach to measuring recovery in injured workers with acute low back pain: Resumption of Activities of Daily Living Scale. *Phys Ther* 1998;78:613–23.

16. McPhillips-Tangum CA, Cherkin DC, Rhodes LA, Markham C. Reasons for repeated medical visits among patients with chronic back pain. *J Gen Intern Med* 1998;13:289–95.

17. Di Fabio RP, Boissonnault W. Physical therapy and health-related outcomes for patients with common orthopaedic diagnoses. *J Orthop Sports Phys Ther* 1998;27:219–30.

18. Masset DF, Piette AG, Malchaire JB. Relation between functional characteristics of the trunk and the occurrence of low back pain. Associated risk factors. *Spine* 1998;23:359–65.

19. Nadler SF, Wu KD, Galski T, Feinberg JH. Low back pain in college athletes. A prospective study correlating lower extremity overuse or acquired ligamentous laxity with low back pain. *Spine* 1998;23:828–33.

20. Friedrich M, Gittler G, Halberstadt Y, Cermak T, Heiller I. Combined exercise and motivation program: effect on the compliance and level of disability of patients with chronic low back pain: a randomized controlled trial. *Arch Phys Med Rehabil* 1998;79:475–87.

21. Loisel P, Abenhaim L, Durand P, et al. A population-based, randomized clinical trial on back pain management. *Spine* 1997;22:2911–8.

22. Gose JC. Continuous passive motion in the postoperative treatment of patients with total knee replacement. A retrospective study. *Phys Ther* 1987;67:39–42.

23. Dore D. Effect of the Medicare prospective payment system on the utilization of physical therapy. *Phys Ther* 1987;67:964–6.

24. Melzack R, Vetere P, Finch L. Transcutaneous electrical nerve stimulation for low back pain. A comparison of TENS and massage for pain and range of motion. *Phys Ther* 1983;63:489–93.

25. Wingate L. Efficacy of physical therapy for patients who have undergone mastectomies. A prospective study. *Phys Ther* 1985;65:896–900.

26. Kolobe THA, Palisano RJ, Statford PW. Comparison of two outcome measures for infants with cerebral palsy and infants with motor delay. *Phys Ther* 1998;78:1062–1072.

27. Warren M. Relationship of constructional apraxia and body scheme disorders in dressing performance in adult CVA. *Am J Occup Ther* 1981;35:431–7.

28. Deitz JC, Crowe TK, Harris SR. Relationship between infant neuromotor assessment and preschool motor measures. *Phys Ther* 1987;67:14–7.

29. Lowe HJ, Barnett GO. Understanding and using the Medical Subject Headings (MeSH) vocabulary to perform literature searches. *JAMA* 1994;271:1103–8.

30. Einstein A, Infield L. *The Evolution of Physics.* New York: Simon and Shuster, 1938.

31. Findley TW. Research in physical medicine and rehabilitation. I. How to ask the question. *Am J Phys Med Rehabil* 1991;70 (Suppl):S11–S16.

CHAPTER
8
Sampling

In the process of defining a research question, the researcher must also decide who will be studied. The goal, of course, will be to make generalizations beyond the individuals studied to others with similar conditions or characteristics. Generalization is basic to all types of research, as scientists continually draw conclusions about human behavior and the environment based on limited experiences and measurements. The purpose of this chapter is to describe how the responses of a small representative group can be used with confidence to make predictions about the larger world.

POPULATIONS AND SAMPLES

The larger group to which research results are generalized is called the **population.** A population is a defined aggregate of persons, objects, or events that meet a specified set of criteria. For instance, if we were interested in studying the effects of various treatments for osteoarthritis, the population of interest would be all people in the world who have osteoarthritis; however, it is not reasonable to test every person who has osteoarthritis. Working with smaller groups is generally more economical, more time efficient, and potentially more accurate than working with large groups because it affords better control of measurement. Therefore, through a process of *sampling,* a researcher chooses a subgroup of the population, called a **sample.** This sample serves as the reference group for estimating characteristics of or drawing conclusions about the population.

Populations are not necessarily restricted to human subjects. Researchers may be interested in studying characteristics of institutions or geographical areas, and these may be the units that define the population. In test–retest reliability studies, the population will consist of an infinite series of measurements. The sample would be the actual measurements taken. An epidemiological study may focus on blood samples. Industrial quality control studies use samples of items from the entire inventory of a particular manufacturing lot. Surveys often sample households from a population of housing units. A population can include people, places, organizations, objects, animals, days, or any other unit of interest.

Sampling Bias

To make generalizations, the researcher must be able to assume that the responses of sample members will be representative of how the population members would respond in similar circumstances. Human populations are, by nature, heterogeneous, and the variations that exist in behavioral, psychological, or physical attributes should also be present in a sample. Theoretically, a good sample reflects the relevant characteristics and variations of the population in the same proportions as they exist in the population.

Although there is no way to guarantee that a sample will be representative of a population, sampling procedures can minimize the degree of bias or error in choosing a sample. It is not so much the size of a sample that is of concern. A small representative sample of 50 may be preferable to an unrepresentative sample of 1,000. For example, in 1968 the Gallup and Harris polls predicted that Richard Nixon would receive 43% and 41% of the popular vote, respectively, based on samples of only 2,000 voters. Nixon actually received 42.9%.[1] In contrast, a 1936 *Literary Digest* poll predicted that Alf Landon would win the presidential election based on the preference of over 2 million voters, chosen from lists of automobile owners and telephone directories. Although 57% of the respondents indicated they would vote for Alf Landon, Franklin Roosevelt was elected by the largest margin in history up to that time. Roosevelt's support came primarily from lower-income voters, most of whom did not own automobiles or telephones. This historical polling blunder has served as a classic example of a *biased* sample.

Sampling bias occurs when the individuals selected for a sample overrepresent or underrepresent certain population attributes that are related to the phenomenon under study. Such biases can be conscious or unconscious. Conscious biases occur when a sample is selected purposefully. For example, a clinician might choose only patients with minimal dysfunction to demonstrate a treatment's effectiveness, eliminating those subjects who were not likely to improve. Unconscious biases might occur if an interviewer, who is interested in studying attitudes of the public toward the disabled, stands on a busy street corner in a downtown area and interviews people "at random" or haphazardly. The interviewer may unconsciously choose to approach only those who look cooperative, on the basis of appearance, sex, or some other characteristics. Persons who do not work or shop in that area will not be represented. The conclusions drawn from such a sample cannot be useful for describing attitudes of the "general public." The validity of generalizations made from a sample to the population depend on the method of selecting subjects. Therefore, some impartial mechanism is needed to make unbiased selections.

Target Populations and Accessible Populations

The first step in planning a study is to identify the overall group of people to which the researcher intends to generalize findings. This universe of interest is the **target population,** or **reference population.** The target population for a study of motor skills could be defined as all children with learning disabilities in the United States today. Because it is not possible to gain access to every child with learning disabilities, some portion of the target population that has a chance to be selected must be identified. This is the **accessible population,** or **experimental population.** For example, an accessible population might include all children identified as having a learning disability in a given city's

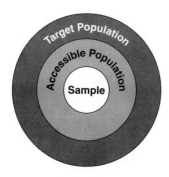

FIGURE 8.1 Levels of the sampling process.

school system. The units within this population are the individual children. The study sample will be chosen from this accessible population (see Fig. 8.1).

Strictly speaking, a sample can only be representative of the accessible population, not necessarily the target population. For example, some school systems may be more proficient at diagnosing children with learning disabilities; others may have more advanced programs that address motor skills. Such differences can complicate generalizations to the target population. When the differences between the target and accessible populations are potentially too great, it is often appropriate to identify a more restricted target population. For example, we could designate a target population of children with learning disabilities who have participated in a comprehensive motor skills program for at least one year. The results of the study would then be applicable only to children meeting this criterion. Because the validity of the accessible population is not readily testable, researchers must exercise judgment in assessing the degree of similarity with the target population.

Inclusion and Exclusion Criteria

In defining the target population, an investigator must first specify selection criteria that will govern who will and will not be subjects. **Inclusion criteria** describe the primary traits of the target and accessible populations that will qualify someone as a subject. The researcher must consider the variety of characteristics present in the population in terms of clinical findings, demographics, and geographic factors, and whether these factors are important to the question being studied. For example, consider a study to look at the effect of physical activity on cognitive performance of students with learning disabilities. The investigator may need to consider the specific type of learning disability, gender and age, or the state or city where subjects will be found. Therefore, a researcher might decide to include only students who have been identified as having dyslexia, only males, and only schools within one town in Massachusetts. The accessible population may be further defined by temporal factors, such as students who were in the school system between 1997 and 1999. It is vitally important to remember, however, that as the researcher restricts the population, and creates a more homogeneous sample, the ability to generalize research findings will also be restricted; that is, the findings will only be applicable to a population with those specific characteristics. Such a scenario may be quite artificial in terms of the patients that are typically seen in the clinic.

Exclusion criteria indicate those factors that would preclude someone from being a subject. These factors will generally be considered potentially confounding to the results; that is, they are likely to interfere with interpretation of the findings. Perhaps students who also have other types of learning disabilities or attention deficit disorders will be excluded. If tests are only given in English, subjects may be excluded if they are not fluent in that language. The researcher may want to eliminate students who have physical disabilities or some other factors that would limit their ability to actively participate in physical exercise programs. Children with asthma may be eliminated, for example. The specification of inclusion and exclusion criteria is an important early step in the research process because it helps to narrow the possibilities for seeking an accessible population. These criteria also define the population.

Subject Selection

Once an accessible population is identified, the researcher must devise a plan for subject selection, inviting members to participate. This process may involve written invitations mailed to potential subjects' homes, telephone calls, or personal contacts in the clinical setting. All members of the subpopulation may be approached, or a smaller group may be selected. Not all of these invited individuals will be interested or willing to participate, and so the sample becomes further reduced to those who agree to participate. With survey questionnaires, many subjects will not respond. In an experimental study, where participants are further divided into groups, subjects may drop out before completion of data collection. In all types of studies, the researcher may have to discard the data of some subjects because of inaccuracies in procedure or missing responses. In the end, the sample used for data analysis may actually be a select subgroup of the population, and is likely to differ from nonparticipants in many ways that could affect the variables being studied.[2-4] The hierarchy that describes the process of sample selection is illustrated in Figure 8.2.

SAMPLING TECHNIQUES

Sampling techniques can be categorized as probability or nonprobability methods. **Probability samples** are created through a process of **random selection.** Random is not the same as haphazard. It means that every unit in the population has an equal chance, or probability, of being chosen. This also means that every unit that is chosen has an equal chance of having some of the characteristics or exposures that are present throughout the population. Therefore, the sample *should* be free of any bias and is considered representative of the population from which it was drawn. Note that we say it is *considered* representative, not that it *is* representative. Because this process involves the operation of chance, there is always the possibility that a sample's characteristics will be different from those of its parent population.

If we summarize sample responses using averaged data, this average will most likely be somewhat different from the total population's average responses, just by chance. The difference between sample averages (called **statistics**) and population av-

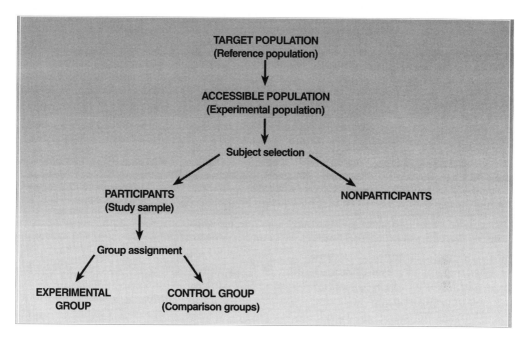

FIGURE 8.2   Hierarchy for selection of a study sample.

erages (called **parameters**) is **sampling error,** or sampling variation. The essence of random sampling is that these sampling differences are due to chance and are not a function of any human bias, conscious or unconscious. Because this process controls for the potential effect of bias, it provides a basis for statistically estimating the degree of sampling error (see Chapter 18). Although it is not perfect, random selection affords the greatest possible confidence in the sample's validity because, *in the long run,* it will produce samples that most accurately reflect the population's characteristics.

The selection of **nonprobability samples** is made by nonrandom methods. The probability of selection is not known, and therefore, the degree of sampling error cannot be estimated. This limits the ability to generalize outcomes beyond the specific sample studied. Nonprobability techniques are probably used more often in clinical research out of necessity, but we recognize that their outcomes require some caution for generalization.

PROBABILITY SAMPLING

The most basic method of probability sampling is through simple random selection, giving every member of a population an equal opportunity, or probability, of being selected; however, this technique is rarely used in practice because of practical difficulties in accessing total populations. For clinical experiments, researchers often use more efficient variations on this theme.

Simple Random Sampling

A random sample is *unbiased* in that each selection is independent, and no one member of the population has any more chance of being chosen than any other member. A random sample is drawn from the accessible population, often taken from a listing of persons, such as membership directories, or institutions, such as lists of accredited hospitals. Often the accessible population is actually defined according to the available listings. For example, if we use a professional membership directory to create a sample of therapists, the accessible population would be defined as therapists who were members. Not all therapists belong to the association, however, and it may not be valid to generalize responses of such a sample to all practicing therapists.

Once a listing is available, a random sampling procedure can be implemented. Suppose we were interested in choosing a sample of 100 occupational therapy students to study their interest in working with the elderly after graduation. We could define the accessible population as the total number of students attending 25 programs in the Northeast. The simplest approach would be to place each student's name on a slip of paper, place these slips into a container, and blindly draw 100 slips. If the accessible population had 56 or fewer elements, we could number them 11 through 66 and choose them on the basis of the throw of two dice.

A more convenient method involves the use of a *table of random numbers,* such as the one given in Table 8.1. Tables of random numbers can be found in most statistics texts. They are generated by computers and comprise thousands of digits (0 to 9) with no systematic order or relationship. The selections made using a table of random numbers are considered unbiased as the order of digits is completely due to chance. To use this system, the accessible population must be in numbered list form, so that every element has a unique number, or identifying code. In this example, if there were a total of 985 students, they would be numbered 001 through 985. Each identification code has the same number of digits, in this case three.

We enter Table 8.1 at random, choosing a starting point using an arbitrary method, such as blindly placing a pencil at a point on the page. For this example, we will start at the seventh digit in row 12. Note that the digits are grouped in twos, but this is just for ease of reading. Some tables group numbers differently. As we are interested in three-digit numbers, we will use the first three digits from our starting point, number 977. Therefore, the student numbered 977 is the first subject selected. We can then move up, down, or across to continue the process. If we choose to move across the row, the next student is number 584, then 160, then 744, and so on, until we choose 100 names. Note that the next number in the series will be 998, a value beyond the range of our accessible population. Any number that comes up out of range is simply ignored and the next three-digit number is used. Similarly, if a student's number should occur again in the list of random numbers, it is also ignored and the next random number is used. This process is called **simple random sampling,** or *sampling without replacement,* as once a unit is selected it has no further chance of being selected.*

---

*Random sampling can also be performed using the technique of *sampling with replacement,* in which each unit that is selected is put back into the pool before the next selection is made. Therefore, each unit truly has an equal chance of being chosen throughout the selection procedure. This method is not used in clinical studies, because subjects cannot represent themselves more than once. Sampling with replacement is used primarily in probability and mathematical studies.

TABLE 8.1   TABLE OF RANDOM NUMBERS

03 47 43 73 86	39 96 47 36 61	46 98 63 71 62	33 26 16 80 45	60 11 14 10 95
97 74 24 67 62	41 81 14 57 20	42 53 32 37 32	27 07 36 07 51	24 51 79 89 73
16 76 62 27 66	59 50 26 71 07	32 90 79 78 53	13 55 38 58 59	88 97 54 14 10
12 56 85 99 26	96 96 68 27 31	05 03 72 93 15	57 12 10 14 21	88 26 49 81 76
55 59 56 35 64	38 54 82 46 22	31 62 43 09 90	06 18 44 32 53	23 83 01 30 30
16 22 77 94 39	49 54 43 54 82	17 37 93 23 78	87 35 20 96 43	84 26 34 91 64
84 42 17 53 91	57 24 55 06 88	77 04 74 47 67	21 76 33 50 25	83 92 12 06 76
63 01 63 78 58	16 95 55 67 19	98 10 50 71 75	12 86 73 58 07	44 39 52 38 79
33 21 12 34 29	78 64 56 07 82	52 42 07 44 38	15 51 00 13 42	99 66 02 79 54
57 60 86 32 44	09 47 27 96 54	49 17 46 09 62	90 52 84 77 27	08 02 73 43 28
18 18 07 92 46	44 17 16 58 09	79 83 86 19 62	06 76 50 03 10	55 23 64 05 05
26 62 38 97 75	84 16 07 44 99	83 11 46 32 24	20 14 85 88 45	10 93 72 88 71
23 42 40 64 74	82 97 77 77 81	07 45 32 14 08	32 98 94 07 72	93 85 79 10 75
52 36 28 19 95	50 92 26 11 97	00 56 76 31 38	80 22 02 53 53	86 60 42 04 53
37 85 94 35 12	83 39 50 08 30	42 34 07 96 88	54 42 06 87 98	35 85 29 48 39
70 29 17 12 13	40 33 20 38 26	13 89 51 03 74	17 76 37 13 04	07 74 21 19 30
56 62 18 37 35	96 83 50 87 75	97 12 25 93 47	70 33 24 03 54	97 77 46 44 80
99 49 57 22 77	88 42 95 45 72	16 64 36 16 00	04 43 18 66 79	94 77 24 21 90
16 08 15 04 72	33 27 14 34 09	45 59 34 68 49	12 72 07 34 45	99 27 72 95 14
31 16 93 32 43	50 27 89 87 19	20 15 37 00 49	52 85 66 60 44	38 68 88 11 80
68 34 30 13 70	55 74 30 77 40	44 22 78 84 26	04 33 46 09 52	68 07 97 06 57
74 57 25 65 76	59 29 97 68 60	71 91 38 67 54	13 58 18 24 76	15 54 55 95 52
27 42 37 86 53	48 55 90 65 72	96 57 69 36 10	96 46 92 42 45	97 60 49 04 91
00 39 68 29 61	66 37 32 20 30	77 84 57 03 29	10 45 65 04 26	11 04 96 67 24
29 94 98 94 24	68 49 69 10 82	53 75 91 93 30	34 25 20 57 27	40 48 73 51 92
16 90 82 66 59	83 62 64 11 12	67 19 00 71 74	60 47 21 29 68	02 02 37 03 31
11 27 94 75 06	06 09 19 74 66	02 94 37 34 02	76 70 90 30 86	38 45 94 30 38
35 24 10 16 20	33 32 51 26 38	79 78 45 04 91	16 92 53 56 16	02 75 50 95 98
38 23 16 86 38	42 38 97 01 50	87 75 66 81 41	40 01 74 91 62	48 51 84 08 32
31 96 25 91 47	96 44 33 49 13	34 86 82 53 91	00 52 43 48 85	27 55 26 89 62
56 67 40 67 14	64 05 71 95 86	11 05 65 09 68	76 83 20 37 90	57 16 00 11 66
14 90 84 45 11	75 73 88 05 90	52 27 41 14 86	22 98 12 22 08	07 52 74 95 80
68 05 51 18 00	33 96 02 75 19	07 60 62 93 55	59 33 82 43 90	49 37 38 44 59
20 46 78 73 90	97 51 40 14 02	04 02 33 31 08	39 54 16 49 36	47 95 93 13 30
64 19 58 97 79	15 06 15 93 20	01 90 10 75 06	40 78 78 89 62	02 67 74 17 33
05 26 93 70 60	22 35 85 15 13	92 03 51 59 77	59 56 78 06 83	52 91 05 70 74
07 97 10 88 23	09 98 42 99 64	61 71 62 99 15	06 51 29 16 93	58 05 77 09 51
68 71 86 85 85	54 87 66 47 54	73 32 08 11 12	44 95 92 63 16	29 56 24 29 48
26 99 61 65 53	58 37 78 80 70	42 10 50 67 42	32 17 55 85 74	94 44 67 16 94
14 65 52 68 75	87 59 36 22 41	26 78 63 06 55	13 08 27 01 50	15 29 39 39 43
17 53 77 58 71	71 41 61 50 72	12 41 94 96 26	44 95 27 36 99	02 96 74 30 83
90 26 59 21 19	23 51 23 33 12	96 93 02 18 36	07 02 18 36 07	25 99 32 70 23
41 23 52 55 99	31 04 49 69 96	10 47 48 45 88	13 41 43 89 20	97 17 14 49 17
60 20 50 81 69	31 99 73 68 68	35 81 33 03 76	24 30 12 48 60	18 99 10 72 34
91 25 38 05 90	94 58 28 41 36	45 37 59 03 09	90 35 57 29 12	82 62 54 65 60
34 50 57 74 37	98 80 33 00 91	09 77 93 19 82	74 94 80 04 04	45 07 31 66 49
85 22 04 39 43	73 81 53 94 79	33 62 46 86 28	08 31 54 46 31	53 94 13 38 47
09 79 13 77 48	73 82 97 22 21	05 03 27 24 83	72 89 44 05 60	35 80 39 94 88
88 75 80 18 14	22 95 75 42 49	39 32 82 22 49	02 48 07 70 37	16 04 61 67 87
90 96 23 70 00	39 00 03 06 90	55 85 78 38 36	94 37 30 69 32	90 89 00 76 33

From Fisher RA, Yates F: *Statistical Tables for Biological, Agricultural and Medical Research,* ed 6. London, Longman Group, 1974, Table XXXIII(I), p 124. Used with permission.

Random selections can be made by computer, using statistical packages, given a numbered list of subjects in a data set. The total data set usually will represent an accessible population. The computer can then generate a random list of any specified size to select the sample.

Systematic Sampling

Random sampling can be a laborious technique, unless the accessible population is organized as a short, prenumbered list. When lists are arranged alphabetically or in some other ordered fashion, an alternative approach can be used that simplifies this procedure, called **systematic sampling.** To use this sampling technique, the researcher divides the total number of elements in the accessible population by the number of elements to be selected. Therefore, to select a sample of 100 from a list of 1,000 students, every tenth person on the list is selected. The interval between selected elements is called the *sampling interval,* in this case 10. The starting point on the list is determined at random, often using a table of random numbers. This approach is usually the least time-consuming and most convenient way to obtain a sample from an available listing of potential subjects. Systematic sampling is generally considered equivalent to random sampling, as long as no recurring pattern or particular order exists in the listing.

Stratified Random Sampling

In random and systematic sampling, the distribution of characteristics of the sample can differ from that of the population from which it was drawn just by chance, because each selection is made independently of all others. It is possible, however, to modify these methods to improve a sample's representativeness (and decrease sampling error) through a process known as **stratification.**

Stratified random sampling involves identifying relevant population characteristics, and partitioning members of a population into homogeneous, nonoverlapping subsets, or **strata,** based on these characteristics. For example, in our study of students' attitudes toward working with the elderly, we may be concerned about the differential effect of level of education. Those who have had more professional education may have different attitudes than those who have not yet been exposed to clinical education. Let us assume that our accessible population consists of 300 freshmen, 300 sophomores, 200 juniors, and 200 seniors. In a simple random sample drawn from the list of 1,000 students, it is possible, just by chance, that the distribution of subjects will not reflect the differential proportions of these classes in the population. To control for this, we can create a **proportional stratified sample,** by first separating the population into the four classes and then drawing random or systematic samples from each class in the proportion that exists in the population. Therefore, to obtain a sample of 100 students, we would choose 30 freshman, 30 sophomores, 20 juniors, and 20 seniors. The resulting sample would intuitively provide a better estimate of the population than simple random sampling.

Stratification increases the precision of estimates only when the stratification variable is closely related to the variables of experimental interest. It would not be of any benefit to stratify subjects on the basis of blood type, for example, in a study of attitudes toward the elderly. It might be important to use variables such as age, gender, or race. National samples for surveys and polls are often stratified by geographic area so that the distribution of regional variables mirrors the population. Stratification can be done on more than one variable when appropriate. Sometimes, however, variables are correlated in such a way that only one variable needs to be the basis for stratification. For instance, age and college class are generally related, and therefore, stratification on class should also control for variations in age.

Although stratified sampling takes additional time, it can actually provide a more representative sample than random sampling, with no sampling error on the stratified variable. Therefore, when relevant strata can be identified, this approach presents an opportunity to strengthen a research design.

Disproportional Sampling

The benefits of stratified sampling can be frustrated when the researcher knows in advance that strata are of greatly unequal size, creating a situation in which one or more strata may provide insufficient samples for making comparisons. Suppose, for example, that we are interested in drawing a sample of 200 therapists from a professional organization with 2,000 members, including 1,700 females and 300 males. Using proportional selection, we would choose 10% of each group, 170 females and 30 males; however, such a small number of males would probably not provide adequate representation for drawing conclusions about that segment of the population.

One way of dealing with this situation is to use a simple random sample and leave the proportional representation to chance; however, unless the sample is unusually large, the differential effect of gender will probably not be controlled. Alternatively, we can adopt a **disproportional sampling** design, in which we select random samples of adequate size from each category. For example, we might select 100 females and 100 males. This sample of 200 cannot be considered random, because each male has a much greater chance (higher probability) of being chosen. This approach creates an adequate sample size, but it presents problems for data analysis, because the characteristics of one group, in this case males, will be overrepresented in the sample. We can control for this effect by weighting the data, so that females receive a proportionally larger mathematical representation in the analysis of scores than males.

To calculate *proportional weights,* we first determine the probability that any one female or male will be selected. For example, to choose 100 females, the probability of any one female being chosen is 100 of 1,700, or 1 of 17 (1/17). The probability of any one male being chosen is 100 of 300, or 1 of 3 (1/3). Therefore, each male has a probability of selection more than 5 times that of any female.

Next we determine the assigned weights by taking the inverse of these probabilities.[2] Therefore, the weight for female scores is $17/1 = 17$, and that for males is $3/1 = 3$. This means that when data are analyzed, each female's score will be multiplied by 17 and each male's score will be multiplied by 3. In any mathematical manipulation of the data, the total of the females' scores would be larger than the total of the males' scores. Therefore, the proportional representation of each group is differentiated in the total data set. Because all subjects in a group will have the same weight, the average scores for that group will not be affected; however, the relative contribution of these scores to overall data interpretation will be controlled. This approach has been used, for example, in large surveys such as the National Health Interview Survey, to ensure adequate representation of minorities in the study sample.

Cluster Sampling

In many research situations, especially those involving large, dispersed populations, it is impractical or impossible to obtain a complete listing of a population. For instance, if we wanted to sample therapists in rehabilitation hospitals across the country, it is unreasonable to expect that we could easily compile such a list. We therefore need some strategy that will allow us to link members of the population to some already established grouping that can be sampled. This approach is called **cluster sampling,** or *multistage sampling.*

Cluster sampling involves successive random sampling of a series of units in the population. For example, suppose we were interested in generating a random sample of American school children by selecting 125 classes, as shown in Figure 8.3. In stage 1, we choose a random sample, or *cluster,* of 5 states. In stage 2, we select a random sample of 5 schools from each state. In stage 3, we randomly select 5 classes from each school.

The advantage of cluster sampling is its obvious convenience and efficiency when dealing with large populations; however, this comes at the price of increased sampling error. Because two or more samples are drawn, each is subject to sampling error, potentially compounding the inaccuracy of the final sample. This disadvantage can be minimized by choosing as large a sample as possible within each cluster and by stratifying within any stage of sampling. For example, Tomblin and coworkers used a stratified cluster sample to screen kindergarten children for speech language impairment across rural, urban, and suburban areas in the Midwest.[5]

Survey researchers often use multistage sampling to generate random samples of households. One technique, called **area probability sampling,** allows a population to be sampled geographically. The total target land area is divided into mutually exclusive sections. A list is then made of housing units in each section, and a sample is drawn from these lists. The final survey may be administered to all selected housing units, or the list may be subdivided further into individuals within households.

Another survey sampling technique, called **random-digit dialing,** involves the random selection of phone numbers based on multistage sampling of area codes and telephone exchanges. Most of us have had experience with this type of survey (usually at dinner time). Many studies in marketing research use this approach. Obviously this method presents problems in that only households with listed telephone numbers have a chance of being selected. In addition, bias may be introduced by timing. Calls made during working hours or weekdays versus weekends may alter the characteristics of sample respondents. For certain research questions, however, random-digit dialing is most useful for generating a sizable sample over a large area.

NONPROBABILITY SAMPLING

In practice, it is sometimes difficult, if not impossible, to obtain a true random sample. Clinical researchers are often forced to use **nonprobability samples,** created when samples are chosen on some basis other than random selection. Because all the elements of

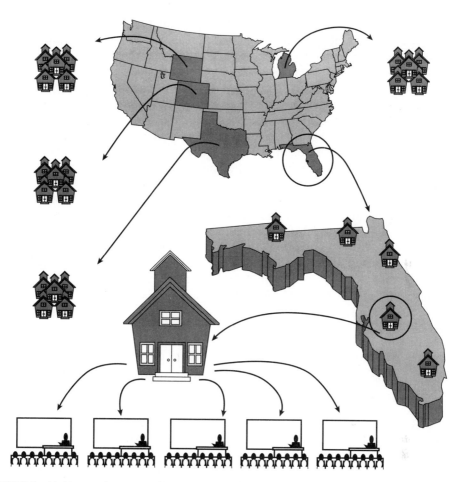

FIGURE 8.3   Multistage cluster sampling process to select a random sample of 125 classes of school children. In stage 1, five states are randomly chosen. In stage 2, five schools are randomly chosen from each state. In stage 3, five classes are randomly chosen from each school. The process is illustrated for one state and one school in that state.

the population do not have an equal chance of being selected under these circumstances, we cannot readily assume that the sample represents the target population. The probability exists that some segment of the population will be disproportionately represented.

Convenience Sampling

The most common form of nonprobability sample is a **convenience sample,** or *accidental sample.* With this method, subjects are chosen on the basis of availability. Perhaps the most used and practical approach to convenience sampling is **consecutive sampling,** which involves recruiting all patients who meet the inclusion and exclusion criteria as they become available. Essentially, a consecutive sample includes the entire accessible population within the defined period of the study. This can be problematic if the study period is too short, and a sufficient number of qualified subjects cannot be obtained, or if the period does not allow a representative group. For example, if we were studying causes of low back pain, and we only included patients who came to the clinic in the summer months, we might miss patients whose pain is caused by shoveling snow or slipping on ice.

The use of volunteers is also a commonly used convenience sampling method because of its expedience. Researchers who post signs in dormitories or hospitals to recruit subjects with specific characteristics are sampling by this method. Polls in magazines or on street corners and most commercial advertisements are based on samples of convenience. The major limitation of this method, however, is the potential bias of **self-selection.** It is not possible to know what attributes are present in those who offer themselves as subjects, as compared with those who do not, and it is unclear how these attributes may affect the ability to generalize experimental outcomes. Those who volunteer may be quite atypical of the target population in terms of such characteristics as age, motivation, activity level, and other correlates of health consciousness.[6, 7] Although all samples, even random samples, are eventually composed of those who participate voluntarily, those who agree to be part of a random sample were not self-selected. Therefore, characteristics of subjects in a random sample can be assumed to represent the target population. This is not necessarily a safe assumption with nonrandom samples.

Quota Sampling

Nonprobability sampling can also incorporate elements of stratification. Using **quota sampling,** a researcher can control for the potential confounding effect of known characteristics of a population by guiding the sampling process so that an adequate number of subjects are obtained for each stratum. This approach requires that each stratum is represented in the same proportion as in the population. For example, using the previous example examining students' attitudes toward the elderly, we could call for volunteers to take the questionnaire and stop the call once we have achieved the proper number of subjects for each class. Although this system still faces the potential for nonprobability biases, it does improve on the process by proportionally representing each segment of the population in the sample.

Purposive Sampling

A third nonprobability approach is **purposive sampling,** in which the researcher handpicks subjects on the basis of specific criteria. The researcher may locate subjects by chart review or interview patients to determine if they fit the study. A researcher must exercise fair judgment to make this process meaningful. For instance, in a study to test the effectiveness of an exercise program, the researcher may choose patients who are likely to be compliant from among the patients seen in his clinic. In studies to establish the validity of newly developed measuring instruments, researchers may want to test a variety of subjects with specifically different degrees of limitation in the variable being measured. Purposive sampling is similar to convenience sampling, but differs in that specific choices are made, rather than simple availability. This approach has the same limitations to generalization as a convenience sample, in that it can result in a biased sample. However, in many instances, purposive sampling can yield a sample that will be representative of the population if the investigator wisely chooses individuals who represent the spectrum of population characteristics.[8] Purposive samples are commonly used in qualitative research to ensure that subjects have the appropriate knowledge and will be a good informant for the study.[9]

Snowball Sampling

Snowball sampling is a useful technique when subjects with specific characteristics are hard to locate. This approach is carried out in stages. In the first stage, a few subjects who meet selection criteria are identified and tested or interviewed. In the second stage, these subjects are asked to identify others who have the requisite characteristics. This process of "chain referral" or "snowballing" is continued until an adequate sample is obtained. The researcher must be able to verify the eligibility of each respondent to ensure a representative group.[10, 11] Snowball sampling is used extensively, for example, in studies involving homeless persons and drug abusers.[11, 12] It is also a practical approach for studies involving infants. For instance, a researcher can identify women in later stages of pregnancy who might have contact with other pregnant women through health plans or childbirth classes. Finding children in specific age groups might be facilitated by parents' contacts through schools, play groups, or day care centers.

RECRUITMENT

The practicalities of clinical research demand that we consider feasibility issues in initial stages of planning a study. One of the most serious of these considerations is how to recruit the sample. Once the inclusion and exclusion criteria have been defined, the researcher begins the process of finding appropriate subjects in sufficient numbers.

Recruitment methods will depend on the research question. Community studies will often involve the use of advertisements, newspapers, or mailings. Large studies may be based on samples derived from telephone listings or membership directories. Health clubs, schools, and day care centers may be helpful. For clinical studies, subjects are often recruited from the patient population in the researcher's facility. Investigators must be aware of the ethical concerns that arise when using their own patients as subjects, including fair descriptions of the study in an effort to gain their trust and secure their participation (see Chapter 3). Subjects may also be recruited from other facilities or agencies, usually through the cooperation of colleagues at those institutions. In this case, the researcher should obtain written endorsements from the appropriate administrative officials to confirm their cooperation and to include with applications for funding.

When subjects are recruited through external agencies, it may be critical to establish who will have access to the data, and who will "own" the data. This is especially important with collaborative efforts. The distinction of data ownership may impact decisions about publication and dissemination of findings.

Researchers should be prepared to give administrative officials a copy of the study proposal, often in abbreviated form. When subjects are patients, researchers must contact the physician in charge of the patient's care. Sometimes it is efficient to work with a particular physician or practice group to recruit patients on an ongoing basis through the practice. Once the physician's approval has been obtained, the researcher can then contact individual patients to secure their participation. This may be done in person or by letter, explaining the purpose of the study and assuring them that their treatment will not be affected regardless of their participation. The consent form will be given to the patients to read and to discuss with the researcher, with a contact number if they have further questions.

Many of the individuals who are contacted will consent to participate in the study, and many others will not. To obtain a sample of sufficient size, it is often necessary to contact a large number of prospective individuals. A question about the number of subjects needed is often the first to be raised. The issue of sample size is an essential one, as it directly affects the statistical power of the study. **Power** is the ability to find significant differences when they exist.[†] With a small sample, power tends to be low, and a study may not succeed in demonstrating the desired effects. As the researcher explores the availability of subjects, we can generally be sure that fewer subjects will agree to enter the study than originally projected (see Fig. 8.2). Every investigator should have a contingency plan in mind, such as recruiting subjects from different sites or expanding inclusion criteria, when the sample size falls substantially short of expectations. For studies that involve the use of questionnaires, sample size is a function of response rate, and should be a factor in deciding how many questionnaires to send out.

Once the study is completed, it is also appropriate to offer to send a summary of the findings to physicians, agencies, and subjects. The results may have an impact on the patient's care or future clinical decisions. Maintaining such contact will often encourage colleagues to be part of future studies as well.

COMMENTARY

Sampling, Like Life, Is a Compromise

Nonprobability samples are used more often than probability samples in clinical research because of the difficulties in obtaining true access to populations. We frequently encounter statements such as "Subjects were selected from the patient population at Hospital X between 1992 and 1994," and "Subjects were volunteers from the senior class at University Y." Most clinical situations require that samples of convenience be used. Patients are often recruited as they become available, making true random selection impossible. Inclusion and exclusion criteria may be made sufficiently broad so that a sample of sufficient size can be obtained within a reasonable amount of time. Recruiting subjects from more than one site can also increase generalizability of findings.

Generalizations of data collected from nonrandom samples must be made with caution; however, this is not to say that studies with nonrandom samples are invalid. The data collected are still meaningful within the confines of the defined group being tested. The researcher must determine if the characteristics of the sample are an adequate representation of the target population. When using conven-

[†]Statistical implications of sample size and power are discussed in Chapter 18 and Appendix C.

ience samples, the researcher has an added responsibility to identify important extraneous variables that might influence the dependent variable. It is important to decide if a restricted sample, with homogeneous subjects, would be more useful, or if the full variation in the population should be represented. The risk of interpretative error can be reduced by comparing sample characteristics to other groups from the population that may be described in the literature, and by replicating studies to show that subjects chosen nonrandomly from different sources respond in a similar way.[13] Sample size is also an important consideration. In qualitative studies, samples may be quite small, as compared with quantitative studies that will require statistical comparisons. Researchers must consider the effect of sample size on their analytic process. Sometimes the restrictions set for inclusion and exclusion criteria must be modified to obtain a large enough sample, and the implications of this process must be considered.

Keppel suggests that researchers can distinguish between statistical and nonstatistical generalizations.[13] Statistical inferences theoretically require random sampling and are based on the validity of representativeness. Strictly speaking, it is inappropriate to apply many inferential statistical procedures to data that were obtained from nonprobability samples, although most researchers are willing to make assumptions about the representativeness of their sample so that the statistical analysis can be carried out. Generalizations from nonprobability samples can be justified on the basis of knowledge of the research topic, experience, the logic of the study, and consistency in replicated outcomes. Often, one can conclude that a convenience sample will provide data that, for all practical purposes, are as "random" as those obtained with a probability sample, especially with relatively small samples.[8] It is important, however, that this determination is critically assessed, not simply assumed, based on the specific circumstances of the study. Researchers must be aware of the limitations inherent in any sampling method and should try to incorporate elements of random sampling whenever possible.

KEY TERMS

population
sample
sampling bias
target population
   (reference population)
accessible population
   (experimental
   population)
inclusion criteria
exclusion criteria
probability sample
random selection

statistic
parameter
sampling error
nonprobability sample
simple random sampling
systematic sampling
stratification
stratified random sample
strata
proportional stratified
   sample
disproportional sampling

cluster sampling
   (multistage sampling)
area probability sampling
random-digit dialing
convenience sample
   (accidental sample)
consecutive sampling
self-selection
quota sampling
purposive sampling
snowball sampling
power

REFERENCES

1. Babbie ER. *Survey Research Methods.* Belmont, CA: Wadsworth, 1973.
2. Friedman LM, Furberg CD, DeMets DL. *Fundamentals of Clinical Trials.* Littleton, MA: PSG, 1985.
3. Wilhelmsen L, Ljungberg S, Wedel H, et al. A comparison between participants and nonparticipants in a primary preventive trial. *J Chron Dis* 1976;29:331–9.
4. Fetter MS, Feetham SL, D' Apolito K, et al. Randomized clinical trials: issues for researchers. *Nurs Res* 1989;38:117–20.
5. Tomblin JB, Records NL, Buckwalter P, Zhang X, Smith E, O'Brien M. Prevalence of specific language impairment in kindergarten children. *J Speech Lang Hear Res* 1997;40:1245–60.
6. Hennekens CH, Buring JE. *Epidemiology in Medicine.* Boston: Little Brown, 1987.
7. Ganguli M, Lytle ME, Reynolds MD, Dodge HH. Random versus volunteer selection for a community-based study. *J Gerontol* 1998;53A:M39–M46.
8. Hahn GJ, Meeker WQ. Assumptions for statistical inference. *Am Statistician* 1993;47:1–11.
9. Morse JM. Strategies for sampling. In: Morse JM, ed. *Qualitative Nursing Research: A Contemporary Dialogue.* Rockville, MD: Aspen, 1989, 117–31.
10. Biernacki P, Waldorf D. Snowball sampling: problems and techniques of chain referral sampling. *Sociol Methods Res* 1981;10:141.
11. Lopes CS, Rodriguez LC, Sichieri R. The lack of selection bias in a snowball sampled case-control study on drug abuse. *Int J Epidemiol* 1996;25:1267–70.
12. Willems JC, Iguchi MY, Lidz V, Bux DAJ. Change in drug-using networks of injecting drug users during methadone treatment: a pilot study using snowball recruitment and intensive interviews. *Subst Use Misuse* 1997;32:1539–54.
13. Keppel G. *Design and Analysis: A Researcher's Handbook.* 2d ed. Englewood Cliffs, NJ: Prentice Hall, 1982.

C H A P T E R

9

Experimental Control

The most rigorous form of scientific investigation for testing hypotheses is the **experiment.** Experiments are based on a logical structure, or *design,* within which the investigator systematically introduces changes into natural phenomena and then observes the consequences of those changes. The purpose of an experiment is to support a **cause-and-effect relationship** between a particular action or condition (the independent variable) and an observed response (the dependent variable).

The essence of an experiment lies in the researcher's ability to manipulate and control variables and measurements, so that rival hypotheses are ruled out as possible explanations for the observed response. These rival hypotheses concern the potential influence of unrelated factors, called **extraneous variables** (also called nuisance variables or intervening variables). An extraneous variable is any factor that is not directly related to the purpose of the study, but that may affect the dependent variable. Extraneous variables can be *extrinsic factors* that emerge from the environment and the experimental situation or *intrinsic factors* that represent personal characteristics of the subjects of the study.

When extraneous variables are not controlled, they exert a **confounding** influence on the independent variable; that is, they contaminate the independent variable in such a way that their separate effects are obscured. For example, if we wanted to examine the effect of cryotherapy for relieving shoulder pain, and our subjects were on pain medication, the medication would be a confounding factor. If we observe a decrease in pain following treatment, we could not determine if the effect was due to the treatment, the medication, or some combination of the two. Other extraneous factors that could interfere with conclusions could be spontaneous healing or other treatments the patient is receiving. Experiments are designed to **control** for this type of confounding.

In reality, of course, clinical experiments seldom have the ability to completely eliminate confounding effects; however, even though causality can never be demonstrated with complete certainty, the experimental method provides the most convincing evidence of the effect one variable has on another. The purpose of this chapter is to examine issues of experimental control that must be addressed if the researcher is to have confidence in the validity of experimental outcomes.

CHARACTERISTICS OF EXPERIMENTS

To be considered a true experiment, a study must have three essential characteristics: The independent variable must be manipulated by the experimenter, the subjects must be randomly assigned to groups, and a control group must be incorporated within the design.

Manipulation of Variables

Manipulation of variables refers to a deliberate operation performed by the experimenter, imposing a set of predetermined experimental conditions (the independent variable) on at least one group of subjects. The experimenter manipulates the levels of the independent variable by assigning subjects to varied conditions, usually administering the intervention to one group and withholding it from another. For example, we might be interested in the effect of medication to reduce hypertension. We can assign subjects to treatment and control groups and measure blood pressure changes that occur following a period of treatment or no treatment. It is possible to manipulate a single variable or several variables simultaneously.

Active and Attribute Variables

Independent variables can be distinguished as either active or attribute factors. An **active variable** is one that is manipulated by the experimenter so that subjects are assigned to levels of the independent variable. For instance, subjects can be assigned to receive medication or a placebo. Therefore, treatment is an active variable. With an **attribute variable** the researcher is not able to assign subjects to groups, but must observe them within natural groupings according to inherent physical, psychological, or personal characteristics. Age group would be an attribute factor, as subjects automatically belong to only one group, with no possibility for assignment. Preexisting characteristics such as gender, occupation, and diagnosis are other examples of attribute variables.

Attribute variables cannot be manipulated by the experimenter. Therefore, when the effect of one or more attribute variables is studied, the research cannot be considered a true experiment. For example, we could look at differences in strength and range of motion across various age groups or between males and females. This approach is considered **ex post facto research,** because all elements of the design have already been determined before the study begins. Ex post facto research allows us to consider relationships, but it does not afford adequate opportunity for control, thereby limiting interpretation of cause and effect. This can be an important consideration for choosing statistical analyses.

It is possible to combine active variables and attribute variables in a single study. For instance, we could look at the effect of medication on hypertension combined with the influence of age. By dividing subjects into four age groups, the subjects within each age group could be assigned to one of the two treatment groups. Even though this study includes an attribute variable, it qualifies as an experiment because the researcher is able to manipulate the assignment of treatment levels for at least one independent variable.

Random Assignment

In Chapter 8 we discussed the importance of random selection for *choosing* subjects, to ensure that a sample was representative of the parent population and that it was not biased. Once a sample is selected, it is important to continue the process of randomization in *assigning* subjects to groups. **Random assignment** means that each subject has an equal chance of being assigned to any group; that is, assignments will be independent of personal judgment or bias. Random assignment is an essential feature of experimental research, providing the greatest confidence that no systematic bias exists with respect to a groups' collective attributes that might differentially affect the dependent variable. If we can assume that groups are equivalent at the start of an experiment, then we can have confidence that differences observed at the end of the study are not due to intersubject variability that existed before the experiment began.

The concept of random assignment refers to groups being considered equivalent. Equivalence does not mean that every subject in one group is exactly equal to another subject in the other group. It does mean that any differences between the groups have been distributed as a function of chance alone. We can think of subjects as composites of personal characteristics such as motivation, intellectual ability, attitude, medical history, and strength. With randomization, subjects with high or low values of these variables are just as likely to be assigned to one group or another. Randomization is also expected to control for random events that might affect subjects during the course of the study; that is, subjects in both groups should be equally likely to experience illness, personal tragedy, happy occasions, or any other nonsystematic event that might affect the dependent variable. Thus, *overall*, intersubject differences should balance out.

Although randomization is the preferred method for equalizing groups for scientific study, it does not guarantee equivalence. The concept of randomization is theoretical in that it applies to the probability of outcomes in the proverbial "long run." In other words, if we use randomization to divide an infinitely large sample, the groups' average scores should not be different; however, because clinical samples tend to be limited in size, randomization can result in groups that are quite disparate on certain important properties. Researchers often use statistical means of comparing groups on initial values that are considered relevant to the dependent variable, to determine if those extraneous factors did balance out. For example, it may be important to determine if relatively equal numbers of males and females were assigned to each group, or if groups are equivalent on age. When randomization does not successfully balance the distribution of intersubject differences, several design variations can be used. These are discussed shortly.

Process of Assigning Subjects

The process of assigning subjects to groups can be carried out in several ways; however, the most effective method involves the use of a table of random numbers, such as the one given in Table 8.1. The procedure for using a table of random numbers was introduced in Chapter 8 in relation to random selection. The reader is encouraged to review that process, as it is applicable for random assignment as well.

Suppose we are interested in comparing the effects of two exercises for strengthening knee extensors against a control group that receives no exercise. We assemble a list of 45 subjects, so that we can assign 15 subjects to each of the three groups. The names are numbered from 01 to 45. Because subjects are numbered with two-digit codes, we would use pairs of digits to identify them from the table. As subjects are chosen, they are assigned to group 1, group 2, or group 3 on a rotating basis, until all subjects have been assigned.

In the assignment process, we designate groups as 1, 2, or 3, not by treatment. A good experimental strategy involves continuing the process of random assignment to assign levels of the independent variable to groups. If each treatment level is given a number, we can use the table of random numbers to carry out this assignment. By employing randomization techniques at each step, we have enhanced the validity of the study and fulfilled an essential requirement of experimental research.

Intention to Treat

After a subject has been randomly assigned to a group, that subject may or may not actually get the treatment that was assigned. This can occur for many reasons. Often, the patient will drop out of the study or terminate treatment before the study is complete. Sometimes a patient's condition changes and the assigned treatment is no longer appropriate. For instance, a study was done to compare use of single-chamber ventricular pacemakers and dual-chamber pacemakers for patients who required cardiac pacing.[1] Patients were randomly assigned to receive one treatment or the other; however, 26% of those who were assigned ventricular pacing experienced symptoms that required changing to the dual-chamber pacemaker, and 2% of those initially assigned to dual-chamber pacing had their pacemakers reprogrammed to ventricular pacing.

In another scenario that often occurs, a patient may initially consent to join a study, knowing that she may be assigned to either group, but after assignment is complete, the patient decides she wants the other treatment. For example, patients were entered into a randomized trial to compare the effects of epidural analgesia with intravenous analgesia on the outcome of labor.[2] The study included 1,330 women, but only 65% of each randomization group accepted the allocated treatment. Ethically, these patients must be allowed to receive the treatment they want. From a research standpoint, however, we do not want to consider these women members of the other group. If every patient chose their own treatment, the two groups would have no basis for equivalence and the comparisons would be fundamentally confounded.

This situation causes a problem for analysis, obviously, as the composition of the groups is biased from the initial assignment, especially if the number of subjects involved is large. There is no clean way to account for this difficulty. At first glance, it might seem prudent to simply eliminate any subjects who did not get their assigned treatment, but this also introduces a bias. First, it may seriously reduce the sample size. Second, if we find group differences, we would not know if they are due to the treatment, or because the healthier or stronger patients remained in one group. Another approach is to analyze subjects according to the treatment they did receive, which is called **on-protocol analysis.** This method will tend to bias results in favor of a treatment effect, often resulting in misleading interpretations.[3,4] A more conservative approach uses a principle called **intention to treat**, which means that data are analyzed assuming each patient receives the treatment to which he was assigned. We analyze the data according to the way we *intended* to treat the subjects, not the way they were actually treated. As might be expected, this approach will make it harder to find significant differences. Many researchers will analyze data both ways. If the two methods yield different results, the conclusions may be suspect. If the outcomes are the same, the researcher will have strong confidence in the study.[5] Various statistical methods have been proposed for evaluating results using intention-to-treat analysis.[6–9]

Control Groups

The most effective design strategy for ruling out extraneous effects is the use of a **control group** against which the experimental group is compared. Subjects in a control group may receive a standard treatment that will act as a basis of comparison for a new intervention, a placebo, or no intervention at all. To draw valid comparisons, we must be able to assume a reasonable degree of equivalence between the control and experimental groups. Then, if we observe a change in the treatment group, but no change in the control group, we can reasonably attribute the change to treatment. If the control group responds similarly to the experimental group, it is likely that the observed changes are due to chance.

The operational definition of a control condition is important to the interpretation of outcomes. The difference between the two groups should be the essential element that is the independent variable. For example, Mulrow and associates studied the effects of physical therapy intervention on mobility in frail elders in a nursing home.[10] The control group did not receive therapy, but instead was assigned "friendly visitors" who visited with the same frequency as treatment was given. The visitors were intended to control for the effects of personal interaction and attention that were necessary parts of the physical therapy treatment, but not the essential component of the intervention.

The use of a control group is often unfeasible in clinical situations, for practical or ethical reasons. Therefore, clinical researchers often evaluate a new experimental treatment against conventional methods of care. This does not diminish the validity or usefulness of the study, but it does change the question that can be asked of the data. Instead of assessing whether the new treatment *works*, this approach assesses whether the new treatment is more effective than standard methods. Unless the standard treatment has previously been tested against an untreated control, this type of question does not allow us to determine if the interventions are actually responsible for observed change. If such a study results in improvement in both groups, it would not be possible to determine if both treatments were equally effective or if both groups would have improved spontaneously without any intervention. It is justifiable to design studies with comparative treatments as controls when previous research has clearly established their effectiveness against a true control group, or when it is considered unreasonable to leave patients untreated.

THE RESEARCH PROTOCOL

To control for the effect of extraneous factors that occur within the experimental situation, the researcher must either eliminate them or provide assurance that they will affect all groups equally. This classical concept of control can truly be realized only in the laboratory, where environmental influences are under maximal control by the experimenter. In field settings, this type of control is more illusive. Clinical situations cannot always be altered to meet experimental requirements, and, indeed, it may be undesirable to do so.[11] To consider it a true experiment, however, the researcher must be able to exercise sufficient control over the experimental situation, so that the effect of confounding variables can be ruled out with confidence. Therefore, the clinical researcher must determine which factors are most likely to contaminate the independent variable and attempt to minimize their effects as much as possible. If they are considered important, the experimenter should attempt to control for environmental confounders such as scheduling, location, lighting, and room noise. For instance, in studies of patients with rheumatoid arthritis, investigators have recommended that the time of day that measurements are taken be kept constant because of circadian rhythms for pain and stiffness.[12]

Although it is impossible to make every subject's experience exactly alike, it is often possible to achieve a reasonable level of constancy for many relevant extraneous variables through delineation of a standardized research protocol. Such reliability must be built into a research design for both the independent and dependent variables; that is, the application of treatment and measurement should be consistent. The protocol should specify the positioning of subjects, the timing of all treatments and measurements, the methods of calibrating equipment, and any other specifications necessary to ensure the most consistent performance of experimental activities. Researchers often read instructions to subjects (or have subjects read them), so that each one receives exactly the same information. Criteria for assessing the dependent variable should be clear, and those performing data collection should be trained and tested for their reliability.

It is necessary to control subjects' activities outside the experimental situation only if those activities are directly related to their performance. For instance, it may or may not be important to control the subjects' diet, activity level immediately prior to testing, or amount of sleep obtained the night before. If these factors *are* important, and if the researcher cannot control them, then these variables represent **limitations** to the study. The experiment goes on despite their potential influence; however, the researcher must monitor and evaluate the impact of these factors. Most often, such problems will not be so serious as to jeopardize the experiment, but they should be taken into account when interpretations are made. If their impact is sufficiently serious to rule out sensible conclusions, the experiment should probably be restructured or abandoned.

The realities of the clinical environment suggest, however, that we should weigh the merits of control over experimental conditions versus relevance to practice.[11] If we design protocols that are more restrictive than typical practice, we may find that results are not readily applicable to real-world situations. This is most pertinent in studies where the essential nature of treatment cannot reasonably be uniform for all patients. Sometimes we must be able to develop specific treatment plans and progress a patient according to individualized goals, or set the dosage of medication for individual needs.[13] In this case, protocols should be made as consistent as possible, providing a standardized set of guidelines that would make it reproducible.[14] For instance, in the study by Mulrow and associates, examining the effect of physical therapy on mobility of nursing home residents, intervention plans were developed by setting specific treatment goals for each patient and organizing all treatments around range of motion, strength, balance, and mobility.[10] This approach resulted in individualized treatment sessions, but used the same decision-making model for all patients, which should be reproducible. The essential element in these situations, of course, is to detail the protocol as much as possible, so that cause-and-effect relationships can be interpreted.

BLINDING

The potential for observation bias is an important concern in experimental studies. The participants' knowledge of their treatment status or the investigator's expectations can, consciously or unconsciously, influence performance or the recording and reporting of outcomes. Protection against this form of bias is best achieved by using a **double-blind study,** where neither the subjects nor the investigators are aware of the identity of the treatment groups until after data are collected.

In its most complete form, a blind design can involve hiding the identity of group assignments from subjects, from those who provide treatment, from those who measure outcome variables, and from those who will reduce and analyze the data. It is useful to insulate each of these components by having different personnel involved at each level. It is also advisable to blind those responsible for treatment and assessment from the research hypothesis, so that they do not approach their tasks with any preconceived expectations and so that such knowledge cannot influence their interactions with the subjects.

The necessity for and feasibility of blinding depends on the nature of the experimental treatment and the response variables. To blind subjects, the experimental treatment must be able to be offered as a placebo. For many rehabilitation procedures this is not possible. In that case, a **single-blind study** can be carried out, where only the investigator or measurement team is blinded.

Some types of response variables are totally objective, so that blinding is not really necessary. For example, studies that examine survival rates look at death as an outcome variable, an assessment that is obviously not prone to bias; however, as assessments become more subjective, the need for blinding increases. To whatever extent is possible within an experiment, blinding will substantially strengthen the validity of conclusions.

The technique of blinding requires that treatments be coded in some way, so that when data collection is complete, the code can be broken and group assignments revealed. Because the potential for biases in data collection is so strong, blindness should be preserved carefully during the course of the study.

DESIGN STRATEGIES FOR CONTROLLING INTERSUBJECT DIFFERENCES

Clinical research is often concerned with measuring changes in behavioral responses that are potentially influenced by personal traits of those being studied. There are several design strategies that can be incorporated into a study that will control for these intrinsic variables. The most fundamental of these is random assignment, which eliminates bias by creating a balanced distribution of characteristics across groups. As we have suggested, however, random assignment is not a perfect system, and may result in groups that are not balanced on important variables. When one or two extraneous factors are of special concern, the researcher may not want to depend on randomization. To be sure that certain variables are distributed equally across experimental conditions,

TABLE 9.1. DESIGN STRATEGIES FOR CONTROLLING INTERSUBJECT DIFFERENCES

1. ***Selection of homogenous subjects:*** Choose only subjects who have the same characteristics of the extraneous variable.
2. ***Blocking:*** Build extraneous attribute variables into the design by using them as independent variables, creating *blocks* of subjects that are homogeneous for the different levels of the variable.
3. ***Matching:*** Match subjects on specific characteristics across groups.
4. ***Using subjects as their own control:*** Expose subjects to all levels of the independent variable, creating a *repeated measures* design.
5. ***Analysis of covariance:*** Select an extraneous variable as a *covariate,* adjusting scores statistically to control for differences on the extraneous variable.

control can be increased by selecting homogeneous subjects, blocking, matching subjects, using subjects as their own control, or by statistical manipulation using analysis of covariance (Table 9.1). Each of these strategies requires that the investigator be able to predict which extraneous factors are relevant to the study in advance. Such predictions may be based on theory, past studies, or simply the researcher's intuition. The extent of control offered by these methods depends on which extraneous factors are measured and how strong the relationship is between those factors and the dependent variable.

Selection of Homogeneous Subjects

When a researcher suspects that specific subject traits may interfere with the dependent variable, the simplest way to control for them is to eliminate them by choosing a sample that is **homogeneous** on those characteristics. In that case, the extraneous variables are not allowed to vary; that is, they are eliminated as variables. For instance, if we think males and females will respond differently to the experimental treatment, we can choose only male subjects for our sample. If age is a potential confounder, male subjects can be restricted to a specific age range, such as between 20 and 30 years of age. Once a homogeneous group of subjects is selected, those subjects can be randomly assigned to treatment conditions. In that way, the effects of sex and age are controlled, with all other characteristics equally distributed.

The major disadvantage of this approach is that the research findings can be generalized only to the type of subjects who participate in the study, in this case to men between 20 and 30 years of age. This often limits the application of results. In addition, the researcher must be able to establish that the restrictions put on the sample have achieved the desired control. For instance, if age influences the dependent variable, the researcher must be sure that within the range 20 to 30 years this effect is constant. If the effect of age varies for those who are 21 versus 28 years old, the attempt at control will be ineffective. Therefore, researchers should be reluctant to use this technique unless the restriction is consistent with the purpose of the experiment.

Blocking

Another means of controlling for extraneous effects of attribute variables is to systematically manipulate them by building them into the experimental design as an independent variable. For instance, if we are concerned with the effect of age, we could divide subjects into three age groups: under 30, 30 to 40, and over 40. Then, in addition to treatment, we would have a second independent variable—age—with three levels. Each category of age is called a *block,* and the attribute variable—age—is called a **blocking variable.** This procedure lets us control for age effects by allowing us to analyze the differential effect of age on treatment within the design.

A block represents a group of subjects who are homogeneous on one particular attribute. When subjects within each block are randomly assigned to treatment groups, the design is called a **randomized block design.** The design can be extended to include several blocking variables, although the analysis and interpretation of data become more complex. For instance, we could look at treatment effects across males and females in different age groups. Randomized block designs are discussed further in Chapter 10.

Matching

Another strategy for dealing with extraneous variables involves **matching** subjects on the basis of specific characteristics. For example, if we were concerned with the effect of sex and age on our dependent variable, we could use a matching procedure to guarantee an equivalent group of males and females within different age ranges in the experimental and control groups. Studies that use twins to compare outcomes are using the ultimate matching process.

Matching is accomplished by finding sets of subjects who have the same characteristics and randomly assigning members of each set to the study groups. When only two groups are involved, the technique is called a **matched pairs design.** Matching can be accomplished by purposefully selecting pairs of subjects (or larger sets if there are more than two treatment groups) within the subject pool that most closely match each other on the characteristics of interest. The subjects within each set are then randomly assigned to the treatment groups. These sets are analogous to blocks in a randomized block design. To facilitate finding appropriate matches, a range of values is usually defined, so that matches are made within predetermined limits. For instance, if we want to match on age, we may be willing to accept a match that falls within ±2 years. The researcher must determine how exact a match is necessary to achieve an acceptable level of control.

When matching is done within a preexisting sample, another strategy involves rank-ordering subjects according to the matching variable. This approach is often employed to match subjects on the basis of pretest scores, to ensure that initial measurements on the dependent variable are equally distributed. The first two subjects (assuming two groups) in the list are randomly assigned to the treatment groups, then the next two, and so on, until all subjects have been assigned. The limitations of this method are that it is difficult to match on more than one variable, and there is no control for the quality of the match. For example, if we were matching on age, and the four oldest subjects in our sample were 46, 35, 32, and 19 years of age, the matches would be 46 with 35, and 32 with 19. Depending on how closely age is correlated with the dependent variable, these matches may provide extremely poor control.

Matching is often a difficult process, especially as the number of matching variables increases. This technique also limits interpretation of research findings because the differential effect of the matching variables cannot be analyzed, as it can in the randomized block design. For example, if we match subjects on age and sex, then we cannot determine if the effect of treatment is different across age ranges or across males and females. For most clinical studies, matching is not recommended when other methods of controlling extraneous variables are appropriate and practical.

Using Subjects as Their Own Control

Research designs can be structured to facilitate comparisons between independent groups of subjects, or they may involve comparisons of responses across treatment conditions within a subject. When the levels of the independent variable are assigned to different groups, with an active or attribute variable, the independent variable is considered an **independent factor.*** For example, if we compare the effect of two types of splints for reducing hand deformities in patients with rheumatoid arthritis, each type of splint would be worn by a different set of patients. Therefore, the variable of "splint" is an independent factor with two levels. If we compare the effect of splints between males and females, "gender" would also be an independent factor.

When all levels of the independent variable are experienced by all subjects, the independent variable is considered a **repeated measure** or a **repeated factor.** For instance, if we look at the effect of splinting over time, measuring each subject at 1-week intervals for 3 weeks, the variable of "time" becomes a repeated factor with three levels. If we were interested in functional abilities using each type of splint, we might allow each subject to use both splints and test specific hand tasks with each one to compare their responses. In this case, type of splint would be a repeated factor because both splints would be worn by all subjects. The use of a repeated measure is often described as *using subjects as their own control.*

A **repeated measures design** is one of the most efficient methods for controlling intersubject differences. It ensures the highest possible degree of equivalence across treatment conditions because subjects are perfectly matched with themselves. We can assume that stable individual characteristics such as gender, intelligence, physical characteristics, and age remain constant for each treatment, so that any differences observed among the treatment conditions can be attributed solely to treatment. Although this assumption is not completely valid for all variables (subjects do differ in mood, hunger, fatigue, and so on, from time to time), the variability of subjects from trial to trial will certainly be minimal compared with differences between independent groups of subjects.

Repeated measures analyses are particularly effective when one is interested in how a subject responds under different conditions or over time. For instance, if we wanted to know how isometric strength of elbow extension varied with the elbow at different angles, we could make those comparisons within a subject. With sufficient rest periods, we could determine which position facilitated the greatest force from the elbow extensors. The repeated measures approach is not appropriate in studies where carryover effects are likely. For instance, if we compared two forms of exercise for increasing elbow flexor strength, it would not make sense to expose each subject to both treatments and expect to be able to determine if their effects differed. Surely we can expect strength gains from

---

*The term *independent factor* should not be confused with *independent variable.* An independent variable can be either an "independent factor" or a "repeated factor" depending on how its levels are defined.

one exercise to carry over to the other exercises. Issues related to the design of repeated measures studies are explored further in Chapter 10.

Analysis of Covariance

The last method of controlling for confounding effects does not involve a design strategy, but instead uses a statistical technique to equate groups on extraneous variables. The **analysis of covariance (ANCOVA)** is based on concepts of analysis of variance and regression, which will be described in Chapters 20 and 24. Without going into details of statistical procedure at this time, we describe the conceptual premise for analysis of covariance for a hypothetical study involving a measure of step length in patients wearing two types of lower extremity orthoses.

Suppose we randomly assign 40 subjects to the two treatment groups, thereby assuming that extraneous factors are equally distributed between the groups. When we compare the subjects' step lengths, we find that the average step for those wearing orthosis A is longer than the average step for those wearing orthosis B. We would like to attribute this difference to the differential effects of the orthoses; however, step length is also related to characteristics such as height and leg length. Therefore, if the subjects in group A happen to be taller than those in group B, the observed difference in step length may be a function of height, not orthosis.

The purpose of the analysis of covariance is to statistically eliminate the influence of extraneous factors, so that the effect of the independent variable can be seen more clearly. These identified extraneous variables are called **covariates.** Conceptually, the ANCOVA removes the confounding effect of covariates by making them artificially equivalent across groups, and by estimating what the dependent variable *would have been* under these equivalent conditions. For instance, if the patients wearing orthosis A are taller than those in the other group, the analysis figures out what the step lengths would most likely have been had the heights been equally distributed. The analysis of differences between the two groups will then be based on these *adjusted scores.*

THREATS TO VALIDITY

The goals of experimental research can be summarized by four major questions: (1) Is there a relationship between the independent and dependent variables? (2) Given that a statistical relationship does exist, is there evidence that one causes the other? (3) Given that a cause-and-effect relationship is probable, to what theoretical constructs can the results be generalized? (4) Can the results be generalized to persons, settings, and times that are different from those employed in the experimental situation? These four questions correspond to four types of design validity that form a framework for evaluating experiments: statistical conclusion validity, internal validity, construct validity, and external validity (Table 9.2).[15]

Statistical Conclusion Validity

- *Is there a relationship between the independent and dependent variables?*

Statistical conclusion validity concerns the potential inappropriate use of statistical procedures for analyzing data, leading to invalid conclusions about the relationship

TABLE 9.2.   THREATS TO DESIGN VALIDITY

1. *Statistical conclusion validity:* Refers to the appropriate use of statistical procedures for analyzing data.

   - Low statistical power
   - Violated assumptions of statistical tests
   - Error rate
   - Reliability
   - Variance

2. *Internal validity:* Refers to the potential for confounding factors to interfere with the relationship between the independent and dependent variables.

   - History
   - Maturation
   - Attrition
   - Testing
   - Instrumentation
   - Regression
   - Selection
   - Interactions with selection: maturation, history, instrumentation
   - Ambiguity about the direction of causal influence
   - Diffusion or imitation of treatments
   - Compensatory equalization of treatment
   - Compensatory rivalry or resentful demoralization of respondents

3. *Construct validity of causes and effects:* Refers to the theoretical conceptualization of the independent and dependent variables.

   - Operational definitions of independent and dependent variables
   - Time frame within operational definitions
   - Multiple-treatment interactions
   - Experimental bias
   - Hawthorne effect

4. *External validity:* Refers to the extent to which results of a study can be generalized outside the experimental situation.

   - Interaction of treatment and selection
   - Interaction of treatment and setting
   - Interaction of treatment and history

---

between independent and dependent variables. Some specific threats to statistical conclusion validity are listed here. Because these threats involve concepts of statistical inference that will be covered later in the text, we provide only brief definitions here.

(1) *Low Statistical Power.* The power of a statistical test concerns its ability to reject the null hypothesis, that is, to document a real relationship between independent and dependent variables. Significant effects may be missed because of inadequate sample size or failure to control extraneous sources of variation.

(2) *Violated Assumptions of Statistical Tests.* Most statistical procedures are based on a variety of assumptions about the experimental data and the sample from which they are collected. If these assumptions are not met, statistical outcomes may lead to erroneous inferences.

(3) *Error Rate.* With certain tests, the probability of drawing incorrect conclusions increases as the number of repeated tests increases. Statistical procedures are generally available to control for this threat.

(4) *Reliability and Variance.* Statistical conclusions are threatened by any extraneous factors that increase variability within the data, such as unreliable measurement, failure to standardize the protocol, environmental interferences, or heterogeneity of subjects. These threats contribute to statistical *error variance,* which is a function of all variance in the data that cannot be explained by treatment effects.

Internal Validity

- *Given a statistical relationship between the independent and dependent variables, is there evidence that one causes the other?*

Internal validity helps us determine if the experimental treatment really caused the observed change in the dependent variable, or if other (extraneous) factors may be responsible for that change. Extraneous variables present threats to internal validity because they offer competing explanations for the observed relationship between the independent and dependent variables; that is, they interfere with cause-and-effect inferences. The control mechanisms we have discussed in this chapter are all aimed at securing the internal validity of a study to rule out these competing explanations. True experiments have a high degree of internal validity because of the controlling properties of randomization and control groups.

Cook and Campbell have identified several types of threats to internal validity that can be experienced in clinical studies.[15]

History

History refers to the confounding effect of specific events, other than the experimental treatment, that occurs after the introduction of the independent variable or between the pretest and posttest. For example, if we study the differential effect of two forms of exercise on knee extensor strength, history effects may include some subjects' participation in other athletic activities or other therapies that affect knee extensor strength. If the clinical staff involved in the study is replaced with new personnel during the course of the study, responses may be affected. History can also refer to more global events. For instance, suppose we were interested in studying the effect of educational programs for increasing the use of seat belts by teenagers. If our state passes a law mandating seat belt use during the course of the study, that represents a history effect.

History may not be as serious a concern in studies where data collection is completed within a short period, such as a single session.[16] For example, if range of motion of shoulder flexion is measured, followed by 10 minutes of mobilization exercises, and then immediately remeasured, there is little opportunity for confounding events to influence the dependent variable. Even in this type of situation, however, the effects of conversation, the subject's moving around, or other disturbances in the environment may introduce history effects.

Maturation

A second threat to internal validity concerns processes that occur simply as a function of the passage of time and that are independent of external events. **Maturation effects** may cause subjects to respond differently on a second measurement because they have grown older, stronger, healthier, more experienced, tired, or bored since the first measurement. For example, if we want to examine the effects of therapy on communications disorders following a stroke, we would have to take into account the fact that spontaneous changes often occur without any intervention.

Maturation is a relevant concern in many areas of clinical research, especially in studies where intervals between measurements are long. Those who study children often encounter physical and mental developmental changes, unrelated to therapeutic intervention, that may influence performance. Wound healing, remission of arthritic symptoms, regeneration in neurological injury, and postoperative recovery are all examples of potential maturation effects.

Attrition

Clinical researchers are often faced with the fact that subjects drop out of a study before it is completed. **Attrition,** also called **experimental mortality,** refers to the differential loss of subjects from comparison groups; that is, dropouts occur for specific reasons related to the experimental situation. For example, suppose we studied two programs of breathing exercises for patients with emphysema, and that random assignment resulted in many sicker subjects being assigned to one group. These subjects may find the exercises more difficult, and may be less motivated, than stronger subjects in the other group. If they drop out, this loss can change the original balance of the experimental groups. If the remaining members of this group do not improve as much as the others, the difference may be an artifact of this bias, not a function of treatment effect.

Researchers should try to determine if attrition occurs for random or biased reasons and if a particular group is affected more than others. It is not the loss of subjects per se that is of concern, but rather the need to determine if randomness has been affected. Unfortunately, it is not sufficient to balance groups by taking out some subjects from another group. The researcher cannot assume such choices will re-create the balance of extraneous factors. Many statistical procedures can accommodate for this situation through application of tests for groups with unequal variances. When subject outcomes can be assessed for those who have dropped out, an **intention-to-treat** analysis should be used (see earlier discussion).

Testing

Testing effects concern the potential effect of pretesting or repeated testing on the dependent variable. In other words, the mere act of collecting data changes the response that is being measured. Testing effects can refer to improved performance or increased skill that occurs because of familiarity with measurements. For example, in educational tests, subjects may actually learn information by taking a pretest, thereby changing their responses on a posttest, independent of any instructional intervention. If a coordination test is given before and after therapy, patients may get higher scores on the posttest because they were able to practice the activity during the pretest. Testing effects also refer to situations when the measurement itself changes the dependent variable. For instance, if we take repeated measurements of range of motion, the act of moving the joint through range to evaluate it may actually stretch it enough to increase its range.

Tests that have the potential for changing the response they are measuring are called **reactive measurements.** Reactive effects occur when the testing process stimulates change, rather than acting as a passive record of behavior. For instance, placing a video camera in a room to record patient–therapist interactions may alter the observed responses because the subjects know they are being watched. This type of testing effect can be minimized by practice sessions and warm-up trials, to make subjects more comfortable in the testing environment. Unobtrusive or passive measures should be used whenever possible to avoid reactive effects.[17] Techniques such as watching subjects through a two-way mirror qualify as unobtrusive.

Instrumentation

Instrumentation effects are concerned with the reliability of measurement. Changes that occur in calibration of hardware or shifts in criteria used by human observers can affect the magnitude of the dependent variable, independent of any treatment effect. Mechanical and bioelectronic instruments can threaten validity if linearity and sensitivity are not constant across the full range of responses and over time. Observers can become more experienced and skilled at measurement between a pretest and posttest. This threat to internal validity can be addressed by calibration and documenting test–retest and rater reliability.

Statistical Regression

Statistical regression is also associated with reliability of a test. When measures are not reliable, there is a tendency for extreme scores on the pretest to regress toward the mean on the posttest. This effect occurs even in the absence of intervention. Extremely low scores tend to increase; extremely high scores tend to decrease; and scores that fall around the average tend to stay the same. Statistical regression (also called *regression toward the mean*) is of greatest concern when groups are selected on the basis of extreme scores. For instance, if we wanted to examine the differential effect of a specific exercise on weaker and stronger patients, we might assign subjects to two groups based on their pretest scores. The effect of regression will be to move both groups toward their combined average in posttests. The amount of statistical regression is directly related to the degree of measurement error in the dependent variable. Therefore, this effect is minimized when reliability is strong. Examples of this concept were presented in Chapter 5.

Selection

Important differences may exist between experimental groups prior to data collection on the basis of differential selection. This **selection effect** is obviously controlled when random assignment is used; however, it becomes an issue when intact groups are used or when the independent variable is an attribute variable. Designs that do not allow randomization are considered quasi-experimental, in that differences between groups cannot be balanced out. There may be several reasons that subjects belong to one group over another, and these factors can contribute to differences in their performance. Researchers can exert some degree of control for this effect when specific extraneous variables can be identified that vary between the groups. The strategy of matched pairs or the analysis of covariance may be able to account for initial group differences.

Interactions with Selection

Some of the foregoing threats to internal validity can interact with selection to produce changes in the dependent variable that may look like treatment effects. When subjects are not randomly assigned to groups or when randomization fails, maturation, history, or instrumentation threats may affect the groups differentially.

Selection–maturation effects occur when the experimental groups experience maturational change at different speeds. For instance, if we compare changes in motor learning skills following a course of therapy in 3- and 10-year-olds, we can expect a different rate of developmental change that could confound treatment effects.

Selection–history effects result when experimental groups come from different settings so that the local history of each group influences responses. This is especially important in multicenter studies or when groups are chosen to represent different geographical areas.

Selection–instrumentation interaction occurs when the average scores for the various groups represent different points on the measuring instrument and when the instrument does not register equal intervals across the full range of measurement. For example, a force gauge may be designed to register linear forces between 50 and 100 kg. Average scores for groups that are very strong (near 100 kg) or very weak (near 50 kg) will not be measured as accurately as those for groups whose average falls between 50 and 100 kg. These effects are often called "floor" and "ceiling" effects because the measurement scale is incapable of accurately recording values above or below a certain level.

Ambiguity about the Direction of Causal Influence

When a researcher is interested in establishing a cause-and-effect relationship between two variables, X and Y, it is necessary to determine the direction of that relationship: Did X cause Y, or did Y cause X? This threat will be minimized in experimental studies where manipulation of the independent variable makes the temporal sequencing of action and response obvious.

Diffusion or Imitation of Treatments

Sometimes the independent variable involves some sort of information that is not intended to be equally available to all experimental groups. For instance, we might want to compare the effect of a nutritional education program on patients' diet and cholesterol levels. The experimental group would attend classes and read packets of information related to diet and food content, while a control group is given a neutral experience involving no diet information. If the two groups have an opportunity to communicate, subjects in one group may learn the information intended for the others. This communication will diffuse the treatment effect and make it impossible to distinguish the behaviors of the two groups.

Compensatory Equalization of Treatments

When an experimental treatment is considered a desirable service or condition, those who work with and care for the subjects may try to even out experiences by providing compensatory services to the control group. For example, suppose we wanted to study the effect of continuous passive motion on knee range of motion following total knee replacement. Therapists who work with the control patients might work extra hard on range of motion exercises or joint mobilization to compensate for their patients' missing out on the "better" treatment. The effect of such compensatory attention will be to make the groups look more alike, and obscure the experimental effects of treatment.

Compensatory Rivalry and Resentful Demoralization of Respondents Receiving Less Desirable Treatments

These two effects represent opposite reactions to the same situation. When one group's assigned treatment is perceived as more desirable than the other's, subjects receiving the less desirable treatment may try to compensate by working extra hard to achieve similar results. This is similar to compensatory equalization, described earlier, except that here the subject is responsible for equalizing effects. As an example, this effect may have been operating in the well-known Multiple Risk Factor Intervention Trial (MRFIT), in which two groups were compared for cardiac mortality.[18] The subjects were randomized to receive either an elaborate intervention of exercise and diet, or a nonintervention control group. In the end the results were unfortunate for the researchers because the control group had a lower mortality rate than the experimental group. Because the nature of the interventions made blinding impractical, control subjects were aware of the interventions, and may have attempted to change their diet and exercise habits.[13]

In an alternative reaction to this type of situation, subjects receiving less desirable treatments may be demoralized or resentful. Their reaction may be to respond at lower levels of performance. The effect of such responses will be to artificially inflate group differences, which may then be incorrectly attributed to a significantly greater treatment effect.

One way to control this effect is to be sure that there is no interaction among subjects. Sometimes this is difficult, depending on the experimental environment. For instance, if a study were designed to compare the effect of early mother-newborn contact and usual care on mother-child bonding, it might be difficult to prevent interaction if those assigned to different groups were on the same hospital floor or in the same room. Their interaction would tend to contaminate the treatment effect.[19] When this effect is a potential threat, the researcher may choose to randomly assign treatments to different floors, rather than to individuals. The researcher would have to weigh the impact of this approach, as this en bloc randomization will control for the compensatory interactions, but may be less desirable in terms of truly balancing individual characteristics.[13]

Ruling Out Threats to Internal Validity

Threats to internal validity are present in every study. As this list suggests, the task of ruling out alternative explanations for observed changes and documenting the effect of the independent variable is not a small one. It can, however, be addressed as a logical process, one that requires insight, subject matter expertise, and the capacity for self-criticism.[20] Many threats, such as history, maturation, selection, statistical regression, testing, instrumentation, and selection interactions, can be ruled out by the use of random assignment and control groups. These issues are canceled out when both groups are equivalent at the start and are equally likely to be affected by events occurring during the course of the study. Random assignment cannot rule out the effects of attrition, imitating treatments, or compensatory reactions. Blinding subjects and investigators, however, will control many of these effects. The researcher must examine all possible threats and eliminate them or recognize their influence when they are inevitable. When they cannot be eliminated, it may not be possible to demonstrate causal relationships.

Construct Validity of Causes and Effects

- *Given that a cause-and-effect relationship is probable, to what theoretical constructs can the results be generalized?*

Threats to validity can also be characterized in terms of the construct validity of the independent and dependent variables. As discussed, constructs are abstract behaviors or events that cannot be directly observed, but that can be inferred from other relevant observable variables (see Chapters 2 and 6). **Construct validity of causes and effects** concerns the theoretical conceptualizations of the intervention and response variables and whether these have been developed sufficiently to allow reasonable interpretation and generalization of their relationship.[15]

Most of the treatments and responses that are used in clinical research are based on constructs that must be conceptualized by the researcher in terms of their operational definitions. The levels of the independent variable and measurement methods for the dependent variable will delimit their relationship. If we study "exercises to improve gait," we must conceptualize these variables in terms of specific activities and measurement tools. Outcomes will be interpreted differently, for example, if we study isometric knee exercises and measure gait speed, than if we study walking as an exercise and measure distance walked. Construct validity concerns the researcher's goals and how well experimental results can be generalized within the desired clinical context. Studies that are internally sound may have no practical application beyond the experimental situation if the researcher has not taken the time to explore conceptual questions and the theoretical basis for asking them.

Threats to construct validity are related to how variables are operationally defined within a study and to potential biases introduced into a study by subjects or experimenters.†

---

† These threats were originally defined by Campbell and Stanley under the category of *external validity.*[17] Cook and Campbell have subdivided that original categorization into construct validity and external validity.[16]

Operational Definitions

Cook and Campbell suggest that full explication of most constructs requires use of multiple treatment methods and multiple measurement methods.[15] When studies incorporate only one form of measurement or examine only one form of treatment, the results will apply only to a limited aspect of the construct. For example, the construct of pain is truly multidimensional. Therefore, if a study addresses only one form of treatment or one form of measurement, generalization of the results of that study is limited. This limitation is increased when some levels of the independent variable interact differently with various types of dependent variables. For instance, if we treat pain using relaxation exercises or transcutaneous electrical nerve stimulation (TENS), measures of success may vary depending on whether we assess pain by using a visual analogue scale (VAS), by measuring range of motion of involved joints, or by observing the efficiency of functional tasks. The VAS reflects the patient's subjective and relative feelings of pain intensity, the ROM test reflects physiological concomitants of pain, and functional evaluation is influenced by personality, attitude, motivation, and lifestyle. Therefore, each of these assessments measures a different aspect of pain that reflects components of the total construct.

Generalization is also limited by the time frame within operational definitions. For instance, if we study the effect of TENS over a 2-week period, we cannot generalize outcomes to events that might occur over a longer period of treatment. If treatment shows no effect within this time frame, we would be inaccurate to conclude that TENS does not work. The element of time cannot be ignored in defining the construct of treatment, and testing may need to be done at various intervals to determine the range necessary to achieve maximal effectiveness.

Construct validity is also affected when a study involves the administration of multiple treatments or multiple measurements. Generalization is limited by the possibility of **multiple-treatment interaction,** creating carryover or combined effects. **Order effects** can result when treatments or measurements are consistently given in the same order, creating possible influences on subsequent responses. The researcher cannot generalize these findings to the situation where only a single treatment or measurement is given; that is, the effect of one response cannot be interpreted out of the context of several responses.

Experimental Bias

A second aspect of construct validity concerns biases that are introduced into a study by expectations of either the subjects or the experimenter. Subjects often try their best to fulfill the researcher's expectations or to present themselves in the best way possible, so that responses are no longer representative of natural behavior. This effect was documented in classical studies performed from 1924 to 1927 at the Hawthorne Works, a division of the Western Electric Company in Chicago.[21] Researchers were interested in studying how various levels of illumination affected workers' output. What they found was that no matter what they did, lowering lights or raising lights, the workers increased production. This phenomenon became known as the **Hawthorne effect,** which is the tendency of persons who are singled out for special attention to perform better merely because of the expectations created by the situation. For example, this effect was probably present in a study involving first-year medical residents, to compare different strategies for reducing the number of radiologic tests ordered.[22] Everyone was aware of the expected outcomes of the study, and all residents showed reductions from baseline, including those in the control group. When the researcher cannot control this effect, it should be acknowledged.

Experimenters may also have certain expectancies that can influence how subjects respond. They may react more positively to subjects in the experimental group or give less attention to those in the control group, because of an emotional or intellectual investment in their hypothesis. Rosenthal described several types of **experimenter effects** in terms of the experimenter's *active behavior* and interaction with the subject, such as verbal cues and smiling, and *passive behaviors*, such as those related to appearance.[23] This threat to construct validity can be avoided by employing testers who are blinded to subject assignment and the research hypothesis.

External Validity

- *Can the results be generalized to persons, settings, and times that are different from those employed in the experimental situation?*

External validity refers to the extent to which the results of a study can be generalized beyond the internal specifications of the study sample. Whereas internal validity is concerned specifically with the relationship between the independent and dependent variables within a specific set of circumstances, external validity is concerned with the usefulness of that information outside the experimental situation. Threats to external validity involve the interaction of treatment with the specific type of subjects tested, the specific setting in which the experiment is carried out, or the time in history when the study is done.

Interaction of Treatment and Selection

One major goal of clinical research is to apply results to a target population, that is, to individuals who are not experimental subjects but who are represented by them. If subjects are sampled according to specific characteristics, those characteristics define the target population. For instance, subjects may be restricted to a limited age range, one sex, a specific diagnosis, or a defined level of function. When samples are confined to certain types of subjects, it is not reasonable to generalize results to those who do not have these characteristics.

External validity is threatened when documented cause-and-effect relationships do not apply across subdivisions of the target population, that is, when specific interventions result in differential treatment effects, depending on the subject's characteristics. For instance, suppose we want to demonstrate the benefits of a particular exercise program for improving function following a stroke. The effect of the program may not be generalizable across groups that exhibit various levels of spasticity, those affected on the left or right, patients of different ages, or those with speech disorders. Studies are especially vulnerable to this threat when volunteers are used as subjects. Those who choose to volunteer may do so because of certain personal characteristics that ultimately bias the sample. When studies demonstrate conflicting results, it is often because of the differences within the accessible populations.

A related effect can occur if subjects do not comply with the experimental protocol. A study that is internally valid may still be compromised in relation to external validity under these circumstances. Researchers should examine **adherence** as they interpret findings, to determine if results are realistic and have clinical applicability.[24] From a sampling perspective, some investigators have begun to screen potential subjects prior to randomizing them to groups, to eliminate those who are not adherent. For example, the Physicians' Health Study, which investigated the effect of aspirin and beta carotene in the prevention of ischemic heart disease, used an 18-week "run-in period" and eliminated 33% of the subjects from the final study.[25] This practice may help to build a compliant study sample, but it may also dilute external validity of the findings.[13] It is the researcher's responsibility to evaluate its potential effect in demonstrating the applicability of the findings.[26]

Interaction of Treatment and Setting

If we demonstrate a causal relationship between an exercise program and functional improvement using patients in a rehabilitation hospital, can we generalize these findings to a nursing home or to home care? This question can only be answered by replicating effects in different settings.

Interaction of Treatment and History

This threat to external validity concerns the ability to generalize results to different periods of time in the past or future. For instance, if we look at the results of nutritional studies for reducing cholesterol in the diet, results may be quite different today from results obtained 20 years ago, when knowledge about the effect of diet and exercise on cardiovascular fitness was less developed, and when society and the media were less involved in promoting fitness and health. This type of generalization is supported when results are replicated in future studies and when previous research corroborates the established causal relationship.

COMMENTARY

The Realities of Clinical Research

Because of the many potential threats to validity, researchers must examine priorities among them. Not all threats to validity are of equal concern in every study. When steps are taken to increase one type of validity, it is likely that another type will be decreased. The specific research situation will dictate how specific extraneous factors impact on a given design. For instance, if we attempt to control for extraneous factors by using a homogeneous sample, we will improve internal validity, but at the expense of external validity. If we increase statistical conclusion validity by limiting variability in our data, the sample will be less representative of a general population. This will probably reduce external and construct validity. Similarly, if we work toward increasing construct validity by operationalizing variables in multiple dimensions, we run the risk of decreasing reliability with an increasing number of measurements. When theoretical issues are of special importance, construct validity should be of great concern. When cause-and-effect relationships are sought, internal validity is of primary importance. Over time, as studies are replicated and modified, all types of validity will eventually be addressed in a particular area of investigation.

After describing all the above threats to experimental validity, the clinical researcher might wonder how it is ever possible to design a completely valid study. In fact, there is no such thing in clinical research. Every study contains some shortcomings. Clinical researchers operate in an environment that demands consideration of ethical and practical issues, as well as the unpredictable and often immeasurable factors of human nature, error, emotion, and thought. The clinical researcher can control neither the environment nor the consistency of a subject's interaction with that environment to the same extent that the laboratory researcher can control an animal's genetic makeup, diet, or physiological characteristics. It is virtually impossible to conduct a clinical experiment so that every facet of behavior, environment, and personal interaction is exactly the same for every subject.

Does this mean that we cannot create experimental situations with sufficient control to be able to make valid judgments about human responses? Not at all. We can still conduct experiments and draw meaningful conclusions from them by adhering to the elements of experimental control with as much rigor as possible, accounting for variations in the experimental situation with every reasonable effort, and ultimately recognizing those factors over which we have no control. Limitations of a study should be discussed in a research report so that readers have a complete understanding of the circumstances in which results were obtained. To have confidence in results, however, the researcher must be able to justify the experimental conditions as a fair test of the experimental treatment. When the researcher can anticipate that important extraneous factors cannot be controlled, to the point that they will have a serious impact on the interpretation of outcomes, it is advisable to consider alternatives to experimental research, such as descriptive or correlational approaches.

KEY TERMS

experiment
cause and effect
extraneous variables
confounding
control
manipulation of variables
active variable
attribute variable
ex post facto research
random assignment
on-protocol analysis
intention to treat
control group
limitations
double-blind study
single-blind study
homogeneous sample

blocking variable
randomized block design
matching
matched pairs design
independent factor
repeated measure
    (repeated factor)
repeated measure design
analysis of covariance
    (ANCOVA)
covariate
statistical conclusion
    validity
internal validity
history effect
maturation effect

attrition (experimental
    mortality)
adherence
testing effect
reactive measurement
instrumentation effect
statistical regression
differential selection
construct validity of causes
    and effects
multiple-treatment
    interaction
order effect
Hawthorne effect
experimenter effect
external validity

▀▀▀ REFERENCES ░░░░░░░░░░░░░

1. Lamas GA, Orav EJ, Stambler BS, et al. Quality of life and clinical outcomes in elderly patients treated with ventricular pacing as compared with dual-chamber pacing. *New Engl J Med* 1998;338:1097–1104.
2. Ramin SM, Gambling DR, Lucas MJ, Sharma SK, Sidawi JE, Leveno KJ. Randomized trial of epidural versus intravenous analgesia during labor. *Obstet Gynecol* 1995;86:783–9.
3. Newell DJ. Intention-to-treat analysis: implications for quantitative and qualitative research. *Int J Epidemiol* 1992;21:837–41.
4. Morales AJ. Study design for the evaluation of treatment. *Semin Reprod Endocrinol* 1996;14:111–8.
5. Motulsky H. *Intuitive Biostatistics.* New York: Oxford University Press, 1995.
6. Peduzzi P, Detre K, Wittes J, Holford T. Intent-to-treat analysis and the problem of crossovers. An example from the Veterans Administration coronary bypass surgery study. *J Thorac Cardiovasc Surg* 1991;101:481–7.
7. Little R, Yau L. Intent-to-treat analysis for longitudinal studies with drop-outs. *Biometrics* 1996;52:1324–33.
8. Hogan JW, Laird NM. Intention-to-treat analyses for incomplete repeated measures data. *Biometrics* 1996;52:1002–17.
9. Lagakos SW, Lim LL, Robins JM. Adjusting for early treatment termination in comparative clinical trials. *Stat Med* 1990;9:1417–24; discussion 1433–7.
10. Mulrow CD, Gerety MB, Kanten D, et al. A randomized trial of physical rehabilitation for very frail nursing home residents. *JAMA* 1994;271:519–24.
11. Fetter MS, Feetham SL, D'Apolito K, et al. Randomized clinical trials: issues for researchers. *Nurs Res* 1989;38:117–20.
12. Bellamy N, Sothern RB, Campbell J, Buchanan WW. Circadian rhythm in pain, stiffness, and manual dexterity in rheumatoid arthritis: relation between discomfort and disability. *Ann Rheum Dis* 1991;50:243–8.
13. Kramer MS, Shapiro SH. Scientific challenges in the application of randomized trials. *JAMA* 1984;252:2739–45.
14. Silverman WA. *Human Experimentation: A Guided Step into the Unknown.* New York: Oxford University Press, 1985.
15. Cook TD, Campbell DT. *Quasi-experimentation: Design and Analysis Issues for Field Settings.* Boston: Houghton Mifflin, 1979.
16. Campbell DT, Stanley JC. *Experimental and Quasi-experimental Designs for Research.* Chicago: Rand McNally, 1963.
17. Webb EJ, Campbell DT, Schwartz RD, Sechrest L. *Unobtrusive Measures.* Skokie, IL: Rand McNally, 1966.
18. Multiple Risk Factor Intervention Trial Research Group. Multiple risk factor intervention trial. Risk factor changes and mortality results. *JAMA* 1982;248:1465–77.
19. Thomson ME, Kramer MS. Methodologic standards for controlled clinical trials of early contact and maternal-infant behavior. *Pediatrics* 1984;73:294–300.
20. Kirk RE. *Experimental Design: Procedures for the Behavioral Sciences.* 2nd ed. Belmont, CA: Brooks/Cole, 1982.
21. Roethlisberger J, Dickson WJ. *Management and the Worker.* Cambridge, MA: Harvard University Press, 1966.
22. Martin AR, Wolf MA, Thibodeau LA, Dzau V, Braunwald E. A trial of two strategies to modify the test-ordering behavior of medical residents. *N Engl J Med* 1980;303:1330–6.
23. Rosenthal R. *Experimenter Effects in Behavioral Research.* New York: Appleton-Century-Crofts, 1966.

24. Guyatt GH, Sackett DL, Cook DJ. Users' guides to the medical literature. II. How to use an article about therapy or prevention. B. What were the results and will they help me in caring for my patients? Evidence-Based Medicine Working Group. *JAMA* 1994;271:59–63.

25. Steering Committee of the Physician's Health Study Research Group. Final report on the aspirin component of the ongoing Physicians' Health Study. *N Engl J Med* 1989;321:129–35.

26. Pablos-Mendez A, Barr RG, Shea S. Run-in periods in randomized trials: implications for the application of results in clinical practice. *JAMA* 1998;279:222–5.

C H A P T E R

10

Experimental Design

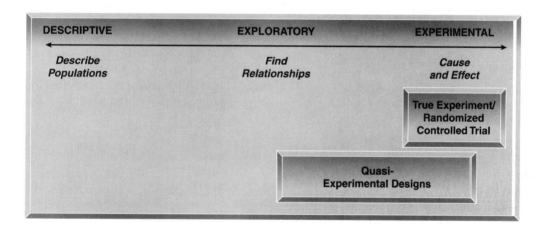

The purpose of an experimental design is to provide a structure for evaluating the cause-and-effect relationship between a set of independent and dependent variables. Within the design, the researcher manipulates the levels of the independent variable and incorporates elements of control, so that the evidence supporting a causal relationship can be interpreted with confidence.

Experimental designs can be described according to several types of design characteristics. A basic distinction among them is the degree of experimental control.[1, 2] In a **true experimental design,** subjects are randomly assigned to at least two comparison groups. A true experiment is theoretically able to exert control over most threats to internal validity, providing the strongest evidence for causal relationships. A **quasi-experimental design** does not meet the requirements of a true experiment, lacking randomization or comparison groups, or both. Even though quasi-experimental designs cannot rule out threats to internal validity with the same confidence as experimental designs, many such designs are appropriate when stronger designs are not feasible. Quasi-experimental designs represent an important contribution to clinical research, because they accommodate for the limitations of natural settings, where scheduling treatment conditions and random assignment are often difficult, impractical, or unethical.[3, 4]

True experimental designs may be differentiated according to how subjects are assigned to groups. In **completely randomized designs,** also called *between-subjects designs*, subjects are assigned to independent groups using a randomization procedure. In a **randomized block design** subjects are first classified according to an attribute variable (a blocking variable) and then randomized to treatment groups. A design in which subjects act as their own control is called a *within-subjects design* or a **repeated measures design.**

Designs can also be described according to the number of independent variables, or *factors,* within the design. *Single-factor designs* have one independent variable with any number of levels. *Multifactor designs* contain two or more independent variables.

Although experimental designs can take on a wide variety of configurations, the important principles can be illustrated using a few basic structures. The purpose of this chapter is to present these basic designs and to illustrate the types of research situations for which they are most appropriate. For each design, we discuss strengths and weaknesses in terms of experimental control and internal and external validity. In addition, we include a short statement suggesting general statistical procedures for analysis. These suggestions do not present all statistical options for a particular design, but they do represent the more commonly used techniques. This information demonstrates the intrinsic relationship between analysis and design, and should serve as a focus for future discussions.

SELECTING A DESIGN

Once a research question is formulated, the researcher must decide on the most effective design for answering it. Although experimental designs represent the highest standard in scientific inquiry, they are not necessarily the best choice in every situation. When the independent variable cannot be manipulated by the experimenter, or when important extraneous factors cannot be controlled, a descriptive or correlational design may be more useful.

When an experimental design is deemed appropriate, the choice of a specific design will depend on the answers to six critical questions about how the study is conceptualized:

1. How many independent variables are being tested?
2. How many levels does each independent variable have, and are these levels experimental or control conditions?
3. How many groups of subjects are being tested?
4. How will subjects be selected, and how will they be assigned to groups?
5. How often will observations of responses be made?
6. What is the temporal sequence of interventions and measurements?

When each of these issues is considered, the range of potential designs will usually be narrowed to one or two appropriate choices. As specific designs are presented, these questions will be addressed within the context of specific research questions.

DESIGN NOTATION

To facilitate explanations of the following designs, we present several diagrammatic representations. For single-factor designs, we have adopted the notation introduced by Campbell and Stanley.[1] An X is used to represent the experimental intervention, or levels of the independent variable. When more than one level of intervention is applied, subscripts are attached, such as X_1 and X_2. A control condition is usually represented by the absence of an X. An O is used to represent an observation or measurement of the dependent variable. Subscripts for observations identify the order of measurements. In these diagrams, rows represent independent groups. When an **R** appears to the left of the design, it indicates that all subjects have been randomly assigned to groups. A dotted line separating rows indicates that the groups have not been randomly assigned.

For multifactor designs, a matrix is used to show the relationship among groups. Uppercase letters, typically A, B, and C, are used to label the independent variables and their levels. For instance, with two independent variables, A and B, we can designate three levels for the first one (A_1, A_2, and A_3) and two levels for the second (B_1, B_2). The application of this notation will become clearer as specific designs are illustrated.

TRUE EXPERIMENTAL DESIGNS

Single-Factor Designs for Independent Groups

A single-factor design, also called a **one-way design,** is used to structure the investigation of one independent variable. The study may include one or more dependent variables.

Design 1: Pretest–Posttest Control Group Design

The **pretest–posttest control group design** is the basic structure of an experiment. It is used to compare two or more groups that are formed by random assignment. One group receives the experimental variable and the other acts as a control. Both groups are tested prior to and following treatment. The groups differ solely on the basis of what occurs between measurements. Therefore, changes from pretest to posttest that appear in the experimental group but not the control group can be reasonably attributed to the treatment. This design is considered the scientific standard in clinical research for establishing a cause-and-effect relationship.[5] The term **randomized controlled trial (RCT)** is often applied to this design.

The pretest–posttest control group design can be configured in several ways. Design 1a illustrates the simplest configuration of the pretest–posttest control group design, with one experimental group and one control group.

Researchers conducted a randomized controlled trial to study the effect of progressive resistance exercises in depressed elders.[6] They studied 35 volunteers who suffered from depression. Subjects were randomly assigned to an exercise group, which met three times per week for 10 weeks, or a control group which met two times per week for an interactive health education program over the same period. The

outcome variables were level of depression, function, and quality of life, using standardized instruments. Pretest and posttest measures were taken for both groups and differences were compared.

Measurements for the control group are taken within intervals that match those of the experimental group. The independent variable has two levels, in this case exercise intervention and control. The absence of experimental intervention in the control group is considered a level of the independent variable. To control for the possibility of social interaction effects during exercise, the control group was given a placebo condition, rather than being told to do nothing.

The pretest–posttest design can also be used when the comparison group receives a second form of the intervention. The *two-group pretest–posttest design* (Design 1b) incorporates two experimental groups formed by random assignment.

Standard clinical practice permits the use of either single-chamber ventricular pacemakers or dual-chamber pacemakers for most patients who require cardiac pacing. Ventricular pacemakers are less expensive, but dual-chamber pacemakers are believed to be more physiologic. Researchers were interested in determining if either type of pacemaker resulted in a superior clinical outcome.[7] They randomly assigned 407 patients to receive either a ventricular or dual-chamber pacemaker. Health-related quality of life was measured before and after a 30-month trial.

Researchers use this approach when a control condition is not feasible or ethical, often comparing a "new" treatment with an "old" standard or alternative treatment. Even though there is no traditional control group, this design provides experimental control because we can establish initial equivalence between groups formed by random assignment. In this example, the ventricular pacing group acts as a control for the dual-chamber group and vice versa. If one group improves more than the other, we can attribute that difference to the fact that one treatment was more effective. This design is appropriate when the research question specifically addresses interest in a difference between two treatments, but it does not allow the researcher to show that treatment works better than no intervention.

The *multigroup pretest–posttest control group design* (Design 1c) allows researchers to compare several treatment and control conditions.

Researchers wanted to evaluate the effectiveness of preventive occupational therapy services specifically tailored for independent-living older adults.[8] They studied 361 volunteers. Subjects were randomized to one of three groups: an occupational therapy group, a generalized social activity group, or a nontreatment control group. Primary outcome measures were functional status, life satisfaction, depression, and overall health status, using standardized instruments. Outcomes were assessed at baseline and following a 9-month treatment period.

In this example, the social activity group also acted as a control, accounting for the effect of social interaction during treatment. In this way, the effect of therapy could be interpreted without bias.

As these examples illustrate, the pretest–posttest control group design can be expanded to accommodate any number of levels of one independent variable, with or without a traditional control group. This design is strong in internal validity. Pretest scores provide a basis for establishing initial equivalence of groups, strengthening the evidence for causal factors. Selection bias is controlled because subjects are randomly assigned to groups. History, maturation, testing, and instrumentation effects should affect all groups equally in both the pretest and posttest. The only threat to internal validity that is not controlled by this design is attrition.

The primary threat to external validity in the pretest–posttest control group design is the potential interaction of treatment and testing. Because subjects are given a pretest, there may be reactive effects, which would not be present in situations when a pretest is not given.

Analysis of Design 1.   Pretest–posttest designs are often analyzed using change scores, which represent the difference between the posttest and pretest.* With interval-ratio data, difference scores are usually compared using an unpaired *t*-test (with two groups) or a one-way analysis of variance (with three or more groups). With ordinal data, the Mann-Whitney *U*-test can be used to compare two groups, and the Kruskal-Wallis analysis of variance by ranks is used to compare three or more groups. The analysis of covariance can be used to compare posttest scores, using the pretest score as the covariate. The design can also be analyzed as a two-factor design, using a two-way analysis of variance with one repeated factor, with treatment as one independent variable and time (pretest and posttest) as the second (repeated) factor. Discriminant analysis can also be used to distinguish between groups with multiple outcome measures.

Design 2: Posttest-Only Design

The **posttest-only design** (Design 2) is identical to the pretest–posttest design, with the obvious exception that a pretest is not administered to either group.

A study was designed to test the hypothesis that high-risk patients undergoing elective hip and knee arthroplasty would incur less total cost and shorter length of stay if inpatient rehabilitation began on postoperative day 3 rather than day 7.[9] Eighty-six patients who were older than 70 years were randomly assigned to begin rehabilitation on day 3 or day 7. The main outcome measures were total length of stay and cost from orthopedic and rehabilitation admissions.

In this study of hospital cost and length of stay, the dependent variables can only be assessed following the treatment condition. This design is a true experimental design, which like the pretest–posttest design, can be expanded to include multiple levels of the independent variable, with or without a control group.

Because this design involves randomization and comparison groups, its internal validity is strong, even without a pretest; that is, we can assume groups are equivalent prior to treatment because they have been randomly assigned to groups. Because there is no pretest score to document the results of randomization, this design is most successful when

---

*See discussion about the reliability of change scores in Chapter 6.

the number of subjects is large, so that the probability of truly balancing interpersonal characteristics is increased.

The posttest-only design can also be used when a pretest is either impractical or potentially reactive. For instance, to study the attitudes of health care personnel toward patients with AIDS, we might use a survey instrument that asks questions about attitudes and experience with this population. By using this instrument as a pretest, subjects might be sensitized in a way that would influence their scores on a subsequent posttest. The posttest-only design avoids this form of bias, increasing the external validity of the study.

Analysis of Design 2.   With two groups, an unpaired *t*-test is used with interval-ratio data, and a Mann-Whitney *U*-test with ordinal data. With more than two groups, a one-way analysis of variance or the Kruskal-Wallis analysis of variance by ranks should be used to compare posttest scores. An analysis of covariance can be used when covariate data on relevant extraneous variables are available. Regression or discriminant analysis procedures can also be applied.

Multifactor Designs for Independent Groups

The designs presented thus far have involved the testing of one independent variable, with two or more levels. Although easy to develop, these single-factor designs tend to impose an artificial simplicity on most clinical and behavioral phenomena; that is, they do not account for simultaneous and often complex interactions of several variables within clinical situations. Interactions are generally important for developing a theoretical understanding of behavior and for establishing the construct validity of clinical variables. Interactions may reflect the combined influence of several treatments or the effect of several attribute variables on the success of a particular treatment.

Design 3: Factorial Design

A **factorial design** incorporates two or more independent variables, with independent groups of subjects randomly assigned to various combinations of levels of the two variables. Although such designs can theoretically be expanded to include any number of variables, clinical studies usually involve two or three at most. As the number of independent variables increases, so does the number of experimental groups, creating the need for larger and larger samples, which are typically impractical in clinical situations.

Factorial designs are described according to their dimensions or number of factors, so that a *two-way* or two-factor design has two independent variables, a *three-way* or three-factor design has three independent variables, and so on. These designs can also be described by the number of levels within each factor, so that a 3×3 design includes two variables, each with three levels, and a $2 \times 3 \times 4$ design includes three variables, with two, three, and four levels, respectively.

A factorial design is diagrammed using a matrix notation that indicates how groups are formed relative to levels of each independent variable. The number of groups is the product of the digits that define the design. For example, $3 \times 3 = 9$ groups; $2 \times 3 \times 4 = 24$ groups. Each cell of the matrix represents a unique combination of levels. In this type of diagram there is no indication if measurements within a cell include pretest–posttest scores or posttest scores only. This detail is generally described in words.

Two-Way Factorial Design. A *two-way factorial design* (Design 3a) incorporates two independent variables.

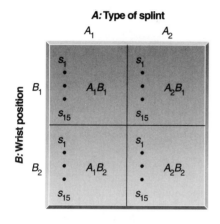

Design 3a

Researchers were interested in studying the effect of dorsal and volar resting hand splints for reducing abnormal tone in patients with neurologic disability. They also wanted to examine the difference in outcome if the splints were applied in a flexed or extended wrist position. Using a 2 × 2 factorial design, 60 patients were randomly assigned to one of four groups, receiving a combination of dorsal or volar splint in a flexed or extended position. The degree of hypertonus was measured before and after a 3-month intervention period.

In this example, the two independent variables are type of splint and wrist position, each with two levels (2 × 2). One group (A_1B_1) will receive the dorsal splint in the flexed position. A second group (A_2B_1) will receive the volar splint in the flexed position. The third group (A_1B_2) will receive the dorsal splint in the extended position, and the fourth group (A_2B_2) will receive the volar splint in the extended position. The two independent variables are *completely crossed* in this design, which means that every level of one factor is represented at every level of the other factor. Each of the four groups represents a unique combination of the levels of these variables, as shown in the individual cells of the diagram. Using random assignment with a sample of 60 patients, we assign 15 subjects to each group.

This design allows us to ask three questions of the data: (1) Is there a differential effect of wearing dorsal versus volar hand splints? (2) Is there a differential effect of positioning the wrist in flexion or extension? (3) What is the interaction between type of splint and wrist position? The answers to the first two questions are obtained by examining the **main effect** of each independent variable, with scores collapsed across the second independent variable, as shown in Figure 10.1. This means that we can look at the overall effect of type of splint without taking into account any differential effect of wrist position. Therefore, with 15 subjects per cell, we would have 30 subjects representing each type of splint. The main effect of wrist position is analyzed without differentiating type of splint. Each main effect is essentially a single-factor experiment. The third question addresses the **interaction effect** between both independent variables. This question represents the essential difference between single-factor and multifactor experiments. Interaction occurs when the effect of one variable varies at different levels of the second variable. For example, we might find that the dorsal splint is more effective, but only with the wrist in extension.

This example illustrates the major advantage of the factorial approach, which is that it gives the researcher important information that could not be obtained with any one

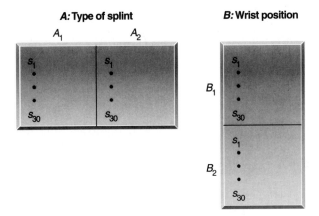

FIGURE 10.1   Main effects for a two-way factorial design (Design 3a).

single-factor experiment. The ability to examine interactions greatly enhances the generalizability of results.

Three-Way Factorial Design.   Factorial designs can be extended to include more than two independent variables. In a *three-way factorial design* (Design 3b), the relationship among variables can be conceptualized in a three-dimensional format. We can also think of it as a two-way design crossed on a third factor.

Design 3b

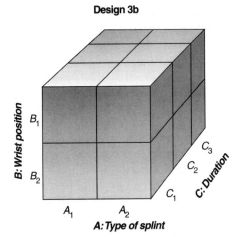

We can expand the splint study to include a third variable, duration of splint use. We could then evaluate the simultaneous effect of splint, wrist position, and use. We assign subjects to wear the splint for 3 hours, 5 hours, or 7 hours daily. Now using a 2 × 2 × 3 randomized factorial design, subjects are randomly assigned to 1 of 12 independent groups.

A three-way design allows several types of comparisons. First, we can examine the main effect for each of the three independent variables, collapsing data across the other two. We can examine the difference between the two splints, regardless of the effect of wrist position or daily use. We can test the difference between the two wrist positions, regardless of type of splint worn or daily use. We can also evaluate the effect of duration of use, regardless of type of splint or wrist position. Each of the three main effects essentially represents a single-factor study for that variable.

Then we can examine three *double interactions:* splint × position, splint × daily use, and position × daily use. For example, the interaction between splint and position is obtained by collapsing data across the three levels of daily use. Each double interaction represents a two-way design. Finally, we can examine the *triple interaction* of splint, position, and daily use. This interaction involves analyzing the differences among all 12 cells.

Many clinical questions have the potential for involving more than one independent variable, because response variables can be influenced by a multitude of factors. In this respect, the compelling advantage of multidimensional factorial designs is their closer approximation to the "real world." As more variables are added to the design, we can begin to understand responses, increasing construct validity of our arguments. The major disadvantages, however, are that the sample must be extremely large to create individual groups of sufficient size and that data analysis can become cumbersome.

Analysis of Design 3.   A two-way or three-way analysis of variance is most commonly used to examine the main effects and interaction effects of a factorial design.

Design 4: Randomized Block Design

When a researcher is concerned that an extraneous factor might influence differences between groups, one way to control for this effect is to build the variable into the design as an independent variable. The **randomized block design** (Design 4) is used when an attribute variable, or *blocking variable,* is crossed with an active independent variable; that is, homogeneous *blocks* of subjects are randomly assigned to levels of a manipulated treatment variable. In the following example, we have a 3 × 4 randomized block design, with a total of 12 groups.

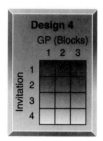

Health researchers were interested in studying methods for improving attendance for screening programs for cervical and breast cancer.[10] They identified over 16,000 eligible women, listed in the rosters of general practitioners (GP), who had indicated their interest in such a program. The women were first grouped according to their GP, and within each GP group they were randomly assigned to four intervention groups, each providing a different form of invitation to the program.

In studying attendance at screening programs, the researchers might be concerned that women's attendance will differ, depending on who they see as their primary care physician. Patients may go to a particular doctor for many reasons that could influence the outcome, or certain physicians may encourage patients more than other physicians. Therefore, we can account for this potential effect by looking at differences across physicians as well as across intervention groups. We can then assume that compliance will not be confounded by variability in physician.

We can think of the randomized block design as three single-factor randomized experiments, with each block representing a different subpopulation. When the design is analyzed, we will be able to examine possible interaction effects between the treatment conditions and blocks. When this interaction is significant, we will know that the effects of treatment do not generalize across the block classifications, in this case across physician groups. If the interactions are not significant, we have achieved a certain degree of generalizability of the results.

For the randomized block design to be used effectively, the blocking factor must be related to the dependent variable; that is, it must be a factor that affects how subjects will respond to treatment. If the blocking factor is not related to the response, then using it as an independent variable provides no additional control to the design, and actually provides less control than had random assignment been used. Therefore, the randomized block design should be used only in those situations when a specific relevant attribute variable has been identified. Randomized block designs can involve more than two independent variables, with one or more blocking variables.

Generalization of results from a randomized block design will be limited by the definition of blocks. For example, classification variables, such as gender or diagnosis, are often used as blocking variables. The number of levels of these variables will be inherent. When the blocking factor is a quantitative variable, however, such as age, two important decisions must be made. First, the researcher must determine the range of ages to be used. Second, the number and distribution of blocks must be determined. Generally, it is best to use equally spaced levels with a relatively equal number of subjects at each level. If the researcher is interested in trends within a quantitative variable, three or more levels should be used to describe a pattern of change. For instance, if four age groups are delineated, we would have a clearer picture of the trends that occur with age than if only two levels were used.

Analysis of Design 4.   Data from a randomized block design can be analyzed using a two-way analysis of variance or multiple regression analysis.

Design 5: Nested Design

To this point, we have described multifactor designs in terms of two or three independent variables that are completely crossed; that is, all levels of variable A have occurred within all levels of variable B. This approach does not fit all multifactor analyses, however, when attribute variables are involved. Sometimes attribute variables cannot be crossed with all levels of other variables. Consider the following example.

> *Clinical researchers were interested in studying rater reliability of range of motion measurements using two types of goniometers. They also wanted to determine if more experienced therapists perform better than less experienced therapists. They selected 10 therapists from one clinic, 5 who had more than 3 years experience, and 5 who had less than 3 years experience. Each therapist measured knee range of motion on the same sample of 25 patients. They used both types of goniometers, in random order.*

To study the reliability of range of motion measurements, we could compare recordings made by 10 therapists, each using both goniometric methods. In a two-way design (10 × 2), we could cross all 10 levels of "therapists" with both levels of "method."

Design 5

	Less experienced					More experienced				
Therapists	1	2	3	4	5	6	7	8	9	10
Methods 1										
Methods 2										

If the main effect of therapists showed a significant difference, the therapists would not be considered reliable, regardless of the method used. If a significant interaction occurred between therapist and method, it would mean that readings taken with a particular goniometer vary depending on which therapist is using it.

If we wanted to follow up on this interaction, we might suspect that less experienced therapists performed better with one type of goniometer. To test this hypothesis, we could divide our sample of therapists into two groups based on their years of experience, and thus introduce a third independent variable, experience, with two levels. These two levels, however, cannot be crossed with the 10 levels of therapists; that is, the same therapist cannot appear in both experience groups. Therefore, "therapists" are *nested* within "experience." All levels of therapist and experience can be crossed with the two methods in this **nested design** (Design 5). Although this design resembles a three-way randomized block design, it must be analyzed differently because the interactions of therapist × experience and therapist × experience × method cannot be assessed.

Most variables in clinical studies can be completely crossed; however, with certain combinations of attribute variables, a nested arrangement is required. Nesting is commonly used in educational studies where classes are nested in schools or schools are nested in cities. For instance, Edmundson and associates studied an educational program to reduce risk factors for cardiovascular disease.[11] They evaluated the effect of the program on 6,000 students from 96 schools in four states. The schools were nested in states. Within each state the schools were randomly assigned to receive the program or a control condition.

Analysis of Design 5. An analysis of variance is used to test for main effects and relevant interactions. The dimensions of that analysis depend on how many variables are involved in the study. Nested designs require a complicated approach to analysis of variance, which goes beyond the scope of this book. See Kirk[12] and Keppel[13] for discussions of analysis of nested designs.

REPEATED MEASURES DESIGNS

All of the experimental designs we have considered so far have involved at least two independent groups, created by random assignment or blocking. There are many research questions, however, for which control can be substantially increased by using a **repeated measures design,** where one group of subjects is tested under all conditions and each subject acts as his own control. Conceptually, a repeated measures design can be considered a series of trials, each with a single subject. Therefore, such a design is also called a *within-subjects design*, because treatment effects are associated with differences observed within a subject across treatment conditions, rather than between subjects across randomized groups.

The major advantage of the repeated measures design is the ability to control for the potential influence of individual differences. It is a fairly safe assumption that important subject characteristics such as age, sex, motivation, and intelligence will remain constant throughout the course of an experiment. Therefore, differences observed among treatment conditions are more likely to reflect treatment effects, and not variability between subjects. Using subjects as their own control provides the most equivalent "comparison group" possible.

One disadvantage of the repeated measures approach is the potential for *practice effects*, or the learning effect that can take place when one individual repeats a task over and over. For instance, practice effects may result in a subject becoming more adept at a task, not because the intervention is improving performance, but because of repeated performance. Another disadvantage is the potential for *carryover effects* when one subject is exposed to multiple-treatment conditions. Carryover can be reduced by allotting sufficient time between successive treatment conditions to allow for complete dissipation of previous effects. For instance, if we study the effect of different forms of heat on intramuscular temperature to relieve pain, we may need to repeat testing on different days to be sure that tissues have returned to resting temperatures. We would also have to be assured that the patient's pain level was constant across these days. Therefore, repeated measures can only be used when the outcome measure will revert to baseline between interventions, and the patient problem will remain relatively stable throughout the study period. There are many treatments for which carryover cannot be eliminated. For example, if we evaluate the effects of different exercise programs for increasing strength over a 4-week period, the effects of each exercise regimen will probably be long lasting, and rest periods will be ineffective for reversing the effect. With variables that produce permanent or long-term physiological or psychological effects, repeated measures designs are not appropriate.

Single-Factor Designs for Repeated Measures

Design 6: One-Way Repeated Measures Design

The simplest form of repeated measures design involves a single-factor experiment, where one group of subjects is exposed to all levels of one treatment variable (Design 6a).

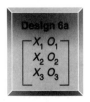

Researchers were interested in the effect of using a cane on the intramuscular forces on prosthetic hip implants during walking.[14] They studied 24 subjects with unilateral prosthetic hips under three conditions: walking with a cane on the side contralateral to the prosthesis, on the same side as the prosthesis, and on the contralateral side with instructions to push with "near maximal effort." They monitored electromyographic (EMG) activity of hip abductor muscles and cane force under each condition.

For the study of cane use, the researchers wanted to examine EMG activity of the hip abductor muscles, with all subjects exposed to all three cane conditions. It would be possible to use a randomized design to investigate this question, by assigning different groups to each condition, but it does not make logical sense. By using a repeated measures format we can be assured that differences across conditions are a function of cane use, and not individual physiological differences. In this example, the independent variable does not present a problem of carryover that would preclude one subject participating at all three levels. This design is commonly referred to as a *one-way repeated measures design.*

The repeated measures design is also naturally suited to assessing performance trends over time (Design 6b).[15, 16]

| Design 6b | Researchers studied the effects of low-impact aerobic exercise on fatigue, aerobic fitness, and disease activity in adults with rheumatoid arthritis.[17] Measures were obtained preintervention, midtreatment (after 6 weeks of exercise), end of treatment (after 12 weeks of exercise), and at a 15-week follow-up. |

$O_1 \: X \: O_2 \: O_3 \: O_4$

In this example, time is the independent variable, not treatment, as every subject receives the treatment. Every subject is evaluated at each time interval, making it a repeated measure. When time is the independent variable, however, this design has limitations. Without a control group, internal validity is a threat, as it is not possible to discern if changes would have occurred over time without the intervention.

Analysis of Design 6.   The one-way analysis of variance for repeated measures is used to test for differences across levels of one repeated factor. When time is the independent variable, analysis will often include polynomial contrasts to describe trends.[16]

Design 7: Crossover Design

Because subjects are exposed to multiple-treatment conditions in a repeated measures design, there must be some concern about the potentially biasing effect of test sequence; that is, the researcher must determine if responses might be dependent on which condition preceded which other condition. Effects such as fatigue, learning, or carryover may influence responses if subjects are all tested in the same order.

Two solutions are available to address this problem of **order effect.** One is to randomize the order of presentation for each subject, often by the flip of a coin, so that there is no bias involved in choosing the order of testing.

Researchers were interested in determining the effect of a wrist orthosis on work performance and pain during specific tasks in patients with rheumatoid arthritis.[18] Forty patients were fitted with a Futuro wrist orthosis. Performance and pain were measured with and without the orthosis, with the order of orthosis versus no orthosis randomly assigned.

In the example of the wrist orthosis, the researchers were concerned that the subjects' responses could be affected if one condition was always tested first. This approach does theoretically control for order effects; however, there is still a chance that some sequences will be repeated more often than others, especially if the sample size is small.

A preferred method is to *counterbalance* the treatment conditions so that their order is systematically varied. This creates a **crossover design** (Design 7), in which half the subjects receive treatment A followed by B, and half receive B followed by A. Two subgroups are created, one for each sequence, and subjects are randomly assigned to one of the sequences.

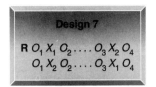

A study was designed to examine the effects of Dantrium on muscle strength, spasticity, and functional status in patients following stroke.[19] Thirty-eight patients were enrolled in the study within 8 weeks of onset of stroke. Patients were randomly assigned to begin a 6-week treatment period with either the active drug or a placebo. This was followed by a 1-week washout period, and then a reversed placebo or drug treatment period for 6 more weeks. Measurements were taken at the start and end of each phase of the study.

A crossover design should only be used in trials where the patient's condition or disease will not change appreciably over time. It is not a reasonable approach in situations when treatment effects are slow, as the treatment periods must be limited. It is similarly impractical when treatment effects are long term and a reversal is not likely. This design is especially useful, however, when treatment conditions are immediately reversible, as in the use of a wrist orthosis. When the treatment has cumulative effects, as in the Dantrium study, a **washout period** is essential, allowing a common baseline for each treatment condition. The washout period must be long enough to eliminate any prolonged effects of the treatment. In this case, 1 week was considered sufficient for removal of drug effects from the patient's system.

Analysis of Design 7.   In the analysis of a crossover design, researchers will usually group scores by treatment condition, regardless of which order they were given. A paired *t*-test can then be used to compare change scores, or a two-way analysis of variance with two repeated measures can be used to compare pretest and posttest measures across both treatment conditions. The Wilcoxon signed-ranks test should be used to look at change scores when ordinal data are used. In some situations, the researcher may want to see if order had an effect on responses, and subjects can be separated into independent groups based on sequence of testing. This analysis may include a two-way analysis of variance with one repeated measure, with sequence as an independent factor and treatment condition as a repeated measure.

Design 8: Latin Square Design

When more than two treatment conditions are used in a study, the number of sequences must be considered. For example, with three treatment conditions there are six possible sequence combinations: 1-2-3, 1-3-2, 2-3-1, 2-1-3, 3-2-1, and 3-1-2. These six sequences represent blocks to which subjects can be assigned at random. This assures that no bias exists in who performs which sequence. These blocks can also be analyzed as an independent variable in the design, to determine if sequence of testing created differences in response patterns.

When the size of the sample does not fit a pattern to accommodate all sequences equally, or when the number of possible sequences is too great, a form of random assignment is needed to select sequence combinations. This can be accomplished by using a **Latin square,** which is a matrix composed of equal numbers of rows and columns, designating random permutations of sequence combinations. For example, with three treatment conditions, we would use a 3 × 3 matrix, as shown in Figure 10.2A.

In this square, rows represent blocks. A block may be composed of one subject or it may represent a group of subjects. Each column in the design represents a testing session. No one treatment condition appears in a column or row more than once. Once the square is configured, with letters assigned to each cell of the matrix, the actual treatment conditions are then randomly assigned to the letter designations, and blocks are randomly assigned to each sequence. Note that not every possible sequence is included; that is, of the six possible sequences, these three were chosen at random.

For instance, suppose we wanted to study the EMG activity of abdominal muscles during sit-ups, with arms crossed, overhead, and outstretched. If we have 30 subjects, we could assign 10 subjects to each of three sequences. Using randomization, we would determine which group was to be designated sequence 1, 2, or 3. Then we would randomly assign each arm position to one letter, A, B, or C. The Latin square would then designate the order of testing for each block: Subjects in block 1 would receive condition A first, followed by condition B, and then condition C. Subjects in block 2 would receive condition B first, followed by condition C, and then condition A, and so on. If the independent variable had four levels, a 4 × 4 Latin square could be constructed, as shown in Figure 10.2B.

With repeated measures, it is not desirable to create a Latin square with a cyclical pattern, where each subsequent row is created by shifting the treatment sequence by one cell, but with the same relative order within each row. The squares in Figures 10.2A and 10.2B are such squares. Treatment B always follows A, D always follows C, and so on. Although the sequences are varied, and no two sequences are the same, the concern for order effects is not adequately addressed. To control for this effect, a *balanced Latin square* must be constructed in which all treatments precede and follow each other only once.[20] The square in Figure 10.2C illustrates this concept.

The methods involved in constructing Latin squares are beyond the scope of this text, but fortunately random permutations of Latin squares of various sizes have been developed.[21] The choice of a particular square for a given size should be made at random. An abbreviated selection of Latin squares is included in Appendix Table A.12.

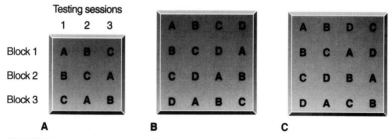

FIGURE 10.2 Examples of three Latin squares: (**A**) 3 × 3; (**B**) 4 × 4; and (**C**) 4 × 4 balanced Latin square.

Multifactor Designs for Repeated Measures

Design 9: Two-Way Design with Two Repeated Measures

Repeated measures can also be applied to studies involving more than one independent variable (Design 9).

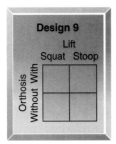

The use of back belts in industry is a subject of controversy. A study was designed to investigate the effect of back belts on oxygen consumption during lifting movements.[22] To study this question, researchers recruited 15 healthy subjects who were fitted with a semi-rigid lumbosacral orthosis. Oxygen consumption was measured while subjects participated in 6-minute submaximal lifting bouts of 10 kg. Each subject performed squat and stoop lifting, with and without the orthosis, for a total of four lifting bouts, in random order.

In the study of back belts, researchers created a 2×2 design with two repeated measures: type of lift (squat or stoop) and wearing of the orthosis (yes or no). Each subject was exposed to four test conditions. This design can also be expanded to include three independent variables.

Analysis of Design 9.   The two-way analysis of variance with two repeated measures is used to analyze differences across main effects and interaction effects.

Design 10: Mixed Design

A **mixed design** (Design 10) is created when a study incorporates two independent variables, one repeated across all subjects and the other randomized to independent groups.

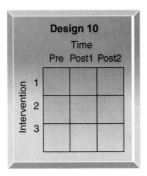

A study was designed to explore whether exercise programs would affect the ability to minimize postural sway in relatively inactive, older subjects.[23] Seventy-two subjects were randomly assigned to a computerized balance training group, a tai chi group, or an educational group serving as a control. Interventions were given over 15 weeks. All subjects were evaluated before, immediately after, and 4 months following their respective interventions. Outcome measures included a series of balance measures and fear of falling.

In the comparison of different balance exercise programs, subjects were randomly assigned to treatment groups. Each subject was tested three times (pretest and two posttests). The variable of exercise program is considered an *independent factor* because its levels have been randomized, creating independent groups. The variable of time is a *repeated factor* because all subjects are exposed to its three levels. Therefore, this design is also called a *two-way design with one repeated measure*, or a 3×3 mixed design. This example illustrates a commonly used approach, where researchers want to establish if the effects of intervention are long lasting, and not just present immediately following completion of the program.

Mixed designs can also be used with attribute variables. For instance, we could look at balance across age groups or between males and females. This would be a special case of a randomized block design, where subjects within a block act as their own controls.

Analysis of Design 10. A two-way analysis of variance with one repeated measure is used to analyze main effects and interaction effects with a two-way design with one repeated factor.

QUASI-EXPERIMENTAL DESIGNS

Although the randomized trial is considered the optimal design for testing cause-and-effect hypotheses, the necessary restrictions of a randomized trial are not always possible within the clinical environment.[24] The specification of inclusion and exclusion criteria will often reduce generalizability and limit the range of patients that can be included. **Quasi-experimental designs** are experiments that do not use random assignment for comparisons. They involve nonequivalent groups that may differ from each other in many ways in addition to differences between treatment conditions.[2] Therefore, the degree of confidence in results is reduced. Many clinical studies incorporate quasi-experimental elements because of the limitations of clinical conditions. These designs present reasonable alternatives to the randomized trial, as long as the researcher carefully documents subject characteristics, controls the research protocol, and uses blinding as much as possible. The conclusions drawn from these studies must take into account the potential biases of the sample, but may provide important information, nonetheless.[25]

One-Group Designs

Design 11: One-Group Pretest–Posttest Design

The **one-group pretest–posttest design** is a quasi-experimental design that involves one set of measurements taken before and after treatment on one group of subjects. The effect of treatment is determined by measuring the difference between pretest (O_1) and posttest (O_2) scores.

A study was designed to examine the effect of electrical stimulation on passive range of motion of wrist extension in 16 patients who suffered a stroke.[26] Researchers studied the effects of treatment on sensation, spasticity, range of motion, and strength in the hand. Subjects were given pretest and posttest measurements before and after a 4-week intervention program. The researchers observed significant reductions in wrist flexion deformities and concluded that the treatment was effective.

We must hold any conclusions drawn from this design as suspect, however. The design is weak because it has no comparison group, making it especially vulnerable to threats to internal validity. Although the researcher can demonstrate change in the dependent variable by comparing pretest and posttest scores, there is always the possibility that some events other than the experimental treatment occurred within the time frame of the study that caused the observed change. This design is particularly threatened by history and maturation effects, as there is no mechanism for evaluating if temporal factors influenced observed outcomes. In addition, the influence of testing, instrumentation, statistical regression, and selection interaction effects cannot be ruled out. External validity is also limited by potential interactions with selection because there is no comparison group.

The one-group pretest–posttest design may be defended, however, in cases when previous research has documented the behavior of a control group in similar circumstances. For instance, other studies may have shown that wrist ROM does not improve in this population over a 4-week period without intervention. On that basis, we could justify using a single experimental group to investigate just how much change can be expected with treatment.[27] This documentation might also allow us to defend the lack of a control group on ethical grounds. The design is reasonable in situations when the experimental situation is sufficiently isolated so that extraneous environmental variables are effectively controlled, and when the time interval between measurements is short so that temporal effects are minimized.[2] In studies where data collection is completed within a single testing session, temporal threats to internal validity will be minimal, but testing effects remain uncontrolled. Under all circumstances, however, this design is not considered an experiment, and should be expanded when possible to compare two groups.

Analysis of Design 11.   A t-test for paired comparisons is typically used to compare pretest and posttest mean scores. With ordinal data, the sign test or the Wilcoxon signed-ranks test can be used.

Multigroup Designs

Design 12: Time-Series Design

Many research questions that deal with the effects of treatment on physiological or psychological variables are concerned with how those effects are manifested over time. **Time-series designs** are based on the application of multiple measurements, before and after treatment, to document patterns or trends of behavior. These designs have been adapted by behavioral analysts for the study of single subjects' responses over time (see Chapter 12). Basic time-series designs have been defined by Cook and Campbell.[2]

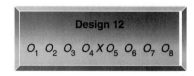

Design 12

$O_1 \; O_2 \; O_3 \; O_4 \; X \; O_5 \; O_6 \; O_7 \; O_8$

Researchers investigated the effects of a new program for improving tactile discrimination in patients who have suffered a stroke.[37] Eight subjects received training in specific, graded discrimination tasks that required feeling different types of surfaces with a finger. Measures were taken using the Tactile Discrimination Test. A series of baseline measures were taken for several weeks prior to starting the intervention, and then continued following introduction of the training program, spanning a 13-week period.

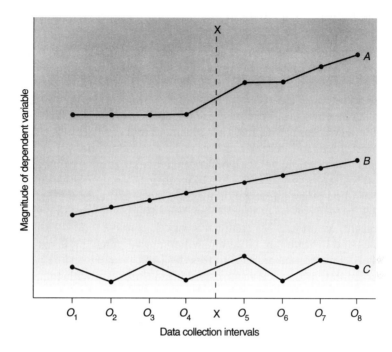

FIGURE 10.3 Illustration of three possible outcome patterns in the interrupted time-series design.

This study is an example of an *interrupted time-series design* (Design 12), so named because it involves a series of measurements over time that are "interrupted" by one or more treatment occasions.[†] It is considered a quasi-experimental design because only one group is studied. The independent variable is time; that is, each measurement interval represents one level of time.[‡] The research question concerns trends across these time intervals. The number of observations can vary, depending on the stability of the dependent variable. In this example, researchers used a predetermined set of 10 measures in the baseline phase, but extended it for 5 more measures for two patients who demonstrated variability within the baseline scores. It is generally advisable to keep intervals equally spaced, to avoid confounding by extraneous temporal factors.

This design may be considered an extension of the one-group pretest–posttest design. It offers more control, however, because the multiple pretests and posttests act as a pseudo-control condition, demonstrating maturational trends that naturally occur in the data or the confounding effects of extraneous variables. To illustrate, consider several possible outcomes for an interrupted time-series design, shown in Figure 10.3. A series of observations

---

[†]Time-series designs are distinguished from repeated measures designs by the large number of measurements that are taken continuously across baseline and intervention phases. See Chapter 12 for a description of time-series experiments as they are constructed for single-subject research.
[‡]The time-series design is distinguished from the one-way repeated measures design in the number of observations over time, and the repetitive monitoring of performance throughout the time frame of the study.

are taken at times 1 through 8 (O_1–O_8), with the introduction of treatment at point X. In all three patterns, a similar increase in the dependent variable is seen from O_4 to O_5. In pattern A we would be justified in assuming that treatment has an effect, as no change occurred prior to intervention. In pattern B, however, it would be misleading to make this interpretation, as the responses are continually increasing within the baseline measures. Although pattern C also shows an increase in the dependent variable from O_4 to O_5, which would look like a treatment effect if these were the only two measurements taken, we can see from the erratic pattern changes before and after treatment that this conclusion is unwarranted.

The greatest threat to internal validity in the time-series design is history. There is no control over the possible coincidental occurrence of some extraneous event at the same time that treatment is initiated. Most other threats to internal validity are, however, fairly well controlled by the presence of multiple measurements; that is, their effects are not eliminated, but we can account for them. For instance, if instrumentation or testing effects are present, we should see changes across the pretest scores. External validity of a time-series design is limited to situations when repeated testing takes place.

Several variations can be applied to this design. Comparisons may include two or more groups. Treatment may be administered one time only with follow-up measurements, or it may be continued throughout the posttest period. In a third variation, treatment may be started after a series of pretest measurements, and then withdrawn after a specified time period, with measurements continuing into the withdrawal period. The *withdrawal design* does help to account for history effects. If the behavior improves with treatment, and reverts to baseline levels when treatment is withdrawn, a strong case can be made that extraneous factors were not operating. In a fourth model, called a *multiple baseline design*, each subject is tested under baseline conditions, and the introduction of treatment is staggered, again controlling for history and maturation effects. These models have been incorporated into single-subject designs (see Chapter 12).

Analysis of Design 12.   Many researchers use graphic visual analysis as the primary means of interpreting time-series data. There is considerable disagreement as to the validity of visual analysis. Statistical techniques for time-series analysis involve complex multivariate methods. The procedure that is most recommended is based on a model called the *autoregressive integrated moving average (ARIMA)*.[9, 10] This technique accommodates for serial scores and weighs heavily on the observations that fall closer to the point at which treatment is introduced (see Chapter 12 for a discussion of serial dependency). It analyzes the trends in data and proposes a model that represents the observed pattern. This model can then be used to describe the behavior of interest. To be effective, the ARIMA procedure requires at least 25 data points in each phase.[38] For a more detailed description of this procedure, consult Cook and Campbell.[2]

Design 13: Nonequivalent Pretest–Posttest Control Group Design

There are many research situations in the social, clinical, and behavioral sciences where groups are found intact or where subjects must be self-selected. The former case is common in a clinic or school where patients or students belong to fixed groups or classes. The latter case will apply when attribute variables are studied or when volunteers are recruited. The **nonequivalent pretest–posttest control group design** (Design 13) is similar to Design 2 except that subjects are not assigned to groups randomly. This design can be structured with one treatment group and one control group or with multiple treatment and control groups.

A study was performed to test the efficacy of a family education program for cystic fibrosis management.[28] Participants were recruited from two health centers. One center provided a comprehensive program for parents and children. The other center provided usual care. Pretest and posttest measures were taken for knowledge, self-efficacy, self-management behavior, health, and quality of life.

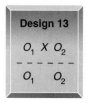

Design 13

$$O_1 \; X \; O_2$$
$$\text{-----}$$
$$O_1 \qquad O_2$$

A study was designed to examine the influence of regular participation in chair exercises on postoperative deconditioning following hip fracture.[29] Subjects were distinguished by their willingness to participate, and could not be randomly assigned to groups. A control group received usual care following discharge. Physiological, psychological, and anthropometric variables were measured before and after intervention.

In the study of family education, the patients are members of intact groups by virtue of the clinic they attend. In the chair exercise study, subjects self-selected their group membership.

Although the nonequivalent pretest–posttest control group design is limited by the lack of randomization, it still has several strengths. Because it includes a pretest and a control group, there is some control over history, testing, and instrumentation effects. The pretest scores can be used to test the assumption of initial equivalence on the dependent variable, based on average scores and measures of variability. The major threat to internal validity is the interaction of selection with history and maturation. For instance, if those who chose to participate in chair exercises were stronger or more motivated patients, changes in outcomes may have been related to physiological or psychological characteristics of subjects. These characteristics could affect general activity level or rate of healing. Such interactions might be mistaken for the effect of the exercise program. These types of interactions can occur even when the groups are identical on pretest scores.

Another strategy for comparing treatments involves the use of **historical controls** who received a different treatment during an earlier time period.

A study was conducted to assess the benefits of moderate hypothermia on patients with anoxic brain injury after out-of-hospital cardiac arrest.[30] Participants were 22 adults who remained unconscious after return of spontaneous circulation following cardiac arrest. This treatment group was studied prospectively, and a control group of 22 similar patients was studied by retrospective chart review. For the experimental subjects, moderate hypothermia (33°C) was induced in the emergency room by means of surface cooling and maintained for 12 hours in the ICU with rewarming to normothermia over 6 hours; control patients had been maintained at normothermia. Outcome measures included changes in pulse rate, arterial blood pressure, serum potassium and pH, number of septic complications, and score on the Glasgow Outcome Coma Scale.

As this example illustrates, a nonconcurrent control group may best serve the purpose of comparison when ethical concerns may preclude a true control group. When the researcher truly believes that the experimental intervention is more effective than standard care, the use of historical controls provides a reasonable alternative.[31] This approach has been used in cancer trials, for example, when protocols in one trial act as a control for subsequent studies.[32] The major advantage of this approach is its efficiency. Because all subjects are assigned to the experimental condition, the total sample will be smaller and the results can be obtained in a shorter period of time.

The disadvantages of using historical controls must be considered carefully, however. Studies that have compared outcomes based on historical controls versus randomly allocated controls have found positive treatment effects with historical controls that randomized trials have not been able to replicate.[33, 34] The most obvious problem, therefore, is the potential for confounding because of imbalances in characteristics of the experimental and historical control groups. For this approach to work, then, the researcher must be diligent in establishing a logical basis for group comparisons. This means that the historical controls should not simply be any patients described in the literature, or those treated at another time or another clinic.[31] It is reasonable, however, as in the hypothermia example, to consider using groups that were treated within the same environment, under similar conditions, where records of protocols were kept and demographics of subjects can be obtained. This approach may prove useful as large clinical databases are accumulated within a given treatment setting.

Analysis of Design 13. Several statistical methods are suggested for use with nonequivalent groups, including the unpaired t-test (with two groups), analysis of variance, analysis of covariance, analysis of variance with matching, and analysis of variance with gain scores.[35] Ordinal data can be analyzed using the Mann-Whitney U-test. Nonparametric tests may be more appropriate with nonequivalent groups, as variances are likely to be unequal. Preference for one approach will depend in large part on how groups were formed and what steps the researcher can take to ensure or document initial equivalence. Regression analysis or discriminant analysis may be the most applicable approach to determine how the dependent variable differentiates the treatment groups. Statistical strategies must include mechanisms for controlling for group differences on identified variables.

Design 14: Nonequivalent Posttest-Only Control Group Design

Nonequivalent designs are less interpretable when only posttest measures are available. The **nonequivalent posttest-only control group design** (Design 14), also called a *static group comparison,* is a quasi-experimental design that can be expanded to include any number of treatment levels, with or without a control group.[1] This design uses existing groups who have and have not received treatment.

Researchers were interested in studying the outcomes of an evaluation and treatment program for patients with cerebrovascular accident that followed a specific frame of reference for decision making.[36] They gathered data from 25 former patients, who served as control subjects, and 25 patients who were admitted after the implementation of the new program. They compared functional status at discharge as well as discharge disposition.

To draw conclusions from this comparison, we would have to determine if variables other than the new treatment paradigm could be responsible for functional status at discharge. Confounding factors such as the patient's physiological function, physical mobility, cardiac status, weight, and age should be identified. Although the static group comparison affords some measure of control in that there is a control group, internal validity is severely threatened by selection biases and attrition. This design is inherently weak because it provides no evidence of equivalence of groups before treatment. Therefore, it should be used only in an exploratory capacity, where it may serve to generate hypotheses for future testing. It is essentially useless in the search for causal relationships.

Analysis of Design 14.   Because this design does not allow interpretation of cause and effect, the most appropriate analysis is a regression approach that compares group membership, such as discriminant analysis. Essentially this design allows the researcher to determine if there is a relationship between the presence of the group attribute and the measured response.

COMMENTARY

Efficacy versus Effectiveness

The importance of understanding concepts of experimental design cannot be overemphasized in the planning stages of an experimental research project. There is a logic in these designs that must be fitted to the research question and the scope of the project, so that meaningful conclusions can be drawn once data are analyzed. Alternative designs should be considered on the basis of their relative validity, and the strongest designs should be chosen whenever possible. The design itself is not a guarantee of the validity of research findings, however. Process must be controlled within the structure. Attention to measurement issues is especially important to ensure that outcomes will be valid. It is also important to note that the strongest design for a given question need not be the most complicated design. In many cases, using the simpler designs can facilitate answering the research question, where a more complex design creates uninterpretable interactions. The choice of a design should ultimately be based on the intent of the research question:

> . . . the question being asked determines the appropriate research architecture, strategy, and tactics to be used—not tradition, authority, experts, paradigms, or schools of thought.[39]

The underlying importance of choosing an appropriate research design relates to consequent analysis issues that arise once data are collected. Many beginning researchers have had the unhappy experience of presenting their data to a statistician, only to find out that they did not collect the data appropriately to answer their research question. Fisher expressed this idea in his classical work, *The Design of Experiments:* "Statistical procedure and experimental design are only two different aspects of the same whole, and that whole comprises all the logical requirements of the complete process of adding to natural knowledge by experimentation."[40]

The relevant point is the need to use a variety of research approaches to answer questions of clinical importance. Although the clinical trial or experiment is considered a "gold standard" for establishing cause and effect, it is by no means the best or most appropriate approach for many of the questions that are most important for improving practice. The real world does not operate with controls and schedules the way an experiment can. There are many examples of good research that use quasi-experimental designs to look at clinical outcomes.

Researchers will often distinguish between efficacy and effectiveness in clinical studies. **Efficacy** is generally defined as the benefit of an intervention as compared to a control or standard program. It provides information about the behavior of clinical variables under controlled, randomized conditions. This lets us examine theory and draw generalizations to large populations. **Effectiveness** refers to the benefits and use of the procedure under "real world" conditions. It is the expectation that when we apply treatments, we do so without being able to control all the circumstances around us, and our results may not be the same as those obtained with a randomized experiment. This distinction helps us understand the situation when the findings of a controlled trial demonstrate that a treatment works, but clinicians find that it does not have the same effect when used on their patients in actual treatment conditions. The efficacious treatment was tested on a specified sample, with inclusion and exclusion criteria, and was applied under controlled and defined conditions. It then becomes imperative to determine if the same result can be obtained when personnel, patients and the environment cannot be manipulated. Quasi-experimental studies, using intact groups or non-random samples, are often used to demonstrate effectiveness. As we continue to examine outcomes as a primary focus of clinical research, we must consider many alternatives to the traditional clinical trial, to discover the most "effective" courses of treatment.

KEY TERMS

true experimental design
quasi-experimental design
completely randomized
    design
between-subjects design
randomized block design
within-subjects design
repeated measures design
one-way design
pretest–posttest design
randomized clinical trial
    (RCT)

posttest-only design
factorial design
main effect
interaction effect
randomized block design
nested design
order effect
crossover design
washout period
Latin square
mixed design

one-group pretest–posttest
    design
time-series design
nonequivalent
    pretest–posttest control
    group design
historical controls
static group comparison
efficacy
effectiveness

REFERENCES

1. Campbell DT, Stanley JC. *Experimental and Quasi-experimental Designs for Research.* Chicago: Rand McNally, 1963.
2. Cook TD, Campbell DT. *Quasi-experimentation: Design and Analysis Issues for Field Settings.* Boston: Houghton Mifflin, 1979.
3. Reilly RP, Findley TW. Research in physical medicine and rehabilitation. IV. Some practical designs in applied research. *Am J Phys Med Rehabil* 1989;68:196–201.
4. Behi R, Nolan M. Quasi-experimental research designs. *Br J Nurs* 1996;5:1079–81.
5. Horowitz RI. The experimental paradigm and observational studies of cause-effect relationships in clinical medicine. *J Chron Dis* 1987;40:91–9.
6. Singh NA, Clements KM, Fiatarone MA. A randomized controlled trial of progressive resistance training in depressed elders. *J Gerontol* 1997;52A:M27–M35.
7. Lamas GA, Orav EJ, Stambler BS, et al. Quality of life and clinical outcomes in elderly patients treated with ventricular pacing as compared with dual-chamber pacing. *New Engl J Med* 1998;338:1097–1104.
8. Clark F, Azen SP, Zemke R, et al. Occupational therapy for independent-living older adults: a randomized controlled trial. *JAMA* 1997;278:1321–6.
9. Munin MC, Rudy TE, Glynn NW, Crossett LS, Rubash HE. Early inpatient rehabilitation after elective hip and knee arthroplasty. *JAMA* 1998;279:847–52.
10. Segnan N, Senore C, Giordano L, Ponti A, Ronco G. Promoting participation in a population screening program for breast and cervical cancer: a randomized trial of different invitation strategies. *Tumori* 1998;84:348–53.
11. Edmundson E, Parcel GS, Feldman HA, et al. The effects of the Child and Adolescent Trial for Cardiovascular Health upon psychosocial determinants of diet and physical activity behavior. *Prev Med* 1996;25:442–54.
12. Kirk RE. *Experimental Design: Procedures for the Behavioral Sciences.* 2d ed. Belmont, CA: Brooks/Cole, 1982.
13. Keppel G. *Design and Analysis: A Researcher's Handbook.* 2d ed. Englewood Cliffs, N.J.: Prentice Hall, 1982.
14. Neuman DA. Hip abductor muscle activity as subjects with hip prostheses walk with different methods of using a cane. *Phys Ther* 1998;78:490–501.
15. Myers JL. *Fundamentals of Experimental Design.* 3d ed. Boston: Allyn and Bacon, 1979.
16. Green SB, Salkind NJ, Akey TM. *Using SPSS for Windows: Analyzing and Understanding Data.* Upper Saddle River, NJ: Prentice Hall, 1997.
17. Neuberger GB, Press AN, Lindsley HB, et al. Effects of exercise on fatigue, aerobic fitness, and disease activity measures in persons with rheumatoid arthritis. *Res Nurs Health* 1997;20:195–204.
18. Pagnotta A, Baron M, Korner-Bitensky N. The effect of a static wrist orthosis on hand function in individuals with rheumatoid arthritis. *J Rheumatol* 1998;25:879–85.
19. Katrak PH, Cole AM, Poulos CJ, McCauley JC. Objective assessment of spasticity, strength, and function with early exhibition of dantrolene sodium after cerebrovascular accident: a randomized double-blind study. *Arch Phys Med Rehabil* 1992;73:4–9.
20. Wagenaar WA. A note on the construction of diagram-balanced Latin squares. *Psychol Bull* 1969;72:384.
21. Fisher RA, Yates F. *Statistical Tables for Biological, Agricultural and Medical Research.* 9th ed. Edinburgh: Oliver & Boyd, 1963.
22. Duplessis DH, Greenway EH, Keene KL, et al. Effect of semi-rigid lumbosacral orthosis use on oxygen consumption during repetitive stoop and squat lifting. *Ergonomics* 1998;41:790–7.

23. Wolf SL, Barnhart HX, Ellison GL, Coogler CE. The effect of Tai Chi Quan and computerized balance training on postural stability in older subjects. *Phys Ther* 1997;77:371–81.

24. D'Agostino RB, Kwan H. Measuring effectiveness. What to expect without a randomized control group. *Med Care* 1995;33:AS95–AS105.

25. Johnston MV, Ottenbacher KJ, Reichardt CS. Strong quasi-experimental designs for research on the effectiveness of rehabilitation. *Am J Phys Med Rehabil* 1995;74:383–92.

26. Baker LL, Yeh C, Wilson D, Waters RL. Electrical stimulation of wrist and fingers for hemiplegic patients. *Phys Ther* 1979;59:1495–9.

27. Cox KR. *Planning Clinical Experiments.* Springfield, IL: Charles C. Thomas, 1968.

28. Bartholomew LK, Czyzewski DI, Parcel GS, et al. Self-management of cystic fibrosis: short-term outcomes of the Cystic Fibrosis Family Education Program. *Health Educ Behav* 1997;24:652–66.

29. Nicholson CM, Czernwicz S, Mandilas G, Rudolph I, Greyling MJ. The role of chair exercises for older adults following hip fracture. *S Afr Med J* 1997;87:1131–8.

30. Bernard SA, Jones BM, Horne MK. Clinical trial of induced hypothermia in comatose survivors of out-of-hospital cardiac arrest. *Ann Emerg Med* 1997;30:146–53.

31. Moser M. Randomized clinical trials: alternatives to conventional randomization. *Am J Emerg Med* 1986;4:276–85.

32. Gehan EA, Freireich EJ. Non-randomized controls in cancer clinical trials. *N Engl J Med* 1974;290:198–203.

33. Sacks HS, Chalmers TC, Smith H, Jr. Sensitivity and specificity of clinical trials. Randomized v historical controls. *Arch Intern Med* 1983;143:753–5.

34. Micciolo R, Valagussa P, Marubini E. The use of historical controls in breast cancer. An assessment in three consecutive trials. *Controlled Clin Trials* 1985;6:259–70.

35. Reichardt CS. The statistical analysis of data from nonequivalent group designs. In: Cook TD, Campbell DT, eds. *Quasi-experimentation: Design and Analysis Issues for Field Settings.* Boston: Houghton Mifflin, 1979,147–205.

36. Gibson JW, Schkade JK. Occupational adaptation intervention with patients with cerebrovascular accident: a clinical study. *Am J Occup Ther* 1997;51:523–9.

37. Carey LM, Matyas TA, Oke LE. Sensory loss in stroke patients: effective training of tactile and proprioceptive discrimination. *Arch Phys Med Rehabil* 1993;74:602–611.

38. Ottenbacher KJ. Analysis of data in idiographic research. *Am J Phys Med Rehabil* 1992;71:202–8.

39. Sackett DL, Wennberg JE. Choosing the best research design for each question. *BMJ* 1997;315:1636.

40. Fisher RA. *The Design of Experiments.* 6th ed. New York: Hafner, 1951.

Sequential Clinical Trials

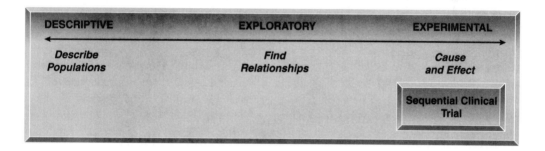

Experimental designs provide a strong foundation for making decisions about the relative efficacy of different treatments; however, clinical realities often create practical and ethical dilemmas that limit the application of experimental methods for research with patients. One problem with group studies is the need to determine a fixed sample size prior to starting an experiment; that is, the experimenter must decide how many subjects will be needed to achieve statistical validity. Sometimes it can take months, even years, to obtain a sufficiently large sample, especially if the disorder being studied is relatively rare.

A second problem concerns how data are analyzed. In group studies, data are collected until all subjects have been treated and tested. Only then can data be analyzed and a decision made about the effect of the experimental treatment. This decision is delayed until the end, even if the experimental treatment turns out to be consistently inferior during the course of the study. In fact, it is generally considered good practice to remain blind to results until the end of data collection, so that the researcher would not know if an inferior treatment was being administered until the experiment was over.

The purpose of this chapter is to introduce an alternative research approach, called the **sequential clinical trial,** that addresses both of these issues.[1] A sequential technique allows for continuous analysis of data as they become available, instead of waiting until the end of the experiment. Results are accumulated as each subject is tested, so that the experiment can be stopped at any point as soon as the evidence is strong enough to determine a significant difference between treatments. Consequently, it is possible that a decision about treatment effectiveness can be made earlier than in a fixed sample study, leading to a substantial reduction in the total number of subjects needed to obtain valid statistical outcomes and avoiding unnecessary administration of inferior treatments.

The special appeal of sequential analysis is that it is more than just a design. It is also a statistical technique for analyzing data; that is, the process involves a system for collecting data and for determining if significant differences exist between treatments. The advantage of this technique is that statistical analysis is based on the use of specially constructed charts that provide visual confirmation of statistical outcomes, without the use of a computer or any calculations on the part of the researcher! Even though it obviates statistical calculations, sequential analysis still requires the application of certain statistical principles in the construction of these charts. Therefore, those who are unfamiliar with concepts of hypothesis testing will find it helpful to review principles of inference in Chapter 18 in conjunction with this discussion.

The idea of sequential analysis was originally developed during World War II for military and industrial applications, and was for a time considered an official secret.[2] Soon after, it was recognized as a useful model for medical research, particularly in clinical trials of pharmacological agents.[3] Even though there are a few examples of its application in rehabilitation literature,[4-6] sequential analysis remains a relatively unknown technique in rehabilitation research. This is unfortunate because the sequential clinical trial is a convenient design that is applicable to many clinical research questions. We hope that once clinicians become familiar with the technique, more instances can be found for its use.

THE DESIGN OF A SEQUENTIAL TRIAL

The specific purpose of a sequential trial is to compare two treatments, a "new" or experimental treatment, usually designated A, and an "old" or standard treatment, designated B. Treatment can also be compared with a control or placebo, which is labeled B. Although these are arbitrary designations, consistency across studies has helped to standardize presentation of sequential data.

As in any other experiment, a research hypothesis must be stated indicating the expected relationship between treatments A and B. The null hypothesis states that both treatments will be equally effective (H_0: A = B). The alternative hypothesis may be stated with or without direction. Explicit operational definitions must be provided for each treatment and for measurement of responses. The research hypothesis will specify the target population to which results will be applied. Specific inclusion and exclusion criteria must be developed for subjects to enter the study.

Once the subjects, treatments, and measurements have been adequately defined, the process begins by admitting the first eligible patient into the study. This patient is assigned to either treatment A or B, using the flip of a coin or some other randomization process. When the next eligible patient is admitted (and this can be months later), she is assigned to the alternate treatment. These two patients now form a *pair*, the results of which can be considered a "little experiment"; that is, we can determine for these two people whether treatment A or treatment B was better. This is considered a *between-subject* comparison.

Alternatively, the comparison between A and B can be made *within* a single subject, with both A and B presented to each subject. This approach is appropriate when carryover effects are not expected from one treatment to the other, and when the manifestations of the disorder being treated are expected to remain fairly constant over time. Usually, alternate pairs are given the two treatments in reverse order, resulting in a **crossover design.** Depending on the nature of the variables being studied, there may need to be a reasonable interval between administrations of the two treatments, to allow for dissipation of effects and to be sure that subjects are starting at the same level for each test. The advantage of a crossover design is that intersubject variability is reduced in analyzing responses, making the design more powerful. The paired scores for each subject constitute the results of a "little experiment."

The whole experiment is a *sequence* of these "little experiments," with each pair representing a comparison. The comparison between A and B can be made in two ways, depending on the type of measurements taken. With continuous variables such as blood pressure, grip strength, and range of motion, the *magnitude* of the difference between A and B can be calculated directly. Most often, however, sequential studies use qualitative measures that indicate *preference* for A or B. Preferences are based on subjective but clearly defined criteria for saying that one treatment is clinically more effective than the other. We focus on the analysis of preferences in this chapter.

The result of each comparison within a pair of subjects is plotted on a *sequential chart*, showing the cumulative results for all comparisons. After each successive "little experiment" is plotted, the researcher stops to consider the results of all the pairs completed thus far and makes one of three decisions: (1) Stop and reject H_0, making a **terminal decision** to recommend A or B; (2) stop the experiment and accept H_0, making a terminal decision that treatments A and B are not different; or (3) continue to collect data because the cumulated data are not yet sufficient to draw a conclusion. This process of considering cumulative results after each pair of subjects has been tested is called **sequential analysis.** The decision to stop or continue will depend on how strong the evidence is to that point in favor of one treatment.

MEASURING PREFERENCES

It is often convenient to evaluate the relative effectiveness of two treatments by collecting a series of qualitative preferences in favor of one or the other.[7] **Preference** is defined on the basis of clinically meaningful differences between two treatments. The specific criteria for expressing preference for one treatment over another can vary in objectivity. At one extreme, the patient can merely express subjective feelings that one treatment seems to work better or is more comfortable than the other. At the other extreme, outcomes can be totally objective, such as death–survival or cured–not cured. In between are many subjective and objective types of measurements. A clinician might express preference based on a subjective evaluation of function or on the patient's general reaction to treatment. It is necessary, of course, to develop reliable criteria for making such dichotomous judgments.

It is also possible to reduce continuous data to a measure of preference. For instance, if we were measuring the effect of two treatments for increasing range of motion, we could specify that treatment A would be preferred if it could produce at least 20 degrees more of an increase in range than treatment B. In other words, any difference smaller than 20 degrees would not be clinically meaningful, and both treatments would be considered equally effective. This is a convenient approach, but the researcher must be

Outcome	Treatment A	Treatment B	Preference
1	Improvement	Improvement	None
2	No improvement	No improvement	None
3	Improvement	No improvement	A
4	No improvement	Improvement	B

FIGURE 11.1 Four possible outcomes for evaluating preferences.

aware that it results in a loss of information by reducing the data to a dichotomous outcome. Any difference greater than 20 degrees would indicate preference, whether that difference was 25 or 100 degrees. If analysis was based on the magnitude of differences, the amount of difference would be taken into account. The researcher must determine if the magnitude of difference is important or if the comparison between treatments is adequately assessed simply by expressing preference.*

When two treatments are compared, there are four possible outcomes for classifying preference, as shown in Figure 11.1. In outcome 1, both treatments are equally successful, in which case we would not be able to specify a preference for A or B. In outcome 2, neither treatment is successful. In either of these two cases, we have no information as to which treatment is superior. These outcomes are considered *ties* and are dropped from the analysis. In outcomes 3 and 4, one treatment is preferred over the other, providing one piece of evidence in favor of either A or B.

SEQUENTIAL PLANS FOR EVALUATING PREFERENCES

The decision to stop or continue a trial is based on a sequential chart that shows the cumulative preferences of each paired "little experiment." An example of such a chart is shown in Figure 11.2. A horizontal line is drawn along the X-axis. The units on this line represent the *number of pairs* (not individuals) that have demonstrated a preference for A or B (excluding tied pairs). This number is designated *n*. The Y-axis represents the direction of preference[†]: Each time a preference for A is expressed, the plot will move one unit in a positive direction; each time preference is expressed for B, the plot will move one unit in a negative direction. Above and below the X-axis, a set of mirrored boundaries are drawn. These upper (U), lower (L), and middle (M) boundaries are used to determine when the trial should be stopped.

For instance, suppose we gathered the hypothetical data shown in Table 11.1. The first pair shows a preference for A. Therefore, on the graph (Fig. 11.2) a dot is placed one unit above the origin at *n* = 1. We draw a line from the origin to this dot. Pair 2 also prefers A. Therefore, we place a second dot one unit above and to the right of the first dot at *n* = 2. Pair 3 demonstrates no preference, and is not included on the graph. Pair 4 prefers B; therefore, from the last plotted point we move down one unit and to the right

---

*In most cases, using the actual magnitude measures with continuous variables will result in a more powerful test. When continuous measures are used in sequential analysis, the test has been called a sequential *t*-test. For guidelines for using continuous measures with sequential analysis, see Armitage, Chapters 5 and 6.
[†]Some sequential charts will use the term *excess preferences* to label the Y-axis.

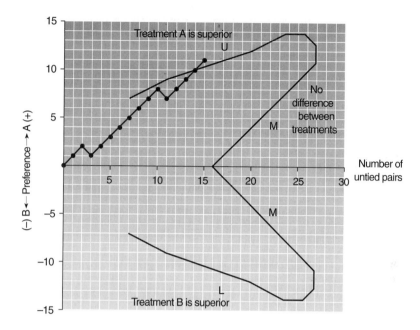

FIGURE 11.2 A sequential plan for evaluating preferences, showing upper (U), lower (L), and middle (M) boundaries. For these hypothetical data, the path of preferences shows a significant difference in favor of treatment A.

at $n = 3$ (there are now three pairs that have shown preferences). Each of these points is connected by a line. For a while, the line zigzags its way in the channels between the boundaries. We continue gathering paired data until the path crosses one of the outer boundaries, indicating that the experiment is finished.

These boundaries represent three **stopping rules:** (1) If the upper boundary (U) is crossed, we can make a terminal decision to recommend A (accept H_1: A > B). (2) If the lower boundary (L) is crossed, we can make a terminal decision to recommend B (accept H_1: B > A). (3) If the middle boundary (M) is crossed (either above or below the origin), there is no preference (accept H_0: A = B). In this example, we continued to test 12 more pairs. At the 16th pair ($n = 15$ because one pair was tied), we crossed the upper boundary, indicating that treatment A is preferred over treatment B. This study required 32 subjects (including one tied pair) to demonstrate a significant difference between treatments.

Choosing a Sequential Plan

The chart shown in Figure 11.2 is one type of **closed sequential plan,** also called a *restricted plan,* which means that the outer boundaries are truncated by allowing them to meet at the far right.[8] This approach is distinguished from *open plans,* which do not close off the outer boundaries, creating the potential for an exceptionally long sample path. For examples of open plans, see Armitage.[7]

Closed sequential plans have been developed by Armitage[7] and Bross.[9] Although their approaches are the same in principle, they do differ in technical details, as well as in their degree of flexibility. As both methods are presented in the literature, we describe examples of each.

TABLE 11.1.   HYPOTHETICAL DATA SHOWING PREFERENCES FOR TREATMENT A OR B

Pair	Preference
1	A
2	A
3	None
4	B
5	A
6	A
7	A
8	A
9	A
10	A
11	A
12	B
13	A
14	A
15	A
16	A

Armitage's Plans

Armitage presents a series of tables that allow the researcher to tailor a restricted sequential plan to a specific research situation; that is, there is no one plan that is appropriate for all studies. The plans differ in the location of the boundary lines and in the minimum and maximum sample sizes that would be needed to reach a boundary (the maximum sample size is designated N). The choice of a particular plan depends on three statistical specifications that must be set by the researcher before data collection begins: effect size (θ_1), Type I error rate, and Type II error rate.[‡] These specifications determine how the boundaries are drawn.

Effect Size

The first specification for choosing a sequential plan is the size of the expected effect for treatment A. Effects for preferences are expressed in terms of a proportion. For instance, for the data in Table 11.1, of the 15 pairs that expressed preferences, 87% of the preferences (13 of 15) were for treatment A and 13% (2 of 15) were for treatment B. Statistically, it is convenient to consistently describe preference according to the proportion in favor of treatment A (the new treatment), given the value θ (theta). Under the null hypothesis, $\theta = 0.50$. This means that, assuming A is not any better than B, we would expect 50% of the preferences to be for A (and 50% for B). Under the alternative hypothesis, θ will be some value greater than 0.50 (more than 50% will prefer A). This value can be designated θ_1. For example, if $\theta_1 = 0.90$, we would expect 90% of the preferences to be for treatment A. The difference between θ and θ_1 is the size of the expected effect for treatment A, called the **effect size.**

[‡]See Chapter 18 for a more complete explanation of these concepts.

Boundaries will be drawn differently depending on the researcher's estimate of θ_1. With a larger expected effect size, fewer subject pairs will be needed to cross a boundary. The estimate of θ_1 can be based on clinical experience or previous research, but it should reflect what the researcher considers a *clinically meaningful difference* between A and B, or the minimal difference that would be important to detect. For instance, if we set $\theta_1 = 0.80$, we are saying that at least 80% of the pairs should find A superior to B before we are willing to recommend treatment A.

Type I Error

A second specification concerns the acceptable risk of recommending one treatment over the other when treatments A and B are not really different. This risk is the probability of committing a **Type I error.** Type I error rate is the probability of incorrectly rejecting the null hypothesis. This risk is symbolized by α (alpha) and is conventionally set at .05. This means that a decision to prefer one treatment over the other will be wrong only 5% of the time, or that there is only a 5% chance of crossing the upper or lower boundaries when in fact the treatments are not different. This is generally considered an acceptable statistical risk. When greater protection is desired against type I error, α can be set to .01.

Alpha can designate a *one-tailed test* (α_1) or a *two-tailed test* (α_2). A one-tailed test is used when a directional research hypothesis has been proposed, when the researcher predicts that one treatment will be superior to the other. A two-tailed test is used when a nondirectional alternative hypothesis has been proposed, when the researcher does not predict which treatment will be superior.

Type II Error

It is also possible to make an error in deciding to accept the null hypothesis; that is, there may really be a difference between A and B, but the analysis of sample data is unable to document that difference statistically. The probability of recommending no preference when one treatment really is better than the other is called **Type II error,** symbolized by β (beta) and conventionally set at values between .05 and .20.

The **power** of a test is its sensitivity, or the probability that a statistical test will be able to detect a true difference between A and B. Power is equal to $1-\beta$. Therefore, if $\beta = .05$, power $= .95$. This means that there is a 95% chance that an outer boundary will be correctly crossed, or a 95% chance the test will result in crossing an outer boundary with an effect equal to θ_1. Power is directly related to both sample size and effect size; that is, power is increased as sample size or effect size increases.

To choose a particular sequential plan, the researcher must make a commitment in setting values of θ_1, α, and β. By tailoring the plan to each specific research situation, the sequential design will be capable of detecting differences with a minimum number of subjects. Armitage provides coordinates for constructing sequential plans for various values of θ_1.[7] Each plan is associated with a different maximum sample size (N), corresponding to the differences in anticipated effect size (θ_1).

The plan in Figure 11.2 is drawn for $\theta_1 = 0.85$, $\alpha = .05$, and $1-\beta = .95$. The coordinates for the upper (U), lower (L), and middle (M) boundaries are shown in Table 11.2. For $\theta_1 = 0.85$, the upper and lower boundaries start at $n = 7$, $Y = +7$ for U, and $Y = -7$ for L. They

TABLE 11.2   COORDINATES FOR UPPER (U), LOWER (L), AND MIDDLE (M) BOUNDARIES FOR CLOSED SEQUENTIAL PLANS FOR PREFERENCES AT DIFFERENT VALUES OF θ_1 (α_2 = .05 AND 1–β = .95)

Coordinates for U and L*	θ_1 = 0.75 N = 62				θ_1 = 0.80 N = 40		θ_1 = 0.85 N = 27		θ_1 = 0.90 N = 19		θ_1 = 0.95 N = 13	
	n	Y	n	Y	n	Y	n	Y	n	Y	n	Y
	9	9	45	19	8	8	7	7	7	7	6	6
	12	10	47	19	11	9	11	9	10	8	11	9
	15	11	50	20	14	10	14	10	14	10	13	9
	18	12	53	21	17	11	17	11	18	12		
	20	12	56	22	20	12	20	12	19	11		
	23	13	58	22	23	13	24	14				
	26	14	60	22	26	14	26	14				
	28	14	61	21	29	15	27	13				
	31	15	62	20	32	16						
	34	16			35	17						
	37	17			38	18						
	39	17			39	17						
	42	18			40	16						

Coordinates for M												
Top			62	18	40	14	27	11	19	9	13	7
X-axis			44	0	26	0	16	0	10	0	6	0
Bottom			62	–18	40	–14	27	–11	19	–9	13	–7

* Values of Y for upper boundary (U) will be positive; values of Y for lower boundary (L) will be negative.
Adapted from Armitage P. *Sequential Medical Trials*, 2d ed. Oxford: Blackwell Scientific, 1975, Table 3.7, p. 56. Used with permission.

end at n = 27, Y = +13 for U, and Y = –13 for L. The lines stop at N = 27, which is the maximum number of pairs that would be needed to cross a boundary for this effect size. The top portion of the middle boundary starts at n = 27, Y = +11, and meets the X-axis (Y = 0) at n = 16. The bottom portion of the middle boundary starts at n = 27, Y = –11, and also meets the X-axis at n = 16. The end points of U and L meet the corresponding middle boundaries, closing off the channels by connecting them with a vertical line at N = 27.

We have included templates for five sequential plans at the end of this chapter (see Addenda). These charts correspond to values of θ_1 from 0.75 to 0.95, at α_2 = .05 and 1–β = .95. Coordinates for boundary lines are given in Table 11.2. Note that for each plan the boundaries start at a different point. This starting point represents the minimum number of pairs that would have to be tested for the path to cross the boundary if all pairs responded with the same preference. Note, too, that as θ_1 increases (a larger expected treatment effect), both the minimum and maximum sample sizes decrease; that is, fewer subjects would be needed to show a significant difference if the treatment effect was strong enough to show consistent preferences. For those interested in more conservative analyses, see Armitage for coordinates of boundary points for plans at α_2 = .01.[7]

In choosing a particular plan, the researcher must balance requirements for statistical power with the desire to economize in sample size. It is difficult to make a rational

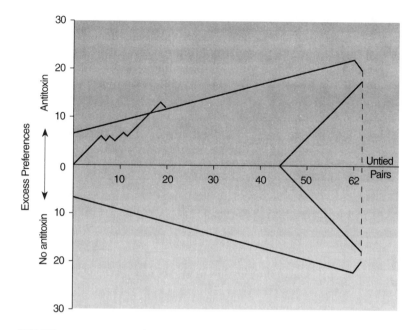

FIGURE 11.3 A restricted sequential plan showing preferences for use of antitoxin in the treatment of clinical tetanus ($\alpha_2 = .05$; $1-B = .95$; $\Theta_1 = 0.75$). (From Brown A, Mohamed SD, Montgomery RD, et al. Value of a large dose of antitoxin in clinical tetanus. *Lancet* 1960; 2:227, p 228, with permission.)

choice unless information is available to estimate θ_1, the proportion of expected preferences for treatment A. Armitage suggests that, when proportions cannot be estimated reliably, the researcher can start the trial without setting boundaries, and draw the boundaries in once the rate of preferences can be estimated from the data.[7]

Examples

The following illustrations help to demonstrate how this design is used. The first study is an early clinical trial examining the effect of antitoxin for treatment of tetanus.[10] The researchers supported the need for the study based on the lack of evidence available at that time to show that antitoxin was effective, the potential hazards of its administration, and its expense. Patients diagnosed as having tetanus were randomly assigned in pairs to receive or not receive the antitoxin. Preference was defined according to survival: If both members of the pair survived, or both died, the pair was tied and eliminated; if one member survived and the other died, preference was charted for the survivor. The researchers estimated that it would be important to recommend using the treatment if at least 75% of the preferences favored the antitoxin ($\theta_1 = 0.75$). Using Armitage's plan, as given in Table 11.2, they developed the sequential chart shown in Figure 11.3.[§] The upper boundary was crossed at the 18th preference (15 of the 18 were in favor of the antitoxin). Therefore, the authors concluded that antitoxin is a valuable remedy in clinical tetanus.

[§]This is the same configuration for a sequential chart as shown in Addendum 11.1

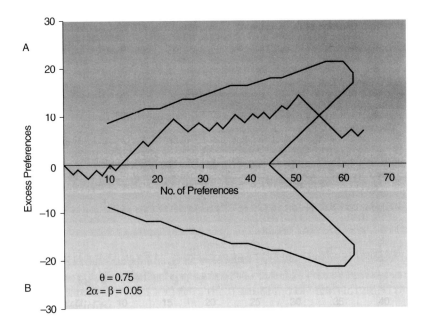

FIGURE 11.4 A restricted sequential plan showing preferences for use of antibiotics in combination with surgery for treatment of septic lesions ($\alpha_2 = .05$, $1–B = .95$, $\Theta_1 = 0.75$). (From Rutherford WH, Calderwood JW, Hart D, et al. Antibiotics in surgical treatment of septic lesions. *Lancet* 1970; 1:1077, Figure 2, p. 1078, with permission.)

In a second example, researchers examined the effect of antibiotics in the surgical treatment of septic lesions.[11] Treatment A consisted of a combination of surgical intervention and antibiotic treatment, and treatment B was surgery only. Preference was defined as a difference in healing time of 3 days or more.[11] These authors also estimated that a preference rate of 75% would be important, and therefore used the same sequential chart format as in the previous illustration. Results are shown in Figure 11.4. After 56 preferences were recorded (31 in favor of treatment A), the plot crossed the middle boundary, showing no significant difference between the two treatments. Note how much longer this path is than that in Figure 11.3, indicating that the treatment effect (effect size) was much stronger for the antitoxin study.

Bross's Plans

Bross has prepared two specially constructed, closed sequential plans, which are based on one-tailed tests at $\alpha_1 = .10$ (plan A) and $\alpha_1 = .05$ (plan B).[9] Although Bross suggests that $\alpha_1 = .10$ is appropriate for many experimental situations, .05 continues to be con-

---

[11]Rutherford et al.[11] also analyzed their data using the sequential *t*-test, which is a form of sequential analysis for use with continuous measurements. They used healing time, in days, as their dependent variable.

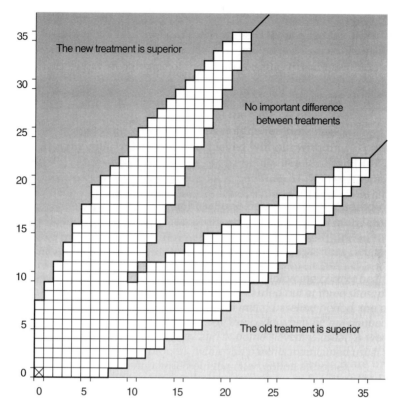

FIGURE 11.5   Bross's sequential plan B for $\alpha_1 = .05$. (From Bross I. Sequential medical plans. *Biometrics* 1952; 8:188, Figure 3, p. 198, with permission.)

sidered the minimum standard for hypothesis testing. Therefore, we have chosen to include only plan B in the present discussion.

Bross uses a different type of diagram than Armitage, as shown in Figure 11.5. In this chart, preferences are plotted along both axes, with the *Y*-axis representing preference for treatment A (the new treatment) and the *X*-axis representing preference for treatment B (the old treatment). The plot begins in the lower left corner square (a free square). As each comparison is made within a pair, an "x" is placed in the square either above the last occupied square (if A is superior) or to the right (if B is superior). If neither treatment is preferred within a pair, nothing is entered. The path continues until one of the boundaries is crossed. If the path goes upward, treatment A is significantly superior; if it goes to the right, treatment B is superior. As in Armitage's design, the middle boundary represents the null hypothesis; that is, if the path moves diagonally, the conclusion is that no difference exists. The longest possible path in this plan is 58 squares (116 patients).

Bross's plan is based on *comparative success rates*, indicating whether treatment A has an "advantage" over treatment B. Bross includes a table that statistically defines "important advantage."[9] For instance, if treatment B is known to "cure" 25% of the patients, treatment A would demonstrate an important advantage over B if it could cure 44%. If B cures 50%, then treatment A would be important if it could cure 70%; if treatment B cures 75%, then treatment A should cure 88% (see Bross's article[9] for additional comparative success rates).[#] The power of this analysis is approximately 86% when treatment A offers an important advantage over B; that is, 86% of the time the upper boundary will be correctly crossed.

Example

To illustrate the application of Bross's design, Light et al. studied the differential effect of low-load prolonged stretch (LLPS) versus the more traditional high-load brief stretch (HLBS) for treating knee flexion contractures in elderly patients.[4] Subjects were admitted to the study based on the presence of bilateral knee flexion contractures of at least 3 months' duration, and at least 30 degrees short of full extension. In addition, subjects had to be unable to walk or pivot transfer without maximal assistance. Subjects acted as their own controls, with limbs randomly assigned to receive either LLPS or HLBS. Treatment was performed twice daily, 5 days a week, for 4 weeks. The investigators provided explicit operational definitions of both stretching procedures.

Preference was defined in terms of change in range of motion from pretest to posttest. A difference of at least 10 degrees was considered an important improvement. Results are shown in Figure 11.6. The first patient tested demonstrated a preference for HLBS, and so the first "×" was placed just above the starting square. All further testing showed a preference for LLPS. Therefore, marks were made in a horizontal direction for all succeeding comparisons. In all, 11 subjects were required to cross the lower boundary, indicating a significantly greater effect for LLPS. Had the first subject also "preferred" LLPS, only 8 subjects would have been needed to demonstrate significance.

Comparing the Armitage and Bross Plans

Two points should be made in comparing the plans described by Armitage and Bross. One concerns the flexibility of plans. Bross does not provide alternative boundaries for different expected effect sizes. Therefore, it will often be possible to achieve significance earlier with one of Armitage's plans, especially with larger effect sizes. A second point concerns the difference between one-tailed and two-tailed tests. Bross's plans are based on one-tailed tests.[**] The probability associated with a two-tailed test is double that of a one-tailed test. Therefore, Bross's plan B would represent a two-tailed probability of .10, which is generally considered too high a risk of Type I error (his plan A would represent a two-tailed probability of .20). The researcher must determine if a one- or two-tailed test is appropriate, based on the research hypothesis and knowledge of the subject matter. Bross's plans are often used inappropriately because they are easier to apply, requiring

---

[#]To demonstrate the correspondence between Bross's and Armitage's plans, a closed sequential plan at $\theta_1 = 0.75$ is comparable to a success rate of 50% for treatment B as compared with 75% for treatment A.[10] Therefore, Bross's plan B offers approximately the same configuration as Armitage's plan for $\theta_1 = 0.75$. Note that the maximum sample size for Bross's plan B is 52, whereas for Armitage's plan the maximum is 62.

[**]There is some consensus that clinical trials should generally be performed using two-tailed tests, based on the practical possibility that experimental results may not support preconceived judgments of treatment effects.[12]

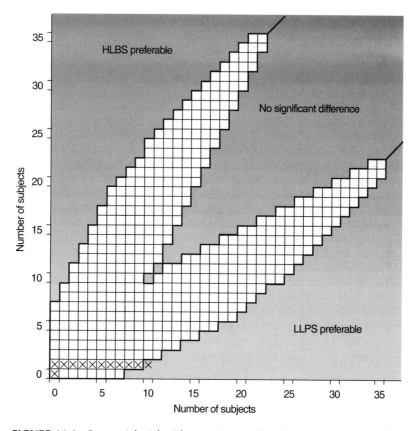

FIGURE 11.6 Sequential trial grid using Bross's plan B, showing preference for low-load prolonged stretch (LLPS) over high-load brief stretch (HLBS) for treatment of knee flexion contractures. (From Light KE, Nuzik S, Personius W, et al. Low-load prolonged stretch vs. high-load brief stretch in treating knee contractures. *Phys Ther* 1984; 64:330, Figure 3, p. 332. Reprinted with the permission of the American Physical Therapy Association.)

no construction on the part of the researcher. The researcher is, however, obliged to consider the specifications that go with a particular plan and to determine if those specifications fit each individual research situation.

LIMITATIONS OF SEQUENTIAL DESIGNS

Although sequential analysis has practical appeal for clinical research, several issues need to be addressed concerning its limitations. One practical disadvantage is the limitation of analysis to two treatments. Many clinical studies involve more than two levels of an independent variable or more than one independent variable. Sequential designs do not provide an opportunity to explore multiple effects or interaction effects. Snell and Armitage have demonstrated the use of sequential analysis with three treatment groups.[13] A separate chart was used for each pair of treatments, so that three comparisons were made. This approach allows for conclusions for each paired comparison, but it does not provide a basis for overall comparisons, in the manner of an analysis of variance (see Chapter 20). Such multiple comparisons using sequential designs are rare in the literature.

Many researchers have looked at more than one dependent variable during the course of a sequential trial. These paths can be plotted on different graphs or combined on one graph to show their relationship. The disadvantage to this approach is that the variables may not demonstrate changes at the same rate or in the same direction; that is, preferences may not be the same for each dependent variable. Therefore, the paths for each dependent variable may cross different boundaries, or they may require a different number of total subjects. When this approach is used, the trial must continue until all variables have crossed a boundary; however, it is often difficult to determine how conflicting preferences should be interpreted.

Sequential plans do not provide an opportunity to control for extraneous variables in an experimental design, except by the nature of randomization of pairs. Some researchers try to match subjects on one or two important variables, but this has limited value as far as creating a representative sample. Many researchers have found it helpful to supplement sequential analysis with other more formal statistical methods, to examine different aspects of the data. For instance, multivariate methods, such as discriminant analysis (see Chapter 27), can be used to study the relationship among several patient characteristics and responses to treatment.

A more theoretical issue arises in the consideration of the effect of ties. When the difference between two treatments within a pair does not meet the criterion for demonstrating preference, that pair of subjects is discarded from the sequential analysis. If many ties occur, the final sample that is used for statistical testing is not a true random sample; that is, it is not a true representation of all tied and untied pairs that were originally chosen.[14] It is useful to keep a record of ties, as they provide information about the similarity of treatments. If the researcher finds that too many pairs result in ties, it might be reasonable to end the trial, as very little information will be gained by continuing to collect data. Such a decision is considered a **conditional decision** (as opposed to a terminal decision that occurs when a boundary is crossed). A conditional decision is rendered without crossing a boundary, but is based on practical considerations and observation of the plotted path.

The issue of random selection may also be of some concern in regard to the essential principle of sequential analysis—the stopping of a trial when a boundary is crossed. In a fixed sample study, a large group is chosen, with randomization promising representative and balanced treatment groups. In a sequential study, however, the patients that are admitted early in the trial are not necessarily representative of a larger population. For instance, they may be sicker patients, those who attend clinics regularly, or those who are more available for treatment. Sequential analysis is inappropriate, therefore, when the purpose of an investigation is specifically to estimate population characteristics. Therefore, the external validity of sequential studies must be supported by replication, using either sequential or nonsequential experiments.

Sequential trials are also somewhat limited by the time frame within which treatment effects can be expected to occur. The response should be observable relatively soon after treatment is begun. The outcome should at least be available within an observation period that is short relative to the total time of the study.[14] Otherwise, at any point in time, there will be a large number of subjects entered into the trial, but only a small proportion of results will be available. For instance, if a treatment effect is not expected for 6 months, within 1 year many subjects may have started treatment, but hardly any results would have been obtained. Consequently, the sequential rationale for economizing on time and subjects is subverted.

COMMENTARY

Try It, You Might Like It!

The sequential clinical trial is one alternative in a wide variety of experimental designs available for clinical research; however, just like any other design, it is not appropriate in every research situation. It is useful in experiments where the format for data collection lends itself to sequential analysis and where it is important to terminate a trial quickly with a minimal sample size.[15] It is also important to consider the rationale behind using a sequential clinical trial, based on the comparison of treatment effects, and not to use this design simply because it offers a nonmathematical approach to statistical testing.

A major advantage of sequential analysis is that it more readily fits a clinical research model, allowing for subjects to enter the study as they are admitted for treatment and providing a structure for administering treatment within a clinical context; that is, the experimental treatments can be applied as they would be during normal practice, without having to create an artificial experimental environment. The sequential trial also provides a useful mechanism for studying qualitative outcomes, using the measure of preferences. In a practical sense, this approach can be quite effective as an adjunct to clinical decision making, because it allows the decision to be based on a variety of empirical criteria.

KEY TERMS

sequential clinical trial	preference	Type I error
crossover design	stopping rule	Type II error
terminal decision	closed sequential plan	power
sequential analysis	effect size	conditional decision

REFERENCES

1. Bross IDJ. Sequential clinical trials. *J Chron Dis* 1958;8:349.
2. Wald A. *Sequential Analysis.* New York: Wiley, 1947.
3. Armitage P. Sequential tests in prophylactic and therapeutic trials. *Q J Med* 1954;23:225.
4. Light KE, Nuzik S, Personius W, et al. Low-load prolonged stretch vs. high-load brief stretch in treating knee contractures. *Phys Ther* 1984; 64:330–3.

5. Bohannon RW. Knee extension torque during repeated knee extension–flexion reversals and separated knee extension–flexion dyads. *Phys Ther* 1985;65:1052–4.
6. Gault SJ, Spyker JM. Beneficial effect of immobilization of joints in rheumatoid and related arthritides: a splint study using sequential analysis. *Arthritis Rheum* 1969;12:34–44.
7. Armitage P. *Sequential Medical Trials.* 2d ed. New York: Wiley, 1975.
8. Armitage P. Restricted sequential procedures. *Biometrika* 1957;44:9.
9. Bross I. Sequential medical plans. *Biometrics* 1952;8:188.
10. Brown A, Mohemed SD, Montgomery RD, et al. Value of a large dose of antitoxin in clinical tetanus. *Lancet* 1960;2:227–30.
11. Rutherford WH, Calderwood JW, Hart D, Merrett JD. Antibiotics in surgical treatment of septic lesions. *Lancet* 1970;1:1077–80.
12. Friedman LM, Furberg CD, DeMets DL. *Fundamentals of Clinical Trials,* 2d ed. Littleton, MA: PSG, 1985.
13. Snell ES, Armitage P. Clinical comparison of diamorphine and pholcodine as cough suppressants, by a new method of sequential analysis. *Lancet* 1957;1:860.
14. Mainland D. Statistical ward rounds 4. *Clin Pharmacol Ther* 1967;8:615.
15. Colton T. A rebuttal of "Statistical ward round 4." *Clin Pharmacol Ther* 1968;9:113–128.

Suggested Additional Readings

Colton T. *Statistics in Medicine.* Boston, Little, Brown, 1974 (Chap. 8: Sequential Analysis, pp. 229–236).
Gonella C. Designs for clinical research. *Phys Ther* 1973;53:1276 (describes the use of clinical trials and sequential trials).
Mainland D. Part II. Dr. Colton's rebuttal of ward rounds 4: comments and more thoughts about sequential trials. *Clin Pharmacol Ther* 1968;9:120 (thoughtful discussion of several issues associated with sequential trials).
Pasternak BS, Shore RE. Group sequential methods for cohort and case–control studies. *J Chronic Dis* 1980;33:365–73.

Additional Examples of Sequential Clinical Trials

Cattaneo AD, Lucchelli PE, Bona N, et al. Sequential experimentation and multivariate analysis in the evaluation of a treatment for postoperative intestinal symptoms. *Clin Pharmacol Ther* 1966;7:429–35 (uses Bross's plans A and B, plus discriminant analysis).
Coninx P, Nasca S, et al. Sequential trial of initial chemotherapy for advanced cancer of the head and neck. *Cancer* 1988;62:1888–92 (uses a closed sequential plan at $\theta_1 = .95$ in a randomized study).
Fearnley ME, Rainer EH, Taverner D, et al. Cervical sympathetic block in treatment of Bell's palsy: a controlled trial. *Lancet* 1964;2:725 (uses Armitage's plan for $\theta_1 = .90$ in a random study comparing treatment against a control).
Jacobs JH, Grayson MF. Trial of an anti-inflammatory agent (Indomethacin) in low back pain with and without radicular involvement. *Br Med J* 1968;3:158–60 (uses a closed plan at $\theta_1 = .85$ in a double-blind study comparing treatment against placebo in two separate trials for different diagnostic categories; preferences plotted based on both subjective and objective criteria).
Kao LC, Warburton D, Cheng M, et al. Effect of oral diuretics on pulmonary mechanics in infants with chronic bronchopulmonary dysplasia: results of a double-blind crossover sequential trial. *Pediatrics* 1984;74:37–44 (double-blind crossover design for preferences using a restricted plan for $\theta_1 = .90$ and $\alpha_2 = .01$).
Smith JM, Devey GF. Clinical trial of disodium cromoglycate in treatment of asthma in children. *Br Med J* 1968;2:340–4 (double-blind crossover study using a restricted sequential plan for preferences).

ADDENDA

Sequential plans for evaluating preferences at $\alpha_2 = .05$ and $1-\beta = .95$ for various levels of θ_1. Boundaries are drawn from coordinates shown in Table 11.2.

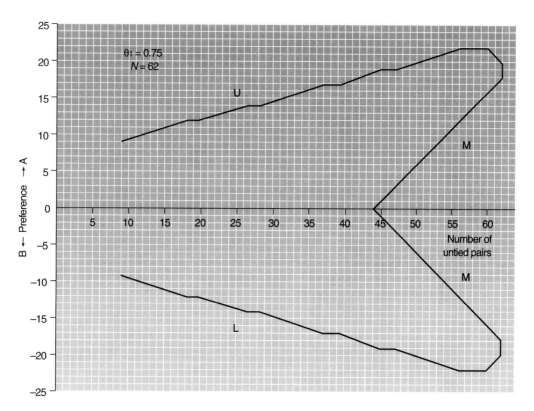

ADDENDUM 11.1

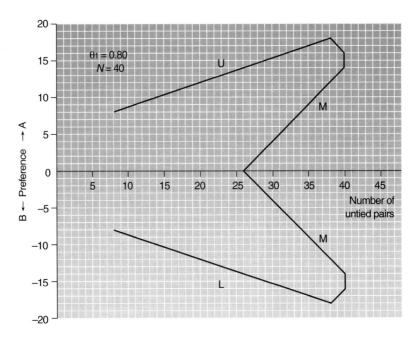

ADDENDUM 11.2

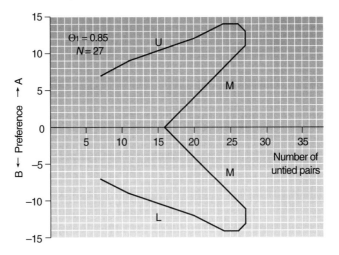

ADDENDUM 11.3

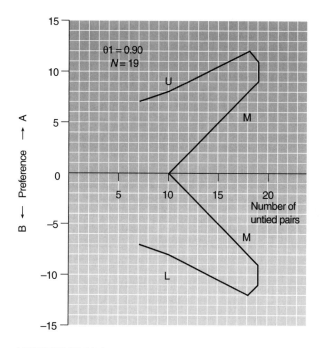

ADDENDUM 11.4

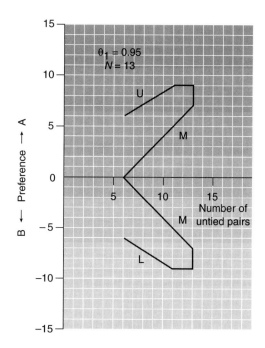

ADDENDUM 11.5

12

Single-Subject Designs

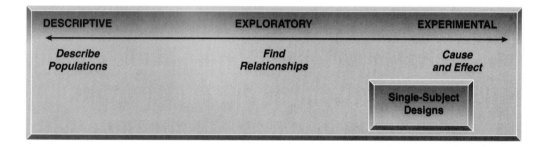

The demands of traditional experimental methods are often seen as barriers to clinical inquiry because of their rigorous structure, requiring control groups and large numbers of subjects. In addition, the experimental model deals with group averages and generalizations across individuals, philosophically conflicting with the clinical appreciation of that which is unique and different in each client or patient. Group data do not allow the researcher to differentiate characteristics of those patients who responded favorably to treatment from those who did not improve. Therefore, although generalizations are important for explaining behavioral phenomena, clinicians understand that group performance is relevant only if it can be used to understand and predict individual performance.

Given the practical and philosophical limitations of traditional experimental research, an alternative approach is needed that will allow us to draw conclusions about the effects of treatment based on the responses of a single patient under controlled conditions. **Single-subject designs,*** derived from applied behavior analysis, were developed for this purpose. Through a variety of strategies and structures, these designs provide a clinically

---

*These designs have also been called *single-system strategies*[1], N of 1 studies,[2] and *time-series designs*.[3] Cook and Campbell describe time-series designs as quasi-experimental designs with multiple measurements over time.[4] They present several variations of these designs, which are analogous to the withdrawal and multiple baseline designs presented in this chapter. The subject or system used most often is a single individual, but the sampling unit may be any unit of interest, such as a small group, a community, a department, or an institution.

viable, controlled experimental approach to the study of a single case or several subjects, and the flexibility to observe change under ongoing treatment conditions. Single-subject designs require the same attention to logical design and control as any other experimental design, based on a research hypothesis that indicates the expected relationship between an independent and dependent variable and specific operational definitions that address reliability and validity. The independent variable is the intervention. The dependent variable is the patient response, defined as a **target behavior** that is observable, quantifiable, and a valid indicator of treatment effectiveness.

Single-subject designs can be used to study comparisons between several treatments, between components of treatments, or between treatment and no-treatment conditions. They can also be used to study sequential activities, such as training strategies or techniques to shape behavioral responses. The purpose of this chapter is to describe a variety of single-subject designs and to explore issues associated with their structure, analysis, and interpretation.

STRUCTURE OF SINGLE-SUBJECT DESIGNS

Single-subject designs are structured around two core elements that distinguish them from a case study or group studies: repeated measurement and design phases.

Repeated Measurement

Single-subject designs involve the systematic collection of *repeated measurements* of a behavioral response over time, usually at frequent and regular intervals, such as at each treatment session (which may be more than once a day, each day, or once a week). These repeated assessments are required to observe trends and patterns in the data and to evaluate variability of the behavioral response over time. This type of variability is obscured in group studies when behavior is measured only before and after treatment. The advantage of repeated assessment is that the researcher can observe response patterns and modify the design as the study progresses to obtain the most meaningful outcome.

Design Phases

The second core element of a single-subject design is the delineation of at least two testing periods, or phases: a **baseline phase,** prior to treatment, and an **intervention phase,** during treatment. The target behavior is measured repeatedly across both baseline and intervention phases. The baseline phase provides information about responses during a period of "no treatment," or a control condition. This initial observation period reflects the natural state of the target behavior over time in the absence of the independent variable. The assumption is that baseline data reflect the ongoing effects of background variables, such as daily activities, other treatments, and personal characteristics, on the target behavior. Therefore, when treatment is initiated, changes from baseline to the intervention phase should be attributable to intervention. Therefore, baseline data provide a standard of comparison for evaluating the potential cause-and-effect relationship between the intervention and target behavior.[5]

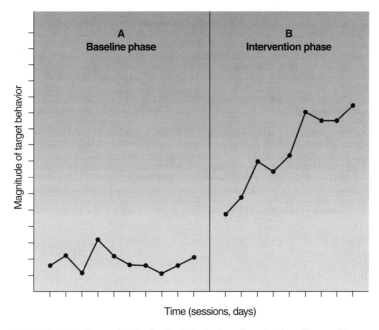

FIGURE 12.1 Example of a basic A–B design, showing baseline and intervention phases.

Design phases are traditionally plotted on a line graph, as shown in Figure 12.1, with magnitude of the target behavior along the *Y*-axis and time (sessions, trials, days, weeks) along the *X*-axis. Using conventional notation, the baseline period is represented by the letter *A* and the intervention period by the letter *B*. To facilitate description, this design, with one baseline phase and one intervention phase, is called an **A–B design.**

The collection of baseline data is the single feature of a single-subject design that particularly distinguishes it from clinical practice, case studies, and traditional experimental designs, where treatment is initiated immediately following assessment. From a research standpoint, the traditional approach makes it impossible to determine which components of treatment actually caused observed changes, or more importantly, if observed changes would have occurred without intervention. Just as we need a control group to validate group comparisons, we must have a control period to make these determinations for a single-subject experiment.

Ethical objections often arise when the baseline concept is introduced, just as they do when a control group is proposed for a group comparison study. Two points must be made in this regard. First, we can argue that it is not unethical to withhold treatment for a relatively short period when we are unsure about the effectiveness of the intervention in the first place. Indeed, it may actually be unethical to continue to provide an inferior or ineffective treatment without testing it experimentally. It is, however, important to realize that this approach is not appropriate for studying every type of intervention, such as treatments for critical or life-threatening situations, when treatment effects are not questioned and withholding treatment would be harmful. Second, collecting baseline data does not mean that the clinician is denying all treatment to the patient. It only means that one portion of the patient's total treatment is being isolated for study while all other treatments and activities are continued as background.

Baseline Characteristics

Two characteristics of baseline data are important for interpretation of clinical outcomes: **stability,** which reflects the consistency of response over time, and **trend,** or slope, which shows the rate of change in the behavior. The most desirable baseline pattern demonstrates a constant level of behavior with minimal variability, indicating that the target behavior is not changing (see Figure 12.2A). Therefore, changes that are observed following intervention can be confidently attributed to a treatment effect. If treatment has no effect, we would expect to see this baseline pattern continue into the intervention phase.

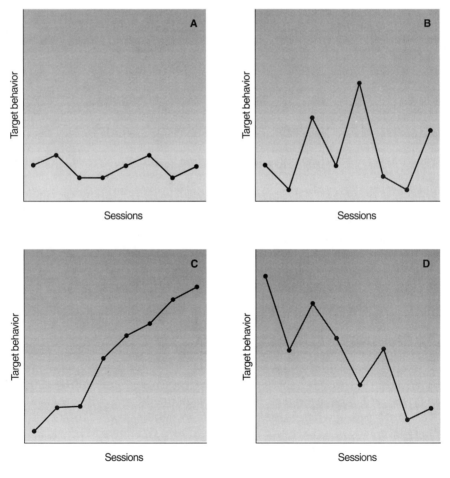

FIGURE 12.2   Types of baselines that may be encountered in single-case designs: (**A**) stable, level baseline, (**B**) variable baseline, (**C**) stable accelerating trend, (**D**) variable decelerating trend.

A variable baseline (Figure 12.2B) can present a problem for interpretation. When this type of pattern emerges, it is generally advisable to continue to collect baseline data until some stability is achieved. With extreme variability, the researcher is obliged to consider what factors might be influencing the target behavior to create such an erratic response. Sometimes cyclical patterns are evident, perhaps with variations corresponding to days of the week, time of day, or regular events occurring in the subject's life. If these factors continue to operate during intervention, they could easily obscure treatment effects.

An *accelerating* baseline (Figure 12.2C) suggests an increasing rate of response; a *decelerating* baseline (Figure 12.2D) suggests a decreasing rate. Either type of trend may represent improvement or deterioration, depending on the target behavior. In either case, a trend in baseline data indicates that a change in the target behavior is occurring without intervention. Trends can also be characterized as stable or unstable; that is, the rate of change may be constant (as in Figure 12.2C) or variable (as in Figure 12.2D). Trends in baseline data must be identified to determine if responses that are observed during the treatment phase logically represent change.

Length of Phases

One of the first questions clinicians ask when planning single-subject experiments concerns the length of phases. Single-subject designs provide some flexibility in these choices, allowing for consideration of the type of patient, the type of treatment, and the expected rate of change in the target behavior. This flexibility differentiates the single-subject design from traditional designs where onset and duration of treatment are established prior to experimentation, regardless of how the patient responds. There are some guidelines that can be followed to assist in these decisions.

It is generally desirable to use relatively equal phase length. It is not uncommon, for example, to find that researchers preset intervals of 1 week for each phase in a design when daily measurements are taken. This practice helps to control for potential time-related factors such as maturation or the motivational influence of continued attention over prolonged treatment periods. Despite these plans, however, it is usually advisable to extend baseline or intervention phases until stability is achieved, or at least until one is sure that responses are representative of the true condition under study. Most importantly, it is essential that the length of time within each phase is sufficient to capture any changes that will occur over time.

Because trend is an important characteristic of repeated measurements, there must be a minimum of three to four data points in each phase. Clearly, the greater the number of data points, the more obvious trends will become. It is useful to remember that the intervals used for repeated measurements may not represent single days. If appropriate, more than one session can be plotted within a day, so that a sufficient number of data points can be obtained in a short period.

TARGET BEHAVIOR

Target behaviors can reflect different response systems and may focus on impairments, functional limitations, or measures of disability. Measurements may deal with overt motor behaviors, such as functional performance, ROM, strength, or gait characteristics. We can also assess physiological reactions, such as blood pressure or exercise responses, and verbal reactions, such as the number of correct responses to specific questions or subjective feelings of pain.[5] Assessment techniques vary, depending on the types of variables designated as target behaviors. One benefit of the single-subject approach is the ability to develop individualized measurement systems that reflect a patient's performance in a clinically relevant way. For instance, specific functional tasks may be emphasized that indicate a patient's major limitations. The choice of a target behavior can be an important first step in making a single-subject study meaningful.

Measuring the Target Behavior

Although many clinical variables are typically assessed using qualitative values, they must be quantified in some way to be used as experimental data. One major advantage of the single-subject approach is that it provides a mechanism for quantifying even the most subjective clinical behaviors. The most common techniques for measuring behaviors within single-subject designs are frequency, duration, and magnitude measures.

Frequency

Behaviors can be measured by counting the number of occurrences of that behavior within a fixed time interval or a fixed number of trials. A *frequency count* is the simplest of all behavioral measures and is an appropriate way to assess discrete clinical behaviors. For example, we can count the number of times a particular gait deviation occurs, the number of times a patient can repeat a certain exercise, or the number of times a patient loses her balance during a treatment session. Operational definitions for frequency counts must specify how the target behavior is distinguished from other responses and exactly what constitutes an occurrence and nonoccurrence of the target behavior. For instance, if a patient attempts an exercise and achieves only partial range, is that counted as an occurrence? If a patient begins to fall over but catches herself by reaching for the wall, is that considered loss of balance?

Frequency counts are not useful when a behavior occurs too often to be counted reliably or when the behavior lasts for a long time, and therefore occurs too seldom to be counted meaningfully. The total time or total number of trials within which the count is made must remain constant across sessions, so that results at each session are comparable. We must also recognize that frequency counts do not reflect the quality of the behavior, but only that it occurred.

Frequency can be expressed as a percentage, by dividing the number of occurrences of the target behavior by the total number of opportunities for the behavior to occur. This method is often used in studies where accuracy of performance (percentage correct) is of primary interest. Percentages are useful in that they are easily understood, are efficient for summarizing large numbers of responses, and can normalize frequency counts obtained during intervals of different lengths. If, however, the actual number of correct responses is an important indicant of the target behavior, percentages can be misleading because they do not provide information about the number of responses observed, the total time period over which the behavior was assessed, or the total number of trials that were attempted.

Frequency counts can also be translated into *rates.* Rate refers to the number of times a behavior occurs within a specified time period. It is calculated by dividing the total number of occurrences of the behavior by the total time (seconds, minutes, or hours) during which the behavior was observed. For example, we can measure ambulation in steps per minute or endurance in repetitions per minute.

Duration

Target behaviors can also be evaluated according to how long they last. *Duration* can be measured either as the cumulative total duration of a behavior during a treatment session or as the duration of each individual occurrence of the behavior. Operational definitions for duration measures must specify criteria for determining when the behavior starts and when it ends. For example, we can measure how long a patient stays in a balanced standing posture within a single trial or over a treatment session, or we can time how long it takes for a patient to complete a specific functional task, such as buttoning a shirt.

Duration can also be reported in terms of percentages. For example, Leiper et al. studied the effects of a head position monitor on head tilt in a group of children with cerebral palsy.[6] They used a stopwatch to measure the amount of time each child was able to maintain his head in the desired angular zone. They then calculated "percentage time in zone" by dividing total time in the desired zone by total time of the training session. This approach is useful for comparisons when the sessions are not of equal length.

Magnitude

Many clinical variables are measured using some form of instrumentation that provides a quantitative score. In psychological and educational studies these types of measures are used less often, but they have a strong place in rehabilitation research as many physical and physiological variables can be measured directly. For example, Laskas et al. used electromyography (measured in microvolts) to monitor the effect of neurodevelopmental treatment on dorsiflexor activity in a 2-year-old boy with cerebral palsy.[7] In another study, Ray et al. measured the amount of saliva collected during drooling following a technique to facilitate mouth closure.[8]

Magnitude measures can also be used to demonstrate change in functional scales. Many instruments provide a quantitative score, which may be a summary score, a subscale score, or a single test value. For example, Tona and Schneck used the Modified Ashworth Score as the target behavior to document the effect of inhibitive casting on resistance to passive motion in a child with upper extremity spasticity.[9] Kaelin et al. evaluated the effect of Ritalin on attention deficit and function in adults with acute brain injury using neuropsychological tests and the Disability Rating Scale score.[10] Function can also be assessed using basic outcome measures such as gait parameters to determine the effectiveness of intervention. For instance, Diamond and Ottenbacher measured velocity, step length, and cadence to evaluate the effects of different ankle-foot orthoses in a patient with right hemiparesis.[11] These examples illustrate the potential for using single-subject designs to study changes in outcomes, including impairments, functional limitations, and disability measures.

Interval Recording for Observational Measures

Target behaviors are generally recorded using either quantitative instrumentation, self-report, or direct observation. The use of instrumentation is appropriate for many magnitude measures and is advantageous in that it is objective. Self-report is often used to monitor activities that occur outside the clinical environment and for which the clinician must depend on the subject's perception of performance. Probably the most common approach is the use of observational measures for assessing behavioral acts.

Observational measures are often recorded using frequency and duration methods to monitor the occurrence or nonoccurrence of the behavior. For instance, Dave studied the effects of vestibular stimulation on stereotypic body-rocking behaviors in three adults with profound mental retardation.[12] Such a behavior is difficult to quantify, except to say that it does or does not occur. One useful approach for measuring this type of repetitive behavior is to break down the measurement period into preset time intervals, and to determine if the behavior occurs or does not occur during each interval. In this example, the author monitored the behavior for a 5-minute period, looking at the occurrence or nonoccurrence of rocking within consecutive 15-second intervals. This procedure is called *interval recording*, or time sampling. The researcher tallied how many of the intervals contain an occurrence of rocking. This tally is the value that is plotted as the frequency of the behavior.

Interval sampling requires dividing the total treatment session into small equal intervals. Measurement may involve simply recording the presence or absence of the target behavior within each interval and then tallying how many intervals contained the behavior, or it may involve recording the frequency or duration of the behavior within each interval. It is important to select a time interval that will best reflect the expected frequency and duration of the target behavior. For example, with short-duration or high-frequency behaviors, smaller time intervals should be used, as in the previous example with rocking behaviors. Some studies use intervals as short as 10 seconds. With long-duration or low-frequency behaviors, longer intervals are necessary, sometimes as long as 10 or 15 minutes.

Interval recording requires the use of some type of signaling device to indicate the start and end of each interval. Researchers have used kitchen timers, prerecorded tones on a tape recorder, timed light cues, and stopwatches for this purpose. It is usually necessary to practice using the signal device, as measurements are taken very quickly. Some researchers use an assistant to provide signaling cues. With auditory cues, many researchers use earphones to minimize reactivity of measurements.

Choosing a Target Behavior

Because patients usually present several clinical problems, choosing one specific problem as the focus of an experiment can be difficult. To focus on one target behavior, it is often necessary to define complex behaviors and determine which component of the behavior is most problematic.[13] It is useful to consider the relative stability with which a behavior is expected to respond. It is also important to establish that a specific intervention is readily available to address the target behavior, that the behavior is a valid indicator of that intervention's effectiveness, and that the treatment will cause an observable change in the behavior. Finally, choice of a target behavior may be influenced by available instrumentation and clinical goals. Researchers can also look at several target behaviors simultaneously, to examine their potential interaction or to document the relationship between impairments and functional measures.

In addition, a measurement method must be chosen that will reflect the element of performance that is of primary concern. Is it how often a patient can perform a particular task, or how long a behavior can be maintained? Is the number of correct responses or incorrect responses of interest? Or is it simply whether or not the behavior occurs? Each measurement method will provide a different perspective of the target behavior, which will obviously influence how the data will be interpreted.

Target behaviors can be defined according to the specific responses that constitute performance, or by delineating functional outcomes. For example, if we wanted to assess the efficacy of a treatment for frozen shoulder, we could look directly at range of motion measurements or we could assess the patient's ability to reach or dress. Functional measures, however, are based on assumptions about the relationship with impairments. For example, Sharpe and Ottenbacher used a single-subject design to study the effect of using elbow restraints on stereotypical involuntary hand movements in a child with Rett syndrome.[14] Because the focus of treatment was an improvement in functional skills, the investigators chose to look at the child's ability to finger-feed cereal from a bowl as the target behavior. The observed experimental effects were smaller than they expected, providing only minimal support for their hypothesis. The authors expressed the reservation that had they measured a more direct aspect of hand movement, results may have been more dramatic. Their result emphasizes the need to choose a target behavior that is sensitive enough to show meaningful change.

This example also demonstrates the utility of single-subject designs for evaluation of the relationship between impairments and functional limitations. More than one target behavior can be examined at the same time, to determine if an intervention affects them differently. For instance, Sharpe and Ottenbacher[14] could have looked at the functional activity of finger-feeding at the same time that they examined specific coordination movements, range of motion, or the ability to touch a target. Had they seen changes in these actions, but not in the functional activity, they would then have to question the relationship between these individual motions and the activity they wanted to encourage. In this way, researchers can examine both the specific impairments, such as range of motion, strength, pain, or coordination, and the functional limitations that we often assume are sequelae of these impairments. This approach provides a useful opportunity to examine the theoretical framework that often guides our clinical thinking.

RELIABILITY

Reliability is important in single-subject research as it is in any form of clinical inquiry. Because the single-subject experiment focuses on observation of behaviors in a clinical setting, reliability is usually assessed concurrently with data collection, rather than in a separate pilot study. Researchers usually report interrater reliability using a measure of percent agreement between observers.[15] Reliability checks are performed by having two testers simultaneously observe the target behavior at several sessions across each phase of the study. An agreement score is obtained for each session, and results are then re-ported as a range of agreement scores or as an average.[†]

Total Reliability

Total reliability reflects reliability of data obtained by two raters during a single trial. To-tal reliability is calculated by dividing the smaller frequency or duration obtained by one observer by the larger value obtained by the other observer, and multiplying by 100. For example, suppose we wanted to measure the interrater reliability of two clinicians recording the total number of steps taken during an ambulation session. If one observer records a total of 25 steps, and the second observer records 28 steps for the same trial, the total reliability for that trial would be $(25/28) \times 100 = 89\%$.

The interpretation of total reliability is limited in that it reflects only the consistency of obtaining a total score for a session, not the reliability of individual observations of behav-ior.[17] Therefore, it is possible that within a single session, two clinicians will actually ob-serve different instances of the target behavior, but agree on a total score. For instance, sup-pose two raters measure the total duration of standing balance (in seconds) over a 2-minute period. Both record 30 seconds. The first rater may have observed the patient in a balanced state during the first 15 seconds and last 15 seconds of the trial, while the second rater recorded the behavior during the middle 30 seconds of the trial. Even though the raters did not agree at all on the actual occurrence of the behavior, their total reliability is 100%. There-fore, measures of total reliability may provide an inflated estimate of reliability.

Point-by-Point Reliability

A more precise measure of agreement focuses on responses during individual time in-tervals, trials, or points in time. Depending on the unit of analysis, this approach has been called interval-by-interval, trial-by-trial, or *point-by-point reliability.*[18] With this ap-proach, the number of occasions on which the observers agree that the behavior either occurred or did not occur is divided by the total number of recording occasions (or the total number of occasions on which they agree and disagree). This value is multiplied by 100 to yield percent agreement. This definition fits the traditional definition of percent agreement used in studies of categorical data (see Chapter 26).

For example, in Sharpe and Ottenbacher's study of finger-feeding, described earlier, the researchers observed 30 trials within a session in which the subject attempted to pick up a piece of cereal and put it in her mouth.[14] Reliability was established by determin-ing how often two observers agreed on the success or failure of each trial. Suppose, for a single session, the two raters agreed on 29 of the 30 trials. Trial-by-trial reliability would then be $(29/30) \times 100 = 97\%$.

In a similar fashion, interval-by-interval reliability is established by looking at agree-ment or disagreement for each interval within a time sample. For instance, McCullough et al. looked at the occurrence of cooperative behaviors in a child with behavior disor-der by dividing hourly sessions into 15-minute intervals.[19] For each interval, observers

---

[†]With magnitude data, reliability can also be established using correlational methods, such as the intraclass cor-relation coefficient (see Chapter 26); however, in an effort to keep single-case research a "people's science," be-havior analysts have traditionally preferred not to use correlational procedures.[16]

TABLE 12.1.   INTEROBSERVER RELIABILITY DATA BASED ON SCORING THE OCCURRENCE (+) OR NONOCCURRENCE (–) OF COOPERATIVE BEHAVIOR

	15-Minute Intervals															
	1	**2**	**3**	**4**	**5**	**6**	**7**	**8**	**9**	**10**	**11**	**12**	**13**	**14**	**15**	**16**
Observer 1	+	–	+	–	+	+	+	–	+	–	–	+	+	–	+	+
Observer 2	+	–	–	–	–	+	+	–	+	–	+	+	+	–	+	+
Agreements	+	–		–		+	+	–	+	–		+	+	–	+	+

scored a plus if the child exhibited cooperative behaviors only and a minus if the child exhibited any uncooperative behaviors. Hypothetical results for this type of reliability check are shown in Table 12.1. Of 16 intervals, the observers disagreed three times, in intervals 3, 5, and 11. Therefore, of 16 occasions, 13 were agreements, resulting in an interobserver reliability of $(13/16) \times 100 = 81\%$.

Occurrence and Nonoccurrence Reliability

Percent agreement is an intuitively useful measure, but it, too, is limited in that it can be artificially inflated by very high or very low response rates. In other words, when a behavior occurs quite often, the chance is much greater that two raters will agree on its occurrence, just because of its increased frequency, even when they are not applying consistent criteria. The same is true of nonoccurrence. As a control for this type of chance agreement, some investigators will focus reliability specifically on occurrences or nonoccurrences of the target behavior.[17]

When a target behavior occurs with low to moderate frequency (less than 75% of the sampled intervals),[20] a reliability test is directed toward agreement on occurrences. *Occurrence reliability* is obtained by dividing the number of intervals in which the observers agreed the behavior occurred by the number of intervals in which one or both of the observers recorded an occurrence. For the data in Table 12.1, one or both observers scored an occurrence in 11 intervals. They agreed that the behavior occurred in 8 of those intervals. Therefore, occurrence reliability is $(8/11) \times 100 = 73\%$. *Nonoccurrence reliability* is of interest when the target behavior occurs with high frequency (greater than 75% of the intervals).[20] It is calculated by dividing the number of agreements on nonoccurrences of the behavior by the number of intervals in which one or both observers scored a nonoccurrence. For the data in Table 12.1, one or both observers scored a nonoccurrence in 8 intervals. They agreed that the behavior did not occur in 5 of these intervals. Therefore, nonoccurrence reliability is $(5/8) \times 100 = 62.5\%$.

Chance Agreement

Issues of chance agreement can also be addressed using procedures that provide formal statistical correction, such as the *kappa* statistic κ, which is a chance-corrected measure of percent agreement.[21,22] Although kappa is obtained easily, it has not been reported with any regularity in the behavioral analysis literature. It is, however, a useful method for summarizing observer consistency. The use of kappa for estimating agreement is described in Chapter 26.

EXPERIMENTAL CONTROL: LIMITATIONS OF THE A–B DESIGN

The element that most clearly characterizes an experimental research design is its ability to control for threats to internal validity (see Chapter 9). Unfortunately, the basic A–B single-subject design is limited in this respect. Consider the following example:

> Researchers explored the relationship between language development and sensory integration using a single-subject experimental study of four aphasic children ranging in age from 4 years, 0 months to 5 years, 3 months.[23] Other agencies had assessed all the children in the area of language development at least 6 months before the start of occupational therapy. Three of the four children had received either speech therapy, special education specific to aphasia, or both, before starting occupational therapy. Additional baseline data on language expression and comprehension, as well as on sensory integrative functioning, were gathered before beginning a year of occupational therapy that involved sensory integration procedures.

Figure 12.3 shows the development of language comprehension in one child for this study. Stable responses were observed over a 9-week baseline phase. Immediately fol-

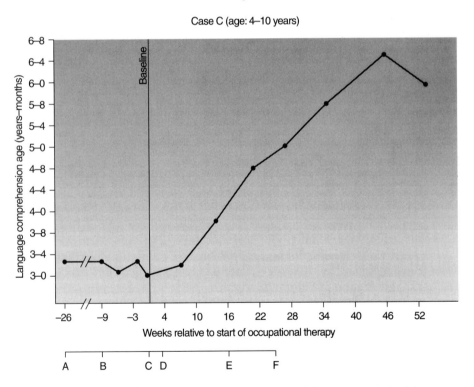

FIGURE 12.3   Example of an A–B design, illustrating potential threats to internal validity: scores on a language comprehension test in an aphasic child before and after the onset of occupational therapy. Relevant events: (A) initial testing, (B) first baseline data gathered, (C) started occupational therapy, (D) started individual speech therapy, (E) entered public school aphasia class, (F) started developmental therapy. (Adapted from Ayres AJ, Mailloux Z. Influence of sensory integration procedures on language development. *Am J Occup Ther* 1981; 35:383–90, Figure 3, p. 187. Copyright 1981 by the American Occupational Therapy Association. Reprinted with permission.)

lowing the onset of occupational therapy, scores rose markedly, suggesting at first glance that the therapy was instrumental in achieving this change. But is this conclusion definitive? Did other events or changes within the subject occur coincidentally at the same time that treatment was initiated that could have accounted for the observed change? In other words, is this conclusion internally valid?

Note that several other events may be associated with this change. Speech therapy was begun 1 week later (D), an aphasia class started at 16 weeks (E), and a developmental therapy program began at 25 weeks (F). With this design, it is impossible to conclude that the occupational therapy treatment was the causative factor in improving language comprehension scores.

To strengthen the control in this design, we must include some other form of evidence that the treatment was indeed responsible for observed changes—evidence that will discredit alternative hypotheses for explaining treatment outcomes. Within a single-subject strategy, this additional control is provided by *replication of effects*, which can be accomplished in several ways. Phases can be repeated by withdrawing and reinstating baseline and treatment conditions or by alternating two or more interventions. For instance, we could have withdrawn the sensory integration therapy in the preceding example after 22 weeks. If the language comprehension scores decreased, we would then have evidence that the treatment was responsible for the observed trend. We can also replicate effects across more than one subject or within one subject across multiple conditions or behaviors. The more often an effect can be replicated within a design, the stronger the design controls against potential threats to internal validity. These strategies form the basis for structuring single-subject designs.

WITHDRAWAL DESIGNS

Experimental control within a single-subject design can be achieved through withdrawal of intervention, to demonstrate that the target behavior occurs only in the presence of treatment. The **withdrawal design** includes a second baseline period, but may also include a second intervention period. Because one series of measurements is taken on one behavior within one individual, these designs are also called *within-series designs*.[3]

A–B–A Design

The **A–B–A design** replicates one baseline phase following intervention. The premise of this design lies in its ability to show that behavioral changes are evident only in the presence of the intervention, during phase B. If changes in the target behavior are not maintained during the second baseline period, one can logically conclude that the treatment was the factor causing the changes observed during the intervention phase. Internal validity is controlled because it is highly unlikely that confounding factors would coincidentally occur at both the onset and the cessation of treatment. If other variables were responsible for changes seen in the target behavior during the first two phases, the behavior would not be expected to revert to baseline levels during the withdrawal phase.

> *Laskas and coworkers examined the immediate effects of four neurodevelopmental treatment (NDT) activities on two dependent variables: dorsiflexor muscle activity during an equilibrium response and frequency of heel contact during movement to a*

standing position.[7] The subject was a 2.5-year-old boy with spastic quadriplegia. During the 7 days of baseline 1, the 9 days of treatment, and the 7 days of baseline 2, dorsiflexor muscle activity was examined using an EMG instrument with surface electrodes (Figure 12.4A). Frequency of heel contact was recorded as the number of times in seven trials that the child came to a standing position with his heel contacting the floor (Figure 12.4B). Conditions were identical across all three phases except that four NDT activities were introduced during the treatment phase and were withdrawn during the second baseline phase.

The results show that dorsiflexor responses were not stable, although it is clear that the level of activity increased with treatment and decreased again when treatment was withdrawn. Changes in frequency of heel contacts were more dramatic, showing distinct changes across all phases. In this particular example, the child was tested over a fixed number of trials for heel contacts at each session, creating a ceiling effect during the intervention period.

There are obvious problems with the A–B–A design. First, for the design to be effective, the behavior must be reversible, which is often not the case. Any response that is learned or that creates permanent change will not show a decrement when treatment is withdrawn. Second, it may be ethically unreasonable, or even dangerous, to withdraw a treatment that is working. In such situations, alternative designs that do not require withdrawal can be used.

A–B–A–B Design

Experimental control and clinical relevance can be strengthened through the use of an A–B–A–B design, which provides initial baseline data and ends on an intervention phase. The major advantage of this design is that it provides two opportunities to evaluate the effects of the intervention. If effects can be replicated during two separate intervention phases, then the evidence is quite strong that behavioral change was directly related to the treatment. This is a form of experimental reliability, demonstrating consistency of response and controlling for internal validity.

Asymmetrical posture during static stance has been identified as a common problem in persons with hemiplegia. Researchers examined the effect of an activity-based therapy regimen on symmetric weight bearing in three adult subjects with hemiplegia.[24] An A–B–A–B single-subject design was used. The intervention program, including playing a bean bag game, was introduced for 30 minutes each day during each intervention phase. Quantitative measurements of weight distribution were taken with the Balance Master System.

Figure 12.5 shows results for one subject for this study. Weight distribution was plotted as a ratio of the percent weight on the affected limb over total body weight; therefore, the goal was to achieve higher ratios. Although performance is variable, there is clearly a declining ratio during both baseline phases, and increases during both intervention phases. The A–B–A–B design faces the same limitations as the A–B–A design, in that behaviors must be reversible to see treatment effects. If, however, the target behavior does not revert to original baseline values, but stays level during the second baseline, the A–B–A–B strategy still makes it possible to demonstrate change if there is further improvement during the second intervention phase.

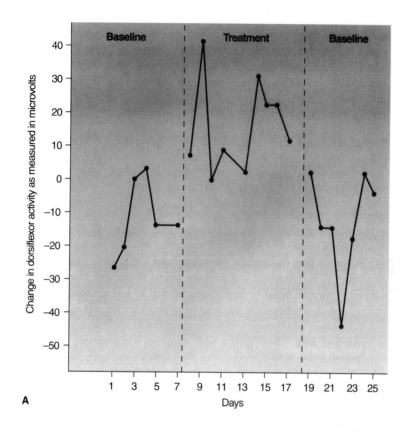

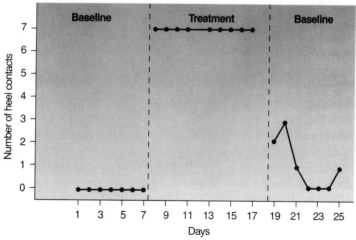

FIGURE 12.4 Examples of an A–B–A design, illustrating the effect of neurodevelopmental treatment on (**A**) changes in dorsiflexor muscle activity and (**B**) frequency of heel contacts, in a child with spastic quadriplegia. (From Laskas CA, Mullen SL, Nelson DL, et al. Enhancement of two motor functions of the lower extremity in a child with spastic quadriplegia. *Phys Ther* 1985; 65:11–16, Figure 2, p. 14; Figure 3, p. 15. Reprinted with permission of the American Physical Therapy Association.)

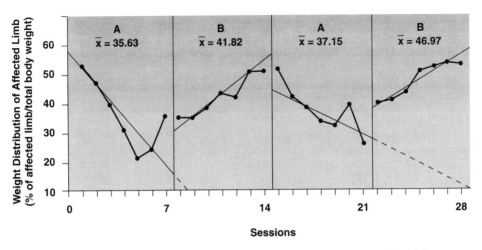

FIGURE 12.5   Example of an A–B–A–B design, showing the effect of an activity-based therapy on weight distribution over the affected leg (percent body weight) during static stance in a patient with hemiplegia. (From Wu S, Huang H, Lin C, and Chen M. Effects of a program on symmetrical posture in patients with hemiplegia: a single-subject design. *Am J Occup Ther* 1996;50:17–23, Figure 1, p. 20. Reprinted with permission of the American Occupational Therapy Association.)

MULTIPLE-TREATMENT DESIGNS

Withdrawal designs represent treatment–no treatment comparisons. Single-subject designs can also be used to compare the effects of two treatments. Using a variation of the withdrawal design, a **multiple-treatment design** typically involves the application of one treatment (B) following baseline, the withdrawal of that treatment, and introduction of another treatment (C). These two interventions can represent two different treatments or one intervention and a placebo. In an A–B–C–B design, assuming the two treatments have independent and differential effects, we should be able to see differences in the target responses across the four phases of the study. By replicating the B phase, we provide the control needed to document differences between the two treatments.

A–B–C–B designs have been used extensively to examine the effects of reinforcement procedures.[5]

Miller et al. studied the effects of monetary reinforcement on alcoholic behavior.[25] The target behavior was blood alcohol level. The first intervention, B, involved reinforcement that was contingent on a negative blood alcohol sample. In the second intervention phase, C, reinforcement was provided regardless of blood alcohol levels. In the fourth phase, contingent reinforcement was reinstated (Figure 12.6).

The results of this study show a marked change in trend when contingent reinforcement was in effect. Interpretation of multiple-treatment data is not always as straightforward as this example might suggest, however. For instance, it is important to remember that changes in the target behavior can be assessed only between *adjacent phases*. Therefore, in this example, we cannot make any statements about the client's performance during treatment C as compared with baseline; that is, we do not know what his performance would have been had treatment B not been instituted first. Often it is helpful to institute

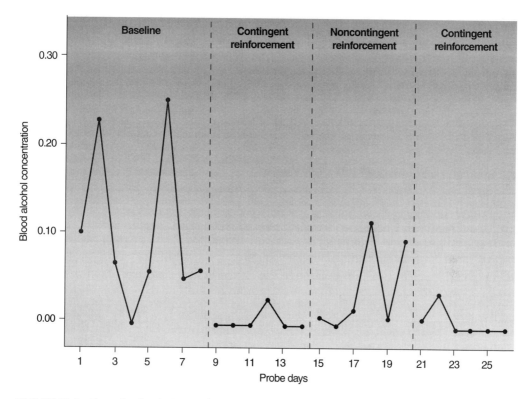

FIGURE 12.6 Example of an A–B–C–B design, showing the effect of contingent and noncontingent rewards on biweekly blood alcohol concentrations in a 48-year-old alcoholic. (From Miller PM, Hersen M, Eisler RM, et al. Contingent reinforcement of lowered blood/alcohol levels in an outpatient chronic alcoholic. *Behav Res Ther* 1974; 12:261–3, Figure 1, p. 262. Reprinted with permission. Copyright 1974 by Pergamon Press Ltd.)

a second baseline period between treatments (A–B–A–C) so that each effect can be evaluated against a "control" condition.

Similarly, it is not obvious how the response during contingent reinforcement would have varied had the noncontingent reinforcement been instituted first, that is, if we had used an A–C–B–C design. The sequence in which treatments are presented and the relative positioning of interventions and baselines can affect how results are interpreted. Order effects can be controlled using a counterbalanced strategy.[26] For instance, we could design an A–B–C–A–C–B strategy to show the sequential relationship between B and C and to examine each treatment effect relative to a baseline. In addition, by introducing each treatment condition twice, we have increased the degree of control built into the design. The second baseline phase also allows for a washout period, so that the effects of treatment C can be observed without the previous effects of treatment B.

Interactive Designs

Single-subject designs can also be used to examine the interactive or joint effect of two or more treatments as they are applied individually or as a treatment package. **Interactive**

designs are based on variations of an A–B–BC strategy (sometimes written A–B–B+C), where BC represents the combined application of interventions B and C. In this design, treatment C is superimposed on treatment B, so that combined and separate effects can be observed. When structuring this type of design, treatment effects should be replicated at least once to achieve internal validity.

> *Agras et al. studied the effects of reinforcement and feedback strategies for increasing weight gain and caloric intake in a subject with anorexia nervosa.[27] They used an A–B–BC–B–BC design, with intervention of reinforcement (B) and reinforcement plus feedback (BC) (Figure 12.7). They monitored caloric intake and weight gain simultaneously over a period of 2 months.*

If we examine caloric intake (dotted lines in Figure 12.7), we see a marked decelerating trend during baseline, followed by only a slight leveling off during reinforcement (B). When feedback was added to reinforcement (BC), however, a sharply increasing trend could be observed. This trend was not maintained when feedback was withdrawn, although responses remained level; that is, there was no withdrawal effect, probably because of carryover from BC to B. Despite the nonreversible nature of the response, we can clearly see that feedback against a background of reinforcement was more effective

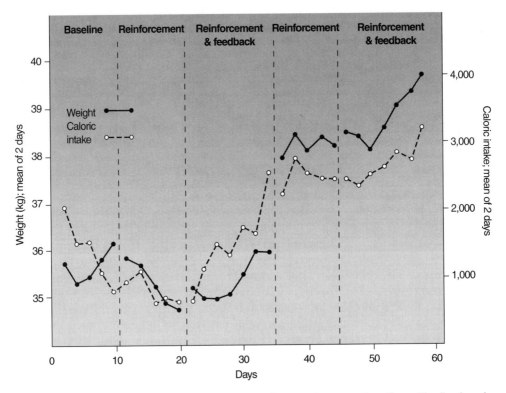

FIGURE 12.7   Example of an A–B–BC–B–BC design, showing the interactive effect of feedback and reinforcement on eating behavior of a patient with anorexia nervosa. (From Agras WS, Barlow DH, Chapin HN, et al. Behavior modification of anorexia nervosa. *Arch Gen Psychiatry* 1974; 30:279–86, Figure 4, p. 283. Reprinted with permission. Copyright 1974, American Medical Association.)

than reinforcement alone, as a marked acceleration in trend occurred once more when feedback was reinstated in the final intervention phase.

Interactive designs provide an opportunity for clinicians to examine combinations of treatments that are used in practice and to attempt to isolate extraneous or therapeutically ineffective components.[28] How the design phases are ordered will influence how these effects are demonstrated. For instance, in the preceding example, it is not possible to determine if feedback would provide a similarly successful outcome without reinforcement, or if the response during reinforcement and feedback (BC) would have been the same had it been done prior to reinforcement (B) being administered alone. It is useful to replicate these types of studies on other subjects using variations of the original design (such as A–BC–B–BC and A–C–BC–C), to determine if one treatment is superior to the other or if their interaction is important.

The study of interactions requires that only one variable be changed at a time from phase to phase, such as BC–B or B–BC, so that changes from isolated to combined conditions can be assessed across adjacent phases. For example, in the study shown in Figure 12.7, alternating from B to BC to B allows the researcher to compare the target behavior in B and BC conditions. If, however, a design such as A–BC–A–B were used, we could not make this comparison. If BC and B phases are not adjacent, we can assess the combined effect of BC only against baseline, not against B alone. Therefore, under these conditions, any interpretation about the interactive effect of the two treatments would be inconclusive.

Alternating Treatment Design

Another strategy for studying multiple treatments involves the **alternating treatment design.** The essential feature of the alternating treatment design is the rapid alternation of two or more interventions or treatment conditions, each associated with a distinct stimulus.[29] Treatment can be alternated within a treatment session, session by session, or day by day. This design can be used to compare treatment with a control or placebo or to compare two different interventions, to determine which one will be more effective. Data for each treatment condition are plotted on the same graph, allowing for comparison of data points and trends between conditions.

Scheduling of alternated "phases" will depend on the time needed to complete the treatment condition at each session and the potential for carryover from trial to trial. Because treatment conditions are continuously alternated, sequence effects are of primary concern. This concern must be addressed either by random ordering of the treatment applications on each occasion or by systematic counterbalancing. In addition, other conditions that might affect the target behavior, such as the clinician, time of day, or setting, should be counterbalanced.

Diamond and Ottenbacher used an alternating treatment design to study the effect of a traditional ankle–foot orthosis (AFO) and a tone-inhibiting dynamic AFO (TIAFO) on gait characteristics of a man with right hemiparesis.[11] They recorded baseline data with the subject barefoot over 5 baseline sessions and then randomly alternated trials with and without the two orthoses within each of 12 measurement sessions.

Figure 12.8 illustrates the outcome for step length, one of the target behaviors in this study. Baseline data indicate a low level of response for the barefoot condition. A marked increase in step length is evident in measurement trials, with the use of the TIAFO consistently resulting in a longer step length. The advantage of using the alternating treatment design over an A–B–A–B design for this type of question is that a prolonged withdrawal is unnecessary, and results can be obtained more quickly.

The alternating treatment design is also called a *between-series strategy*, indicating that analysis is not specifically concerned with trends within treatments, but that the primary focus is comparison of data points between treatment conditions. For instance, in Figure 12.8 we see that the barefoot condition improved slightly with an increasing trend across the measurement sessions; even so, on each occasion, data points demonstrate a longer step length with the orthoses than without them, and consistently higher scores with the TIAFO. Therefore, this design will work even under conditions when responses are very variable or when treatment conditions exhibit similar trends.

It is actually unnecessary to include a baseline phase in an alternating treatment design, just as a control group may not be included in group designs in which two treatments are compared. Baseline data can, however, be useful in situations when both treatments turn out to be equally effective, to show that they are better than no treatment at all.

Because target behaviors are measured in rapid succession, the alternating treatment design is appropriate when treatment effects are immediate and when behavior is a clear consequence of one specific intervention. The target behavior must be capable of changing quickly, and the interventions must be able to trigger those changes as they are

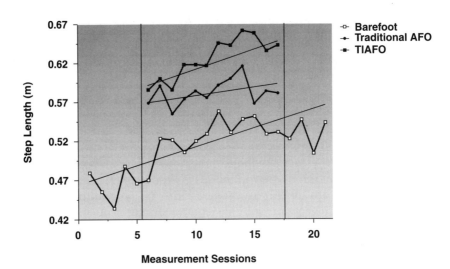

FIGURE 12.8 Example of an alternating treatment design, comparing the effects of walking barefoot, wearing a prefabricated ankle–foot orthosis, and wearing a tone-inhibiting ankle–foot orthosis on step length in a subject with hemiparesis. (From Diamond MF, Ottenbacher KJ. Effect of a tone-inhibiting dynamic ankle–foot orthosis on stride characteristics of an adult with hemiparesis. *Phys Ther* 1990;70: 423–30, Figure 3, p. 427. Reprinted with permission of the American Physical Therapy Association.)

applied and withdrawn. The alternating treatment design is not useful in situations when behavior takes time to change, when learning effects or physiological changes are cumulative and long term, or when multiple-treatment interference is likely. In those situations, it would be difficult to separate out the effects of each intervention in alternated trials. The major advantage of the alternating treatment design is that it will usually provide answers to questions of treatment comparison in a shorter time frame than designs that require introduction and withdrawal of multiple-treatment phases over time.

MULTIPLE BASELINE DESIGNS

The use of withdrawal and alternating treatment designs is limited in situations when ethical considerations of withdrawal prevail and when behaviors are either nonreversible or prone to carryover effects. When practical replication cannot be achieved either within or between series, a **multiple baseline design** can be used, where effects are replicated either across subjects, across treatment conditions, or across multiple target behaviors. The multiple baseline approach allows for use of the basic A–B format, as well as withdrawal variations and multiple-treatment strategies.

The multiple baseline design demonstrates experimental control by first requiring the concurrent collection of baseline data across a minimum of three data series. When all baselines exhibit sufficient stability, the intervention is applied only to the first series, while the other baselines are continued. When the first series achieves stability during treatment, intervention is introduced into the second series. Stability can be achieved either as a constant trend (acceleration or deceleration) or as a level response. This process is repeated on a staggered basis for all remaining baselines. By allowing each baseline to run for a different number of data points, systematic changes in the target behavior that are correlated with the onset of intervention can be reliably attributed to a treatment effect. Experimental control is strengthened by demonstrating that baselines are independent; that is, change is observed only when intervention is applied and does not occur during baseline periods. This process can be explained by example.

Multiple Baseline Design across Subjects

In a *multiple baseline design across subjects,* one intervention is applied to the same target behavior across three or more individuals who share common relevant characteristics. Figure 12.9 illustrates this design using an A–B configuration.

> *Four retarded adults were tested on their ability to use a communication board by pointing to correct letters.[29] During baseline, the subjects were tested one to three times daily. After observing stable responses over 11 sessions, the investigators introduced a process of coordination training for Jill, while baseline measures were continued for the other subjects. Once Jill's responses stabilized (and the other baselines remained stable), Pete began training after 17 baseline sessions. Similarly, Robert started training after 22 sessions, and Victor after 30 sessions.[‡]*

[‡]It is not uncommon to delay the start of baseline for those subjects who will receive treatment last, to reduce the potential reactive effects of a prolonged baseline period.

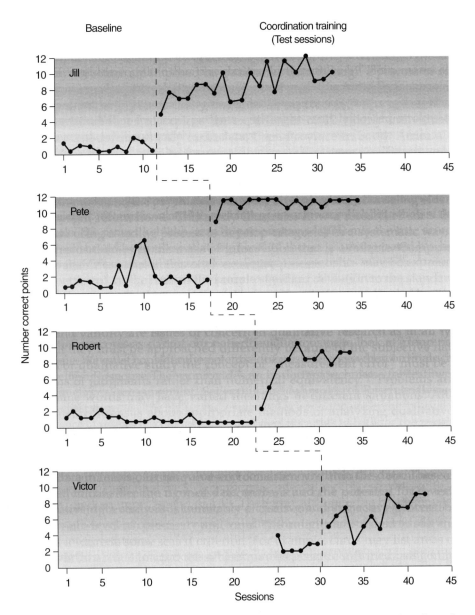

FIGURE 12.9   Example of a multiple baseline design across subjects, showing the effect of a training program on ability to point to specific blocks on a communication board using a head pointer. Subjects were four nonvocal retarded adults. (From Reid DH, Hurlbut B. Teaching nonvocal communication skills to multihandicapped retarded adults. *J Appl Behav Anal* 1977; 10:591–603, Figure 1, p. 597, with permission.)

With all four subjects, noticeable changes occur with the onset of intervention. Note that the phases are not staggered at equal intervals; that is, the sequential introduction of treatment is based on achieving stability in the data, not on predetermined schedules. If we had used the A–B format with only one of these subjects, these results would not have been so definitive because of potential threats to internal validity; however, because the results have been replicated across four people at staggered times, it is highly unlikely that external factors could have coincidentally occurred at the time each treatment was initiated to cause the response change. One major advantage of the multiple baseline approach is that replication and experimental control can be achieved without withdrawal of treatment.

Multiple Baseline Design across Conditions

In the *multiple baseline design across conditions,* one behavior is monitored on one individual, with the same treatment applied sequentially across two more environmental conditions. These may include different treatment settings, different instructional arrangements, or different clinicians.

> *Researchers were interested in the effect of praise for reinforcing correct head posture in a child with cerebral palsy.[30] The intervention was carried out at three sites: physical therapy, speech therapy, and home. Following an initial baseline period, the physical therapist began a systematic process of praising the child when he maintained correct head posture. Activities in speech therapy and at home stayed as usual. A week later, the speech therapist began a similar process, while the parents maintained usual care at home. Finally, the child's parents carried out the intervention at home.*

Experimental control in this design can be demonstrated only if the target behavior is independent of the environment. Therefore, behavioral change in one environment will not influence behavior in other settings. Such control will be evidenced by maintained baselines in settings that have not yet begun to address the target behavior.

Multiple Baseline Design across Behaviors

Sometimes it is of interest to study the effect of one intervention on several related clinical behaviors. In the *multiple baseline design across behaviors,* the researcher monitors a minimum of three similar yet functionally independent behaviors in the same subject that can be addressed using the same intervention. Each target behavior is measured concurrently and continuously, until a stable baseline is achieved. The intervention is then introduced sequentially across the different behaviors.

> *Warren and coworkers studied the effect of an interactive teaching approach on the acquisition of prelinguistic skills in a child with Down syndrome and language delay.[31] They focused on three specific components of communication: prelinguistic requesting, vocal imitation, and commenting. They measured the subject's responses, tallying the number of appropriate responses observed during each session. After an initial baseline period of six sessions, the researchers instituted a training program to facilitate the child requesting toys within the environment. They continued to monitor vocal imitation and commenting during this time, but no training was focused on these behaviors. After session 17, training strategies were offered for both requesting and vocal imitation, while baseline continued for commenting behaviors. Finally, training strategies directed at commenting were instituted starting after session 39.*

The results, shown in Figure 12.10, demonstrate treatment effects most clearly for commenting behavior, with moderate gains in vocal imitation and dramatically variable changes in requests. Obviously, the multiple baseline design across behaviors requires that the targeted behaviors are similar enough that they will all respond to one treatment approach, and that they are functionally independent of one another so that baselines will remain stable until treatment is introduced. With many social and physical variables, this assumption can be problematic. For instance, if we monitored a patient's ability to learn three different self-care skills using peer modeling, we might find a covariation across behaviors; that is, as the patient becomes proficient in one activity, her motivation, physical skill, and understanding of the required tasks could improve so that the other behaviors demonstrate improvement before they are modeled. In that case, it would probably be more appropriate to test each behavior separately using a multiple baseline design across subjects.

Nonconcurrent Multiple Baseline Design

A basic premise of the multiple baseline design across subjects is that baseline data are available for all subjects simultaneously so that temporal effects cannot contaminate results. A more recent variation of this design has been proposed as an alternative, to account for the common clinical situation in which similar subjects are not available for concurrent monitoring.[32] In the *nonconcurrent multiple baseline design* across subjects, the researcher arbitrarily determines the length of several baselines, such as 5, 10, and 15 days. When a subject who matches the study criteria becomes available, he is randomly assigned to one of the predetermined baseline lengths. Baseline data are collected, and treatment is introduced at the appropriate time, assuming baselines are sufficiently stable. If baseline data are too variable, the subject is dropped from the study. As other subjects become available, they are randomly assigned to the remaining baselines.

The benefit of this approach is obvious in terms of practical research requirements; however, it is a weaker design than the standard multiple baseline approach because external factors related to the passage of time may be different for each baseline. For instance, patients may be tested during different seasons of the year, or the clinical environment may change over time. Therefore, the nonconcurrent multiple baseline design should be used only when a sufficient number of subjects are not available for concurrent study. Because of this potential weakness as an experimental design, the number of subject replications should be increased as an additional element of control.

CHANGING CRITERION DESIGN

The **changing criterion design** is a useful strategy for assessing interventions that are geared toward the gradual development or shaping of a target behavior.[33] Clinical goals often focus on accelerating or decelerating behaviors, such as improving endurance, decreasing abnormal movements in patients with neurological deficits, or increasing strength or range of motion. Very often, treatment techniques involve setting criteria or goals for performance that change over time, as the patient becomes more proficient at the target behavior. As the criterion changes, the patient must work harder to attain the new goal, and the behavior progresses.

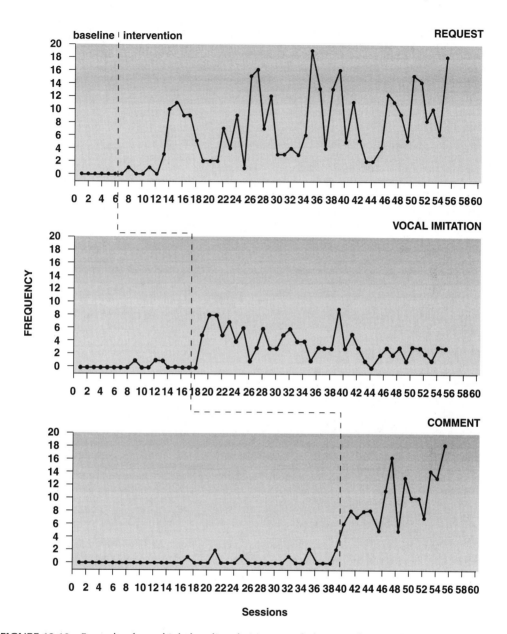

FIGURE 12.10   Example of a multiple baseline design across behaviors, showing the effect of an interactive teaching approach on the frequency of requests, vocal imitations, and comments by a child with Down syndrome and language delay. (From Warren SF, Yoder PJ, Gazdag GE, Kim K, Jones HA. Facilitating prelinguistic communication skills in young children with developmental delay. *J Speech Hear Res* 1993; 36:83–97, Figure 1, p. 88. Reprinted with permission of the American Speech-Language-Hearing Association.)

The changing criterion design begins with a baseline phase that establishes initial observations of the target behavior. The intervention is then applied in a series of phases, each one associated with a specific stepwise performance criterion for the target behavior. At each phase, the target behavior must meet the preset criterion and achieve some stability before the next criterion level is applied. This process continues until the final goal is reached. Essentially, each phase acts as a baseline for the following phase. When the rate of change in the target behavior varies in accordance with the stepwise changes in the criterion, experimental control is demonstrated.[33]

Foxx and Rubinoff studied the effect of behavioral reinforcement (monetary rewards) on reducing intake of excess caffeine.[34] The treatment goal was to reduce daily caffeine intake from baseline level to 600 mg (less than five cups). The difference between baseline levels and this goal was divided by 4 to yield four stepwise criteria to be used during treatment. For instance, one subject started the study drinking an average of 1008 mg of caffeine per day (Figure 12.11). Therefore, to get down to 600 mg the subject had to achieve a total decrease of at least 408 mg. This amount was divided into four intervals of 100 mg each. In the first treatment phase, the criterion for reward was set at 900 mg: If the subject maintained caffeine intake at that level, she would receive the reward; if she exceeded this level, she forfeited part of her reward. Once performance stabilized at this level, the criterion for reward was dropped to 800 mg. This procedure continued in two more steps, resulting in the subject's reducing her intake of caffeine to 357 mg in the final phase.

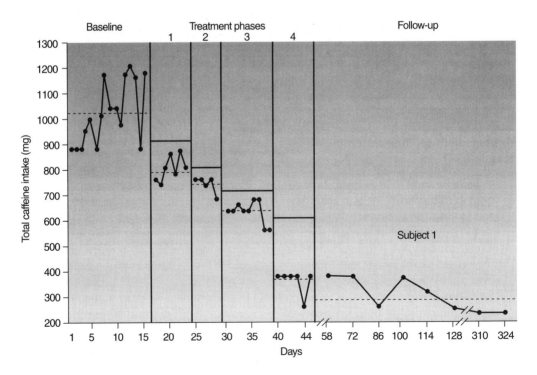

FIGURE 12.11 Example of a changing criterion design, showing the effect of monetary rewards for reducing caffeine intake. Solid horizontal lines indicate the criterion level for each phase. Broken horizontal lines indicate the mean for each condition. (From Foxx RM, Rubinoff A. Behavioral treatment of caffeinism: reducing excessive coffee drinking. *J Appl Behav Anal* 1979; 12:335–44, Figure 1, p. 339, with permission.)

This example documents the appropriate use of this design, where the performance of the target behavior is tied to the criterion level. These data suggest that this reinforcement technique seems to be a reasonable method for reducing excess caffeinism.

Three major concerns are addressed in the planning of a changing criterion design: the length of baseline and treatment phases, the number of criterion changes, and the magnitude of criterion steps.[34] The baseline phase should be long enough to establish stability or to show a definite trend in the direction opposite the desired change. The length of treatment phases will also depend on the stability of response. Achieving stabilization at each criterion level prior to introduction of the next criterion level is crucial to being able to demonstrate experimental control. For behaviors that are slow to change, treatment phases will have to be longer to document the effect of the criterion level. Hartmann and Hall suggest, however, that clinicians must also remain sensitive to clients' needs and not hold them at a criterion longer than would be wise therapeutically.[33] They also suggest that, at minimum, two criterion changes are necessary to show a clear relationship between criterion and behavior, although more are usually necessary.

When the target behavior does not change in clear response to changing the criterion, a withdrawal phase can be included in the design, in which the criterion is returned to a lower step and then returned to a higher level.[35] If the behavior mimics the change in criterion, the treatment effect is strengthened. For example, if the criterion for caffeine level was returned to 900 mg after the second treatment phase, and the subject's caffeine intake increased accordingly, the effect of setting the criterion level becomes even clearer. This strategy is also useful for examining potential confounding by temporal factors. For instance, suppose we wanted to increase a patient's ability to ambulate long distances, and set progressive distance requirements. If the patient's condition is naturally improving over time (a maturation effect), she may be able to walk further simply because she feels better, not because of any motivation to achieve a certain criterion. In that case, withdrawal of the criterion should not have a decelerating effect; that is, even if we set a distance requirement at a lower level, the patient will still be able to walk longer distances.

The magnitude of stepwise changes in the criterion should be related to the length and number of treatment phases. Steps can be determined according to the total length of treatment, or according to the difference between baseline and final goal (as in the caffeine example). The size of each step should be large enough to ensure that changes in the target behavior can be seen. Therefore, with variable responses, larger criterion steps will be needed. At the same time, with behaviors that are difficult to change, steps should be small enough that changes can be observed. The researcher must achieve a practical balance in making these decisions.

Changing criterion designs are applicable in a wide range of clinical situations where response changes are expected to follow performance criteria and where steplike changes in behavior are identifiable. Treatments that involve motivational factors or shaping procedures, such as biofeedback and behavior modification, would be responsive to changing criterion methods.

DATA ANALYSIS IN SINGLE-SUBJECT RESEARCH

Data analysis in single-subject research is based on evaluation of measurements within and across design phases, to determine if behaviors are changing and if observed changes during intervention are associated with the onset of treatment. *Visual analysis* of the graphic display of data is the most commonly used method. *Statistical analysis* provides a more quantitative approach to determine whether observed changes are real or chance occurrences. In this section we examine both approaches and discuss some of the more commonly used methods for analyzing data from single-subject experiments.

Visual Analysis

Visual analysis is used most often to analyze single-subject data because it does not require mathematical operations, and because it is intuitively meaningful. With basic information, researchers can accurately describe outcomes using this method.[36] Data collected in a single-subject experiment can be analyzed in terms of within-phase and between-phase characteristics. Data within a phase are described according to **stability,** or variability, and **trend,** or direction of change. An analysis of changes between phases is used to evaluate the research hypothesis. *Phase comparisons can be made only across adjacent phases.* These comparisons are based on changes in three characteristics of the data: level, trend, and slope. Figure 12.12 shows several common data patterns that reflect different combinations of these characteristics.

Changes in **level** refer to the value of the dependent variable, or magnitude of performance, at the point of intervention. It is judged by comparing the value of the target behavior at the last data point of one phase with its value at the first data point of the next adjacent phase. For example, Figures 12.12A and 12.12B show a change in level from the baseline to the intervention phase.

Level can also be described in terms of the *mean* or average value of the target behavior within a phase. This value is computed by taking the sum of all data points within a phase and dividing by the number of points. Mean levels can be compared across phases, as a method of summarizing change. For instance, in Figure 12.11, mean levels for each condition in the changing criterion design are shown by dotted lines. Means are useful for describing stable data that have no slope, as stable values will tend to cluster around the mean; however, when data are highly variable or when they exhibit a sharp slope, means can be misleading. For example, in Figure 12.12C, the dotted lines represent the mean score within each phase. On the basis of these values, one might assume that performance did not change once intervention was introduced. Obviously, this is not the case. Mean values should always be shown on a graph of the raw data to reduce the chance of misinterpretation.

Trend refers to the direction of change within a phase. Trends can be described as accelerating or decelerating and may be characterized as stable (constant rate of change) or variable. Trends can be linear or curvilinear. Changes in linear trend across phases are displayed in Figures 12.12A and 12.12C. In Figure 12.12D, no trend is observed during baseline, and a curvilinear trend is seen in the intervention phase; that is, the data change direction within the intervention phase.

A trend in baseline data does not present a serious problem when it reflects changes in a direction opposite to that expected during intervention. One would then anticipate a distinct change in direction once treatment is initiated; however, it is a problem when the baseline trend follows the direction of change expected during treatment. If the improving trend is continued into the intervention phase, it would be difficult to assess treatment effects, as the target behavior is already improving without treatment. It is im-

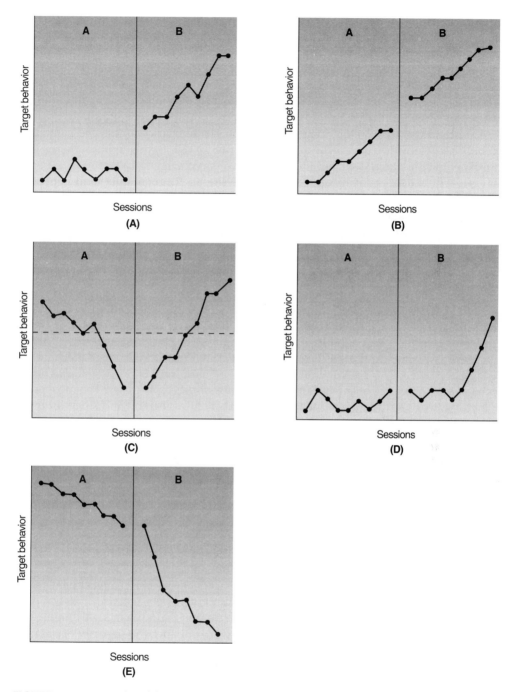

FIGURE 12.12 Examples of data patterns across baseline and intervention phases, showing changes in level and trend: (**A**) change in level and trend; (**B**) change in level, no change in trend; (**C**) change in trend; (**D**) change in trend, with a curvilinear pattern during *B*; (**E**) no change in level or trend, but a change in slope.

portant to consider what other factors may be contributing to this improvement. Perhaps changes reflect maturation, a placebo effect, or the effect of other treatments. Instituting treatment under these conditions would make it difficult to draw definitive conclusions. When trends occur in the baseline, it is usually advisable to extend the baseline phase, in hopes of achieving a plateau or reversal in the trend, and to try to identify causative factors. Those factors may be useful interventions in their own right and may provide the basis for further study.

The **slope** of a trend refers to its angle, or the rate of change within the data. Slope can only be determined for linear trends. In Figure 12.12B, trends in both phases have approximately the same slope (although their level has changed). In Figure 12.12E, both phases exhibit a decelerating trend; however, the slope within the intervention phase is much steeper than that in the baseline phase. This suggests that the rate of change in the target behavior increased once treatment was initiated.

Data analysis in single-subject research has traditionally focused on visual interpretation of these characteristics. Unfortunately, as examples throughout this chapter have shown, real data tend to be sufficiently variable that such subjective determinations are often tenuous and unreliable.[37,38] For instance, review the baseline data in Figure 12.11 for level of caffeine. Although it is relatively easy to determine that the level of response changed between the baseline and the first treatment phase, it would not be so easy to determine the trend or slope in these data based solely on visual judgment.

Although interrater reliability of visual analysis is not necessarily strong,[38,39] the reliability of assessing trend is greatly enhanced by drawing a straight line that characterizes rate of change.[36,40–42] Several procedures can be used for this purpose. Lines drawn freehand are generally considered unacceptable for research purposes. The most popular method involves drawing a line that represents the linear trend and slope for a data series. This procedure results in a **celeration line,** which describes trends as accelerating or decelerating. Linear regression procedures can be used to draw a *line of best fit*, although this technique is used less often (see Chapter 24).

Celeration Line

A celeration line is used to estimate the trend within a data series. We demonstrate the steps in drawing a celeration line using the hypothetical data shown in Figure 12.13. Although we will go through the process for the baseline phase only, in practice a separate celeration line can be computed for each phase in the design. Celeration lines are illustrated in Figures 12.5 and 12.8. Some advocates of this procedure suggest using semilogarithmic units to plot data.[43] On a semilogarithmic chart, the X-axis (time) is plotted in equal intervals, and the Y-axis (magnitude of behavior) is drawn in logarithmic units. The use of semilogarithmic charts has been shown to enhance the linearity of data and to flatten trends;[40] however, the technique can be used just as effectively with ordinary graph paper with equal intervals, as we illustrate here.[43]

The first step is to count the number of data points in the phase and then to divide those points into two equal halves along the X-axis. A vertical line is drawn to separate the two halves, as shown by the dotted line in Figure 12.13B. This example shows 10 baseline data points. Therefore, 5 points fall in each half of the phase. If an odd number of data points were plotted, the line would be drawn directly through the middle point.

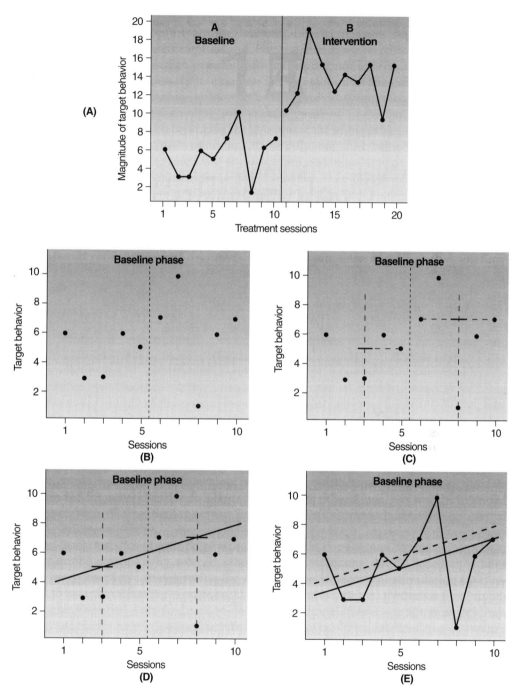

FIGURE 12.13 Computation of the split-middle line, or celeration line, for baseline data only: (**A**) Original data, showing baseline and intervention series. (**B**) Baseline points are divided in half along the *X*-axis. (**C**) Baseline points in each half-phase are divided in half again (broken lines); median values for each half-phase are marked with horizontal lines. (**D**) Celeration line is drawn. (**E**) Celeration line (broken line) is adjusted downward to represent the split-middle line (solid line).

The second step is to divide these halves in half again, as shown by the broken vertical lines in Figure 12.13C. With 5 data points, the line is drawn through the third point in each half. If there were an even number of data points in each half, the line would be drawn between the two middle points.

The next step is to determine the *median score* for each half of the phase (using the halves created by the dotted vertical line). The median score divides the data in half along the Y-axis. This point is obtained by counting from the bottom up toward the top data point within each half-phase. The point that divides the series in half vertically is the median score. For instance, in Figure 12.13B, there are five data points in the first half of the phase. Therefore, the third score will divide the series in half. Counting from the bottom up, these scores are 3, 3, 5, 6, and 6. The median score is 5. For the second half of the phase, scores are 1, 6, 7, 7, and 10, with a median of 7. If there were an even number of points, the median would be midway between the two middle points. A horizontal line is then drawn through each median point until it intersects the broken line, as shown in Figure 12.13C. Finally, a straight line is drawn connecting the two points of intersection. This is the celeration line, shown in Figure 12.13D.

Split-Middle Line

The celeration line demonstrates trend in the data. The line can also be used to represent a measure of central tendency using the split-middle technique. The **split-middle line** divides the data within a phase into two equal parts; therefore it represents a median point within the phase. To make the celeration line a split-middle line, the final step is to count the number of points on or above and on or below the line, and then to adjust the celeration line up or down to a point where the data are equally divided. The adjusted line must stay parallel to the original line; that is, the slope of the line does not change. In many cases, the line will not have to be adjusted. In the example in Figure 12.13, however, there are six points below the celeration line and four points above it. Therefore, we must adjust the line downward. Figure 12.13E shows the original celeration line (broken) and the adjusted split-middle line (solid), which now has four points above it and four points below it (two points are directly on the line).

The split-middle line is useful as an estimate of trend, but its interpretation is limited as a descriptor of clinical change because it is relatively insensitive to the magnitude of extreme scores. For instance, if the first data point in Figure 12.13 were changed to 20 and the second data point to 1, the split-middle line (and its slope) would not be affected; that is, the median points would remain unchanged. Therefore, the split-middle line should not take attention away from the clinical interpretation of data patterns using visual assessment of the raw data.

Calculating Slope

The slope of the celeration line can be calculated to estimate the rate of change in the target behavior. Slope is computed by taking Y values on two points along the celeration line, usually spaced 1 week apart (although any relevant time period can be used). The numerically larger value is divided by the smaller value to determine the slope. For example, in Figure 12.13E, the adjusted line is at 4 on day 3 and at 7 on day 10. Therefore, the slope of the line is $7/4 = 1.75$. By looking at the direction of the trend line, we can determine that this target behavior is increasing at an average rate of 1.75 times per week. Slopes can be calculated for each phase in the design, and compared to determine if the rate of change in the target behavior is accelerating or decelerating. The difference between slopes of adjacent phases can be used to provide a numerical estimate of how intervention changes the rate of response.

Statistical Analysis

Many researchers prefer to use a form of statistical analysis to corroborate visual analysis of time-series data, to determine whether differences between phases are meaningful or if they could have occurred by chance alone. Several authors have described methods for analyzing these designs.[43–45] The two most commonly used procedures include a test of the split-middle line and the two standard deviation band method.

Test of Significance Using the Split-Middle Line

The split-middle line can be used to compare the trend of data across two adjacent phases.[§] Wu and colleagues used this method in their study of activity-based therapy and weight distribution, shown earlier in Figure 12.5.[24] To illustrate this method, we have taken the split-middle line that was drawn for baseline data in Figure 12.13, and re-created it in Figure 12.14. The line has been extended from the baseline phase into the intervention phase. If there is no difference between the phases, then the split-middle line for baseline data should also be the split-middle line for the intervention phase. Therefore, 50% of the data in the intervention phase should fall on or above that line, and 50% should fall on or below it. If there is a difference, and treatment has caused a real change in observed behavior, then the extended baseline trend should not fit this pattern. Statistically, we propose a null hypothesis (H_0), which states that there is no difference across phases; that is, any changes observed from baseline to the intervention phase are due to chance, not treatment. We also propose an alternative to H_0, which can be phrased as a nondirectional or directional hypothesis; that is, we can state that we expect a difference between phases (nondirectional) or that responses will increase (or decrease) from baseline (directional). For the example shown in Figure 12.14, assume that we propose an increase in response with intervention.

To test H_0, we apply a procedure called the **binomial test,** which is used when outcomes of a test are dichotomous, in this case data points are either above or below the split middle line. To do the test, we count the number of points in the intervention phase that fall above and below the extended line (ignoring points that fall directly on the line). In our example, one point falls below the line and nine points fall above the line. Clearly, this is not a 50–50 split. On the basis of these data, we would like to conclude that the treatment did effect a change in response; however, we must first pose a statistical question:

[§]The celeration line can be limited as a means of analysis if the data within a phase are not linear. Ottenbacher recommends using an alternative approach to account for nonlinear trends in data called the *running medians procedure*.[44] This procedure breaks the data within a phase into three segments, so that nonlinear trends can be observed. Refer to Ottenbacher's informative paper for a clear description of this method.

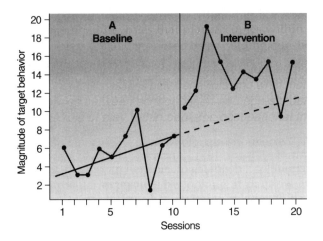

FIGURE 12.14 Celeration line for baseline and intervention phases. The split-middle line for the baseline data is extended into the intervention phase to test the null hypothesis.

Could this pattern, with one point below and nine points above the line, have occurred by chance? Or can we be confident that this pattern shows a true treatment effect?

We answer this question by referring to Appendix Table A.9, which lists probabilities associated with the binomial test. Two values are needed to use this table. First, we find the appropriate value of n (down the side), which is the total number of points in the intervention phase that fall above and below the line (not counting points on the line). In this case, there are a total of 10 points. We then determine if there are *fewer* points above or below the extended celeration line. In our example, there are fewer points (one) below the line. The number of fewer points is given the value x; therefore, $x = 1$. The probability associated with $n = 10$ and $x = 1$ is .011, that is, $p = .011$.

The probabilities listed in Table A.9 are *one-tailed probabilities*, which means they are used to evaluate directional alternative hypotheses, as proposed in this example. If a nondirectional hypothesis is proposed, then a *two-tailed test* is performed, which requires doubling the probabilities listed in the table.

The probability value obtained from the table is interpreted in terms of a conventional upper limit of $p = .05$. Probabilities that exceed this value are considered *not significant;* that is, the observed pattern could have occurred by chance. In this example, the probability associated with the test is less than .05 and, therefore, is considered significant. The pattern of response in the intervention phase is significantly different from baseline. The concept of probability testing and statistical significance is covered in detail in Chapter 18.

Two Standard Deviation Band Method

Another useful method of analysis is the **two standard deviation band method.** This process involves assessing variability within the baseline phase by calculating the mean and standard deviation of data points within that phase (see Chapter 17 for calculation

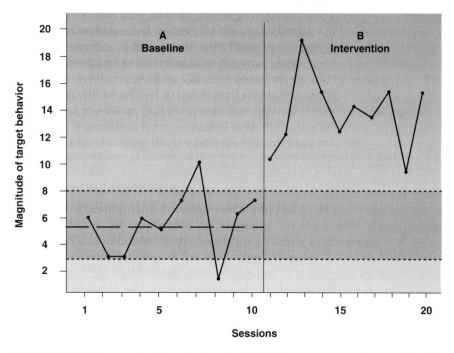

FIGURE 12.15   Two standard deviation band method, showing mean performance level for baseline (dashed line) and shaded area two standard deviations above and below the mean. Because points in the intervention phase fall out of this band, the difference between phases is considered significant.

methods for these statistics). To illustrate this procedure, we have again taken the hypothetical data from Figure 12.13, this time reproduced in Figure 12.15. The dashed line represents the mean level of performance for the baseline phase, and the shaded areas above and below this line represent two standard deviations above and below the mean. As shown in the figure, these lines are extended into the intervention phase. If at least two consecutive data points in the intervention phase fall outside the two standard deviation band, changes from baseline to intervention are considered significant.[1,46] In this example, the mean response for baseline is 5.4, with a standard deviation of 2.55. All points in the intervention phase fall above the shaded two standard deviation band. Therefore, we would conclude that there was a significant change from baseline to the intervention phase.

Time-Series Analysis

It is also possible to use conventional statistical tests, such as the *t*-test and analysis of variance (see Chapters 19 and 20), with time-series data; however, these applications are limited because these tests are not useful in situations where data points are interdependent, as is often the case in single-subject research.[47,44] This interdependence is called **serial dependency,** which means that successive observations in a series of data points are related or correlated; that is, knowing the level of performance at one point in time allows the researcher to predict the value of subsequent points in the series. Serial dependency can interfere with several statistical procedures, and may also be a problem for making inferences based on visual analysis.[48]

The degree of serial dependency in a series is reflected by the **autocorrelation** in the data, or the correlation between data points separated by different intervals, or lags. For example, a lag 1 autocorrelation is computed by pairing the first data point with the second, the second with the third, and so on for the entire series. Using lag 2, the first data point is paired with the third, the second with the fourth, and so on. The higher the value of autocorrelation, the greater the serial dependency in the data. Ottenbacher presents a method for computing autocorrelation by hand,[1] but the process is easily performed by computer, especially with large numbers of data points.

When serial dependency is an issue, a statistical technique called *time-series analysis* can be used to make inferences about changes in trend and level across phases.[49] This analysis involves a complex process whereby a statistical model is created to adjust for autocorrelation, so that differences between phases can be analyzed. The procedure that is most recommended is based on a model discussed in Chapter 10, the *autoregressive integrated moving average (ARIMA)*.[44,50] The technique accommodates for serial scores and weighs heavily on the observations that fall closer to the point at which treatment is introduced. It analyzes the trends in the data and proposes a model that represents the observed pattern. This model can then be used to describe the behavior of interest. A more detailed description of this procedure is beyond the scope of this book.

GENERALIZATION OF FINDINGS

The special appeal of single-subject research is that it focuses on clinical outcomes and can provide data for clinical decision making. With this intent, then, it is not sufficient to demonstrate these outcomes during an experimental period. It is also necessary to show that improvements or changes in behavior will be sustained under conditions that differ from experimental conditions and after the intervention has ended.

To establish carryover outside the experimental setting, researchers try to establish that the responses observed during the study can be generalized to nontraining conditions.[51] For example, in a study by Renne and Creer, children who suffered from asthma were tested for their ability to use inhalation equipment.[52] They were given specific rewards for proper use of the equipment within special training sessions, and demonstrated successful learning. It would then be of interest to establish that the children could maintain their performance when they were actually exhibiting asthmatic symptoms. To evaluate this generalization, the investigators told the children that the "intervention," the reward strategies, would continue if they used the equipment properly whenever it was really needed. Follow-up data provided by the nursing staff supported the generalization of the target behavior to actual treatment situations.

The term **generalization** is used in this sense to represent a limited form of external validity for the single case. Generalization can be demonstrated in a variety of ways. For instance, the target behavior can be monitored in different settings than the original study; different clinicians, support personnel, or family members can perform the intervention; the treatment may be given at different times of day; or different types of equipment may be used. The continued success of intervention under these changed conditions provides strong evidence supporting application of the treatment under clinical conditions that typically cannot incorporate experimental controls.

We can also incorporate a *follow-up* or *maintenance* phase in a single-subject design, which involves monitoring the target behavior after the intervention is stopped, often weeks or months later. For example, Foxx and Rubinoff, in their study of caffeine intake, continued to monitor their clients' coffee drinking by contacting a family member every 2 weeks for several months after intervention was stopped (see Figure 12.11).[34] Follow-up is important when the intent of treatment is to effect a permanent change in behavior.

External Validity

For clinical research findings to have broad applicability, they must be externally valid, beyond the behavior of a single individual. Single-subject designs are often challenged on this basis, with claims that no one subject can be considered representative of a larger group and that significant effects on a single patient provide no "proof" that a treatment will work for others. Although this is logically true, it is not unreasonable to assume that the treatment will work for other patients with similar characteristics. The important contribution of single-subject research is that the specific characteristics of the treatment and the circumstances in which the treatment is successful can be delineated, so that this assumption can be tested. This type of data is not available from group studies. Group averages do not allow us to distinguish those who reacted positively to treatment from those who did not. In addition, visual inspection of individual performance allows the researcher to observe clinically strong effects that would not necessarily have been statistically significant (and would therefore have been ignored). Therefore, the argument can be made that generalization from the single case is actually more realistic and has greater direct clinical value than generalization from group studies.

To demonstrate external validity in single-subject research, it is necessary to replicate the results of single-subject experiments on other subjects with similar characteristics in different settings. This replication is the only method by which the clinical researcher can maintain a focus on the individual and still establish generality of findings for others. Over time, three types of replication strategies should be employed to support a given hypothesis.

Direct Replication

Direct replication is performed by applying the same procedures across several subjects or repeating the study on the same subject. The setting, treatment conditions, and patient characteristics should be kept as constant as possible. External validity becomes stronger as results accumulate across subjects, establishing what types of patients respond favorably to the treatment. Barlow and Hersen have suggested that one successful experiment and three successful replications are usually sufficient to demonstrate that findings are not a result of chance.[5] Multiple-baseline designs provide direct replication.

When results are not consistent, patient characteristics can be examined to determine which factors might distinguish successful and unsuccessful subjects. For those who do not respond favorably, the investigator can modify the design and manipulate the intervention in an attempt to change the target behavior. If the modified treatment is successful, it can then be investigated in other similar subjects. This flexibility adds a dimension to single-subject research that is not possible with group experimental designs.

Systematic Replication

Systematic replication is used to demonstrate that findings can be observed under conditions different from those encountered in the initial experiment. Systematic replication should occur after generalization across subjects has been established through direct replication. The purpose of systematic replication is to define the conditions under which the intervention will be successful or fail. It is, in essence, a search for exceptions.[5] It involves the variation of one or two variables from the original study in an attempt to generalize to other similar, but not identical, situations.

Clinical Replication

Although we have attempted to define the process of single-subject research using a clinical model, in reality the fit is less than perfect. Treatment plans are not developed around isolated patient problems, nor are they based on partitioned treatment components. In the long run, then, the true applicability of research data will depend on our ability to demonstrate that treatment packages can be successfully applied to patients with multiple behaviors that tend to cluster together. Barlow and Hersen have called this process **clinical replication**.[5] Such a procedure may be considered field testing; that is, clinical replication becomes one with actual practice.

Clinical replication is an advanced replication procedure, which can occur only after direct replication and systematic replication have supplied the researcher with well-defined relationships between treatment components and patient characteristics. After testing these relationships one at a time, the researcher can begin to build clinical strategies by combining and recombining successful treatments for coexisting problems. For example, consider the multitude of problems inherent in disorders such as stroke, cerebral palsy, autism, and low back dysfunction. Many of the "treatments" that are used to address these problems incorporate a variety of techniques, with expected overlapping and combined effects. In fact, these treatment programs are not always successful. A comprehensive process of clinical replication is really the only way to establish the conditions under which we can expect positive results.

Social Validation

Beyond the question of external validity, which concerns generalization of findings to different subjects and settings, behavioral analysts are also interested in the social validity of applied research, which concerns the importance of treatment effects within a social context. Wolf suggests that there are three levels of **social validation**—goals, procedures, and effects—each addressing a different set of issues in clinical practice.[53]

Setting treatment goals involves concern for the social importance of the target behavior to the patient; that is, goals should be established within the context of the patient's present and future functional requirements and environment. These goals may be evaluated by those who are in a position to judge the patient's needs, including the patient, family, or care provider, or they may be defined with reference to a peer group's functional level.

The second level of social validation is concern for the appropriateness and *acceptability of treatment procedures* for changing the target behavior. Interventions should be chosen on the basis of patient preferences, comfort, and safety, as well as cost and simplicity of application.[35] Procedures that are intrusive, threatening, obscure, or impractical are less likely to be used and, therefore, less important to study.

The third level of social validation concerns the *magnitude of treatment effects,* or the optimal levels of performance required for the behavior to be considered valuable. This is a practical issue, based on whether training has changed the target behavior sufficiently to be functional. Treatments can cause marked changes in behavior, but if those behaviors are still too weak or too strong (in the case of negative behaviors) to accomplish required tasks, the observed changes will not be practically useful. Investigators must be able to identify necessary limits of behavior to define socially valid standards for which they can aim.[54] Standards of performance can be established by subjective evaluation, by use of normative data, or by assessment of the performance of individuals who are judged to be competent in the behavior of interest.

Although social validation is not required for establishing treatment effectiveness, it has always been recognized as an important element of treatment planning and decision making, and serves an important function in the interpretation of clinical research findings. Measures of social validation should be encouraged as a critical link between single-subject research and the treatment planning process.

COMMENTARY

It's a Start

The maturation of single-subject research methodology has been an important step in the development of clinical research. It provides an opportunity for the practitioner to evaluate treatment procedures within the context of clinical care, and to share insights about patient behavior and response that are typically ignored or indiscernible using traditional group research approaches. The process of single-subject research should eventually diminish the role of trial and error in clinical practice and provide useful guidelines for making clinical choices. The underlying message in all of this is that the clinician, working in the practice setting, is uniquely qualified to perform these studies, especially in terms of the importance of clinical replication.

Statistical procedures can be a useful adjunct to visual analysis for interpreting the results of single-subject experiments, most importantly in situations when data variability makes subjective assessments of change difficult and inconsistent. Behavioral analysts will probably continue to debate the benefits of using statistics for studying single organisms. Because many analysis procedures are available, clinical researchers must be able to decide what type of documentation is appropriate for a particular study. This decision must be based on the nature of the target behavior, the expected direction of change, variability in the data, the extent of treatment effects, and the way clinical outcomes will be interpreted.

Of course, single-subject designs are not a panacea for all clinical research woes. Many research questions cannot be answered adequately using these designs. Single-subject designs can be limited in that they require time to document outcomes. They are not readily applicable to acute situations where baseline periods are less reasonable and treatment does not continue for long periods. In addition, researchers often find that patient responses are too unstable, making attempts at analysis very frustrating. Nonetheless, single-subject designs serve a distinct purpose in the ongoing search for scientific documentation of therapeutic effectiveness. They offer a practical methodology for exploring cause-and-effect relationships in clinical phenomena and for sorting out the effects of individual patient characteristics on treatment outcomes.

These designs are flexible enough to provide opportunities for examining the relationships among impairments, functional limitations, and disability measures. As the emphasis on outcomes continues in rehabilitation research, the single-subject strategy provides a unique opportunity to explore these relationships and to ask questions about those factors that may impact on these relationships. Group designs will often hide these factors or cancel their effect, giving us no information with which to critically examine the differences among our patients. Because of the emphasis on visual presentation and continuous description of responses over time, single-subject experiments can be the source of empirical hypotheses that lead to new avenues of study and to the discovery of clinical implications that would not otherwise be seen or shared. This process will force us to challenge clinical theories and to document the benefits of our interventions in a convincing scientific way, for ourselves and for others.

KEY TERMS

single-subject designs
target behavior
baseline phase (A)
intervention phase (B)
A–B design
stability
trend
withdrawal design
A–B–A design
multiple-treatment design

interactive design
alternating treatment
    design
multiple baseline design
changing criterion design
level
slope
celeration line
split-middle line
binomial test

two standard deviation
    band method
serial dependency
autocorrelation
generalization
direct replication
systematic replication
clinical replication
social validation

REFERENCES

1. Ottenbacher KJ. *Evaluating Clinical Change: Strategies for Occupational and Physical Therapists.* Baltimore: Williams & Wilkins, 1986.
2. Hasson S. Guest Editorial: Making a case for single-case research. *J Orthop Sports Phys Ther* 1996;24:1–3.
3. Hayes SC. Single-case experimental design and empirical clinical practice. *J Consult Clin Psychol* 1981;49:193–211.
4. Cook TD, Campbell DT. *Quasi-experimentation: Design and Analysis Issues for Field Settings.* Boston: Houghton Mifflin, 1979.
5. Barlow DH, Hersen M. *Single Case Experimental Designs: Strategies for Studying Behavior Change.* 2d ed. New York: Pergamon Press, 1984.
6. Leiper CI, Miller A, Lang J, Herman R. Sensory feedback for head control in cerebral palsy. *Phys Ther* 1981;61:512–8.
7. Laskas CA, Mullen SL, Nelson DL, Willson-Broyles M. Enhancement of two motor functions of the lower extremity in a child with spastic quadriplegia. *Phys Ther* 1985;65:11–6.

8. Ray SA, Bundy AC, Nelson DL. Decreasing drooling through techniques to facilitate mouth closure. *Am J Occup Ther* 1983;37:749–53.

9. Tona JL, Schneck CM. The efficacy of upper extremity inhibitive casting: a single-subject pilot study. *Am J Occup Ther* 1993;47:901–10.

10. Kaelin DL, Cifu DX, Matthies B. Methylphenidate effect on attention deficit in the acutely brain-injured adult. *Arch Phys Med Rehabil* 1996;77:6–9.

11. Diamond MF, Ottenbacher KJ. Effect of a tone-inhibiting dynamic ankle–foot orthosis on stride characteristics of an adult with hemiparesis. *Phys Ther* 1990;70:423–30.

12. Dave CA. Effects of linear vestibular stimulation on body-rocking behavior in adults with profound mental retardation. *Am J Occup Ther* 1992;46:910–5.

13. Hawkins RP. Who decided *that* was the problem? Two stages of responsibility for applied behavior analysis. In: Wood WS, ed. *Issues in Evaluating Behavior Modification.* Champaign, IL: Research Press, 1975, 95–214.

14. Sharpe PA, Ottenbacher KJ. Use of an elbow restraint to improve finger-feeding skills in a child with Rett syndrome. *Am J Occup Ther* 1990;44:328–32.

15. Kelley MB. A review of the observational data-collection and reliability procedures reported in the *Journal of Applied Behavior Analysis. J Appl Behav Anal* 1977;10:97.

16. Hawkins RP, Fabry BD. Applied behavior analysis and interobserver reliability: a commentary on two articles by Birkimer and Brown. *J Appl Behav Anal* 1979;12:545.

17. Hawkins RP, Dotson VA. Reliability scores that delude: an Alice in Wonderland trip through the misleading characteristics of interobserver agreement scores in interval recording. In: Ramp E, Semb G, eds. *Behavioral Analysis: Areas of Research and Application.* Englewood Cliffs, NJ: Prentice-Hall, 1975.

18. Birkimer JC, Brown JH. A graphical judgmental aid which summarizes obtained and chance reliability data and helps assess the believability of experimental effects. *J Appl Behav Anal* 1979;12:523.

19. McCullough JP, Cornell JE, McDaniel MH, Mueller RK. Utilization of the simultaneous treatment design to improve student behavior in a first-grade classroom. *J Consult Clin Psychol* 1974;42:288.

20. Tawney JW, Gast DL. *Single Subject Research in Special Education.* Columbus, OH: Charles E. Merrill, 1984.

21. Cohen J. A coefficient of agreement for nominal scales. *Educ Psychol Meas* 1960;20:37.

22. Cohen J. Weighted kappa: nominal scale agreement with provisions for scale disagreement or partial credit. *Psychol Bull* 1968;70:313.

23. Ayres AJ, Mailloux Z. Influence of sensory integration procedures on language development. *Am J Occup Ther* 1981;35:383–90.

24. Wu S, Huang H, Lin C, Chen M. Effects of a program on symmetrical posture in patients with hemiplegia: a single-subject design. *Am J Occup Ther* 1996;50:17–23.

25. Miller PM, Hersen M, Eisler RM, Watts JG. Contingent reinforcement of lowered blood-alcohol levels in an outpatient chronic alcoholic. *Behav Res Ther* 1974;12:261–3.

26. Hains AH, Baer DM. Interaction effects in multielement designs: inevitable, desirable, and ignorable. *J Appl Behav Anal* 1989;22:57–69.

27. Agras WS, Barlow DH, Chapin HN, Abel GG, Leitenberg H. Behavior modification of anorexia nervosa. *Arch Gen Psychiatry* 1974;30:279–86.

28. Barrios BA. Single-subject strategies for examining joint effects: a critical evaluation. *Behav Assess* 1984;6:103.

29. Reid DH, Hurlbut B. Teaching nonvocal communication skills to multihandicapped retarded adults. *J Appl Behav Anal* 1977;10:591–603.

30. Martin JE, Epstein LH. Evaluating treatment effectiveness in cerebral palsy. Single-subject designs. *Phys Ther* 1976;56:285–94.

31. Warren SF, Yoder PJ, Gazdag GE, Kim K, Jones HA. Facilitating prelinguistic communication skills in young children with developmental delay. *J Speech Hearing Res* 1993;36:83–97.

32. Watson PJ, Workman EA. The noncurrent multiple baseline across individuals design: an extension of the traditional multiple baseline design. *J Behav Ther Exp Psychiatry* 1981;12:257.

33. Hartmann DP, Hall RV. The changing criterion design. *J Appl Behav Anal* 1976;9:527–32.

34. Foxx RM, Rubinoff A. Behavioral treatment of caffeinism: reducing excessive coffee drinking. *J Appl Behav Anal* 1979;12:335–44.

35. Kazdin AE. *Single-Case Research Designs: Methods for Clinical and Applied Settings.* New York: Oxford University Press, 1982.

36. Bobrovitz CD, Ottenbacher KJ. Comparison of visual inspection and statistical analysis of single-subject data in rehabilitation research. *Am J Phys Med Rehabil* 1998;77:94–102.

37. DeProspero A, Cohen S. Inconsistent visual analysis of intrasubject data. *J Appl Behav Anal* 1979;12:573.

38. Ottenbacher KJ. Reliability and accuracy of visually analyzing graphed data from single-subject designs. *Am J Occup Ther* 1986;40:464–9.

39. Harbst KB, Ottenbacher KJ, Harris SR. Interrater reliability of therapists' judgements of graphed data. *Phys Ther* 1991;71:107–15.

40. Bailey DB. Effects of lines of progress and semilogarithmic charts on ratings of charted data. *J Appl Behav Anal* 1984;17:359.

41. Hojem MA, Ottenbacher KJ. Empirical investigation of visual-inspection versus trend-line analysis of single-subject data. *Phys Ther* 1988;68:983–8.

42. Johnson MB, Ottenbacher KJ. Trend line influence on visual analysis of single-subject data in rehabilitation research. *Int Disabil Stud* 1991;13:55–9.

43. Kazdin AE. Statistical analyses for single-case experimental designs. In: Barlow DH, Hersen M, eds. *Single Case Experimental Designs: Strategies for Studying Behavior Change.* New York: Pergamon Press, 1984, p. 285–324.

44. Ottenbacher KJ. Analysis of data in idiographic research. *Am J Phys Med Rehabil* 1992;71:202–8.

45. Edgington ES. Statistics and single case analysis. In: Hersen M, Eisler RM, Monti PM, eds. *Progress in Behavior Modification.* 16 vol. New York: Academic Press, 1984.

46. Gottman JM, Leiblum SR. *How to Do Psychotherapy and How to Evaluate It.* New York: Holt, Rinehart & Winston, 1974.

47. Jones RR, Baught RS, Weinrott MR. Time-series analysis in operant research. *J Appl Behav Anal* 1977;10:151.

48. Jones RR, Weinrott MR, Vaught RS. Effects of serial dependency on the agreement between visual and statistical inference. *J Appl Behav Anal* 1978;11:277.

49. Hartmann DP, Gottman JM, Jones RR. Interrupted time-series analysis and its application to behavioral data. *J Appl Behav Anal* 1980;13:543.

50. McCain LJ, McCleary R. The statistical analysis of the simple interrupted time-series quasi-experiment. In: Cook TD, Campbell DT, eds. *Quasi-experimentation: Design and Analysis Issues for Field Settings.* Boston: Houghton-Mifflin, 1979, p. 233–93.

51. Stokes TF, Baer DM. An implicit technology of generalization. *J Appl Behav Anal* 1977;10:349.

52. Renne CM, Creer TL. Training children with asthma to use inhalation therapy equipment. *J Appl Behav Anal* 1976;9:1–11.

53. Wolf MM. Social validity: the case for subjective measurement or how applied behavior analysis is finding its heart. *J Appl Behav Anal* 1978;11:203.

54. Van Houten R. Social validation: the evolution of standards of competency for target behaviors. *J Appl Behav Anal* 1979;12:581.

13

Descriptive and Exploratory Research

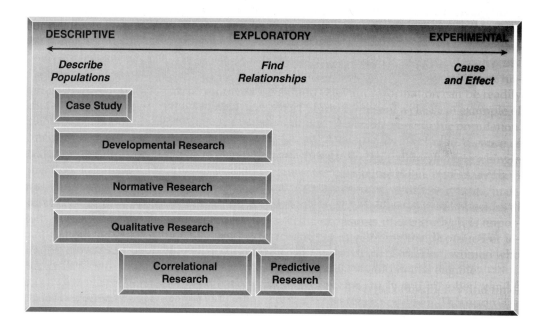

Many important questions in clinical inquiry reflect the scientist's need to understand clinical phenomena. This understanding must start with the description of a phenomenon and an exploration of those factors that influence and interact with it. Valid interpretation of clinical outcomes depends on our ability to develop a clear picture of those we treat, their characteristics and performance under different conditions. Studies that help us gather this information are considered descriptive or exploratory. **Descriptive research** is designed to document conditions, attitudes, or characteristics of individuals or groups of individuals. **Exploratory research** focuses on the relationships among these factors. As our diagram of the continuum of research shows, however, descriptive and exploratory elements are commonly combined, depending on how the investigator conceptualizes the research question. These research approaches are also considered *observational* or *nonexperimental* because data are collected as they naturally exist, rather than through manipulation of variables as in experiments. For example, researchers have used descriptive studies to describe gait characteristics of patients with specific disorders,[1] biomechanical parameters of wheelchair propulsion,[2] factors that influence pain threshold in children,[3] and the course of recovery of functional skills in adults with severe head injuries.[4]

Several types of research can be categorized as descriptive or exploratory. These include case studies, descriptive analyses, developmental research, normative research, qualitative research, and correlational and predictive research. The purpose of this chapter is to describe these designs and their various configurations.

RETROSPECTIVE AND PROSPECTIVE RESEARCH

Descriptive and exploratory studies can be carried out retrospectively or prospectively. **Retrospective research** involves the examination of data that have been collected in the past,* often obtained from medical records or surveys. As an example, Sellers and coworkers were interested in developing criteria to predict prolonged ventilator dependence in patients who have experienced severe burns.[5] They reviewed medical records of patients who had been admitted over a 4-year period who required ventilator support, and successfully documented a series of objective factors that were effective predictors. Inferences from retrospective research must be viewed within the constraints of the data, however. The researcher cannot control operational definitions of variables or the reliability with which data were collected. Data will often be missing or incomplete. Therefore, both the accuracy and the credibility of the data source are important considerations. Retrospective data, however, represent an important source of information because many research questions can only be answered using data that have already been collected. The availability of data through clinical databases will usually qualify as retrospective study.

In **prospective research,** variables are measured through direct recording in the present. The researcher follows patients as they progress through their treatment or evaluation. For example, Cerhan et al. were interested in the relationship between physical activity and the development of breast cancer.[6] Their study followed a cohort of over 1,000 women from 1973 to 1993, during which time they collected data on the incidence of breast cancer as well as activity level, medical history, education, and other developmental variables to determine which factors were related. Prospective studies are more reliable than retrospective studies because of the potential for greater control of data collection methods. The major disadvantage of prospective studies is the time and expense associated with long periods of data collection.

---

*Retrospective studies are a form of *ex post facto research,* which means the researcher does not have direct control of the variables under study because they have occurred in the past or they represent attribute variables that cannot be manipulated.[54]

DESCRIPTIVE RESEARCH

Descriptive studies document the nature of existing phenomena and describe how variables change over time. They will generally be structured around a set of guiding questions or research objectives to generate data or characterize a situation of interest. Often this information can be used as a basis for formulation of research hypotheses that can be tested using exploratory or experimental techniques. The descriptive data supply the foundation for classifying individuals, for identifying relevant variables, and for asking new research questions.

Case Studies

Clinicians and researchers have long recognized the importance of the **case study** for developing a clinical knowledge base. A description of interesting, new, and unique cases is necessary to build a foundation for clinical science and as a means of sharing special information among professional colleagues. Typically, case studies involve the in-depth description of an individual's condition or response to treatment; however, case studies can also focus on a group, institution, or other social unit, such as a particular school, community, or family. A *case series* is an expansion of a case study, in which observations of several similar cases are reported.

Most often, case studies emphasize unusual patient problems or diagnoses that present interesting clinical challenges. As an example, Gann and Nalty highlighted the unusual diagnosis of a patient with a vertical patellar dislocation.[7] The case was remarkable because the injury occurred without trauma. The authors documented their findings as a contribution to understanding mechanisms of patellar injury. Alternatively, case reports will focus on innovative approaches to treatment. For instance, LaPier and colleagues documented the case of a patient with chronic multisystem impairments, and their nontraditional treatment approach using an aerobic exercise program.[8]

A case study is an intensive investigation designed to analyze and understand those factors important to the etiology, care, and outcome of the subject's problems. It is a comprehensive description of the subject's background, present status, and responses to intervention. A case study begins with a full history, delineating problems, symptoms, and prior treatments, as well as demographic and social factors that are relevant to the subject's care and prognosis. Elements of a treatment plan should be delineated, and expectations should be presented as justification for the treatment approach chosen.[9] Where relevant, literature should be cited to support the rationale for treatment and interpretation of outcomes. Documentation of all interventions, the subject's responses, and any follow-up should be complete. Data may be qualitative or quantitative, and may be obtained using both objective and subjective methods of observation. If special assessments are used, they should be described in pertinent detail. Some case studies are actually geared to describing the applicability of new or unusual assessment instruments for diagnosing certain problems.[10]

The major contribution of the case study to research is its ability to provide information that can be used to generate inductive hypotheses. Because the case study allows for a thorough analysis of a single situation, it often leads to the discovery of relationships that were not obvious before. As more and more cases are reported, a form of "case law" gradually develops, whereby empirical findings are considered reasonable within the realm of accepted knowledge and professional experience.[9] Eventually, with successive documented cases, a conceptual framework forms, providing a basis for categorizing patients and for generating hypotheses that can be tested using exploratory or experimental methods.

The case study is probably the most practical approach to research because of its direct applicability to patient care, but it is also the least rigorous approach because of its inherent lack of control and limited generalizability. The interaction of environmental and personal characteristics and the effect of multiple interventions make the case study weak in internal validity. Generalization from one case to a larger population is also limited because the responses of one individual or social unit may bear little resemblance to those of others in similar circumstances. In addition, case studies are often concerned with exceptional situations or rare disorders, and subjects are generally not representative of the "typical" patient seen in the clinic. Therefore, external validity is also limited.

The validity of inferences from a case study can be enhanced, however, by taking steps to objectify treatment effects and to demonstrate them under different conditions.[10,11] For instance, interpretations can be made stronger by direct quantified observation and by taking repeated measurements over the course of treatment. Treatment effects can be further supported by using multiple dependent variables and by choosing outcome measures that show large and immediate changes. Generalization can be enhanced by documenting the subject's behavior in more than one setting and by including information from follow-up visits to establish the long-range success of treatment. Literature should be used to demonstrate how results support a particular theoretical approach to treatment.

Perhaps the greatest advantage of the case study as a form of clinical investigation is that it provides an opportunity for understanding the totality of an individual's experience. Rather than simply recording behavior, the depth of the case study allows the researcher to explore the subject's condition, emotions, thoughts, and past and present activities as they relate to the focus of the study. The researcher tries to determine what variables might be important to the subject's development or behavior, in an effort to understand why the subject responds or changes in a particular way or why certain outcomes were achieved and others were not. The case study also provides an opportunity for presentation of unique or special circumstances that would generally be missed in a group study.

Developmental Research

Concepts of human development, whether they are related to cognition, perceptual-motor control, communication, physiological change, or psychological processes, are important elements of a clinical knowledge base. **Developmental research** involves the description of developmental change and the sequencing of behaviors in people over time. Developmental studies have contributed to the theoretical foundations of clinical practice in many ways. For example, the classic descriptive studies of Gesell and Amatruda[12] and McGraw[13] provide the basis for much of the research on sequencing of motor development in infants and children. Erikson's studies in life span development have contributed to an understanding of psychological growth through old age.[14]

Developmental studies can be characterized by the method used to document change. The longitudinal method involves collecting data over an extended period, to document behaviors as they vary over time. With the cross-sectional method, the researcher studies various developmental levels (usually age levels) within a particular cohort of subjects and describes differences among those levels as they exist at a single point in time.

Longitudinal Method

In a **longitudinal study** the researcher follows a cohort of subjects over time, performing repeated measurements at prescribed intervals. Because the same individuals are tested throughout the study, personal characteristics remain relatively constant, and differences observed over time can be interpreted as developmental change.

One of the earliest studies of this type was actually a case report of data collected between 1759 and 1777, chronicling the physical growth of a child at 6-month intervals, from birth to 18 years. These data still represent one of the most famous records of human growth.[15] Intellectual growth has been the subject of many longitudinal studies, in children[16] and adults.[17] Changes that occur in biological and physiological processes with aging are also best described using longitudinal research. For example, researchers have described the sequencing of the development of head, upper extremity, and lower extremity extension in the prone extension posture in healthy full-term infants, followed from 8 to 28 weeks of age.[18] At the other end of the spectrum, research has documented the development of personality through late adulthood[19] and cognitive effects of aging.[20] Longitudinal studies may focus on the progression of disease states. For example, Munsat and coworkers followed patients with amyotrophic lateral sclerosis over 6 years, to document the rate and pattern of motor deterioration.[21] They described a linear and symmetric rate of motor neuron loss, with slower deterioration in the leg than in the arm. The authors suggested that this information will be important in the design of clinical trials and the generation of hypotheses about the etiology of the disease.

The advantage of the longitudinal method is its ability to accumulate data through intensive documentation of growth and change on the same individuals; however, researchers using this approach face many practical difficulties, most notably the extended obligation to a single project, requiring long-term commitment of funds and resources. Once a longitudinal study is begun, it cannot be changed without jeopardizing the validity of all previous data. Subjects cannot be replaced, and their compliance must be ensured. Measurement of a given variable should not be altered unless the characteristics of that variable change over time in such a way as to make the earlier measure inappropriate. For example, measures of cognitive and motor development for infants and children will generally not involve the same performance variables. Internal validity of longitudinal studies can be threatened by testing effects because subjects are tested repeatedly, by attrition because of the long data collection time, and by confounding variables that may coincidentally affect the developmental sequence that is being evaluated.

Cross-Sectional Method

In a **cross-sectional study,** the researcher studies a stratified group of subjects at one point in time and draws conclusions about development within a population by comparing the characteristics of those strata. For example, Zamboni et al. described the effects of aging on body fat distribution and cardiovascular risk factors across age groups representing individuals from 18 to 72 years.[22] In another example, Marsala and VanSant studied toddlers as they rose to a standing position from the floor in a sample of 60 children aged 15 to 47 months.[23] They classified movement patterns of the upper and lower extremities and trunk across different age groups. In both of these studies, the investigators chose to examine the characteristics of a broad sample at one time, rather than follow a group over several years.

The cross-sectional approach has been used more often than the longitudinal study because of its obvious efficiency. In addition, cross-sectional studies are not threatened by testing or history effects because subjects are tested only once, and all subjects are tested at the same time. The major threat to validity in cross-sectional studies is selection; that is, it is difficult to know to what extent results reflect the effects of age or the passage of time versus the effects of extraneous sampling variables.

Many of the extraneous variables that interfere in cross-sectional studies pertain to **cohort effects,** that is, effects that are not age specific but are due to a subject's generation or time of birth. Subjects can differ in quality, style, or duration of education, exposure to information about health, or historical events that influenced life choices and practices. For example, suppose we were interested in studying the development of cardiovascular risk factors using a cross-sectional approach. We include present-day elders who were born at the beginning of the 20th century, adults who were born after World War II, and younger subjects born after 1960. We might observe significant variation across the three age groups; however, based on this evidence alone we cannot conclude that these factors normally change with age. The differences may have some age-related basis, but it is also likely that life experiences play an important role. For instance, the elders did not have the benefits of growing up in a world of improved medical technology and media campaigns about physical fitness and diet. Therefore, conclusions about age effects may be threatened by the extraneous effects of cohort differences.

Developmental research provides an invaluable source of information for the production of correlational and experimental hypotheses. A foundation of descriptive data is needed for the generation of developmental theories and determination of which variables are most important for studying treatment effects. Cross-sectional data are most effective when the primary interest in a developmental study is the description of typical individuals at various stages of life or the description of existing groups in contemporary society. The cross-sectional method will provide a greater possibility of sampling large representative groups for such assessments. If, however, the primary interest is the study of patterns of change, the longitudinal method is preferred, as only this method can establish the validity of temporal sequencing of behaviors and characteristics.

Normative Studies

The utility of evaluative findings in the assessment of a patient's problems is based on the comparison of those findings with known standards of performance. For example, gait deviations are evaluated by comparison with "normal patterns,"[24] joint motion is compared with ranges "within normal limits,"[25] and nerve conduction velocities are interpreted with reference to "normal values."[26] Clinicians need these standards as a basis for documenting the existence and severity of weakness, limitations, and patient problems and as a guide for setting goals.

The purpose of **normative research** is to describe typical or standard values for characteristics of a given population. Normative studies are often directed toward a specific age group, gender, occupation, culture, or disability. For example, researchers have established normative values for speech perception capacity in children aged 5 to 10 years,[27] gait characteristics of patients with above-knee amputations,[28] strength of elite soccer players,[29] and performance on neuropsychological tests in English- and Spanish-speaking elders.[30]

Norms are usually expressed as an average, or mean, within a range of acceptable values. Therefore, the normal nerve conduction velocity of the ulnar nerve is expressed as 57.5 meters/sec, with a normal range of 49.5 to 63.6 m/s.[31] The normal cadence of women walking with high heels is given as 117 steps per minute, with a range from 100 to 133 steps/minute.[32] Average values are often given with a standard deviation.[†] Therefore, we can describe normal knee range for healthy adults during free speed walking as 60 ± 7 degrees.[33] Norms can also represent standardized scores that allow interpretation of responses with reference to an arbitrary "normal" value. For example, IQ scores are "normed" against a mean of 100.

The importance of establishing the validity of normative values is obvious. The estimation of "normal" behavior or performance is often used as a basis for prescribing corrective intervention or for predicting future performance. If the interpretation of assessments and the consequent treatment plan are based on the extent of deviation from "normal," the standard values must be valid reflections of this norm. Because no characteristic of a population can be adequately described by a single value, normal values are often established with reference to concomitant factors. For instance, Molnar and Alexander studied muscle strength in children and established varied norms based on age, gender, height, and weight.[34] Horowitz and colleagues established normative data for grip strength in older persons, and distinguished typical performance by gender and level of fitness activity.[35]

There is still a substantial need for normative research in health-related sciences. As new measurement tools are developed, research is needed to establish standards for interpretation of their output. This is especially true in areas where a variety of instruments are used to measure the same clinical variables, such as function and health status assessments. For example, health status instruments, such as the SF-36, have published norms that help health care providers and clients assess health in several domains.[36] It is also essential that these norms be established for a variety of diagnostic populations and age groups, so that appropriate standards can be applied in different clinical situations. For example, the functional reach test has been used extensively as a measure of stability in the elderly.[37] It has also been tested as a balance assessment for patients with spinal cord injury,[38] and age-related normative values have been determined for children without disabilities, aged 5 to 15 years.[39]

Researchers should be aware of the great potential for sampling bias when striving to establish standard values. Samples for normative studies must be large, random, and representative of the population's heterogeneity. The specific population of interest

---

[†]Standard deviation is a measure of variability within a distribution. A standard deviation expressed as ± estimates the range of scores above and below the average score within which the majority of the population (68%) will fall (see Chapter 17).

should be delineated as accurately as possible. Replication is essential to this form of research, to demonstrate consistency and, thereby, validate findings.

Qualitative Research

Methods of data collection in clinical research vary in their degree of precision and objectivity. At one extreme, researchers employ strictly *quantitative* methods, such as measurement of physiological and physical properties. Quantitative methodology is linked to the philosophy of **logical positivism,** in which human experience is assumed to be limited to logical and controlled relationships between specific measurable variables. The rationale for studying these relationships can be defined in advance, based on hypotheses that guide the methods of data collection. Accordingly, variables can be operationalized and assigned numerical values, independent of historical, cultural, or social contexts within which performance is observed.[40] For example, many quality of life assessments, by virtue of their list of questions, are based on assumptions about measurable behaviors that reflect health status. By using a predetermined rating scale, investigators demonstrate the reductionist premise of quantitative research—that experience and clinical phenomena can be reduced to a set of specific questions and variables.

The essence of the qualitative method, on the other hand, obliges the researcher to understand the patient's perspective first. **Qualitative research** seeks to describe the complex nature of humans and how individuals perceive their own experiences within a specific social context. Qualitative methodology uses the subject's own words and narrative summaries of observable behavior to express data, rather than numbers. The qualitative approach emphasizes an understanding of human experience, exploring the nature of people's transactions with themselves, others, and their surroundings. Questions that lend themselves to qualitative inquiry are generally broad, seeking to understand why something occurs, what certain experiences mean to a patient or client, or how the dynamics of an experience influence subsequent behaviors or decisions. For example, Oiler has suggested that the term "phantom pain" for discomfort following limb amputation is not sufficient to describe the reality of that experience by the patient, but provides only a label that others can use to classify it.[41] Therefore, a qualitative investigation into this phenomenon might try to uncover the meaning of this sensation to those who experience it and how it affects their behavior, emotions, body image, self-esteem, and interactions. The purpose of qualitative inquiry is to examine such experiences using a holistic approach that is concerned with the true nature of "reality" as the participants understand it. Qualitative methodology has been a cornerstone of research in sociology and anthropology and has more recently received attention by clinical researchers.

Qualitative research is not simply a description of a particular situation. To qualify as a research method, such inquiry must be tied to understanding, explanation, or the development of theory about an observed phenomenon. From such insightful description, relevant variables can be uncovered, and questions can then be asked to look at more quantitative aspects of those variables in controlled settings. Qualitative and quantitative aspects can also be combined within one study, to measure certain components of behavior and to see how such measurements relate to the nature of the experience.[42] For example, Danigelis and colleagues studied factors related to compliance with breast screening practices in a sample of African-American women, using both surveys and focus groups.[43]

Perspectives in Qualitative Research

Phenomenology. The tradition known as **phenomenology** seeks to draw meaning from complex realities through careful analysis of narrative subjective materials.[44,45] The researcher begins this type of inquiry by identifying the clinical phenomenon to be studied. Terminal illness, childbirth, or physical disability are examples of phenomena that have been explored by health professionals. For instance, Whalley et al. studied 50 patients with rheumatoid arthritis to describe how the disease affects their life, including moods and emotions, social life, hobbies, everyday tasks, personal and social relationships, and physical contact.[46] This study grew out of the belief that appropriate measures of quality of life for these patients must be based on a better understanding of their disease experience, and that the meaning of that disease experience must be interpreted by the individual who has lived it.

In the phenomenological perspective, experience is constructed within the individual's social context and is, therefore, intersubjective.[47] To illustrate this concept, Gravelle explored the daily experiences of parents who cared for a child with a life-threatening illness at home.[48] She conceptualized their experiences as an ongoing process of "facing adversity," based on their need to constantly redefine their roles as the child's disease progressed. The true depth of the dimensions of feelings, thoughts, and behaviors that are part of this experience could only be investigated by questioning and observing parents who were in that environment.

Ethnography. A second common perspective, called **ethnography,** is the study of the social milieu of a specific cultural group of people. Ethnographic research examines the attitudes, beliefs, and behaviors of sociological units. In ethnographic studies, the researcher becomes immersed in the subjects' way of life to understand the cultural forces that shape behavior and feelings. Questions often emerge as data are collected. The ethnographer begins this type of inquiry by identifying the setting or culture to be studied and may specify the types of phenomena that will be observed. For example, this approach has been used to study the manner in which individuals from different cultures experience and describe pain,[49] and traditional beliefs and practices related to pregnancy and childbirth among Native American women.[50] Classic examples of ethnographic research are found in the well-known anthropological works of Margaret Mead[51,52] and the poignant study, *Number Our Days*, by Barbara Myerhoff, which chronicles the life histories and community experience of elderly Eastern European Jews living in Venice, California.[53] Studies that describe the behaviors and values of a specific professional group can also be considered ethnographic. For instance, Mello and Jenkinson explored decision-making practices of physicians and nurses concerning "Do-Not-Resuscitate" orders in British and American hospitals, and found different attitudes related to autonomous decision making and family involvement.[54]

Grounded Theory. One unique feature of qualitative methodology is that it allows the researcher to develop research hypotheses as the data unfold using inductive processes. Because it is an exploratory technique, qualitative research will not always begin with predetermined expectations. Instead, the researcher can use the data to develop a theory that will explain what is observed. This approach is called **grounded theory research,**

in which the researcher collects, codes, and analyzes data simultaneously, identifying relevant variables, which may lead to the development of theoretical concepts that are "grounded" in the observations.[55] These concepts are not based on preconceived hypotheses, but instead grow out of an ongoing, dynamic analysis. Each interview or observation builds on the previous ones until the data being collected become repetitious and no longer produce new information. As this process progresses, interrelationships emerge that lead to the development of theoretical concepts. The **constant comparative method** is an inductive process that is often used in the grounded theory approach. It calls for continual testing of the theory as the data are examined.[56] As data are collected and coded, each idea or theme is compared with others to determine where they agree or conflict. At any point in the study, if data do not support the theory, they are not discarded, but the theory is refined so that it fits the existing data. This method requires a sophisticated approach to coding and categorizing data.

Methods of Qualitative Data Collection

Because qualitative data can come from a wide variety of sources and take many different forms, the methods of data collection are also quite varied. The most common forms of data collection are interviews and observation.

Interviews.   Interviews involve a form of direct contact between the researcher and the subjects within the subjects' natural environment. Interviews are used to gather information, with the researcher asking questions that probe the subject's experiences and perceptions. For example, Davis used interview techniques to develop a model of empathy by asking therapists to recount experiences with patients in which they believed empathic interactions had taken place.[57] Through their descriptions, she was able to identify three overlapping stages of empathy. McCann interviewed a sample of health professionals and spouse caregivers of elderly chronically ill individuals in an effort to understand the perspectives of each group on long-term home care.[58] She explored the caregivers' motivations, worries, daily activities, and feelings about their role and the impact of their caregiving role on their own lives. The professionals were asked about their perceptions of the caregivers' concerns and what factors contribute to positive or negative outcomes of home care.

Interviews should be approached with a broadly structured script that will guide the discussion and provide a basis for comparing responses; however, they must also be flexible enough to allow the interviewer to probe and ask follow-up questions that are relevant to the specific individual's circumstances. For example, an interviewer might simply ask, "Tell me what it's been like for you to know you have cancer?" Such a question might be followed by additional probes to elicit the full richness of the data. This process requires that the interviewer have expertise in the subject matter that will be discussed, so that the appropriate follow-up questions will be asked. The quality of the data collected will depend on the knowledge and skill of the interviewer. Therefore, interviewers should be trained in both interviewing and observation skills, and must be sensitive to the issues that will be raised by respondents.

Observation.   The interview approach is potentially limiting as a singular data collection strategy in that it may not reflect the feelings and actions that actually occur during the subjects' interactions, but only the subjects' memory of them.[59] In addition, the social context within which feelings and actions took place is not clearly defined in an interview. These limitations can be addressed by combining both observation and interview as a method of data collection. For example, Scully and Shepard examined the process of clinical education in a field study where they observed clinical teachers during the course of their work, recording what they did, when, with whom, and in what circumstances.[60] Interviews supplemented these data, as a way of probing reasons for observed actions. By synthesizing these two sources, the authors were able to identify two components of the clinical education process, one involving the organizational and human factors that influence the teaching situation and the other related to the teaching tools used by the clinical teachers.

Observational techniques are most useful when the researcher wants to document actual behaviors. Researchers can use a range of experiences to try to draw inferences about subjects' behaviors. At one end of the range, the researcher can be a complete observer, simply watching and recording the subjects' responses and reactions. There are, however, situations for which this approach is restrictive in that the researcher's analysis of responses is limited by the context within which the researcher interprets those responses; that is, the researcher can only understand outcomes using a personal frame of reference, not the subjects' "reality." The essence of qualitative research is that the individual's experience should be described as it is lived by that individual. Therefore, at the other end of the range, the researcher can become one of the members of the group that is being observed, using a technique called **participant observation.** With this method, the researcher actually becomes a participant in the activities of the study group, so that observation of behaviors can be appreciated from the standpoint of those who are being observed. Although this technique is inherently biased by the researcher's own preconceptions, it provides a mechanism for the researcher to describe the interactions of individuals within a social context and to analyze behaviors as a function of the subjects' personal realities. The researcher is then in a position to recognize feelings and thoughts that emerge from the subjects' frame of reference. For example, Hasselkus studied the meaning of daily routines and activities at a day care center for persons with Alzheimer disease, as experienced by the staff.[61] Data collection included interviews and participant observation, by working directly with the staff. Through this experience, the researcher determined that the foremost guiding principle for all activities during the day was prevention, that is, to prevent participant behavior that would be harmful to self or to others. In another study, May explored the involvement of fathers during pregnancy by participating in child birth classes and clinics.[62] Participant observer is a complex role, but one that is believed to enhance the validity of qualitative observations.[63]

Data Analysis and Interpretation

Qualitative data analysis is primarily an inductive process, with a constant interplay between observed reality and theoretical conceptualization of that reality. Therefore, the process of analysis is ongoing as data are collected. Because observational and interview responses are recorded as narratives, qualitative data are typically voluminous. Data will usually be recorded through written notes and on audio or videotape. The specific techniques of data analysis can vary from purely narrative descriptions of observations to quantitative descriptions of the frequency of certain behaviors or characteristics in the sample.

Order and structure are imposed on qualitative data through a process of **content analysis.** As an example, Mavundla designed a study to evaluate the experience of leaving home by an elderly person and going into an institution.[64] The researchers used semistructured interviews to explore the experiences of 12 elderly individuals who resided in a home for the elderly in Eastern Cape Province in South Africa. Content analysis of the interviews revealed four types of factors that were significantly related to the decision concerning institutionalization: physical, psychological, psychosocial, and social. The researchers discussed the implications of these factors for the role of the community health nurse and the psychiatric nurse for screening and counseling elderly residents who might return home. This study illustrates how a researcher sorts through narrative data using a coding process to develop categories in a systematic way, to uncover patterns or themes in the mass of information that is available. Computer programs are available to assist in this often extensive process.

Reliability and Validity

Reliability and validity are issues of concern in qualitative research as in all types of research, but they must be approached differently because of the subjective nature of the data.[65] For qualitative study the concept of "measurement error" must be examined in terms of judgments rather than numerical equivalency.[66] Problems arise because the same words may have varied meanings in different situations. Although there is limited consensus about appropriate methods of analyzing qualitative data, such analyses are always grounded in the data. They involve iterative procedures that result in the development and refinement of typologies, analogies, and other forms of concepts to make sense of data.[67] Lincoln[68] and Guba[69] have described credibility of qualitative data in terms of truth value and consistency within the data. These criteria reflect a need to consider the rigor of data analysis and the potential for investigator bias. Qualitative data analysis is inevitably a creative and subjective process, but can achieve a certain level of objectivity and validity through careful definitions and confirmation of interpretations.

Triangulation refers to a process whereby concepts are confirmed using more than one source of data. The concept actually originated as a technical term in surveying, to demonstrate how two visible points could be used to locate a third point. In social sciences the concept has been adopted to reflect multiple methods of data collection to substantiate an outcome. For instance, the researcher may identify a specific concept through information obtained from a subject's interview responses, by direct observation of group performance, and by analysis of written materials. If comparable conclusions are drawn from each method, the validity of the interpretation is considerably strengthened.

The validity of research findings can also be supported by a clear description of the thought processes used to interpret the data. This process is referred to as an **audit trail,** allowing those who read the research to follow the investigator's logic. This provides an opportunity for others to agree or disagree with conclusions. Other strategies for improving accuracy include the involvement of more than one investigator to confirm ideas, and confirmation of conclusions with the subject of the study.[70]

Sampling

Sampling is another issue that can affect validity of a qualitative study. How the researcher selects subjects for study will obviously have a significant impact on the outcome. For the most part, subject selection proceeds in a purposeful way, as the investigator must locate subjects who will be effective informants, and who will provide a rich source of information.[71] Coyne distinguishes this from a process where a few subjects may be initially chosen because they belong to a certain group, but further subjects are recruited based on their fit with theory that emerges from the initial data.[72] This process, termed **theoretical sampling,** is based on the need to collect data to examine emerging categories and their relationships, and not on identifying specific age, gender, or other characteristics of subjects.[73]

Sample size remains an important consideration.[74] Samples that are too small will not support claims of having reached a point of saturation in the data, where no new information is obtained. Samples that are too large will not permit the in-depth analysis that is the essence of qualitative inquiry. Sandelowski suggests that determining adequate sample size in qualitative research is a matter of judgment and experience in evaluating the quality of the information collected and the purpose of the research.[74]

We recognize that this brief introduction to qualitative analysis is by no means sufficient to demonstrate the scope of data collection and analysis methods that have been developed. This approach has great promise for generating understanding of health and how it is evaluated. Those interested in pursuing qualitative research are urged to read the classic work of Glaser and Strauss[55] and other references in this chapter. We also suggest reading professional literature to gain an appreciation for the breadth of qualitative research and to develop familiarity with the techniques and terminology of qualitative methodology. Sandelowski has discussed a method for using the principles of meta-analysis with qualitative studies, to demonstrate broader applicability of findings.[75]

EXPLORATORY RESEARCH

The complexity of human behavior and clinical phenomena present a considerable challenge to the clinician and researcher. In many situations, the impetus for a research study is the need to understand how human attributes and environmental characteristics interact to control behavioral responses. As clinical scientists continue to question how we can achieve optimal outcomes under defined clinical conditions, we must examine the multiple factors that influence our patients' lives. **Exploratory research** is the systematic investigation of relationships among two or more variables. Researchers use this approach to describe relationships, to predict the effect of one variable on another, or to test relationships that are supported by clinical theory. This type of research is usually guided by a set of hypotheses that help to structure measurements and interpretation of findings.

Correlation and Regression

The foundation of exploratory study is the process of *correlation*, a measure of the degree of association among variables. Correlation is a function of *covariation* in data, that is, the extent to which one variable varies directly or indirectly with another variable. We measure the strength of this relationship using a correlation statistic. There are many forms of correlational analysis. The reader is referred to Chapters 23, 24, and 27 for descriptions of specific statistical methods. In summary, correlational statistics produce a coefficient ranging between −1.00 and +1.00. The strength of the relationship is indicated by how close the correlation coefficient is to ±1.00. A negative correlation indicates that variable X increases as variable Y decreases; a positive correlation indicates that variable X increases as variable Y increases. A *regression* procedure is used when the researcher wants to predict the score on an outcome variable by knowing values on other variables. Correlational models can be *bivariate*, including only two variables, or *multivariate*, incorporating several variables.

In exploratory studies, researchers do not attempt to control or manipulate the variables under study, only to measure how they vary with respect to each other. Therefore, exploratory studies are not used to test differences between groups or to establish the presence of cause-and-effect relationships between independent and dependent variables. This distinction is important when interpreting correlational outcomes. There may appear to be a strong correlation between two variables, X and Y, because actually some third variable, Z, causes both X and Y. For instance, we might find that the inability to climb stairs is correlated with poor knee strength in patients with osteoarthritis; however, the cause of the functional limitation may actually be knee pain, which is also related to measurable weakness in knee muscles. Exploratory research will often provide evidence of a relationship that can then be tested using experimental techniques to determine if one variable can be considered the cause of the other.

Correlational and Predictive Studies

The purpose of **correlational research** is to describe the nature of existing relationships among variables. Data from this type of study often provide the rationale for clinical decisions or the generation of hypotheses. Researchers will often look at several variables simultaneously to determine which ones are related. For instance, in a prospective study, Higgins examined the perception of fatigue in chronically ill patients who were undergoing long-term mechanical ventilation.[76] She examined the effect of nutritional status, depression, and sleep on fatigue, and found a strong relationship only between fatigue and depression. Knowledge of this relationship can be used to foster appropriate interventions for this population.

Predictive research studies are designed to predict a behavior or response based on the observed relationship between that behavior and other variables. Predictive designs can be used to develop models that can serve as a basis for decision making. For example, in determining criteria for the presence of weakness, researchers have examined a variety of factors that are related to strength. In one study, researchers investigated the relationship between knee strength and height, weight, age, gender, thigh girth, and percent body fat to establish muscle strength goals for rehabilitation.[77]

Predictive studies are also often used for validation of a measurement tool. For example, Rutledge et al. identified problems in using the Glasgow Coma Scale (GCS) in intubated patients, because the scale requires verbal responses that are blocked by intubation.[78] The purpose of their study, therefore, was to develop a basis for predicting the verbal score using only the motor and eye responses of the scale. The authors used a multiple regression procedure to determine if these variables were strong predictors of the verbal score (see Chapter 27). The following regression equation was developed for the relationship between verbal score and the motor and eye scores:

$$\text{Verbal Score} = 2.3976 + (0.9253 \times \text{GCS motor}) + (-0.9214 \times \text{GCS eye})$$
$$+ (0.2208 \times \text{GSC motor}^2) + (0.2318 \times \text{GSC eye}^2)$$

We could take a single subject's eye and motor scores and, by substituting them in the equation, predict the expected verbal score. The predicted value will not be totally accurate; that is, the equation has some degree of error. We can look at the actual verbal score for that subject and determine the difference between the observed and expected values. A strong model will demonstrate little discrepancy between these values. In this study, the accuracy of the model was extremely high, predicting 83% of the variance in the verbal score. The ultimate purpose of developing the model is to extend its use to a different set of subjects. Therefore, the model must be validated by testing it on different groups. For example, Meredith et al. tested this equation using a retrospective sample of over 14,000 patients taken from a trauma registry by comparing their predicted and actual GCS scores.[79] Their findings supported the use of the prediction model, confirming the ability to determine an accurate GCS score in the absence of the verbal component.

Prediction has become an important research goal in outcomes research as well, with a focus on determining those factors that contribute to or detract from successful clinical outcomes. As an example, Heinemann et al. examined length of stay and motor and cognitive scores on the Functional Independence Measure (FIM) in over 27,000 rehabilitation patients.[80] They hypothesized that admission FIM scores would predict discharge scores and length of stay. Using length of stay as an outcome measure, the investigators concluded that functional measures were useful for predicting resource use by these patients. In another example, researchers studied the contribution of neuromuscular impairments to physical function in 148 patients with lumbar spinal stenosis.[81] They measured function using the physical dimension of the Sickness Impact Profile (P-SIP), and correlated it to the presence of comorbidities and impairments of pin sensation, strength, deep tendon reflexes, and vibration. They determined that neuromuscular deficit (as defined by this set of variables) had little to do with physical functional status in these patients, but that pain, depression, employment status, and comorbidities were important predictors. As clinicians continue to explore the disablement model, these types of studies will prove essential for testing assumptions about the relationships among pathology, impairments, functional limitations, and disabilities.

Theory Testing

Another purpose for correlational study is the testing of theory. With this approach, the researcher chooses specific variables for study, based on expected relationships derived from deductive hypotheses. The evaluation of theory can require elaborate analysis procedures, depending on the nature of the variables and the complexity of the hypotheses drawn from the theory. Multivariate statistical techniques are often used in this type of study (see Chapter 27).

This approach is illustrated in a study by Case-Smith et al., who used correlational data to test the ontogenetic principle that the development of proximal postural stability is a prerequisite for the development of distal fine motor control.[82] They investigated the relationship between proximal and distal motor function in normal infants and anticipated strong correlations between assessments of postural stability and fine motor performance if the hypothesis was true. They used a technique called *partial correlation*, which establishes the relationship between two variables with the effect of a third, potentially confounding variable, statistically removed (see Chapter 27). In this case, the authors observed a high correlation between their assessments and chronological age and, therefore, tested the hypothesis that proximal and distal motor functions would correlate when the effect of age was controlled. If this control had not been used, the distal and proximal assessments might have appeared highly correlated because of their mutual relationship with age, even if they were not related to each other. On the basis of the partial correlations, the authors observed weak relationships that were considered too low to support the theoretical premise.

Advantages and Disadvantages of Exploratory Research

Even though exploratory studies are not able to establish cause-and-effect relationships, they play an important role in clinical research, especially considering the lack of documented evidence that exists concerning most clinical phenomena. Before one can begin to investigate causal factors for behaviors and responses using experimental methods, one must first discover which variables are related and how they occur in nature. For many phenomena, we will probably never be able to establish causality and can move ahead in our critical inquiry only if we can understand how those phenomena manifest themselves with regard to concurrent variables.

Many correlational studies are based on variables that have been measured in the past or that represent attributes of individuals that are beyond the control of the investigator. Under these conditions, exploratory research is limited in its interpretation because of the potential bias that exists in the data. Many secondary analyses are performed on databases that offer a great deal of information, but without the benefit of controlling measurement and operational definitions (see Chapter 16 for a discussion of secondary analysis). The researcher is obliged to consider the implications of these potential biases when interpreting the outcomes of correlational analyses.

Finally, the complex nature of clinical phenomena and the intricate interrelationships that exist among attitudes, behaviors, physical and psychological characteristics, and the environment present special interpretive problems for correlational analysis. It is often very difficult to establish that two variables are associated without considering the multitude of other variables that would have to enter into any predictive or theoretical relationship. Correlational studies compel us to contemplate the theories that would help explain observed relationships, and to approach analyses from a *multivariate* perspective. This means that analyses can become quite complex, but at the same time, it also presents exciting opportunities for exploring alternative explanations for our clinical observations.

COMMENTARY

First Things First

The purpose of descriptive research is to characterize phenomena so that we know what *exists*. Without this fundamental knowledge, it would be impossible to ask questions about behaviors or treatment effects or to propose theories to explain them. This approach is clearly contrasted with traditional experimental research, which seeks to determine what *will happen* in a given set of controlled circumstances.

Although descriptive studies do not strive for the degree of control found in experimental studies, descriptive research serves an important role within the spectrum of research designs. The state of knowledge in the rehabilitation professions is relatively immature, and we still face the need to define clinical behaviors so that we can begin to explore them. Just like a child must first learn to crawl before it can walk, clinical scientists must first discover how the world around them naturally behaves before they can manipulate and control those behaviors to test methods of changing them.

Despite the fact that descriptive studies do not involve manipulation of variables or randomization, descriptive research still requires rigor in defining and measuring variables of interest, whether they emerge as narrative descriptions or quantitative summaries. Unfortunately, there is a tendency to view conclusions from descriptive studies as weaker than conclusions from experimental studies, but this is true only in the context of establishing cause-and-effect relationships. Descriptive findings can be strong and meaningful as a basis for explanation and characterization of variables when they are the result of a well-designed study and when they are interpreted within the context of an appropriate research question. The results of descriptive studies may provide essential information for understanding of the benefits of clinical trials, and for describing or explaining why some subjects respond differently than others.

Experimental designs will not necessarily be "better" if the research question focuses on the development of understanding of clinical phenomena or if the study variables represent constructs that are poorly developed. With so many behavioral and clinical concepts not yet fully understood, descriptive research presents an extraordinary and vital challenge to the clinical researcher.

KEY TERMS

descriptive research
exploratory research
retrospective research
prospective research
case study
developmental research
longitudinal study
cross-sectional study
cohort effects

normative research
logical positivism
qualitative research
phenomenology
ethnography
grounded theory
constant comparative
    method
participant observation

content analysis
triangulation
audit trail
theoretical sampling
correlational research
predictive research

REFERENCES

1. Lechner DE, McCarthy CF, Holden MK. Gait deviations in patients with juvenile rheumatoid arthritis. *Phys Ther* 1987;67:1335–41.
2. Shimada SD, Robertson RN, Bonninger ML, Cooper RA. Kinematic characterization of wheelchair propulsion. *J Rehabil Res Dev* 1998;35:210–8.
3. Hogeweg JA, Kuis W, Oostendorp RA, Helders PJ. The influence of site of stimulation, age, and gender on pain threshold in healthy children. *Phys Ther* 1996;76:1331–9.
4. Panikoff LB. Recovery trends of functional skills in the head-injured adult. *Am J Occup Ther* 1983;37:735–43.
5. Sellers BJ, Davis BL, Larkin PW, Morris SE, Saffle JR. Early prediction of prolonged ventilator dependence in thermally injured patients. *J Trauma* 1997;43:899–903.
6. Cerhan JR, Chiu BC, Wallace RB, et al. Physical activity, physical function, and the risk of breast cancer in a prospective study among elderly women. *J Gerontol* 1998;53A:M251–M256.
7. Gann N, Nalty T. Vertical patellar dislocation: a case report. *J Orthop Sports Phys Ther* 1998;27:368–70.
8. LaPier TLK, Sirotnak N, Alexander K. Aerobic exercise for a patient with chronic multisystem impairments. *Phys Ther* 1998;78:417–424.
9. Bromley DB. *A Case-Study Method in Psychology and Related Disciplines.* New York: John Wiley, 1986.
10. Kratochwill RT, Mott SE, Dodson CL. Case study and single-case research in clinical and applied psychology. In: Bellack AS, Hersen M, eds. *Research Methodology in Clinical Psychology.* New York: Pergamon Press, 1984.
11. Kazdin AE. Drawing valid inferences from case studies. *J Consult Clin Psychol* 1981;49:183–92.
12. Gesell A, Amatruda CS. *The Embryology of Behavior.* New York: Harper & Brothers, 1945.
13. McGraw MB. *The Neuromuscular Maturation of the Human Infant.* New York: Hafner, 1963.
14. Erikson EH. *Childhood and Society.* 2d ed. New York: Norton, 1963.
15. Tanner JM. Physical growth. In: Mussen PH, ed. *Carmichael's Manual of Child Psychology.* 3d ed. New York: Wiley, 1970.
16. Honzik MP, MacFarland JW, Allen L. The stability of mental test performance between two and eighteen years. *J Exp Educ* 1949;17:309.
17. Horn JL, Donaldson G. Cognitive development: II. Adulthood development of human abilities. In: Brim OG, Kagan J, eds. *Constancy and Change in Human Development.* Cambridge, MA: Harvard University Press, 1980.
18. Horowitz L, Sharby N. Development of prone extension postures in healthy infants. *Phys Ther* 1988;68:32–9.
19. Livson FB. Patterns of personality developement in middle-aged women: a longitudinal study. *Int J Aging Hum Dev* 1976;7:107–15.
20. Starr JM, Deary IJ, Inch S, Cross S, MacLennan WJ. Age-associated cognitive decline in healthy old people. *Age Ageing* 1997;26:295–300.
21. Munsat TL, Andres PL, Finison L, Conlon T, Thibodeau L. The natural history of motoneuron loss in amyotrophic lateral sclerosis. *Neurology* 1988;38:409–13.
22. Zamboni M, Armellini F, Harris T, et al. Effects of age on body fat distribution and cardiovascular risk factors in women. *Am J Clin Nutr* 1997;66:111–5.
23. Marsala G, VanSant AF. Age-related differences in movement patterns used by toddlers to rise from a supine position to erect stance. *Phys Ther* 1998;78:149–59.
24. Murray MP. Studies of normal and abnormal locomotion. *Int J Rehabil Res* 1979;2:510–2.
25. Norkin CC, White DJ. *Measurement of Joint Motion: A Guide to Goniometry.* 2d ed. Philadelphia: FA Davis, 1995.
26. Delisa JA, Lee HJ, Baran EM, Lai K. *Manual of Nerve Conduction Velocity and Clinical Neurophysiology.* 3d ed. New York: Raven Press, 1994.

27. Hnath-Chisolm TE, Laipply E, Boothroyd A. Age-related changes on a children's test of sensory-level speech perception capacity. *J Speech Lang Hear Res* 1998;41:94–106.

28. Murray MP, Mollinger LA, Sepic SB, Gardner GM, Linder MT. Gait patterns in above-knee amputee patients: hydraulic swing control vs constant-friction knee components. *Arch Phys Med Rehabil* 1983;64:339–45.

29. Wisloff U, Helgerud J, Hoff J. Strength and endurance of elite soccer players. *Med Sci Sports Exerc* 1998;30:462–7.

30. Stricks L, Pittman J, Jacobs DM, Sano M, Stern Y. Normative data for a brief neuropsychological battery administered to English- and Spanish-speaking community-dwelling elders. *J Int Neuropsychol Soc* 1998;4:311–8.

31. McQuillen MP, Gorin FJ. Serial ulnar nerve conduction velocity measurements in normal subjects. *J Neurol Neurosurg Psychiatry* 1969;32:144–8.

32. Murray MP, Kory RC, Sepic SB. Walking pattern of normal women. *Arch Phys Med Rehabil* 1970;51:637–50.

33. Brinkmann JR, Perry J. Rate and range of knee motion during ambulation in healthy and arthritic subjects. *Phys Ther* 1985;65:1055–60.

34. Molnar GE, Alexander J. Development of quantitative standards for muscle strength in children. *Arch Phys Med Rehabil* 1974;55:490–3.

35. Horowitz BP, Tollin R, Cassidy G. Grip strength: collection of normative data with community dwelling elders. *Phys Occup Ther Geriatr* 1997;15:53–64.

36. Ware JE, Snow KK, Kosinski M, et al. *SF-36 Survey: Manual and Interpretation Guide.* Boston: The Health Institute, New England Medical Center, 1993.

37. Duncan PW, Weiner DK, Chandler J, Studenski S. Functional reach: a new clinical measure of balance. *J Gerontol* 1990;45:M192–M197.

38. Lynch SM, Leahy P, Barker SP. Reliability of measurements obtained with a modified functional reach test in subjects with spinal cord injury. *Phys Ther* 1998;78:128–33.

39. Donahoe B, Turner D, Worrell T. The use of functional reach as a measurement of balance in boys and girls without disabilities ages 5 to 15 years. *Ped Phys Ther* 1994;6:189–93.

40. Leininger MM. *Qualitative Research Methods in Nursing.* Orlando, FL: Grune & Stratton, 1985.

41. Oiler C. The phenomenological approach in nursing research. *Nurs Res* 1982;31:178–81.

42. Goering PN, Streiner DL. Reconcilable differences: the marriage of qualitative and quantitative methods. *Can J Psychiatry* 1996;41:491–7.

43. Danigelis NL, Roberson NL, Worden JK, et al. Breast screening by African-American women: insights from a household survey and focus groups. *Am J Prev Med* 1995;11:311–7.

44. Beck CT. Phenomenology: its use in nursing research. *Int J Nurs Stud* 1994;31:499–510.

45. Jasper MA. Issues in phenomenology for researchers of nursing. *J Adv Nurs* 1994;19:309–4.

46. Whalley D, McKenna SP, de Jong Z, van der Heijde D. Quality of life in rheumatoid arthritis. *Br J Rheumatol* 1997;36:884–8.

47. Anderson JM. The phenomenological perspective. In: Morse JM, ed. *Qualitative Nursing Research: A Contemporary Dialogue.* Rockville, MD: Aspen, 1989, 15–26.

48. Gravelle AM. Caring for a child with a progressive illness during the complex chronic phase: parents' experience of facing adversity. *J Adv Nurs* 1997;25:738–45.

49. Moore R. Ethnographic assessment of pain coping perceptions. *Psychosom Med* 1990;52:171–81.

50. Long CR, Curry MA. Living in two worlds: Native American women and prenatal care. *Health Care Women Int* 1998;19:205–15.

51. Mead M. *Coming of Age in Somoa.* New York: Morrow, 1928.

52. Mead M. Ethnological aspects of aging. *Psychosomatics* 1967;8 (Suppl):33–7.

53. Myerhoff B. *Number Our Days.* New York: EP Dutton, 1978.

54. Mello M, Jenkinson C. Comparison of medical and nursing attitudes to resuscitation and patient autonomy between a British and an American teaching hospital. *Soc Sci Med* 1998;46:415–24.

55. Glaser B, Strauss A. *The Discovery of Grounded Theory.* Chicago: Aldine Publishing, 1967.

56. Simms LM. The grounded theory approach in nursing research. *Nurs Res* 1981;30:356–9.

57. Davis CM. What is empathy, and can empathy be taught? *Phys Ther* 1990;70:707–11.

58. McCann JJ. Long term home care for the elderly: perceptions of nurses, physicians, and primary caregivers. *QRB Qual Rev Bull* 1988;14:66–74.

59. Guccione AA. Commentary: What is empathy, and can it be taught? *Phys Ther* 1990;70:712.

60. Scully RM, Shepard KF. Clinical teaching in physical therapy education. An ethnographic study. *Phys Ther* 1983;63:349–58.

61. Hasselkus BR. The meaning of activity: day care for persons with Alzheimer disease. *Am J Occup Ther* 1992;46:199–206.

62. May KA. Three phases of father involvement in pregnancy. *Nurs Res* 1982;31:337–42.

63. Kielhofner G. Qualitative research: Part two. Methodological approaches and relevance to occupational therapy. *Occup Ther J Res* 1982;2:150.

64. Mavundla TR. Factors leading to black elderly persons' decisions to seek institutional care in a home in the Eastern Cape. *Curationis* 1996;19:47–50.

65. Beck CT. Reliability and validity issues in phenomenological research. *West J Nurs Res* 1994;16:254–62.

66. Brink PJ. Issues in reliability and validity. In: Morse JM, ed. *Qualitative Nursing Research: A Contemporary Dialogue.* Rockville, MD: Aspen, 1989, 151–68.

67. Fitzpatrick R, Boulton M. Qualitative research in health care: I. The scope and validity of methods. *J Eval Clin Pract* 1996;2:123–30.

68. Lincoln YS, Guba EG. *Naturalistic Inquiry.* Newbury Park, CA: Sage, 1985.

69. Guba EG. Criteria for assessing the trustworthiness of naturalistic inquiries. *Educ Commun Technol J* 1981;29:75–92.

70. DePoy E, Gitlin LN. *Introduction to Research: Multiple Strategies for Health and Human Services.* St. Louis: Mosby, 1993.

71. Patton MQ. *Qualitative Evaluation and Research Methods.* 2d ed. Newbury Park, CA: Sage, 1990.

72. Coyne IT. Sampling in qualitative research. Purposeful and theoretical sampling; merging or clear boundaries? *J Adv Nurs* 1997;26:623–30.

73. Chenitz WC, Swanson JM. *From Practice to Grounded Theory: Qualitative Research in Nursing.* Menlo Park, CA: Addison-Wesley, 1986.

74. Sandelowski M. Sample size in qualitative research. *Res Nurs Health* 1995;18:179–83.

75. Sandelowski M, Docherty S, Emden C. Focus on qualitative methods. Qualitative metasynthesis: issues and techniques. *Res Nurs Health* 1997;20:365–71.

76. Higgins PA. Patient perception of fatigue while undergoing long-term mechanical ventilation: incidence and associated factors. *Heart Lung* 1998;27:177–83.

77. Gross MT, McGrain P, Demilio N, et al. Relationship between multiple predictor variables and normal knee torque production. *Phys Ther* 1989;69:54–62.

78. Rutledge R, Lentz CW, Fakhry S, Hunt J. Appropriate use of the Glasgow Coma Scale in intubated patients: a linear regression prediction of the Glasgow verbal score from the Glasgow eye and motor scores. *J Trauma* 1996;41:514–22.

79. Meredith W, Rutledge R, Fakhry SM, Emery S, Kromhout-Schiro S. The conundrum of the Glasgow Coma Scale in intubated patients: a linear regression prediction of the Glasgow verbal score from the Glasgow eye and motor scores. *J Trauma* 1998;44:839–44.

80. Heinemann AW, Linacre JM, Wright BD, Hamilton BB, Granger C. Prediction of rehabilitation outcomes with disability measures. *Arch Phys Med Rehabil* 1994;75:133–43.

81. Stucki G, Liang MH, Lipson SJ, Fossel AH, Katz JN. Contribution of neuromuscular impairment to physical functional status in patients with lumbar spinal stenosis. *J Rheumatol* 1994;21:1338–43.

82. Case-Smith J, Fisher AG, Bauer D. An analysis of the relationship between proximal and distal motor control. *Am J Occup Ther* 1989;43:657–62.

14

Surveys

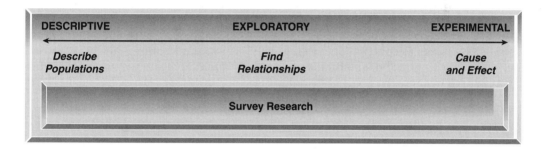

DESCRIPTIVE	EXPLORATORY	EXPERIMENTAL
Describe Populations	*Find Relationships*	*Cause and Effect*

Survey Research

One of the most popular methods for collecting descriptive data is the survey approach. A survey is composed of a series of questions that are posed to a group of subjects, and may be conducted as an oral interview or a written questionnaire. Sometimes the data are intended for generalization to a larger population; other times they may be intended as a description of a particular group. Surveys in clinical research are often concerned with describing attitudes and values, levels of knowledge or experience, current practices, or characteristics of specific groups. For example, survey questionnaires have been used to probe reasons why women who have a mastectomy decide whether to have breast reconstruction,[1] to determine the extent of use of electrical stimulation by clinicians,[2] to examine the utilization of hand splints by occupational therapists treating patients who have had a stroke,[3] and to describe functional characteristics of individuals with spinal cord injury following in-patient rehabilitation.[4] Standardized questionnaires are also used extensively as instruments for assessing outcomes related to function and quality of life.

The purpose of this chapter is to present an overview of the structure of survey instruments. We discuss essential elements of survey design, question writing, and some special assessment techniques associated with surveys, including several measurement scales.

INTERVIEWS AND QUESTIONNAIRES

Interviews

In an **interview** the researcher asks respondents specific questions and records their answers for later analysis. Interviews can take a few minutes or several hours, depending on the nature of the questions and the respondent's willingness to share information. Interviews can be conducted face to face or over the telephone, although face-to-face interviews tend to be more effective for establishing rapport between the interviewer and the respondent. This interaction can be important for eliciting forthright responses to questions that are of a personal nature. The advantage of the interview approach is the opportunity for in-depth analysis of respondents' behaviors and opinions because the researcher can probe responses and directly observe respondents' reactions. The major disadvantages of interviews include cost and time, need for personnel to carry out the interviews, scheduling, and the lack of anonymity of the respondents.

Most interviews are *structured* in that they consist of a standardized set of questions that will be asked. In this way, all respondents are exposed to the same questions, in the same order, and are given the same choices for responses. In an *unstructured* interview, the interviewer does not have a fixed agenda, and can proceed informally to question and discuss issues of concern. This format is typically conversational and is often carried out in the respondent's natural setting. Many qualitative studies use the unstructured interview approach to generate data.

Questionnaires

Questionnaires are structured surveys that are self-administered using pen and paper. The advantages of using questionnaires are many. They are generally more efficient than interviews because respondents complete them on their own time. Data can be gathered from a large sample in a wide geographical distribution in a relatively short time. Written forms are standardized, so that everyone is exposed to the same questions in the same way, reducing potential bias from interactions with an interviewer. Respondents to questionnaires can take time to think about their answers and to consult records for specific information. Questionnaires also provide anonymity, encouraging honest and candid responses. Questionnaires are particularly useful as a research method for examining phenomena that can be assessed through self-observation, such as attitudes, values, and perceptions. They are not as useful for studying behaviors that require objective observation. The primary disadvantages of the written questionnaire are the potential for misunderstanding or misinterpreting questions or response choices, and unknown accuracy or motivation of the respondent. In interviews, the researcher can clarify such misinterpretations.

The most common method of distributing questionnaires is through the mail, although many research situations allow for in-person distribution. Mailed questionnaires are economical and can reach a large population in a relatively short period; however, another major disadvantage of this approach is that the return rate is often quite low. Responses from 60% to 80% of a sample are usually considered excellent. Realistically, researchers can expect return rates between 30% and 60% for most studies. Actual response rates are lowered further by having to discard returns that are incomplete or incorrectly filled out. Low returns can severely limit the external validity of survey results. Therefore, survey samples are usually quite large so that a sufficient percentage of usable responses will be obtained.

Self-Report

Survey data that are collected using either an oral interview or a written questionnaire are based on a form of **self-report;** that is, the researcher does not directly observe the respondent's behavior or attitudes, but only records the respondent's report of them. There is always some potential for bias or inaccuracy in self-reports, particularly if the questions concern personal or controversial issues. The phenomenon of **recall bias** can be a problem when respondents are asked to remember past events, especially if these events were of a sensitive nature. Research has shown, however, that self-report measures are generally valid. For instance, variables such as function,[5] hypertension,[6] and smoking habits[7, 8] have been reported accurately, although a few studies have found poorer accuracy, such as self-report of function in patients over 75 years old.[9] These differences point out the need to understand the target population and the respondents' abilities to answer the questions posed. For many variables, however, such as perceptions, fears, motivations, and attitudes, self-report is the only direct way to obtain information. Data obtained from standardized questionnaires that evaluate health and function must be interpreted as the respondent's perception of those characteristics, rather than performance measures.

DESIGN OF SURVEYS

The process of developing a survey instrument is perhaps more time consuming than most people realize. It involves several stages, within which the instrument is written and revised, until it is finally ready for use as a research tool.

The Research Question

The first consideration in every research effort is delineation of the overall research question (see Chapter 7). The research problem must be identified with reference to a target population. These decisions will form the structure for deciding the appropriate research design. A survey is appropriate when the question requires obtaining information from subjects, rather than measuring performance.

Guiding Questions

As with any other research approach, validity is a major concern in the design of a survey instrument; that is, the questionnaire or interview must measure what it was intended to measure. Questions are not asked out of casual interest or curiosity, but because they reflect specific pieces of information that taken as a whole will address the proposed research question. Therefore, the first step in developing the survey is to define its purpose through a series of **guiding questions,** or objectives that delineate what the researcher is trying to find out. The guiding questions may reflect purely descriptive interest, or they may address expected relationships among variables. For example, Couch and colleagues examined the roles that play occupies within occupational therapy practice with preschoolers.[10] They proposed three guiding questions for their study:

1. *How do occupational therapists incorporate play into their practice?*
2. *Do occupational therapists assess play behaviors and what methods do they use?*
3. *Are there differences between school-based and non-school-based settings that influence the role of play within pediatric occupational therapy?*

These types of questions focus the content of a questionnaire.

Hypotheses

Survey instruments can also be designed to examine relationships. Some researchers will, therefore, specify hypotheses in addition to guiding questions. Hypotheses are important to direct statistical analyses and conclusions. To illustrate, Rozier and coworkers looked at the relationship between gender and career success factors in physical therapists.[11] One of the several guiding questions they posed was, "Are perceptions of career success different for male versus female physical therapists?" They proposed a series of hypotheses to answer this question, such as:

Men and women will differ with respect to perceptions of career success.

    a. *Men will rate themselves higher in career success compared with women.*

    b. *Men will report greater importance of salary and position compared with women.*

By delineating the specific variables and expected outcomes, the authors were able to clearly structure the questions, analysis and discussion of their findings.

Questionnaire Outline

Once the guiding questions or hypotheses are formulated, the researcher must develop a detailed outline, listing each item of information that will be needed to answer the guiding questions. Each item should relate back to at least one of the study's objectives. Often, more than one item will be needed to address a single question or hypothesis.

Stating useful guiding questions that support an overall research question requires that the researcher have a clear conceptualization of the phenomenon or characteristics being studied. If the phenomenon is poorly understood, it will be hard to construct questions that explore its component behaviors. In the study by Couch, it would not be possible to ask questions that allow the researchers to determine if play was truly part of a therapist's practice without a good concept of "play."[10] In Rozier's study, the elements of career success must be understood to compare opinions of male and female respondents.[11] Each individual question in a questionnaire should add to a larger informational context that will answer the guiding questions.

Typically, researchers also include questions about important demographic information in a survey. Couch et al. asked occupational therapists about their academic degrees, years of experience, and practice setting.[10] Rozier et al. asked their sample for information about age, employment setting, length of employment, and family responsibilities.[11] If practice setting is important, a survey may ask about the size of a facility, such as number of beds or number of clinicians. Studies will also often include items related to income, race, marital status, living situation, and so on as relevant. This type of information is needed to describe the characteristics of the respondents, to compare the characteristics of the sample with those of the population to which the results will be generalized, and to interpret how personal characteristics are related to the subject's responses on other questions. Guiding questions should be included to reflect how this information will be related to the overall research question.

It is essential, therefore, that the researcher develop a questionnaire around a model that provides a framework for operational definitions, for selecting a particular target population, and for choosing those variables that are most relevant.

Review of Existing Instruments

An early step in questionnaire development should be to review existing instruments, to determine if they are applicable or adaptable for the study. Many investigators have developed and validated instruments for a variety of purposes. For example, instruments have been developed for exploring attitudes,[12] health behaviors,[13] and functional status.[14, 15] Often these instruments can be used as is, or they can be modified to fit new research situations, saving a great deal of time. It is not wise to adopt previously used surveys blindly, without considering differences in populations being studied, the specific objectives of the instrument, or how changes may affect validity. It is, however, always possible to benefit from the review of literature and insights into development or validation issues that the creator of such an instrument can provide.

Designing the Instrument

The researcher begins to design a survey by writing a series of questions that address each behavior, knowledge, skill, or attitude reflected in the guiding questions. Questions should be grouped and organized to reflect each category or topic. The first draft of a questionnaire should include several questions for each topic, so that these can eventually be compared and weeded out. Content should flow so that the respondent's thought processes will follow a logical sequence. Questions should proceed from the general to the specific. The format of questions will vary, depending on how the survey will be administered, that is, by phone or personal interview, or questionnaire. The initial questions should pique the respondent's interest, or at least be "neutral." Sensitive questions should come later. Some researchers put demographic questions at the beginning, but many prefer to keep these less interesting questions for the end.

The organization of the survey is extremely important to the success of its application. Respondents can easily be turned off by a format that is complicated or confusing. The document should be presented in as "friendly" a format as possible. The page should be uncluttered, printed in laser-quality print, and aligned so that it is easy to find the next question. The font size should be at least 11 or 12 point. The font should be simple to read, not fancy or unusual. Some researchers like to use colored paper, rather than white, to make the survey stand out.

Preliminary Drafts

The preliminary draft of the survey should now be distributed to a panel of colleagues who can review the document and identify problems with questions, including wording and organization. Ask for criticism and suggestions for constructive change. No matter how carefully the survey has been designed, the researcher is usually too close to it to see its flaws. Provide the panel with the study's guiding questions. Based on the panel's comments, the survey should be revised, and then presented to the panel again for further comment. The revision process should continue, with additional feedback from evaluators, until the researcher is satisfied that the instrument is concise, clear, and serves its intended purpose. This process is indeed time consuming, but necessary, and helps to establish the content validity of the instrument.

Pilot Testing and Revisions

The revised questionnaire should then be pilot tested on a small representative sample, perhaps 5 to 10 individuals from the target population. The researcher should interview these respondents to determine where questions were unclear or misleading. If the researcher is unsure about the appropriateness of specific wording, several versions of a question can be asked to elicit the same information in different ways, and responses can be compared for their reliability. Look for missing answers and inconsistencies. It is also useful to monitor the time it takes for respondents to complete the questionnaire. It may be helpful to administer the survey to this group on two occasions, perhaps separated by several days, to see if the responses are consistent, as a way of estimating test–retest reliability. Based on the results of pilot testing, the questionnaire will again be revised and retested until the final instrument attains an acceptable level of validity.

A major concern during this process will be the length of the survey. More often than not, the initial versions will be too long. Long questionnaires are less likely to maintain the respondent's attention and motivation, resulting in potentially invalid or unreliable responses or, in the case of mail surveys, nonresponses. The importance of each item for the interpretation of the study should be examined, and only those questions that make direct and meaningful contributions should be retained. Researchers have shown that shorter questionnaires are often more valid than longer ones, as items generally have some redundancy built into them.[16]

If the study involves the use of interviewers, a formal training process should be incorporated once the questions have been finalized. Interviewers must be consistent in how they present the survey, how questions are asked, and how probing follow-up questions are used (if they are to be allowed). They should be briefed on the purpose of the study, and their presentation should convey the proper attitude. The interviewers must understand the process of recording responses, an important skill when open-ended questions are used.

Administration of the Survey

Before the survey can be administered, the researcher must choose a sample. An accessible population must be identified. As much as possible, a probability sample should be selected. Stratified sampling is often used to control for variations within the sample, such as geographical area when national samples are used. Cluster sampling may be used to increase accessibility of respondents.

For interview surveys, the respondents will typically be within a local geographic area, and may be recruited from agencies or clinics. Before an interview is administered, the potential respondents should be contacted to elicit their cooperation. For telephone interviews, it is appropriate to send advance notice in the mail that the phone call will be coming as a means of introduction and as a way of establishing the legitimacy of the phone call. For mail surveys, the accessible population may be quite dispersed, and may be limited only by the availability of mailing addresses. Mailings lists can be purchased from professional associations or organizations. Published lists of schools or hospitals can usually be obtained from libraries or professional organizations.

Survey respondents should be given an introduction to the survey so that they understand its purpose and how the data will be used. They should be given an idea of how long it will take to complete the survey. In a mail questionnaire, this information will be included in the cover letter. A self-addressed stamped envelope must also be included in a mail survey. It is appropriate to ask respondents if they would like a copy of the study results when it is completed. Because the survey will typically be anonymous, a separate form can be included for respondents to send back with their name and address for this purpose.

Because of low response rates in mail surveys, the researcher should plan to follow up on those who do not respond. To maintain anonymity, researchers will often code the back of the return envelope, so they can keep a record of who has returned the questionnaire. It is appropriate to send out reminders, either postcards, letters, or phone calls, about 2 weeks after the initial mailing to encourage a reply. Many people will have just put the survey aside and forgotten about it. Others will have misplaced it or thrown it out, and it may be helpful to send another copy of the instrument in the follow-up mailing. In the follow-up letter, emphasize the importance of their response to the success of your study. Although the majority of responses will be obtained within the first 2 weeks, a reasonable improvement can usually be obtained through follow-up.

Cover Letter

Mail questionnaires must include a cover letter that orients the respondents to the survey and politely requests their participation. Because a questionnaire can easily be tossed away, the cover letter becomes vitally important to encourage a return. An example of a cover letter is shown in Figure 14.1. The letter should include the following elements:

1. Start with the purpose of the study, including its importance. If the research is sponsored by an agency, this information should be included. If the project is a thesis or student project, the respondents should know this.
2. Indicate why the respondent has been chosen for the survey.
3. Assure the respondents that the survey will be anonymous. Encourage them to be honest in their answers, and assure them that they can refuse to answer any questions that make them uncomfortable.
4. Suggest how long it will take to complete the questionnaire.
5. Ask them to respond by sending back the survey in the enclosed self-addressed stamped envelope. Provide a deadline date. It is reasonable to give 2 to 3

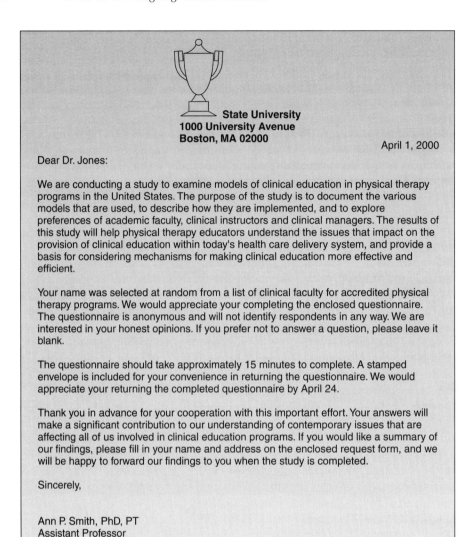

State University
1000 University Avenue
Boston, MA 02000

April 1, 2000

Dear Dr. Jones:

We are conducting a study to examine models of clinical education in physical therapy programs in the United States. The purpose of the study is to document the various models that are used, to describe how they are implemented, and to explore preferences of academic faculty, clinical instructors and clinical managers. The results of this study will help physical therapy educators understand the issues that impact on the provision of clinical education within today's health care delivery system, and provide a basis for considering mechanisms for making clinical education more effective and efficient.

Your name was selected at random from a list of clinical faculty for accredited physical therapy programs. We would appreciate your completing the enclosed questionnaire. The questionnaire is anonymous and will not identify respondents in any way. We are interested in your honest opinions. If you prefer not to answer a question, please leave it blank.

The questionnaire should take approximately 15 minutes to complete. A stamped envelope is included for your convenience in returning the questionnaire. We would appreciate your returning the completed questionnaire by April 24.

Thank you in advance for your cooperation with this important effort. Your answers will make a significant contribution to our understanding of contemporary issues that are affecting all of us involved in clinical education programs. If you would like a summary of our findings, please fill in your name and address on the enclosed request form, and we will be happy to forward our findings to you when the study is completed.

Sincerely,

Ann P. Smith, PhD, PT
Assistant Professor

FIGURE 14.1   Sample cover letter for a mailed questionnaire.

weeks for a response. A shorter time is an imposition, and longer may result in the questionnaire being put aside and forgotten.

6. Thank respondents for their cooperation. Stress the importance of their response for your work. Provide an opportunity for them to receive a summary of the report.

7. Sign the letter, including your name, degrees, and affiliation. If there are several investigators, it is appropriate to include all signatures.

The cover letter should be no longer than one page, typed neatly. If the research is being conducted as part of a professional role, the organizational letterhead should be used. If possible, the letter should be personally addressed to each individual respondent. This is easily accomplished through mail merge programs.

CONSTRUCTING SURVEY QUESTIONS

Two types of questions can be asked in a survey: open-ended and closed-ended questions. **Open-ended questions** ask respondents to answer in their own words. **Closed-ended questions** provide multiple response choices.

Open-Ended Questions

Open-ended questions are useful for probing respondents' feelings and opinions, without biases or limits imposed by the researcher. For example, "What aspects of your job are most satisfying to you?" would require the respondent to provide specific examples of job characteristics. This format is useful when the researcher is not sure of all possible responses to a question. Therefore, respondents are given the opportunity to provide answers in their own words and from their own perspective. Sometimes researchers will use open-ended questions in a pilot study to determine a range of responses which can then be converted to a multiple-choice item.

Open-ended questions are, however, difficult to code and analyze because so many different responses can be obtained. If open-ended questions are misunderstood, they may elicit answers that are essentially irrelevant to the researcher's goal. Respondents may not want to take the time to write a full answer, or they may answer in a way that is clear to them but uninterpretable, vague, or incomplete to the researcher. For instance, a question such as, "What types of exercise do you do regularly?" could elicit a long list of specific movements or a general description of an exercise routine. If the purpose of the question is to find out if the respondent engages in particular exercise activities, it would be better to list certain exercises and ask if they are done. Open-ended questions can be effective in interviews because the interviewer can clarify the respondent's answers by follow-up questions. Open-ended questions are generally avoided in questionnaires, except where responses are fairly objective, such as asking for a person's yearly income, or where the researcher's purpose is to explore respondents' motivations or behaviors without presenting a predefined list of choices.

Closed-Ended Questions

Closed-ended questions ask respondents to select an answer from among several choices that are provided by the researcher.

> Which of the following aspects of your job do you find most satisfying?
>
> [ ] patient contact
> [ ] intellectual challenge
> [ ] interaction with other medical personnel
> [ ] opportunities for educational growth

This type of question is easily coded and provides greater uniformity across responses. Its disadvantage is that it does not allow respondents to express their own personal viewpoints and, therefore, may provide a biased response set. The list of choices may overlook some important responses, or they may bias answers by presenting a particular attitude.

There are two basic considerations in constructing closed-ended questions. First, the responses should be *exhaustive*; that is, they should include all possible responses that can be expected. As a protection, it is often advisable to include a category for "not applicable (NA)," "don't know," or "other (please specify _____)." In the preceding example, for instance, it is likely that respondents will have other reasons for job satisfaction that have not been listed. Second, the response categories should be *mutually exclusive*; that is, each choice should clearly represent a unique answer. The preceding example is inadequate on this criterion. For example, a respondent may see "intellectual challenge" and "opportunities for educational growth" as elements of the same concept. When only one response is desired, it may be useful to add an instruction to the question asking respondents to select the *one best answer* or the answer that is most important; however, this technique does not substitute for carefully worded questions and choices.

There should also be a rationale for ordering response choices. Sometimes there is an inherent hierarchy in the responses, so that choices can be given in order of increasing or decreasing intensity or agreement. When there is no purposeful order, the researcher must be careful to avoid "leading" the respondent to a particular choice by the order or phrasing.

Sometimes the researcher is interested in more than one answer to a question. For instance, we might want to know all the reasons for a person's job satisfaction. Instructing the respondent to mark "all that apply" creates an interpretation problem in that the respondent may not choose a particular item because it does not apply, because it was not clear, or because it was missed. In addition, it is difficult to code multiple responses. When multiple choices are of interest, it is better to ask respondents to mark each choice separately, as in the following example:

Which of the following aspects of your job do you find satisfying?			
	Yes	No	Unsure
patient contact	[ ]	[ ]	[ ]
intellectual challenge	[ ]	[ ]	[ ]
interaction with other medical personnel	[ ]	[ ]	[ ]
opportunities for educational growth	[ ]	[ ]	[ ]

Format of Closed-Ended Questions

Two common formats are used to list choices to closed-ended questions: (1) using brackets, as just presented, where respondents are asked to check the appropriate response, or (2) asking respondents to circle the number or letter that appears before the answer, as shown next.

The simplest form of closed-ended question is one that presents two choices, or *dichotomous* responses:

> Are you presently enrolled in a degree program?
>
> a. Yes
> b. No

When questions address a characteristic that is on a continuum, such as attitudes or quality of performance, it is more useful to provide a range of responses, so that the respondent can find a choice that represents the appropriate intensity of response. Usually, three to five multiple-choice options are provided. An option for "Don't know" or "Unsure" should always be included.

> How important do you think it is to include a research course in your professional program?
>
> a. Very important
> b. Important
> c. Somewhat important
> d. Not important
> e. Unsure

When a series of questions use the same format, a *grid* or checklist can provide a more efficient presentation. With this approach, instructions for using the response choices need only be given once, and the respondent can quickly go through many questions without reading a new set of choices. For example, Figure 14.2 shows a checklist for a question concerning patients' level of knee pain during different activities.

For each of the following activities, please indicate the level of knee pain you have experienced during the past week:				
	No pain	Minimal	Moderate	Severe
Walking a short distance				
Walking a long distance				
Ascending stairs				
Descending stairs				

FIGURE 14.2 Example of a grid for using one set of response choices for a series of questions.

An alternative question format is the *rank-order* question, where the respondent is presented with a series of responses and is asked to rank the responses on an ordinal scale.

The following are some of the reasons applicants choose to attend a particular school. Please order them in terms of importance, from 1 (most important) to 5 (least important).

_____ location
_____ faculty reputation
_____ length of program
_____ affiliation with a medical center
_____ research opportunities

Some question sequences try to follow up on specific answers with more detailed questions, using a technique called *branching.* Depending on the response to an initial question, the respondent will be directed to answer additional questions or to skip ahead to a later question.

1. Do you perform any clinical consulting activities?

    a. No ⇒ Skip to Question 3
    b. Yes

2. Approximately how many hours per week do you work as a consultant? _____

This process saves time by avoiding questions that are irrelevant to a specific respondent.

Wording Questions

Simplicity is a key to good questionnaires. Sentences should be succinct and grammatically correct. Respondents will not be inclined to ponder the meaning of a long, involved question. They will read and answer questions quickly and choices should be understood at a glance. Questions should be written in common language for the lowest educational level that might be encountered. Generally, shorter questions and responses are more likely to be understood and to keep the respondent's attention. The length of the question is not, however, the determining factor in the clarity of the question. Sometimes, longer questions are needed to provide sufficient information to elicit the appropriate response.[17]

Language may be an issue if respondents do not speak English or English is a second language. The researcher must know the sample well enough to use appropriate wording. Idioms or subtle cultural expressions should be carefully avoided. The researcher may have the questionnaire translated into another language for specific sample groups. The translation must account for cultural biases.

It goes without saying that survey questions must be clear and unambiguous. Questions that require subtle distinctions to interpret responses are more likely to be misunderstood. For example, consider the question, "How many different sports do you participate in?" There are two ambiguous terms here. First, there may be different ways to define sports. Some may include any form of physical activity, including riding a stationary bicycle; others may include only legitimate field sports. Second, what constitutes participation? Does it have to be an organized schedule of play, or can it mean throwing a basketball in your yard on weekends or playing golf once a year? This type of ambiguity can be corrected by providing the respondent with appropriate definitions, as in the following example:

Do you participate in any of the following team sports on a regular basis as part of amateur league play?

	Yes	No
softball	[ ]	[ ]
basketball	[ ]	[ ]
football	[ ]	[ ]
soccer	[ ]	[ ]
hockey	[ ]	[ ]

Double-Barreled Questions

Each question should be confined to a single idea. Surveys should avoid the use of **double-barreled questions,** using "or" or "and" to assess two things within a single question. For instance, "How many times a week do you jog or ride a stationary bicycle?" It is obviously possible to perform both of these activities at different rates, making it impossible to answer the question. It is better to ask two questions to assess each activity separately.

Frequency and Time Measures

Researchers are often interested in quantifying behavior in terms of frequency and time. For example, it might be of interest to ask, "How many alcoholic drinks do you consume each day?" or "How many patients do you treat per day?" These types of questions may be very difficult to answer because the frequency of the behavior may vary greatly from day to day, month to month, or even season to season. The researcher should determine exactly what aspect of the behavior is most relevant to the study and provide an appropriate time frame for interpreting the question. For instance, the question could ask about a particular period, such as the maximum number of patients seen within the last week, or the respondent can be asked to calculate an average daily value. This assumes, of course, that this time period is adequately representative for purposes of the study. Alternatively, the question could ask for an estimate of "typical" or "usual" behaviors.

This approach makes an assumption about the respondent's ability to form such an estimate. Some behaviors are much more erratic than others. For example, it may be relatively easy to estimate the number of patients treated in a day, but it may be more difficult to estimate typical behavior in consuming alcoholic beverages. Estimates of "typical" will also tend to ignore extremes, which may or may not be important to the purpose of the study.

Questions related to time should also be specific. A question such as, "Has your back pain limited your ability to work?" may be difficult to answer if it is not a consistent problem. It is better to provide a time frame for reference. For example, "Has your back pain limited your ability to work within the past month?" Many function, pain, and health status questionnaires specify time periods within the last month, last week, or last 24 hours.[18, 19]

Dealing with Sensitive Questions

Questionnaires often deal with sensitive or personal issues that can cause some discomfort on the part of the respondent. Although some people are only too willing to express personal views, others are hesitant, even when they know their responses are anonymous. Some questions may address social behaviors that have negative associations, such as smoking, sexual practices, and drinking alcohol; others may inquire about behaviors that respondents are not anxious to admit to, such as ignorance of facts they feel they should know, or compliance with medications or exercise programs. Sensitive questions may also be subject to recall bias. For example, respondents may be selective in their memory of risk factors for disease or disability. Respondents should be reminded in the introduction to the survey that they may refuse to answer any questions.

Sensitive questions should be phrased to put the respondent at ease. It may be useful to preface such questions with a statement as in these examples: "Many people forget to take their medications from time to time." "It is often very difficult for people to fit exercise sessions into their daily routines." "Clinicians are faced with a tremendous task in keeping up with the variety of treatment approaches that are being developed for low back pain. Depending on experience and practice, some clinicians have had an opportunity to learn these techniques more than others." These statements tell the respondent that it is okay if they fit into that category.

Phillips suggests that questions that ask respondents to admit to socially unacceptable behaviors should be phrased in a manner that assumes the respondent engages in the behavior.[20] For instance, rather than asking,

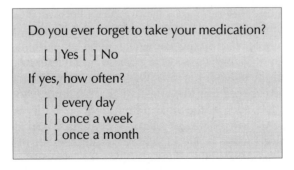

we could ask one question:

> How often do you forget to take your medication?
>
> [ ] every day
> [ ] once a week
> [ ] once a month
> [ ] never

SCALES

A **scale** is an ordered system based on a series of questions or items that provide an overall rating, representing the degree to which a respondent possesses a particular attitude, value, or characteristic. The purpose of a scale is to distinguish among people who demonstrate different intensities of the characteristic that is being measured. Scales have been developed to measure attitudes, function, health and quality of life, pain, exertion, and other physical, physiological, and psychological variables.

Categorical scales are based on nominal measurement. A question asks the respondent to assign himself according to one of several classifications. This type of scale is used with variables such as gender, diagnosis, religion, or race. These data are expressed as frequency counts or percentages.

Most scales represent a characteristic that exists on a continuum. **Continuous scales** may be measured using interval or ratio values, such as age, blood pressure, or years of experience. An ordinal scale requires that a continuous variable be collapsed into ranks. For instance, pain can be measured as "minimal, moderate, severe," or function as "independent, minimal assist, moderate assist, maximal assist, dependent." Scale items should represent the full range of values that indicate the characteristic being measured.

Scales are created so that a *summary score* can be obtained from a series of items, indicating the extent to which an individual possesses the characteristic of interest. Because item scores are combined to make this total, it is important that the scale is structured around only one dimension; that is, all items should reflect different elements of a single characteristic. A **summative scale** is one that presents a total score with all items contributing equal weight to the total. A **cumulative scale** demonstrates an accumulated characteristic, with each item representing an increasing amount of the attribute being measured.

We will describe several scaling models used to summarize respondent characteristics: Likert scales, the semantic differential, visual analogue scales, Guttman scales, and Rasch models.

Likert Scales

A **Likert scale** is a summative scale, most often used to assess attitudes or values. A series of statements is presented expressing a viewpoint, and respondents are asked to select an appropriately ranked response that reflects their agreement or disagreement with each one. For example, Figure 14.3 shows a set of statements that evaluate students' opinions about including a research course in an entry-level professional curriculum. Likert's original scale included five categories: strongly agree (SA), agree (A), neutral

For each statement given below, please indicate whether you strongly agree (SA), agree (A), are neutral (N), disagree (D), or strongly disagree (SD):

		SA	A	N	D	SD
a.	Knowledge of research principles is important for the practicing clinician.	☐	☐	☐	☐	☐
b.	Research and statistics should be taught in entry-level professional programs.	☐	☐	☐	☐	☐
c.	Participation in a research project should be a requirement.	☐	☐	☐	☐	☐

FIGURE 14.3 A 5-point Likert scale.

(N), disagree (D), and strongly disagree (SD).[21] Many modifications to this model have been used, sometimes extending it to seven categories (including "somewhat disagree" and "somewhat agree") or four categories (eliminating "neutral"). There is no consensus regarding the number of response categories that should be used. Some researchers believe the "neutral" option should be omitted so that the respondents are forced to make a choice, rather than allowing them an "out" so that they do not have to take sides on an issue. Others feel that respondents who do not have strong feelings should be given a viable option to express that attitude. When the forced choice method is used, responses that are left blank are generally interpreted as "neutral."

Each choice along the scale is assigned a point value, based on the degree to which the item represents a favorable or unfavorable characteristic. For example, we could rate $SA = 5, A = 4, N = 3, D = 2, SD = 1$, or we could use codes such as $SA = 2, A = 1, N = 0, D = -1, SD = -2$. The actual values are unimportant, as long as the items are consistently scored; that is, agreement with favorable items should always be scored higher than agreement with unfavorable items. Therefore, if positively phrased items are coded 5 through 1, then negatively phrased items must be coded 1 through 5.

An overall score is computed for each respondent by adding points for each item. Creating such a total assumes that the items are measuring the same things and that each item reflects equal elements of the characteristic being studied; that is, one item should not carry any more weight than the others.

Constructing a Likert scale requires more than just listing a group of statements. A large pool of items should be developed, usually 10 to 20, that reflect an equal number of both favorable and unfavorable attitudes. It is generally not necessary to include items that are intended to elicit neutral responses, because these will not help to distinguish respondents. The scale should be validated by performing item analyses that will indicate which items are truly discriminating between those with positive and those with negative attitudes. The basis of the item analysis is that there should be correlation between an individual's total score and each item response. Those who score highest should agree with positively worded statements, and those who obtain the lowest total scores should disagree. If respondents are equally likely to agree with both favorable and unfavorable statements, then the scale is not providing a valid assessment of their feelings about a particular issue. Those items that generate agreement from both those with high and low scores are probably irrelevant to the characteristic being studied, and should be omitted.

Semantic Differential

Attitudes have also been evaluated using a technique called the **semantic differential**.[22] This method tries to measure the individual's feelings about a particular object or concept based on a continuum that extends between two extreme opposites. For example, we could ask respondents to rate their feelings about natural childbirth by checking the space that reflects their attitude on the following scale:

Good |____|____|____|____|____|____|____| Bad

The semantic differential is composed of a set of these scales, using pairs of words that reflect opposite feelings. Typically a 7-point scale is used, as just shown, with the middle representing a neutral position. This scale is different from the Likert scale in two ways. First, only the two extremes are labeled. Second, the continuum is not based on agree/disagree, but on opposite adjectives that should express the respondent's feelings about the concept. Figure 14.4 illustrates a semantic differential to explore self-image in a group of elderly women who reside in a nursing home.

Research has demonstrated that the adjective pairs used in this scale tend to fall along three underlying dimensions, which have been labeled evaluation, potency, and

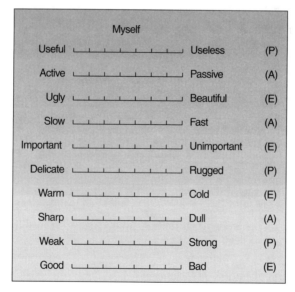

FIGURE 14.4 Example of a semantic differential for testing self-image. Dimensions of evaluation (E), potency (P), and activity (A) are indicated, although these designations would not appear in an actual test.

activity.[22, 23] *Evaluation* is associated with adjectives such as nice–awful, good–bad, clean–dirty, valuable–worthless, and helpful–unhelpful. Some concepts that lie on the positive side of this dimension are doctor, family, peace, success, and truth. Negative evaluation concepts include abortion, disease, war, and failure. *Potency* ideas are big––little, powerful–powerless, strong–weak, large–small, and deep–shallow. Strong potency concepts include bravery, duty, law, power, and science. Negative concepts include baby, love, and art. The *activity* dimension is characterized by fast–slow, alive–dead, noisy–quiet, young–old, active–passive, and sharp–dull. Strong activity concepts are danger, anger, fire, and child. Concepts that lie toward the negative activity side are calm, death, rest, and sleep. The ratings shown in Figure 14.4 are labeled according to their respective dimensions. It is a good idea to mix up the order of presentation of the dimensions in listing the scales.

The semantic differential is scored by assigning values from 1 to 7 to each of the spaces within each adjective pair, with 1 representing the most negative response and 7 indicating the positive extreme. To avoid biases or a tendency to just check the same column in each scale, the order of negative and positive responses should be randomly varied. For instance, in Figure 14.4, ratings of weak–strong, slow–fast, and ugly–beautiful place the negative value on the left; all other scales have the positive value on the left. A total score can be obtained by summing the scores for each rating. Lower total scores will reflect generally negative feelings toward the concept being assessed, and higher scores represent generally positive feelings. Statistical procedures, such as factor analysis, can be applied to the scale ratings to determine if the evaluation, potency, and activity ratings tend to go together (see Chapter 27 for a description of factor analysis). In this way, the instrument can be used to explore theoretical constructs.

Visual Analogue Scales

A **visual analogue scale (VAS)** is one of the simplest methods to assess the intensity of a subjective experience. A line is drawn, usually fixed at 100 mm in length, with word anchors on either end that represent extremes of the characteristic. The intermediate levels along the line are not defined. Respondents are asked to place a mark along the line corresponding to their perceived level for that characteristic. The VAS is scored by measuring the distance of the mark from the left-hand anchor in millimeters. This method has also been used to measure a variety of characteristics, most extensively for pain, as shown in Figure 14.5.[24, 25] The VAS can be used to evaluate a variable at a given point in time or its degree of change over time.

The scores obtained with a VAS have generally been treated as ratio level data, measured in millimeters.[26, 27] This assumption permits VAS scores to be added to obtain a mean and subjected to parametric statistical procedures. Others have argued that the

Describe the level of your back pain at this moment:

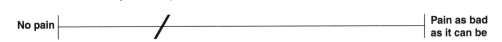

FIGURE 14.5 A 100-mm visual analogue scale for pain, showing a mark at 29 mm.

scores are only pseudo-ratio, and should be treated as ordinal, handled with nonparametric statistics.[28] They suggest that the person marking the line is not truly able to appreciate the full continuum, evidenced by ceiling effects[29] and a tendency to cluster marks at certain points.[25, 30] Therefore, even though the actual readings from the scale are obviously at the ratio level, the true measurement properties may be less precise. This dilemma will continue to emerge in studies using the VAS.[31]

The simple format of the VAS continues to make it a popular method for assessing unidimensional characteristics. This points out one disadvantage of the technique, however, in that each VAS is only capable of evaluating one dimension of a trait. Researchers often incorporate several VAS lines, each with different anchors, to assess related aspects of the characteristic being measured.[32, 33]

Guttman Scales

In a summative scale, several item scores are added to create a total score. One limitation of this type of measure is that the total score can be interpreted in more than one way. Suppose we have a scale, scored from 0 to 100, that measures physical function, including elements related to locomotion, personal hygiene, dressing, and feeding. Two individuals who achieve a score of 50 may have obtained this score for very different reasons. One may be able to walk, but is unable to perform the necessary movements for self-care. Another may be in a wheelchair, but is able to take care of his personal needs. Therefore, a summed score can be ambiguous. This potential outcome reflects the fact that the items within the scale actually reflect different components or dimensions of the trait being measured, in this case physical function, which are not all equal.

Guttman scales provide an alternative approach using a cumulative scale, wherein a set of statements is presented that reflects increasing intensities of the characteristic being measured. Guttman's technique is designed to ensure that there is only one dimension within a set of responses; that is, there is only one unique combination of responses that can achieve a particular score.[34] For instance, in a cumulative scale a respondent who agrees with item 2 will also have had to agree with item 1; one who agrees with item 3 will have had to agree with items 1 and 2; and so on. Therefore, although there may be several combinations of responses that will result in a total score of 10 for a summative scale, there is only one way to achieve that score on a Guttman scale. Consider the following statements which were included in a self-assessment interview of elderly people concerning their functional health status.[35]

1. I can go to the movies, church, or visiting without help.
2. I can walk up and down to the second floor without help.
3. I can walk half a mile without help.
4. I am not limited in any activities.
5. I have no physical conditions or illnesses now.
6. I am still healthy enough to do heavy work around the house without help.

If these items represent a cumulative scale, then all those who can walk half a mile can also climb stairs to the second floor and go out visiting. Those who cannot walk half a mile should not be able to do heavy housework and probably have some limiting illness or physical condition. The development of this scale is, therefore, based on a theoretical premise that there is a hierarchy to this dimension of health.

Each item in the cumulative scale is scored as 1 = agree or 0 = disagree. A total cumulative score is then computed for all items. The maximum score will be equal to the number of items in the scale. A statistical technique, called *scalogram analysis,* can then be used to determine whether a unidimensional scale structure exists among the set of items. For instance, if the scale is cumulative, then a respondent who achieves a score of 2 in the scale would have had to agree only with items 1 and 2. If he agreed with items 1 and 3 only, the scale would be faulty because the set of statements would not constitute a hierarchy in terms of the characteristic being assessed. In reality, such scales are not free of error, and some of the subjects can be expected to present inconsistent patterns of response. In the analysis of the response categories for functional health, researchers found that most of their subjects could participate in social activities (86%) and that the fewest could do heavy work around the house, such as shoveling snow and washing walls (21%).[35] The frequencies for other responses ranged between these two extremes, supporting the Guttman scale. A scalogram analysis will provide an analysis of the error rate within the scale. In the preceding example, the level of error was 9%, which is extremely low.

Guttman scales require a large number of respondents to assess patterns adequately. It is usually necessary to start with a large pool of statements, to weed out those statements that do not contribute to the scale. Guttman scales are also sample dependent, which means that one set of respondents may demonstrate cumulative scores whereas another might not.[36] The technique is appealing, however, for many clinical situations where it would be interesting to document hierarchical skills or behaviors to provide useful models for sequencing treatment goals.

Rasch Analysis

The issues of hierarchical assessment extend to many of the instruments that have been developed to assess functional and health outcomes. In most such scales, items are marked using ordinal values, and a total score is generated. For example, we could ask elderly patients if their health limits their function based on several ADL items, as follows:

	(1) Limited a Lot	(2) Limited a Little	(3) Not Limited
Eating	○	○	○
Walking indoors	○	○	○
Climbing stairs	○	○	○

Although this is an obviously abbreviated scale for the sake of example, a person who is independent in all three items would obtain a total score of 9. A person who is severely limited in all three tasks would receive a total score of 3. For this total score to be meaningful, however, three criteria must be met. First, the scale items must reflect a unidimensional construct. For instance, the ability to eat is not necessarily related to the ability to climb stairs or walk indoors; that is, these items may be part of different dimensions of function.[37] If so, the sum of scores on these items would not reflect a unified construct—sort of adding apples and oranges. Therefore, two patients who obtain a score of 5 may not demonstrate the same functional profile.

Second, the items must progress hierarchically from easy to difficult, so we can determine if someone has more or less of the trait.[38] This would also mean that the order of difficulty for the items is consistent for all patients, and that the range of the scale incorporates the extremes.[39] Therefore, if our sample functional scale was properly arranged, eating would be easier than walking indoors, and walking indoors would be easier than climbing stairs for everyone.

Third, we need a scale that will allow us to measure change within and across patients. As we have noted before, ordinal values may present problems in this regard because they have limited sensitivity and precision. A patient might improve in his ability to climb stairs, but not enough to be scored at a higher level of function. Therefore, for a score to be meaningful, units of measurement must have equal intervals along the scale to account for magnitude of change.[40, 41] These objectives can be achieved using a technique called **Rasch analysis,** which statistically manipulates ordinal data to create a linear measure on an interval scale.[42–46]

We can describe this process using items from the Functional Independence Measure (FIM), a popular instrument for assessing function in rehabilitation settings. The FIM is an 18-item scale designed to evaluate the amount of assistance a patient needs to accomplish activities of daily living (ADLs).[47] The items measure both motor and cognitive functions. Each item is scored on an ordinal scale from 1 (total assist) to 7 (total independence). The larger the total score, the less assistance the patient requires. Theoretically, then, if the scale represents a singular construct of function, the total score should reflect an "amount" of independence; that is, we can think of individuals as being "more" or "less" independent.

The Rasch Model

Now let us conceive of function as a line, representing a continuum, as shown in Figure 14.6. For this example we will use the five items in the cognitive subscale of the FIM, listed in Table 14.1* We construct the line using items in the scale, with easier items at the base, and harder items at the top. Using data from a patient sample and specialized computer programs,[50, 51] the Rasch analysis determines the order of difficulty of the items, and locates them along this continuum, to show how they fit a unidimensional model of cognitive function. The analysis will also calculate the patients' abilities on the set of items, and position the patients along this line according to "how much" or "how little" cognitive function they have. The arrangement of items in Figure 14.6 illustrates these concepts based on a study by Heinemann et al. who performed a Rasch analysis on the cognitive portion of the FIM.[49] The figure illustrates two facets of this scale: on the right, the items are ranked in relation to their difficulty; and on the left, the patients are positioned relative to their abilities.[40] The more difficult items have a higher score, and patients who have these abilities (they are more independent) will also be placed near the top of the scale. Patients who are less functional are placed towards the bottom of the scale, as they are only able to complete the easier items. In Figure 14.6, patient 5 was only able to achieve the auditory comprehension and verbal expression items, while patients 1 and 2 were able to achieve all five items.

---

*Some researchers have distinguished the motor and cognitive portions of the FIM as separate scales based on Rasch analysis.[48, 49] For purposes of illustration, then, it is reasonable to consider the items on cognitive function as a separate scale.

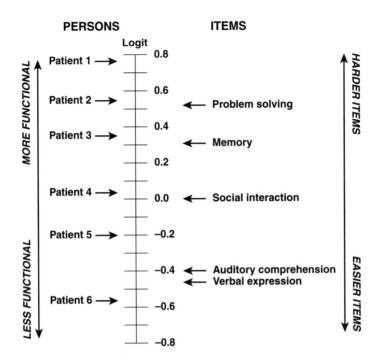

FIGURE 14.6   Example of a two-facet linear functional scale (based on the cognitive items of the FIM), showing the placement of scale items and patients according to a Rasch analysis (Based on data from Heinemann AW, Linacre JM, Wright BD et al. Relationships between impairment and physical disability as measured by the Functional Independence Measure. *Arch Phys Med Rehabil* 1993;74:566–573.)

If the scale truly represents one functional construct, it should meet three measurement principles.[13, 40] First, the total score should reflect level of function implied by the items; second, the items should range in difficulty; and third, the rank order of difficulty should not change from person to person. The results of the computerized Rasch analysis will show where each individual patient fits along the continuum; the level of difficulty achieved by each item on an interval scale; and goodness-of-fit of the model, showing how well each item matches the cumulative scale.[13]

Measurement Criteria

Several criteria are used to judge the adequacy of fit of the data to a Rasch model:

1. *Item difficulty* refers to the position of items within the hierarchical scale. It is expressed as a *logit*[†], or log-odds unit, with a central zero point, allowing items to be scaled

---

[†]To determine the position of an item along an interval scale, each item is examined for the probability that a person with a given level of ability will pass or fail, creating an odds ratio. These odds are then transformed to a logarithmic scale, creating a value called a *logit* that will range from minus to plus infinity. The logit is defined as the mean of the natural logarithm of the odds that the average ability patient will transition from one category to the next higher one (from a rating of 1 to 2, 2 to 3, etc.). It is considered an equal-interval measure, thereby creating an interval scale that has additive properties.

TABLE 14.1. ITEMS FROM THE COGNITIVE SUBSCALE OF THE FUNCTIONAL INDEPENDENCE MEASURE

Item	Logit
1. Problem solving	0.53
2. Memory	0.30
3. Social interaction	0.00
4. Auditory comprehension	−0.40
5. Verbal expression	−0.45

Source: Heinemann AW, Linacre JM, Wright BD, Hamilton BB, Granger C. Relationships between impairment and physical disability as measured by the Functional Independence Measure. *Arch Phys Med Rehabil* 1993;74:566–73.

as positive or negative. The items are ordered so that the degree of function becomes systematically greater as the items become harder; that is, patients who have greater functional ability will "pass" the more difficult items. Therefore, it becomes possible to determine how close or far apart items are in difficulty, not just their rank order of difficulty. Ideally items are positioned equally across the scale, not leaving large gaps. As shown in Table 14.1 and Figure 14.6, the five items on the FIM cognitive subscale range in difficulty from–0.45 to 0.53 logits, with a reasonable spread of scores. The most difficult item is problem solving, and the easiest item is verbal expression. If gaps are identified, they suggest where items need to be added to the scale to better reflect the continuum.

2. *Item fit* is the extent to which the individual scale items conform to a unidimensional model. *Person fit* represents the extent to which individuals fit the model. If we look at the continuum for the construct of cognitive function, for example, a good fit means that each item represents a level on the scale that will discriminate between those who are independent and those who require more assistance. Patients who are less functional will be placed toward the bottom, and those who are more functional will be placed toward the top; that is, the more functional individual will pass more of the items (and more of the difficult items), and the less functional individual will fail more of the items.

The Rasch analysis develops a probability model that predicts what the scores should be for each item and person. When expected relationships are not found, the items are considered a *misfit.*[‡] For example, a Rasch analysis for the entire FIM scale showed that combining all 18 items resulted in a large proportion of misfitting items; that is, some of the more difficult items and more functional patients were not placed at the top (supporting the separation of motor and cognitive subscales).[49]

Fit statistics are calculated for each item to reflect how well the items conform to the hierarchical model. These statistics are expressed as a *mean square residual (MNSQ),* which is the difference between the observed scores and the scores expected by the model. If the observed and expected values are the same, the MNSQ will equal 1.0.[§] Higher MNSQ values indicate greater discrepancy from the model; that is, the item is

---

[‡]Each item in the scale should reflect a given level of function. For a good fitting item, 50% of the sample at that functional level should "pass" that item.[44]

[§]The significance of item fit can be derived using the *t* statistic, testing the difference of the mean square residual from 1.0.[52]

not consistent in its level of difficulty across patients.** It would then be reasonable to consider revising the scale, either by eliminating the item or rewording it to remove ambiguity. If patients are misfit, the researcher must examine their characteristics, potentially identifying subgroups in the population. In the study by Heinemann and colleagues, for example, several patient groups were evaluated, demonstrating that differently ordered cognitive scales were needed to represent groups with and without brain dysfunction.[49] For instance, patients with right- and left-sided strokes did not demonstrate similar difficulty with verbal expression.

3. *Item separation* reflects the spread of items, and *person separation* represents the spread of individuals along the scale. Ideally, the analysis will show that items can be separated into at least three *strata* that represent low, medium, and high difficulty, although a good scale may actually delineate many strata to clarify the construct.[53] Statistically, this spread of items is related to measurement error or reliability; that is, the more reliable a scale, the more likely the item or person score represents the true score. Measurement error should be small so that segments of the scale are separated by distances greater than their measurement error alone. Separation statistics may be expressed as a reliability coefficient, or the ratio of the sample standard deviation to the standard error of the test.[44] Conceptually, this is a ratio of the true spread of scores divided by the measurement error. ‖

An understanding of measurement principles applied to questionnaires is essential if we want to use scores as part of our patient evaluations or to look at group performance over time. We must consider the potential for misinference when ordinal scales are used. Rasch Item Response Theory provides an important technique for testing our assumptions in clinical measurement. Several useful examples of Rasch analysis can be found in the literature.[33, 39, 44, 53–56]

Q-SORT

The **Q-sort** is an analytic technique used to characterize attitudes, opinions, or judgments of individuals through a process of comparative rank ordering.[57] The technique involves presenting an individual with a set of cards containing a series of written items such as statements, ideas, phrases, or pictures. The individual is asked to sort the cards into piles according to some scaled criterion. For example, cards may list areas of clinical research in rehabilitation, and the subject may be asked to sort the cards according to high versus low priority. The criterion is defined on a discrete continuum, such as an 11-point scale, with 0 representing no interest at all and 10 representing the highest priority. Scales of different widths may be appropriate for different variables; however, a wide enough continuum is necessary to see a clear distribution.

**Two indicators of fit may be reported.[39] *Infit* is sensitive to erratic response patterns for items that are close to a patient's functional level. Therefore, a large infit would indicate a problem with the item's fit with the unidimensional model. *Outfit* reflects the occurrence of extremely unexpected or rare responses. A large outfit value would indicate that some patients have unique patterns of impairment and probably reflect a different population.

‖ Items may be considered in distinct strata if their item separation, based on standard error, is greater than ±0.15 logits.[53]

The subject must sort through the cards and place them in piles representing each rank along the continuum; however, the researcher specifies how many cards are to go into each pile, so that the subject is faced with forced choices. For example, we could present a deck of 60 cards, each with a topic of clinical research, and ask a subject to form piles according to the distribution shown in Table 14.2. The subject would be instructed to read through the entire set of cards, and to place in pile 0 the one card containing the single least important topic and in pile 10 the single topic of highest priority. Then, from the remaining 58 cards, the subject would place the two least important items in pile 1 and the two most important in pile 9. This process continues for piles 2 and 8, 3 and 7, and 4 and 6. The remaining 12 cards are placed in pile 5, essentially a neutral pile. The subjects are free to replace or move any card to another pile at any time during the sorting procedure until they are satisfied with results. Although Q-distributions are essentially arbitrary, for statistical convenience the distribution is usually arranged to resemble a normal distribution, with fewer and fewer items toward the extremes. Although the number of cards used will vary according to the research question, Q-sorts generally range from a low of 60 to a high of 100 to 120 items. Too large a deck is difficult to sort through, and too small a deck will not provide sufficient stability for statistical reliability.

Q-methodology provides an empirical basis for exploring abstract ideas and theories, generally with good reliability. It can be applied to a variety of research questions and is quite flexible. It is possible to use the technique to answer questions that require the use of two or more related sets of items, or a single set of items can be sorted on more than one scale. For instance, Biddle et al. used a Q-sort to establish key characteristics of effective primary care training experiences for third-year medical students.[58] The students completed a Q-sort using three sets of items: preceptor characteristics, site characteristics, and a combination of the two.

The approach to analysis of Q-sort data will depend on the research question. For some purposes, descriptive statistics, such as averages, percentages, and simple tallies of rank orderings, will be sufficient. For example, Q-sort has been used to rank applicants to a physical therapy program.[59] More complex statistical procedures can also be applied to the Q-methodology. Correlations are often used to determine if the sorts of several subjects are related, usually using a nonparametric procedure for correlating ranks. For instance, Kovach and associates studied employees in long-term care facilities to describe factors that facilitate positive change in the care of patients with dementia.[60] The employees were asked to rank personal factors and facility factors. Using Spearman correlation coefficients, the researchers found little congruence between real and ideal facility characteristics, but a strong relationship between real and ideal personal characteristics. Factor analysis and content analysis are also used to uncover underlying themes in the Q-sort. For example, in the study of medical students' perceptions of clinical experiences, Biddle et al. used content analysis to group responses into

TABLE 14.2.   DISTRIBUTION OF 60 CARDS FOR A Q-SORT

| | Low priority | | | | | | | | High priority | | |
	0	1	2	3	4	5	6	7	8	9	10
Number of cards	1	2	4	7	10	12	10	7	4	2	1

six categories, namely patients, staff characteristics, preceptor's personal characteristics, programmatic issues, educational opportunities, and the strongest theme around preceptor teaching characteristics.[58]

The Q-sort is limited in its generalizability because subjects are not randomly chosen. Samples tend to be small because of the logistic difficulties administering the technique. Replication of Q-sorts over many samples is necessary to demonstrate validity of findings. Use of already established Q-sorts (sets of items) is helpful to validate findings by replication. When Q-sorts do not exist, the researcher must establish the content validity of items used.

DELPHI SURVEY

Many questions of interest in medical and social sciences are related to practice, values, or standards, and are best answered by developing consensus around a specific issue. In a **Delphi survey,** a panel of experts is asked to complete a series of questionnaires to identify their opinions.[61, 62] The Delphi technique differs from typical questionnaires in several ways. The most distinguishing difference is the use of several rounds of questionnaires, typically two or three. In each round, the researcher reviews and collates the results, and then distributes these findings to the panel for their response. This process generally continues until the responses are consistent with the previous round, demonstrating consensus.

This technique was used, for example, in a study of opinions of physical therapy education program directors on essential functions for physical therapy students.[63] In a first round, the panel was asked to respond to a list of essential functions, modifying or adding items. The results of this first round were summarized and categorized, with four items added and wording modified in four other items. In the second round, panel members were asked to rank the importance of each item on an ordinal scale. The third round incorporated these results, including the median response for each item. The respondents then had the opportunity to change their ratings for any item. The final results showed strong agreement among panel members concerning the functions needed for effective practice.

The Delphi survey has great potential for planning and problem solving for a variety of practice issues. Investigators have used this technique to establish consensus on decision-making criteria for diagnosis of acoustic tumors,[64] core curricula for allied health programs,[65] content validity of motor function assessments for children with cerebral palsy,[66] and priorities in professional ethical issues.[67] It is an efficient method because the members of the panel do not need to come together, making large response groups feasible, including individuals at a distance. Consensus is developed without interaction among respondents, avoiding the potential for group biases, such as one dominant individual swaying others in the group. Responses are shared without any one individual being challenged by the group. The anonymity offered by this method will also encourage honest responses from the panel. The disadvantages include the cost of printing and mailing, and the need to maintain a commitment by the panel members over several rounds. Researchers will generally use follow-up reminders to encourage full participation.

ANALYSIS OF SURVEY DATA

The first step in the analysis of survey data is to collate responses and enter them into a computer. Each item on the survey is a data point, and must be given a variable name, often the item number. The researcher must sort through each questionnaire as it is returned, or through all responses from an interview, to determine if responses are valid. In many instances, the respondent will have incorrectly filled out the survey, and that respondent may have to be eliminated from the analysis. Some questions may have to be eliminated from individual questionnaires because they were answered incorrectly, such as giving two answers for a question that asked for a single response. The researcher must keep track of all unusable questionnaires, to report this percentage in the final report.

Responses to closed-ended questions are *coded*; that is, responses are given numeric codes that provide labels for data entry and analysis. For instance, sex can be coded 0 = male, 1 = female. We could code hospital size as 1 = less than 50 beds, 2 = 50 to 100 beds, and 3 = over 100 beds. These codes are entered into the computer to identify responses. Using codes, the researcher can easily obtain frequency counts and percentages for each question, to determine how many subjects checked each response.

The analysis of survey data may take many forms. Most often, descriptive statistics are used to summarize responses. When quantitative data such as age are collected, the researcher will usually present averages. With categorical data, the researcher reports the frequency of responses to specific questions. These frequencies are typically converted to a percentage of the total sample. For example, a researcher might report that 30% of the sample was male and 70% was female, or in a question about opinions, that 31% strongly agree, 20% agree, 5% disagree, and so on. Percentages should always be accompanied by reference to the total sample size, so that the reader can determine the actual number of responses in each category. Percentages are usually more meaningful than actual frequencies because sample sizes may differ greatly among studies.

Another common approach to data analysis involves the description of relationships between two or more sets of responses. For instance, a survey might contain a question asking a person's gender, and other questions might ask about attitudes toward abortion. The researcher can then examine the frequency of responses to the attitude questions in relation to each respondent's sex. **Cross-tabulations** are usually presented, showing the number of males and females who answered positively or negatively to each attitude question. The *chi-square* test (χ^2) can be used to examine this relationship statistically, to determine if there is a significant relationship between the two variables (see Chapter 25).

When questionnaires include a scale, researchers may want to look at sums as a reflection of the respondents' answers. These sums may be presented for the entire scale, or subscales may be analyzed. Measurement properties of such scales must be considered, such as the potential need for weighting items differently within a scale, or the decision on which items belong to a subscale.

Depending on the length and complexity of the questionnaire, researchers may present response percentages for all questions on the survey, or they may simply summarize the more important relationships that were studied. Some reports present purely narrative descriptions of the results; others include tables showing the responses to each question. The author must determine which type of presentation will be most effective for the data.

If a questionnaire is developed for the purpose of assessing a particular characteristic, such as function or pain, the researcher should evaluate the reliability and validity of the instrument. Different types of reliability and validity should be tested, depending on the type of questions and purpose of the assessment (see Chapters 5 and 6). The examination of an instrument's measurement properties is essential if the instrument will be used by others.

INFORMED CONSENT

Even though interviews or questionnaires do not require physical interaction with subjects, these studies must go through a formal process of review and approval by an institutional review board (IRB) (see Chapter 3). Researchers must be able to demonstrate the protection of subjects from psychological risk and the guarantee of confidentiality. Surveys will often receive expedited reviews by a review board.

Individuals who participate in face-to-face interviews can be given an informed consent form to sign in the presence of the interviewer and a witness. Consent to participate in telephone interviews is implied by the individual's participation. The researcher is obliged to give telephone respondents full information at the beginning of the call, so that they can decide whether they want to continue with the interview. Similarly, consent for mail questionnaires is implied by the return of the questionnaire. The cover letter provides the information needed.

COMMENTARY

They Have a Thousand and One Uses

Survey research represents a technique of data collection that can actually be applied across a wide range of research designs and approaches. Surveys may be purely descriptive, or they may be focused on variables that are expected to demonstrate specific relationships. Surveys and interviews can be the main form of data collection in quantitative or qualitative studies. They may be included as part of the data collection in an experimental study, to gather demographic information as part of the study, or they can be used as an outcome instrument. Surveys can be used for retrospective or prospective studies as well. Most often, surveys are based on a cross-sectional sample, meaning that a large group of respondents are tested at relatively the same point in time. Surveys can, however, be used in longitudinal studies by giving follow-up interviews or questionnaires to document changes in attitudes or behaviors.

Although surveys seem relatively easy to use as a research tool, this approach carries with it methodological problems. For descriptive studies, the researcher must construct a new measuring tool. This is no small accomplishment, and requires attention to principles of reliability and validity. Item reliability of questions, rater reliability for interviewers, and content and construct validity are all concerns for survey researchers. Generalizability issues are potentially of serious concern, especially when response rates are low. The researcher usually tries to determine if there is a difference between the characteristics of those who did respond and the characteristics of those who did not. For example, depending on the type of information available, it may be possible to determine the ages, sex distribution, or occupational characteristics of nonrespondents.

If a questionnaire is being used as an outcome instrument, the examination of its measurement properties must be extensive. We have described the validity issues involved in measuring change (see Chapter 6) and developing scales. The professional literature abounds with examples of the process of establishing validity for many of the currently used health status and functional scales, demonstrating the comprehensive approach that is necessary.

Those who are interested in pursuing the survey approach are encouraged to consult researchers who have had experience with surveys, as well as several informative texts listed at the end of this chapter.

KEY TERMS

interview	double-barreled question	semantic differential
questionnaire	scale	visual analogue scale (VAS)
self-report	categorical scale	Guttman scale
recall bias	continuous scale	Rasch analysis
guiding questions	summative scale	Q-sort
open-ended question	cumulative scale	Delphi survey
closed-ended question	Likert scale	cross-tabulation

REFERENCES

1. Reaby LL. Reasons why women who have mastectomy decide to have or not to have breast reconstruction. *Plast Reconstr Surg* 1998;101:1810–8.
2. Amrein L, Garrett TR, Martin GM. Use of low-voltage electrotherapy and electromyography in physical therapy. *Phys Ther* 1971;51:1283–7.
3. Neuhaus BE, Ascher ER, Coullon BA, et al. A survey of rationales for and against hand splinting in hemiplegia. *Am J Occup Ther* 1981;35:83–90.
4. Pajareya K, Anannontsak A, Paileeklee S. Functional skills after rehabilitation for patients with spinal cord injury. *J Med Assoc Thai* 1998;81:310–5.
5. Jette AM. Functional Status Index: reliability of a chronic disease evaluation instrument. *Arch Phys Med Rehabil* 1980;61:395–401.
6. Giles WH, Croft JB, Keenan NL, Lane MJ, Wheeler FC. The validity of self-reported hypertension and correlates of hypertension awareness among blacks and whites within the stroke belt. *Am J Prev Med* 1995;11:163–9.

7. Wills TA, Cleary SD. The validity of self-reports of smoking: analyses by race/ethnicity in a school sample of urban adolescents. *Am J Public Health* 1997;87:56–61.

8. Willemsen MC, Brug J, Uges DR, Vos de Wael ML. Validity and reliability of self-reported exposure to environmental tobacco smoke in work offices. *J Occup Environ Med* 1997;39:1111–4.

9. Sinoff G, Ore L. The Barthel activities of daily living index: self-reporting versus actual performance in the old-old (> or = 75 years). *J Am Geriatr Soc* 1997;45:832–6.

10. Couch KJ, Deitz JC, Kanny EM. The role of play in pediatric occupational therapy. *Am J Occup Ther* 1998;52:111–7.

11. Rozier CK, Raymond MJ, Goldstein MS, Hamilton BL. Gender and physical therapy career success factors. *Phys Ther* 1998;78:690–704.

12. Shaw ME, Wright JM. *Scales for the Measurement of Attitudes.* New York: McGraw-Hill, 1967.

13. McDowell I, Newell C. *Measuring Health: A Guide to Rating Scales and Questionnaires.* 2d ed. New York: Oxford University Press, 1996.

14. Kantz ME, Harris WJ, Levitsky K, Ware Jr. JE, Davies AR. Methods for assessing condition-specific and generic functional status outcomes after total knee replacement. *Med Care* 1992;30:MS240–MS252.

15. Dodds TA, Martin DP, Stolov WC, Deyo RA. A validation of the Functional Independence Measurement and its performance among rehabilitation inpatients. *Arch Phys Med Rehabil* 1993;74:531–6.

16. Katz JN, Larson MG, Phillips CB, Fossel AH, Liang MH. Comparative measurement sensitivity of short and longer health status instruments. *Med Care* 1992;30:917–25.

17. Converse JM, Presser S. *Survey Questions: Handcrafting the Standardized Questionnaire.* Beverly Hills, CA: Sage Publications, 1986.

18. McHorney CA, Ware Jr. JE, Lu JF, Sherbourne CD. The MOS 36-item Short-Form Health Survey (SF-36): III. Tests of data quality, scaling assumptions, and reliability across diverse patient groups. *Med Care* 1994;32:40–66.

19. Fairbank JC, Couper J, Davies JB, O' Brien JP. The Oswestry low back pain disability questionnaire. *Physiotherapy* 1980;66:271–3.

20. Phillips BS. *Social Research: Strategy and Tactics.* 2d ed. New York: MacMillan, 1971.

21. Likert R. A technique for the measurement of attitudes. *Arch Psychol* 1932;140:5–55.

22. Osgood CE, Suci GJ, Tannenbaum RH. *The Measurement of Meaning.* Urbana, IL: University of Illinois Press, 1957.

23. Heise DR. Semantic differential profiles for 1,000 most frequent English words. *Psychol Monogr* 1965;70:8.

24. Guyatt GH, Townsend M, Berman LB, Keller JL. A comparison of Likert and visual analogue scales for measuring change in function. *J Chronic Dis* 1987;40:1129–33.

25. McCormack HM, Horne DJ, Sheather S. Clinical applications of visual analogue scales: a critical review. *Psychol Med* 1988;18:1007–19.

26. Price DD, Harkins SW, Baker C. Sensory-affective relationships among different types of clinical and experimental pain. *Pain* 1987;28:291–9.

27. McGuire DB. The measurement of clinical pain. *Nurs Res* 1984;33:152–6.

28. Huskisson EC. Measurement of pain. *J Rheumatol* 1982;9:768–9.

29. Fernandez E, Nygren TE, Thorn BE. An 'open-transformed scale' for correcting ceiling effects and enhancing retest reliability: the example of pain. *Percept Psychophysics* 1991;49:572–8.

30. Dixon JS, Bird HA. Reproducibility along a 10 cm vertical visual analogue scale. *Ann Rheum Dis* 1981;40:87–9.

31. Sim J, Waterfield J. Validity, reliability and responsiveness in the assessment of pain. *Physiother Theory Pract* 1997;13:23–38.

32. Streiner DL, Normal GR. *Health Measurement Scales: A Practical Guide to Their Development and Use.* 2d ed. New York: Oxford Press, 1995.

33. Thomee R, Grimby G, Wright BD, Linacre JM. Rasch analysis of Visual Analog Scale measurements before and after treatment of Patellofemoral Pain Syndrome in women. *Scand J Rehabil Med* 1995;27:145–51.

34. Nunally JC. *Psychometric Theory.* 2d ed. New York: McGraw-Hill, 1978.

35. Rosow I, Breslau N. A Guttman health scale for the aged. *J Gerontol* 1966;21:556–9.

36. Kempen GI, Myers AM, Powell LE. Hierarchical structure in ADL and IADL: analytical assumptions and applications for clinicians and researchers. *J Clin Epidemiol* 1995;48:1299–305.

37. Dickson HG, Kohler F. The multi-dimensionality of the FIM motor items precludes an interval scaling using Rasch analysis. *Scand J Rehabil Med* 1996;28:159–62.

38. Mitchell J. *An Introduction to the Logic of Psychological Measurement.* Hillsdale, NJ: Erlbaum, 1990.

39. Heinemann AW, Harvey RL, McGuire JR, et al. Measurement properties of the NIH Stroke Scale during acute rehabilitation. *Stroke* 1997;28:1174–80.

40. Wright BD, Linacre JM. Observations are always ordinal; measurements, however, must be interval. *Arch Phys Med Rehabil* 1989;70:857–60.

41. Merbitz C, Morris J, Grip JC. Ordinal scales and foundations of misinference. *Arch Phys Med Rehabil* 1989;70:308–12.

42. Rasch G. *Probablistic Models for Some Intelligence and Attainment Tests.* Chicago: University of Chicago, 1980.

43. Wright BD, Masters G. *Rating Scale Analysis: Rasch Measurements.* Chicago: MESA, 1982.

44. Fisher AG. The assessment of IADL motor skills: an application of many-faceted Rasch analysis. *Am J Occup Ther* 1993;47:319–29.

45. Andrich D. *Rasch Models of Measurement.* Beverly Hills, CA: Sage Publications, 1988.

46. Chang W, Chan C. Rasch analysis for outcomes measures: some methodological considerations. *Arch Phys Med Rehabil* 1995;76:934–9.

47. UDS Data Management Service. *Guide for the Use of the Uniform Data Set for Medical Rehabilitation Including the Functional Independence Measure (Version 3.0).* Buffalo, NY: Uniform Data System for Medical Rehabilitation, The Buffalo General Hospital, 1990.

48. Linacre JM, Heinemann AW, Wright BD, Granger C, Hamilton BB. *The Functional Independence Measure as a Measure of Disability. Research Report 91-01.* Chicago: Rehabilitation Services Evaluation Unit, Rehabilitation Institute of Chicago, 1991.

49. Heinemann AW, Linacre JM, Wright BD, Hamilton BB, Granger C. Relationships between impairment and physical disability as measured by the Functional Independence Measure. *Arch Phys Med Rehabil* 1993;74:566–73.

50. Wright BD, Linacre JM. *BIGSTEPS: A Rasch-Model Computer Program.* Chicago: MESA Press, 1991.

51. Linacre JM. *FACETS Computer Program for Many-Faceted Rasch Measurement.* Chicago: MESA, 1988.

52. Wright BD, Stone MH. *Best Test Design.* Chicago: MESA Press, 1979.

53. Silverstein B, Fisher WP, Kilgore KM, Harley JP, Harvey RF. Applying psychometric criteria to functional assessment in medical rehabilitation: II. Defining interval measures. *Arch Phys Med Rehabil* 1992;73:507–18.

54. Haley SM, McHorney CA, Ware JE. Evaluation of the MOS SF-36 Physical Functioning Scale (PF-10): I. Unidimensionality and reproducibility of the Rasch Item Scale. *J Clin Epidemiol* 1994; 47: 671–84.

55. Campbell SK, Kolobe TH, Osten ET, Lenke M, Girolami GL. Construct validity of the test of infant motor performance. *Phys Ther* 1995;75:585–96.

56. Ryd JL, Rheault W. Rasch analysis of the Dizziness Handicap Inventory. *J Rehabil Outcomes Meas* 1998;2:17–24.

57. Stephenson W. *The Study of Behavior: Q Technique and Its Methodology.* Chicago: University of Chicago Press, 1975.

58. Biddle WB, Riesenberg LA, Darcy PA. Medical students' perceptions of desirable characteristics of primary care teaching sites. *Fam Med* 1996;28:629–33.

59. Trotter MJ, Fordyce WE. A process for physical therapist student selection. The Q-technique. *Phys Ther* 1975;55:151–6.

60. Kovach CR, Krejci JW. Facilitating change in dementia care. Staff perceptions. *J Nurs Adm* 1998;28:17–27.

61. Moore C. *Group Techniques for Idea Building.* Beverly Hills, CA: Sage Publications, 1987.

62. Delbecq A, Van de Ven A, Gustafson D. *Group Techniques for Program Planning.* Middleton, WI: Green Briar Press, 1986.

63. Ingram D. Opinions of physical therapy education program directors on essential functions. *Phys Ther* 1997;77:37–45.

64. Mangham CA. Expert opinion on the diagnosis of acoustic tumors. *Otolaryngol Head Neck Surg* 1997;117:622–7.

65. Elder Jr. OC, Nick TG. Moving toward a core curriculum in schools of the allied health professions: knowledge and skills considered important by department chairs in four disciplines. *J Allied Health* 1997;26:51–6.

66. Palisano R, Rosenbaum P, Walter S, Russell D, Wood E, Galuppi B. Development and reliability of a system to classify gross motor function in children with cerebral palsy. *Dev Med Child Neurol* 1997;39:214–23.

67. Triezenberg HL. The identification of ethical issues in physical therapy practice. *Phys Ther* 1996;76:1097–1107.

C H A P T E R

15

Epidemiology

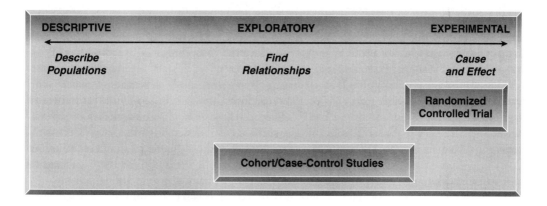

The ultimate goal in the field of epidemiology is to improve the health of populations. A simple, yet comprehensive definition of epidemiology is the study of health and disease, and includes (1) determining the frequencies of diseases and health states and their trends; (2) determining the factors that effect the development of a particular disease or health state and why; (3) predicting the occurrence and distribution of various diseases and health states; and (4) determining the factors which prevent disease, prolong life with a disease, or improve health status.

Classically, the field of **epidemiology** is concerned with the study of the distribution and determinants of disease, injury, or dysfunction in human populations. Epidemiology literally began as the study of "epidemics," concerned primarily with mortality and morbidity from acute infectious diseases. Many of the health standards we take for granted today, such as clean water supplies, treatment of sewage, and food refrigeration, can be credited to discoveries made through epidemiological investigations. Epidemiologists try to identify those who have a specific disorder, when and where the disorder developed, and what exposures are associated with its presence. Epidemiological questions often arise out of clinical experience, laboratory findings, or public health concerns

The authors wish to acknowledge the substantial contribution of Diane Jette, DSc, PT, to this chapter.

about the relationship between societal practices and disease outcomes. Through the analysis of health status indicators and population characteristics, epidemiologists try to identify and explain the causal factors in disease patterns.

As medical cures and treatments have been developed to control many of these problems, and as patterns of disease have changed, the scope of epidemiology has broadened. Today epidemiology includes the study of chronic disease, disability, and health status. Diseases include conditions such as AIDS and chronic conditions such as cardiac disease, arthritis, cancer, and back pain, as well as traumatic injuries and birth defects. This approach fits with the World Health Organization's definition of health which encompasses social, psychological, and physical well-being.[1]

The focus on **exposures,** or causal factors, also takes a broader view that reflects contemporary concerns, including lifestyle practices such as smoking, substance abuse, drinking alcohol or coffee, and eating foods high in cholesterol or salt; occupational hazards, such as repetitive tasks, heavy lifting, and operating computers; environmental influences, such as second-hand smoke, toxic waste, and sunlight; and specific interventions, such as exercise, medications, and treatment modalities. These exposures are considered **risk factors** that increase or decrease the likelihood of developing certain disorders or influence the ultimate outcome of a disorder. For example, smoking and sunlight are considered risk factors that increase the chance of developing cancer.[2,3] Wine may be a preventive factor (negative risk factor) for heart disease.[4]

Epidemiology is distinguished as a research approach because of its unique concern with the identification of health status, risk factors for disability and disease, and the control of these disorders or improvement of health status through policy and intervention.[5] In epidemiology large populations are traditionally studied or inferences are made from large samples of individuals to a population. The population of interest, however, may be defined in many ways. Often, epidemiological principles can be applied to a clinical group of interest rather than to a large general population.[6] Epidemiologic studies are generally distinguished as experimental, quasi-experimental, or observational. In **observational studies** there is no artificial manipulation of any of the study factors. Observational studies are categorized as *descriptive* or *analytic*. Descriptive studies are concerned with the distribution and patterns of disease or disability in a population. These studies are carried out when there is little knowledge about the state of health or frequency of disease. Analytic studies test hypotheses to determine if specific exposures are related to the health status or disease occurrence.

Information from epidemiological research can have direct influence on practitioners' day-to-day choices of interventions and structure of a patient's treatment program. Examples of clinically related questions which can be answered using epidemiological approaches are:

1. What frequency and duration of treatment can be expected to facilitate the most effective return of function in patients who have had a stroke?
2. Which subgroups of patients with myocardial infarction are most likely to have the best outcomes from exercise programs?
3. Is there a difference in the effectiveness of home exercise programs as compared with outpatient therapy for reducing symptoms of low back pain?
4. What are the costs associated with improvements in health-related quality of life following pulmonary rehabilitation?
5. What is the relationship between impairments and the development of disability in elders?

The purpose of this chapter is to describe epidemiologic research approaches, to illustrate research designs that incorporate epidemiologic principles, and to present measures of disease frequency that are used to estimate health risks. Because we are often concerned with functional problems as well as disease states, we facilitate this discussion by using the terms *disease, disorder,* and *disability* interchangeably to represent health outcomes, including illness, injury, and physical, psychological, or social dysfunction.

DESCRIPTIVE EPIDEMIOLOGY

Descriptive studies are done when little is known about the occurrence or determinant of health conditions. The purpose of descriptive studies is to describe patterns of health, disease, and disability in terms of *person, place,* and *time:*

1. *Who* experiences this disorder? Relevant characteristics might include age, sex, religion, race, cultural background, education, socioeconomic status, occupation, and so on. This is the *demography* of the disorder. Epidemiologists try to determine if individuals with certain characteristics are more at risk for a particular disorder than others.
2. *Where* is the frequency of disorder highest or lowest? Epidemiologists may be concerned with identifying restricted areas within a city or large geographic areas in which disease or exposures are commonly found. They may look at environmental factors such as weather, local industry, water source, and lifestyle as potential causative factors.
3. *When* does the disorder occur most or least frequently? The epidemiologist will compare the present frequency of a disorder with that of the past. When the frequency of occurrence varies significantly at one point in time, some specific time-related causative factor is sought. Seasonal variations may become obvious, or trends may be related to other historical factors.

Descriptive Studies

Descriptive studies will often provide information that can be used to set priorities for health care planning, and will generate hypotheses that can be studied using analytic methods. Descriptive studies can be presented as case reports, correlational studies, or cross-sectional surveys.

Case Reports

An epidemiologic **case report,** or case series, is a description of one or more individuals, documenting a unique or unusual occurrence or medical condition. The purpose of the case study is to present as complete a picture as possible about the characteristics of, and exposures faced by, that individual, often resulting in the presentation of a hypothesis about the causal factors that might account for the observed outcome. Many notable examples of this approach exist, such as the single case report in 1961 of a 40-year-old premenopausal woman who developed a pulmonary embolism 5 weeks after starting to use oral contraceptives;[7] the report of the death of a young woman from toxic shock syndrome, which was associated with the use of a particular tampon;[8] and a series of reports documenting the first cases of AIDS in five young previously healthy homosexual males in Los Angeles.[9] These case studies led to the formulation of analytic hypotheses that have since been tested and supported.[10,11]

As is true with clinical case reports, case studies in epidemiology do not provide sufficient control to allow for generalizations or conclusions about causality. They can only act as a catalyst for further study; however, as the preceding examples illustrate, case reports can be vitally important for identifying new health hazards and facilitating further analytic research.

Correlational Studies

In a **correlational study,** the researcher tries to establish a relationship between a disease or disability and particular exposures by looking at patterns within populations. The advantage of this type of study is that researchers can routinely use available data from large databases developed by government and private health agencies. For instance, the National Center for Health Statistics publishes several statistical surveys, such as the Health Interview Survey and the National Long Term Care Survey, that document social, demographic, and economic aspects of illness, disability, and utilization of medical services.[12] The Centers for Disease Control provide statistics on the incidence of specific diseases and mortality rates.[13] These and many other such surveys provide a wealth of information about specific high-risk groups, and have the advantage of being able to sample large representative segments of the population on an ongoing basis.

The major limitation of any correlational study is the inability to draw conclusions about cause and effect based on clinical correlates (see Chapters 13 and 23). In epidemiology this limitation is often compounded by the inability to link the exposure and disease in any one individual. For example, in the 1960s, researchers documented increased mortality from coronary heart disease (CHD) in states where per capita cigarette sales were highest;[14] however, this relationship is based on a correlation of the total population's rate of CHD and cigarette sales. Therefore, we cannot determine a direct causal link because we cannot know if those who died of CHD were the same individuals who smoked. Other factors that are associated with smoking may have influenced the mortality rate. Epidemiologic correlational studies are, therefore, primarily useful for providing evidence to formulate hypotheses that can then be tested using analytic methodology.

Cross-Sectional Studies

A **cross-sectional study** involves the simultaneous assessment of exposures and disease in a given population. These studies are often called "snapshots" because they sample data at a single point in time. A cross-sectional survey may cover a specific time period, such as a given calendar year, or it may focus on a relative time period within the lives of the population, such as the first month of life or the first week of employment. The major purpose of the cross-sectional approach is to describe the frequency of a disorder within an identified group in an efficient manner.

Like other descriptive methods, a cross-sectional study is unable to establish causality. Because the sample is measured at one point in time, it is not possible to determine if the exposure to a risk factor preceded the disorder, a necessary point if etiology is to be determined. A second limitation is that the cross-sectional study is not sensitive to duration of a disorder or disease; that is, there is no discrimination between diseases that are long standing versus those that are of brief duration. Therefore, diseases of shorter duration tend to be underrepresented in cross-sectional data. A third limitation is the focus of cross-sectional surveys on survivors in a population. The presence of a disease can only be assessed in those who are still living. Therefore, if many have died, the frequency of the disease may be inaccurately reflected in a one-time estimate.

Measures of Disease Frequency

The statistical measures used to describe epidemiologic outcomes focus on quantification of disease occurrence. The simplest measure of disease frequency would be a count of the number of affected individuals; however, meaningful interpretation and comparisons of such a measure would also require knowing how many people there were in the total population who could have gotten the disease and the length of time over which the occurrence of the disease was monitored. Therefore, measures of disease frequency will always include reference to population size and time period of observation. For example, we might document 35 cases of a disease within 1 year in a population of 3,200 people, or 35/3,200/year. Typically, population size is expressed in terms of thousands, such as 1,000 (10^3), 10,000 (10^4), or 100,000 (10^5). For instance, the preceding values would be expressed as 10.94 cases per 1,000 per year. To make estimates more useful, such rates are usually calculated in whole numbers, such as 1,094/100,000/year.

The number of cases of a disease that exist in a population reflects the risk of disease for that group. It describes the relative importance of the disease and can provide a basis for comparison with other groups who may have different exposure histories. The two most common measures of disease frequency are prevalence and incidence.

Prevalence

Prevalence is a proportion reflecting the number of *existing* cases of a disorder relative to the total population at a given point in time. It provides an estimate of the probability that an individual will have a particular disorder at that time. Prevalence (P) is calculated as

$$P = \frac{\text{number of existing cases of a disease at a given point in time}}{\text{total population at risk.}} \quad (15.1)$$

For example, the Health Interview Survey in 1977 found that the number of noninstitutionalized elderly who were totally physically dependent was 3,276 out of a sample of 11,698.[15] The prevalence of total dependency in this population is expressed as

$$P = \frac{3,276}{11,698} = \frac{28,005}{100,000} = 28\%$$

Thus, there is a 28% probability that any randomly selected individual from this population would be physically dependent. Because this value reflects the cross-sectional status of the population at a single point in time, it is also called *point prevalence.* Prevalence can be established for an absolute calendar time, as in the preceding example, or it may be relative to a period in time. For example, data obtained from a random sample of 973 newspaper employees found that the number of individuals categorized as having upper limb musculoskeletal complaints after 1 year was 395.[16] The estimate of the prevalence of upper limb musculoskeletal complaints in this population during a 1-year period is, therefore, 41% (395/973). This measure, combining existing with new cases of the disorder during the period of 1 year, is referred to as *period prevalence*.

Prevalence is most useful as an indicator for planning health services, because it reflects the impact of a disease on the population. Therefore, a measure of prevalence can be used to project requirements such as health care personnel, specialized medical equipment, and number of hospital beds. Prevalence should not, however, be used as a basis for examining etiology of a disease because it is influenced by the length of survival of those with the disorder; that is, prevalence is a function of both the number of individuals who develop the disease and the duration or severity of the illness. Because this estimate looks at the total number of individuals who have the disease at a given time, that number will be large if the disease tends to be of long duration.

Incidence

The measure of *incidence* quantifies the number of *new* cases of a disorder or disease in the population during a specified time period and, therefore, represents an estimate of the risk of developing the disease during that time. Incidence discounts the effect of duration of illness that is present in prevalence measures. By examining incidence rates for subgroups of the population, such as age groups, ethnic groups, and geographic locations, the researcher can identify those groups that demonstrate higher disease rates and target them to investigate specific exposures. Incidence can be expressed as cumulative incidence or incidence rate.

Cumulative incidence (CI) quantifies the number of individuals who become diseased during a specified time period:

$$CI = \frac{\text{number of new cases during given time period}}{\text{total population at risk}} \qquad (15.2)$$

For example, the cumulative incidence of low back pain among novice golfers was examined over a 1-year period.[17] One hundred ninety-six men who had recently taken up golf were followed over that 1-year period. During that time, 16 new cases of back pain were identified. The 1-year cumulative incidence of first-time back pain for this cohort was 8% (16/196). The specification of the time period of observation is essential to the interpretation of this value. The number of cases would be perceived differently if subjects were followed for 1 or 10 years. Other issues that require consideration in interpreting a measure of cumulative incidence include the possibility that the number of individuals at risk in the cohort will vary over time, and the possibility that the condition under study is caused by other, competing risks.

Measuring the total population at risk for cumulative incidence assumes that all subjects were followed for the entire observation period; however, some individuals in the population may enter the study at different times, some may drop out, and others who acquire the disease are no longer at risk. Therefore, the length of the follow-up period is not uniform for all participants. To account for these differences, *incidence rate (IR)* can be calculated:

$$IR = \frac{\text{number of new cases during given time period}}{\text{total person–time}} \qquad (15.3)$$

As in cumulative incidence, the numerator for this estimate represents the number of new cases of the disorder; however, the denominator is the sum of the time periods of observation for all individuals in the population at risk during the study time frame, or *person-time*. For example, in the Nurses' Health Study, 121,700 female nurses were enrolled in 1976. During the period of 1976 to 1992, investigators identified 3,603 new cases of breast cancer.[18] Of the women originally enrolled, some left the study as a result of death or loss to follow-up at various times during the period, and some developed breast cancer after different amounts of time, contributing different amounts of time to the denominator. In other words, one woman who died in 1977 in an automobile crash would have contributed 1 person-year to the denominator, whereas two women who developed breast cancer in 1990 would have contributed 28 person-years to the denominator.

Researchers totaled the amount of time each subject was *known to be at risk* between 1976 and 1992, and obtained the total person-years observed; in this case there were 1,794,565 person-years of observation. The incidence rate was, therefore, 3,606/1,794,565 person-years, or 2 cases per 1,000 person years. Incidence rate is often a more efficient measure than cumulative incidence, as it allows for inclusion of all subjects, regardless of the amount of time they were able to participate. Cumulative incidence assumes that all subjects were available for the entire study period.

The relationship between incidence and prevalence is a function of the average duration of the outcome of interest. If the incidence of the disorder is low (few new cases occur), but the duration of the disorder is long, then the prevalence, or proportion of the population that has the disease at a given point in time, may be large. If, however, incidence is high (many new cases of the disease occur), but the disorder is manifest for a short duration (either by quick recovery or death), the prevalence may be low.

Vital Statistics

Epidemiologists often use incidence measures to describe the health status of populations in terms of birth and death rates that inform us about the consequences of disease. The **birth rate** is obtained by dividing the number of live births during the year by the total population at midyear. The **mortality rate** quantifies the incidence of death in a population by dividing the number of deaths during a specific time period by the total population at the midpoint of the time period. These data are generally available through records of state vital statistics reports, census data, and birth and death certificates.

The mortality rate can reflect *total mortality* for the population from all causes of death in the *crude mortality rate,* in which the total number of deaths during the year is divided by the average midyear population. This value is usually expressed as the number of deaths per 100,000 population; however, when different categories within the population differentially contribute to this rate, it may be more meaningful to look at category-specific rates. A **cause-specific rate** looks only at the number of deaths from a particular disease or condition within a year divided by the average midyear population. For instance, rates may reflect mortality specifically resulting from diseases such as cancer and heart disease or from motor vehicle accidents. The **case-fatality rate** is the number of deaths from a disease relative to the number of individuals who had the disease during a given time period.

Other commonly used categories are age, sex, and race. **Age-specific rates** are probably most common because of the differential occurrance of many diseases across the life span. For example, if one looks at the death rate for cancer across age groups, we would find that mortality was higher for older age categories. Therefore, it may be more meaningful to present age-specific mortality rates for each decade of life, rather than a crude mortality rate; however, this results in a long list of rates that may not be useful for certain comparisons. An overall rate would be more practical, but it would have to account for the variation in rates across age categories. For instance, if we compare the crude cancer mortality rate for today versus the crude rate from 50 years ago, we would have to account for the fact that a larger proportion of the total population now falls in the older age range. Therefore, epidemiologists will often report *age-adjusted mortality rates* that reflect different weightings for the uneven age categories. Methods for calculating adjusted rates are described in most epidemiology texts.

ANALYTIC DESIGNS: OBSERVATIONAL STUDIES

Observational analytic designs are distinguished from descriptive studies in that they are used when enough is known about a condition to allow testing of hypotheses about the association of specific risk factors and outcomes. These designs include an explicit comparison group, and are able to document a temporal sequence of exposure and disease. Analytic designs allow the investigator to determine if the disease rate is different for those exposed or unexposed to the factor of interest and, thus, to establish that certain exposures either increase or decrease one's risk of developing that disease. In observational studies the investigator records data based on observed characteristics of subjects and their experiences. No interventions are applied. Observational studies are of two types, case-control and cohort studies.

Case-Control Studies

A **case-control study** is a method of epidemiologic investigation in which groups of individuals are selected on the basis of whether they have the disorder under study. *Cases* are those classified as having the disorder, and *controls* are chosen as a comparison group without the disorder. The investigator then looks backward in time, via direct interview, mail questionnaire, or chart review of previously collected data, to determine if the groups differ with respect to their exposure histories or the presence of specific characteristics that may put a person at risk for developing the condition of interest. The assumption is that differences in exposure histories should explain why the cases experienced the outcome and the controls did not. For example, classically trained professional and student musicians were contacted in the province of Ontario.[19] From this group, those with playing-related musculoskeletal disorders were identified according to an operational definition of the disorder (cases). Musicians with no playing-related musculoskeletal disorder were also identified (controls). Analyses were done to determine whether a variety of factors such as gender, type of instrument played, and warming up (exposures or risks) were related to having the disorder. Statistical estimates are used to quantify the risk associated with the exposure, by determining if a higher percentage of cases were exposed than controls. In this example, females and string players were found to be at higher risk for musculoskeletal disorders. Procedures for calculating these estimates are described later in this chapter.

The advantage of the case-control design is that samples are relatively easy to gather. Therefore, case-control studies are useful for studying disorders that are relatively rare, because they start by finding cases in a systematic manner. Case-control methods are especially applicable for analyzing diseases with long latency periods, where longitudinal studies would require years to identify those who developed the disease. One disadvantage of case-control studies is the potential for uncertainty in the temporal relationship between exposure and disease and for biases in the design. In addition, the proportion of cases and controls in the study is not related to the proportion of cases in the population. Therefore, findings must be subjected to scrutiny in terms of the potential for bias or confounding that may interfere with their validity; however, results of case-control studies provide estimates that, taken with other evidence, may support a causal relationship between specific risk factors and the presence or absence of disease.

Selection of Cases and Controls

The validity of case-control studies is dependent on several design issues. Perhaps most obvious are the effects of case definition and case selection. **Case definition** refers to the diagnostic and clinical criteria that identify someone as a case. These criteria must be comprehensive and specific, so that cases are clearly distinguished from controls and so that the study sample is homogeneous. Case definitions for many diseases have been developed by the Centers for Disease Control and the World Health Organization. At times, these definitions are revised to reflect recent medical findings, as in the increasingly comprehensive definition of AIDS. Clinical diagnoses are sometimes more difficult to define or control. For instance, disorders such as birth defects, hemiplegia, cerebral palsy, and low back pain can be manifested in many different forms. Therefore, the specific characteristics that qualify an individual as having the disease or disability for a specific study must be spelled out in detail. The population to which results will be generalized is defined according to these characteristics.

Selection of Cases.   Once the case definition is established, criteria for *case selection* must be developed. Cases may be identified from all those who have been treated for the disorder at a specific hospital or treatment center, or they may be chosen from the larger general population of those with the disorder. A **population-based study** involves obtaining a sample of cases from the general population of those with the disorder. In a **hospital-based study,** cases are obtained from patients in a medical institution. The latter approach is more common because samples are relatively easy to recruit and subjects are easy to contact. The population-based study affords greater generalizability, but is often too expensive and logistically unfeasible. Cases do not need to represent the entire range of characteristics in the population. For instance, within the scope of the research question, cases may be drawn from a restricted age range, only males or females, or only those who live within a defined area.

The researcher must also determine whether the study should include incident or prevalent cases. The difference, of course, is that with prevalent cases duration of illness is not accounted for. If the duration of a condition is not related to exposure, then a case-control study using prevalent cases is justifiable. If exposure affects duration of the condition, however, then results from a case-control study are more difficult to interpret. In general, it is preferable to use new or incident cases or to restrict cases to those who were diagnosed within a specific period.

Selection of Controls.   The most serious challenge to the researcher in designing a case-control study is the choice of a control group. The purpose of a case-control study is to determine if the frequency of an exposure or certain personal characteristics are different for those who did and did not develop the disease. Therefore, for the comparison to be fair, the controls should be drawn from the population of individuals who would have been chosen as cases had the disease been present. Any restrictions or criteria used to select cases must also be used to select controls. Often, researchers match cases and controls on a variety of relevant factors, such as age, race, gender, occupation, or other variables that could influence the disease status.

Controls can be obtained from several sources. They are often recruited from the same hospital or institution as the cases, from those who have been admitted for conditions other than the disease of interest. The advantage of this process is that hospitalized patients are readily available and similarly motivated. The disadvantage, of course, is that they are ill and, therefore, potentially different from healthy subjects who might be exposed to the same risk factors. In addition, studies have shown that hospitalized patients are more likely to smoke cigarettes, use oral contraceptives, and drink more alcohol than nonhospitalized individuals.[20,21] Therefore, if these risk factors are being studied or if they are related to the disease being studied, they could bias the results. It is also important to determine what disorders other than the case disorder are represented among controls. If the risk factors being studied are associated with these other disorders, the estimate of their effects on cases will be minimized. Despite the disadvantages, however, hospital controls are often used because of the convenience they offer.

Controls can also be obtained from the general population by a variety of sampling methods, such as random-digit dialing, or by using available lists such as voter registration and membership directories. Specific segments of the population may be sampled from special lists. For instance, in a case-control study to establish the risk of hip fracture associated with the use of psychotropic drugs, controls were selected from elderly Medicaid enrollees.[22] Sometimes special groups can be contacted to provide controls, such as family members and friends of those with the disease. These controls provide some comparability in ethnic and lifestyle characteristics.

Analysis Issues

The analysis of results of case-control studies requires attention to bias in the selection and classification of subjects and in the assessment of exposure status. Because subjects are purposefully selected for case-control studies on the basis of their having or not having a disease, **selection bias** is of special concern. Cases and controls must be chosen regardless of their exposure histories. If cases and controls are differentially selected on some variable that is related to the exposure of interest, it will not be possible to determine if the exposure is truly related to the disease. When samples are composed of subjects who have consented to participate, self-selection biases can also occur.

An additional source of bias is introduced if subjects are misclassified, that is, if those who have the disease are put in the control group or those who do not really have the disease are considered cases. If this **misclassification** is random, and equally present in both groups, it is considered *nondifferential misclassification,* which will tend to minimize the relationship between the exposure and disease. With *differential misclassification,* however, when groups are not affected equally, the results may overestimate or underestimate that relationship.[5] For example, in a study evaluating risk factors associated with falling in hospitalized elderly, cases were identified from incident reports of a geriatric rehabilitation hospital for a 1-year period, and controls were selected at random from patients who were "nonfallers," that is, for whom incident reports had not been filed.[23] There may, however, have been cases of falling that were not reported, or nurses may have filed incident reports even when the patient was carefully lowered to the ground by a staff member, if they felt weak while ambulating. In either case, patients would have been misclassified, and in the former situation, some cases may have been chosen as controls.

Observation bias occurs when there is a systematic difference in the way information about disease or exposure is obtained from the study groups. **Interviewer bias** is introduced when the individual collecting data elicits, records, or interprets information differentially from controls and cases. For instance, an interviewer may be aware of the research hypothesis and might ascertain different levels of information from subjects to support the hypothesis. Because so many epidemiologic studies involve an interview or observation, this type of bias must be explicitly addressed by efforts to improve tester reliability, by blinding interviewers to group and hypothesis, and by making data collection as objective as possible.

Recall bias occurs when subjects who have experienced a particular disorder remember their exposure history differently from those who are not affected. This bias may result in an underestimate or an overestimate of the risk of association with a particular exposure. It is not unusual for individuals who have a disease to analyze their habits, past experiences, or recent changes in their lives with greater depth or accuracy than those who are healthy. When cases are selected from hospitalized patients and controls are drawn from the general population, the problem of recall bias may be especially relevant. For example, elderly individuals who fall and require hospitalization may be more likely to remember the circumstances of the fall than those who trip and fall but do not have any serious injury.

A third factor that may interfere with analytic interpretations of case-control data is the confounding effect of extraneous variables that are related to the exposure of interest and, independently, affect the risk of developing the disease. For example, we might try to establish that age is a risk factor related to the incidence of hip fracture, documenting a larger number of such fractures in the elderly. This relationship may be confounded, however, if a third variable, osteoporosis, is related to the exposure (age) and is an independent risk factor for the disease (hip fracture); that is, we might conclude that age is a causal factor in predicting the incidence of hip fracture when actually it is the presence of osteoporosis. Investigators must examine the potential contribution of confounders by collecting data on them and analyzing their association with both the exposure and disease. Strategies for evaluating confounding are described later.

Cohort Studies

In clinical research, a cohort is defined as a group of individuals who are followed together over time. In a **cohort study** (also called a follow-up study), the researcher selects a group of subjects who do not yet have the outcome of interest and follows them to see if they develop the disorder. A cohort study may also include two or more groups who do not have the outcomes of interest but differ according to characteristics or exposures that are considered potential determinants of the outcome. Subjects are interviewed or observed to determine the presence or absence of certain exposures, risks, or characteristics. Cohort studies may be purely descriptive, with the intent of describing the natural history of a disease. More often, however, they are analytic, identifying the risk associated with these exposures by comparing the incidence of specific outcomes in those who were and were not exposed.

One advantage of a cohort study over a case-control study is the ability to determine the incidence of the condition. Another advantage of cohort studies is the ability to establish a temporal sequence for the relationship between exposure to risk factors and development of a particular outcome. This sequence is necessary for drawing inferences about causative factors. The disadvantage of cohort studies is that they are not useful for studying disorders that are uncommon in the population. If the disorder is rare, a large number of subjects would have to be followed for a long time to document a sufficient number of cases for analysis. In this situation, case-control studies would be more appropriate; however, cohort studies are useful when exposures are rare because the cohort can be assembled and classified according to their exposure status (where case-control subjects were classified according to disease status). Cohort studies are also very effective for studying multiple disorders.

One of the more well-known cohort studies is the Framingham Heart Study, which involved an original cohort of over 5,200 adults from Framingham, Massachusetts. The study began in 1948 and is still in progress. These individuals have been examined every 2 years to explore the relationships of a wide variety of risk factors with coronary heart disease.[24] This type of longitudinal study allows researchers to examine consistency of patterns and to evaluate predictive factors. This cohort has expanded as children of the original group have also been included. In addition, data have been used to evaluate many other risk factors, including those related to physical disability,[25–27] stroke,[28,29] and intermittent claudication[30] as outcomes related to a variety of exposures.

Cohort studies can be either prospective or retrospective, depending on the time sequencing of development of the disorder with respect to the start of the study. The basis for distinguishing between prospective and retrospective designs is where the investigator initiates entry into the exposure-disease cycle. If the investigator studies individuals who have already been exposed to risk factors and have already developed the disease, the study is considered retrospective. If the investigator contacts the subjects after the exposure, but before the disorder has developed, it is considered prospective.

The main advantage of the prospective design is the ability to control and monitor data collection and to measure variables completely and accurately. This approach is most useful in situations when the disease of interest occurs frequently, and subjects can be readily obtained. The disadvantage of this approach is that it is expensive and time consuming, and subjects are often lost to follow-up.

The retrospective cohort study uses a cohort that has already been assembled (usually for other reasons), and looks at how variables occurred over time in relation to specific outcomes. Retrospective designs tend to be cheaper and faster than prospective designs, and they are more efficient with diseases of long latency. If a disease takes years to manifest following exposure to a risk factor, a prospective study will have to go on for a long time to document it. The disadvantage of retrospective designs is that they may have to deal with incomplete or inadequate data from medical records, the subject's memory, or the memories and perspectives of family members or caregivers.

Selection of Subjects

The selection of subjects for a cohort study must be appropriate for the research question. For purely descriptive studies, the sample must be representative of the target population to which results will be generalized. Probability samples would be ideal, but are rarely used because of expense and limited accessibility. Even with random selection, not all those who are invited to participate in the study will consent. For analytic studies, two groups must be identified: those who have been exposed and those who have not been exposed to the risk factors. The most important consideration is that the exposed group be of sufficient numbers to obtain meaningful outcome measures; that is, there must be enough subjects who eventually develop the disease.*

The group that has been exposed to the risk factors may come from several sources. For relatively common exposures, a large number of individuals may be available from the general population. Often, accessible groups such as nurses in the previously mentioned Nurses' Health Study,[18] residents of defined geographical areas, or employees of a specific company are targeted as a cohort, not necessarily because of their exposure histories, but because they can be followed easily and relevant information can be readily obtained. The subjects in the Framingham Heart Study represent a classical example of this type of cohort, chosen because of the accessibility of a stable geographic population. When exposures are rare in the population, special cohorts may be chosen because of their unique exposure histories. For example, to study the relationship of extremely vigorous physical activity and exercise to development of musculoskeletal injuries, a cohort was comprised of young men in Army infantry basic training.[31]

The comparison cohort must be as similar as possible to the exposed cohort in all factors related to the disease except for the specific exposures under study. It is important that all subjects who are chosen have a chance of developing the disorder. For instance, if one were studying risks associated with abnormal menstruation, women who have had hysterectomies or who have passed menopause would not be eligible.

In some situations, a general cohort can be chosen for study and members can be classified as exposed or unexposed, creating an *internal comparison group*. This approach was taken in the Framingham Heart Study. When special cohorts are chosen because of unique exposures, an unexposed comparison group may be difficult to locate within the same environment. Therefore, an *external comparison group* must be established, perhaps

---

*Researchers can perform a power analysis when planning a study, to determine how many subjects should be included. The sample size determinations are based on the expected outcome, that is, the degree of association expected between the exposure and the disease. This expected relationship is called the *effect size*. The larger the effect size (a stronger relationship), the fewer subjects would be needed. For a fuller discussion of the concept of effect size, see Appendix C.

including individuals who work at different but similar occupations or residents of the community in which the exposed cohort works. Control for this approach can be improved by establishing that mortality and morbidity rates are similar for the exposed and unexposed cohorts.

Analysis Issues

The results of a cohort study will clearly be influenced by the misclassification of either exposure or disease. The issues related to misclassification were described in the section on case-control studies. Bias is less of a concern in prospective cohort studies than in case-control or retrospective studies, because classification of exposure is made independently of knowledge about the subject's disease status.

Because of the longitudinal nature of prospective cohort studies, they are especially prone to attrition. The researcher must determine the validity of the study based on whether the loss of subjects is related to either the exposure, the disease, or both. Researchers generally take great pains to ensure good rapport with participants, and must be aggressive in maintaining contact with them.

ANALYTIC DESIGNS: CLINICAL TRIALS

The *clinical trial,* or *intervention study,* is the most common type of experimental design in epidemiology and presents the strongest evidence for causality of any epidemiologic approach. A clinical trial is a prospective study comparing the effect of an intervention against a control. In a **randomized clinical trial (RCT),** the investigator randomly allocates the exposure, or intervention, to an experimental group and gives a placebo or no treatment to a control group. Both groups are followed to determine the outcome. The use of blind or double-blind strategies, and the control of threats to internal and external validity, are also applicable to clinical trials (see Chapters 9 and 10). The most important feature of this design, which is not present in case-control or cohort studies, is the ability to randomly select subjects and randomly allocate treatments, strengthening the internal and external validity of the study. As an example, Kelsen et al. performed a multisite randomized trial comparing preoperative chemotherapy followed by surgery with surgery alone for patients with operable esophageal cancer.[32] Subjects were randomly allocated—213 to the preoperative chemotherapy group and 227 to undergo immediate surgery. After a median of almost 5 years, there were no differences in survival rate for the two groups.

Nonrandomized clinical trials are often used to assess community intervention, where the intervention is provided to well-defined, naturally occurring groups in order to address primary prevention. Nonrandomized trials may also involve the comparison of an intervention group with historical controls who have received standard treatment, but this approach will often show that the new intervention is better than the standard treatment.[33] Because there is no way to establish the true equivalence of historical controls with the intervention group, this approach provides limited confidence in outcomes.

Clinical trials can be clinically based or community based, depending on how samples are chosen. To ensure that results will be powerful enough to show differences, clinical trials are generally designed on a large scale, often involving subjects from a range of geographic areas or from several treatment centers. The cost of such trials is understandably great and usually necessitates substantial funding. Accordingly, the feasibility, ethics, and public health benefits of the study should be considered when designing a clinical trial. The concern about denying a potentially beneficial treatment to one group must be satisfied by the impact of the study on health care and public interests.

Clinical trials can be classified as either therapeutic or preventive. *Therapeutic trials* examine the effect of a treatment or intervention on a particular disease. For example, clinical trials in the 1970s began to show that radical mastectomy was not necessary for reducing the risk of recurrence or spread of breast cancer, and that limited resection was equally effective in terms of recurrence and mortality.[34,35] A *preventive trial* evaluates whether a procedure or agent reduces the risk of developing a disease. One of the most famous preventive trials was the field study of poliomyelitis vaccine in 1954, which covered 11 states.[36] The incidence of poliomyelitis in the vaccinated group was over 50% less than among those children who received the placebo, establishing strong evidence of the vaccine's effectiveness.

Selection of Subjects

Before a sample can be selected for a clinical trial, the target population, also called the *reference population,* must be identified. This is the group to which the results of the study will be generalized. The target population may be restricted to specific population groups, such as males between 30 and 80, or it may have a wider reference, such as all adults or all children. The *experimental* or accessible population is the group from which subjects are actually chosen. This group may be composed of patients with a certain diagnosis at several medical centers, a specific community, or members of a particular professional group. For example, in the Physician's Health Study, researchers examined a group of male physicians aged 40 to 84 years to determine the effect of aspirin taken every other day on the incidence of cardiovascular mortality.[37] Subjects were accessible because of their professional affiliations. The experimental population should be representative of the target population to protect external validity. Therefore, in the Physician's Health Study, the target population should be specified as adult males, and one would question the external validity of the project in terms of adult females.

The validity of the trial depends on three major concerns.[5] First, the size of the experimental population must be large enough to ensure adequate numbers of participants who meet study criteria. Second, the researcher must identify a group for which it is likely that a sufficient number of outcome measures will be achieved. For example, in the study of aspirin, one reason that males were studied was because the incidence of cardiovascular disease is relatively low for middle-aged women. Third, the experimental population should be one that is likely to remain accessible for the duration of the study. For instance, college students are often too mobile to ensure a stable sample if the study will extend over several years.

Once the experimental population is designated, subjects must be invited to participate in the trial. They should be given information about the purpose of the study, the procedures that will be used, the potential risks and benefits, and the fact that they will be randomly assigned to either a treatment or a control group. Depending on the nature of the study, those who agree to participate may be screened to see if they meet inclusion and exclusion criteria for the study. The final study sample will typically be a relatively small subgroup of the experimental population. For example, in a large multicenter study to determine the effect of self-education programs on health care utilization, researchers mailed invitations to 11,090 households constituting the enrollment of a health maintenance organization (HMO).[38] Only 2,833 (25.5%) indicated a willingness to participate. Then, after information about the program was sent out, along with an informed consent form, 1,625 households ultimately participated. The questions to be asked, of course, are whether those who eventually became subjects are different from those who did not, and are these differences related to the outcomes being studied. This situation is often the case.[39] Those willing to participate or to volunteer in clinical trials often exhibit lower morbidity and mortality than nonparticipants, regardless of their group assignment in the trial.[40] These differences will not necessarily affect the internal validity of the study, but will reduce generalizability.

Analysis Issues

Once a study sample is identified, subjects must be allocated to intervention and control groups, preferably using a randomization scheme. This is the single most important element of the design for eliminating bias as a cause of differences observed after treatment. In addition, strategies such as double blinding and stratification, or blocking, should be incorporated into the design to reduce the effects of bias and confounding variables (see Chapter 9).

One source of bias that is of particular concern in clinical trials is noncompliance, whether it be from attrition, subjects' forgetting to follow the protocol, or researchers' losing contact with the subjects. Compliance can be monitored during the course of the study by contacting subjects by phone, using monetary incentives, offering free medical care, or asking subjects to keep a log. The study protocol should be relatively easy to follow and cause minimal inconvenience to subjects. Information should be examined for those lost to the study to determine if different characteristics are evident in those who belonged to the two study groups. Analysis must account for dropouts and should be based on the intention-to-treat principle (see Chapter 9).

An important ethical consideration in medical trials is the need to consider the well-being of the study participants. Data are often monitored periodically by individuals external to the study (to respect blinding), to assess if strong statistical relationships have been established. Where clear evidence of benefits can be demonstrated before the projected study time is complete, the study may be discontinued. For example, in a study that looked at the effects of warfarin on the risk of stroke, an interim analysis demonstrated that there was an 81% reduction in risk, which prompted the investigators to discontinue the placebo group.[41]

Data analysis for clinical trials is usually performed using tests of statistical significance, such as *t*-tests or analyses of variance, confidence intervals, or multivariate logistic regression. These topics are covered in Chapters 19, 20, and 27.

MEASURES OF ASSOCIATION

The primary goal of observational analytic studies is to test hypotheses about the relationship between specific exposures or characteristics and disease. These tests will establish if an association exists and the strength of that association. If an association does exist, we say that the specific exposure represents a **risk factor** for the disease.

Analyses of association are based on a measure of effect that looks at the frequency of disease among those who were and were not exposed to the risk factor. A *relative effect* is a ratio that describes the risks associated with the exposed group as compared with the unexposed. An *absolute effect* is the actual difference between the rate of disease in the exposed and unexposed groups, or the difference in the risk of developing the disease between these two groups. To illustrate the concepts of relative and absolute effect, suppose we purchased two books, one costing $3 and the other $6. The absolute difference is $3, whereas the relative difference is that the second book is twice as expensive as the first. Therefore, the relative effect is based on the absolute effect, but takes into account the baseline value. Analogously, we can use measures of incidence of disease in exposed and unexposed groups to determine both relative and absolute effects of particular exposures.

The simplest type of analyses are based on *crude* data. These are data concerning the exposure status and outcome status of all subjects regardless of any other risks or characteristics of the subjects. Although analyses based on crude data are often reported in the literature, most studies also require more complicated analyses to evaluate the role of other factors in the relationship of exposure and outcome. These analyses are accomplished through stratification or multivariate methods and provide *adjusted* measures of association.

Relative Risk

The most common measure of relative effect is **relative risk (RR),** which indicates the likelihood that someone who has been exposed to a risk factor will develop the disease, as compared with one who has not been exposed. Relative risk is defined as the ratio of incidence of disease among the exposed subjects to the incidence of disease among the unexposed.

To determine risk, data are usually organized in a 2 × 2 table, called a **contingency table,** as shown in the Figure 15.1. The vertical columns in the table represent the classification of disease status, and the horizontal rows represent exposure status. To facilitate consistency in presentation and calculation, the cells in the table are designated *a, b, c,* and *d,* as shown in the figure. Therefore, cell *a* represents those who have the disease and were exposed, cell *b* represents those who do not have the disease and were exposed, and so on. The marginal totals for each row and column represent the total numbers of individuals who were exposed ($a + b$) and were not exposed ($c + d$), and the total

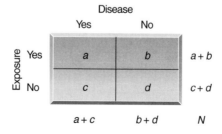

FIGURE 15.1   General format for a 2 × 2 contingency table, showing frequencies for disease and exposure.

numbers who have the disease $(a + c)$ and do not have the disease $(b + d)$. The sum of all four cells is the total sample size (N).

For a cohort study, we can obtain cumulative incidence estimates for the exposed (CI_E) and unexposed (CI_0) groups. The cumulative incidence for the exposed group is the number of cases of the disease among the total exposed sample, or $a/(a+b)$. The cumulative incidence for the unexposed group is the number of cases of the disease among the total unexposed sample, or $c/(c+d)$.[†] Therefore,

$$ RR = \frac{CI_E}{CI_0} = \frac{a/(a + b)}{c/(c + d)} \tag{15.4} $$

If the incidence rates of the outcome are the same for the exposed and nonexposed groups, the relative risk is 1.0, indicating that the exposure presents no excess risk for the outcome. Therefore, a relative risk greater than 1.0 indicates an increased risk, and a relative risk less than 1.0 means that the exposure decreases the risk of developing the disorder.

To illustrate this application, consider the data shown in Table 15.1 for a cohort study of the incidence of functional dependence in relation to the number of predisposing factors for functional dependence among the participants (the exposure).[42] Elders were followed for 1 year. At the start of the study subjects were classified according to their number of risk factors (sensory impairment, affective impairment, and limb impairments). The researchers established that 278 people had none of the risk factors and 83 had three or more risk factors. Over the study period, 69 people within these two classifications became functionally dependent, and 292 did not. The relative risk associated with these data is calculated as follows:

$$ RR = \frac{a/(a + b)}{c/(c + d)} = \frac{50/83}{19/278} = 8.9 $$

This tells us that the incidence of functional dependence among elders with three or more risk factors is almost 9 times that of elders with none of the risk factors; that is, those who have three or more risk factors have almost 9 times the risk of being functionally dependent as compared with those who have no risk factors.

Odds Ratio

In a case-control study we cannot use relative risk because we cannot accurately calculate cumulative incidence. Subjects are purposefully chosen for case-control studies based on the presence or absence of disease, and therefore, we cannot determine the rate of incidence of the disease. The relative risk can, however, be estimated using an **odds ratio (OR),** which is calculated with the formula

$$ OR = \frac{a/c}{b/d} = \frac{ad}{bc} \tag{15.5} $$

[†]This calculation for relative risk is based on the assumption that all subjects in the cohort were followed for the same amount of time. When follow-up time differs, it is the person-time for exposed and nonexposed groups that should be used for marginal totals, rather than just the total number of subjects in each category.

TABLE 15.1. DATA FOR A COHORT STUDY SHOWING THE RELATIONSHIP BETWEEN NUMBER OF RISK FACTORS AND FUNCTIONAL DEPENDENCE IN THE ELDERLY

	Functional Dependence		
	Yes	No	Total
Risk factors			
≥3	50	33	83
None	19	259	278
Total	69	292	361

Source: Tinetti ME, Inouye SK, Gill TM, Doucette JT. Shared risk factors for falls, incontinence, and functional dependence: unifying the approach to geriatric syndromes. *JAMA* 1995; 273:1348–53.

Consider the data shown in Table 15.2. These data are from a case-control study which examined the risk for tuberculosis associated with HIV infection.[43] One hundred fifty-one cases and 545 control subjects were identified. Among the cases, 4 individuals were seropositive for HIV; among the controls, 3 subjects were seropositive. The crude odds ratio for these data is

$$OR = \frac{ad}{bc} = \frac{(4)(542)}{(3)(147)} = 4.92$$

This means that the *odds* of having tuberculosis are almost 5 times greater for those who have HIV infection than for those who do not.

Attributable Risk

It is also useful to examine the public health impact, or the absolute effect of a specific exposure, by looking at the differences in frequency of disease for those who are exposed and unexposed. When we examine outcome data, we find that some individuals who were not exposed to the risk factor still developed the disorder; that is, the disorder would have occurred anyway from other causes. Therefore, if we look at the difference between the incidence of disease in the exposed and nonexposed groups, we obtain an estimate of "excess risk," called **attributable risk (AR),** or risk difference:

$$AR = I_E - I_0 \tag{15.6}$$

TABLE 15.2. CASE-CONTROL DATA SHOWING THE RELATIONSHIP BETWEEN HIV SEROPOSITIVITY AND TUBERCULOSIS

	Tuberculosis		
	Yes	No	Total
HIV seropositivity			
Yes	4	3	7
No	147	542	689
Total	151	545	696

Source: Buskin SE, Gale JL, Weiss NS, Nolan CM. Tuberculosis risk factors in adults in King County, Washington, 1988 through 1990. *Am J Public Health* 1994; 84:1750–6.

where I_E is the incidence of disease for the exposed, and I_0 is the incidence for the unexposed group. For cohort studies, attributable risk is calculated using cumulative incidence or incidence rate.

For example, in the study of number of risk factors and functional dependence in elders (Table 15.1) attributable risk would be

$$AR = CI_E - CI_0 = \frac{a}{a+b} - \frac{c}{c+d}$$

$$= \frac{50}{83} - \frac{19}{278} = 0.3384 = 0.534 = 534/1{,}000$$

This estimate reflects the number of cases of elders with functional dependence that *could be eliminated* if we could control or prevent the risk factors. Among the group with three or more risk factors, we can attribute 534 cases of functional dependence per 1,000 people to having three or more risk factors.

If the incidence of disease is the same for exposed and unexposed groups, we would obtain AR = 0. When attributable risk is above zero, we can estimate how much risk we face over and above the risks provided by other causes of the disease.

We can convert this estimate to a proportion by expressing AR as a percentage, or *attributable proportion* (AR%):

$$AR\% = \frac{AR}{I_E} \times 100 = \frac{I_E - I_0}{I_E} \times 100 \tag{15.7}$$

For the data on falls in elders,

$$AR\% = \frac{0.534}{50/83} \times 100 = 88.7\%$$

Assuming that having three or more risk factors is a cause of functional dependence, we could eliminate 88.7% of the cases of functional dependence in those with three or more risk factors if we could control or prevent the risks.

For case-control data, incidence rates are usually not available, and we cannot compute AR directly. We can calculate AR% using the formula[44]

$$AR\% = \frac{OR - 1}{OR} \times 100 \tag{15.8}$$

where OR is the odds ratio.

For the case-control data in Table 15.2,

$$AR\% = \frac{4.92 - 1}{4.92} \times 100 = 79.7\%$$

Thus, if being HIV seropositive does contribute to developing tuberculosis, almost 80% of tuberculosis among individuals *could be attributed* to having HIV, or could be eliminated if HIV infection were prevented.

TABLE 15.3.   CASE-CONTROL DATA SHOWING THE ASSOCIATION BETWEEN THE USE OF ORAL CONTRACEPTIVES AND THE RISK OF MYOCARDIAL INFARCTION, WITH CONFOUNDING BY AGE

		Myocardial Infarction			Odds
	Exposure	Cases	Controls	Total	Ratio
Total sample	OC user	39	24	63	2.2
	Nonuser	114	154	268	
	Total	153	178	331	
< 40 years old	OC user	21	17	38	2.8
	Nonuser	26	59	85	
	Total	47	76	123	
≥ 40 years old	OC user	18	7	25	2.8
	Nonuser	88	95	183	
	Total	106	102	208	

Source: Mann HI, Inman WHW, Thorogood M. Oral contraceptive use in older women and fatal myocardial infarction. *Br Med J* 1968;2:193–9.

Measures of relative risk and attributable risk provide very different types of information about the association between exposure and disease. The relative risk (or odds ratio) estimates the strength of an association. Attributable risk measures are based on the assumption that there is a causal relationship, and provide information about the impact of the exposure on exposed individuals.

Evaluating the Effect of Confounding

Measures of association must be interpreted in terms of the potential for confounding effects of extraneous variables in the design. **Confounding** is introduced when extraneous variables interfere with the observed association between the exposure and outcome. A *confounder* is a variable that is (1) associated with the exposure, (2) independently of the exposure, is a risk factor for the disease, and (3) is not part of the causal link between the exposure and the disease.

To illustrate this concept, consider the data shown in Table 15.3 for a study of the relationship between use of oral contraceptives (OC) and myocardial infarction (MI).[45] The odds ratio for the total sample was 2.2. Therefore, women who use OC have greater than twice the risk of MI over those who do not use OC; however, the researchers questioned the potential confounding effect of age in the analysis. First, we know that age is generally a risk factor associated with MI. In fact, in this study, among the nonusers of OC, the proportion of cases is greater for older subjects ($88/183 = 0.48$) than for younger subjects ($26/85 = 0.31$). This suggests that age is a risk factor for MI independent of OC use. Second, the data also show that some relationship exists between age and use of OC; that is, among the controls, there is a higher proportion of OC users in the younger age category ($17/76 = 0.22$) as compared with the older category ($7/102 = 0.07$). Third, age cannot be considered a causal link between use of OC and MI. Therefore, age meets the three criteria for a confounding factor.

We can evaluate the possible confounding by age in the analysis of the data by stratifying the sample into younger and older age groups: under 40 and 40 to 44 (the oldest subject was 44). By doing so, we find that the odds ratio for each age group is 2.8. Each stratum shows the same risk associated with OC use regardless of age. The individual estimates for each group are considered "unconfounded" for age; however, these unconfounded estimates are different from the overall or *crude odds ratio* of 2.2. This difference tells us that age does affect the risk estimate; that is, age is a confounding variable. Because OC users tend to be younger, and younger women tend to have fewer MIs, the crude odds ratio was an underestimate of the risk of MI associated with OC use. When age is taken into account, the actual risk is higher. If there was no discrepancy between the crude and unconfounded estimates, there would be no confounding. The degree of discrepancy is indicative of the extent to which age confounded the original data.

To evaluate the effect of confounding in an analysis, the researcher must collect information on the potentially confounding variable. If the investigator in this example had not collected data on the subjects' ages, the preceding analysis would not have been possible. Therefore, the researcher must be able to predict what variables are possible confounders. It is conceivable that several confounding factors will be operating in one study. In addition to controlling for confounding in the analysis, researchers can use design strategies, such as matching or homogeneous subjects, to control for these effects. For instance, if we were to restrict the subjects to women under 40, age could not be a confounding factor.

Effect Modification

Confounding variables can be thought of as nuisance variables. They may or may not be present, depending on the source population and how subjects are chosen. Sometimes, however, a third factor will *interact* with the exposure and disease variables in such a way as to present a constant effect. Such a variable is called an **effect modifier,** which is a natural phenomenon that exists independent of the study design and will always be a factor in interpretation of risk. Effect modifiers tend to be biologically related to the variables being studied. For example, suppose we wanted to look at the association between exposure to asbestos and development of lung cancer. We follow a group of asbestos workers and a group of workers in a different industry for 15 years. Assume we found that asbestos is a risk factor for lung cancer, with a relative risk of 4.5. We might consider collecting data on the subjects' smoking habits as well, because we know that smoking is also a risk for lung cancer. We can stratify our subjects according to smokers and nonsmokers and look at the relative risk associated with asbestos exposure for each group. Suppose we find that the risk associated with asbestos for smokers is 5.0, whereas the risk for nonsmokers is 1.3. This would tell us that smoking is an effect modifier—that the effect of asbestos is exacerbated for a smoker in terms of the risk for lung cancer. The fact that the stratum-specific risk estimates are different for smokers and nonsmokers indicates that smoking interacts with asbestos as an effect modifier. Note that this is not the case with a confounding variable, as illustrated in the previous example of MI and OC use.

Researchers attempt to cancel the effect of a confounding variable in the design or analysis of a study. In contrast, effect modifiers are studied so they can be reported. Data are stratified to evaluate and *remove* confounders. They are stratified to *explain* effect modification.[46] Researchers must consider the potential influence of confounding and effect modification in all analyses and account for them in the design or analysis of data as much as possible.

Pooled Risk Estimates

When data are stratified, and separate risk estimates are calculated for each stratum, it is possible to report each estimate; however, it is usually more useful to calculate a single over-all estimate that reflects the association between exposure and disease with the confound-ing factor taken into account. Several statistical techniques can be used to accomplish this, although the most commonly used procedures belong to a set of estimates proposed by Mantel and Haenszel.[47] The **Mantel-Haenszel pooled risk estimate** provides a weighted summary value that can be used to report the relative risk associated with a specific expo-sure *adjusted* for the confounding variable. When the Mantel-Haenszel estimate differs from the crude risk estimate, it is the Mantel-Haenszel estimate that should be reported. It is most appropriately used when the stratum-specific relative risks are uniform, that is, when there is no effect modification. Formulas used to calculate Mantel-Haenszel estimates of relative risk for case-control and cohort studies are given in Table 15.4. The numerators and denominators in these formulas represent the sum of the expressions for each stratum.

Confidence Intervals

An important assumption in any research study is that we can draw reasonable infer-ences about population characteristics based on sample data. This assumption holds true for epidemiologic studies as well. When a risk estimate is derived from a particular set of subjects, the researcher will use that estimate to make generalizations about ex-pected behaviors or outcomes in others who have similar exposure histories. The statis-tical problem with this process is based on the fact that sample data may differ from pop-ulation data because of chance variations; that is, just by chance, the overall responses of the sample subjects may not be truly representative of the population.

Traditional statistical testing attempts to account for the role of chance by using *prob-ability* (*p* values) to indicate if an observed relationship is "real" (significant) or more likely to be a function of chance variation (not significant) (see Chapter 18). Unfortu-nately, such analyses are often misleading because they are reflective of both the magni-tude of the observed effect and the sample size. Consequently, larger samples will tend

TABLE 15.4.   MANTEL-HAENSZEL POOLED ESTIMATES FOR RELATIVE RISK FOR COHORT AND CASE-CONTROL STUDIES

Cohort Study (with count denominators)

$$RR_{MH} = \frac{\sum \frac{a(c + d)}{N}}{\sum \frac{c(a + b)}{N}}$$

Case-Control Study

$$RR_{MH} = \frac{\sum \frac{ad}{N}}{\sum \frac{bc}{N}}$$

to demonstrate significant outcomes even when the observed differences are very small, and, conversely, large differences may not be significant if the sample is too small.

To overcome this dilemma, Rothman suggests looking at epidemiologic problems as measurement problems, rather than decision-making problems.[46] This means that the purpose of looking at relative risk statistically is not to determine if the observed value is "significant," but rather to *measure a true effect;* that is, sample values are used to estimate population values.

The best estimate for a population value (called a parameter) is the single value obtained from the sample data (called a statistic). Therefore, if we obtain a relative risk of 3.0 in a particular study, we will estimate that this is the associated risk present in the population. This estimate is not considered wholly reliable, however, as there are many variations in the sample that cannot be accounted for. Therefore, to estimate relative risk for the population, it seems more reasonable to propose a range of possible values for the parameter. This range is called a **confidence interval (CI).**

For example, with an observed relative risk of 3.0, we might define a confidence interval from 1.2 to 7.5. This interval represents a range of values within which the true population effect is expected to lie. The specific limits of the interval are determined according to the variability present in the data and the *level of confidence* we want to assign to it.[‡] For instance, we might say that we want to be 95% confident that the interval we calculate really contains the population value. This means that if we could collect data on 100 samples and calculate a confidence interval for each one, in 95 of these samples the confidence intervals would indeed contain the population value. Five of the intervals would not contain the population value. Therefore, for any one interval we actually create, we have a 95% chance that the population parameter is contained within it. Confidence intervals can also be created at 90% or 99% levels; however, the higher the level of confidence, the wider the interval will be.

For instance, a research paper might report a relative risk of 0.73 for the relationship between moderate alcohol consumption and myocardial infarction. Because this estimate is less than 1.0, it suggests that those who drink moderate amounts of alcohol have a reduced risk of having an MI as compared with those who do not drink alcohol. Suppose the report also presented the 95% confidence interval for this estimate, with a lower bound of 0.47 and an upper bound of 1.13. Therefore, although the best estimate of the decreased risk of MI associated with moderate alcohol is 0.73, we are 95% confident that the true relative risk is not less than 0.47 and not greater than 1.13.

Confidence intervals can also be used to provide information about statistical significance. If the null value for an estimate (1.0 for relative risk) is included within the 95% confidence interval, then the corresponding p value is greater than .05, and the estimate is not considered significant. If the null value is not contained within the interval, the p value is less than .05, and the estimate is considered significant. In the preceding example, the 95% confidence interval is 0.47 to 1.13. As this contains the null value of 1.0, we would conclude that the observed association is not statistically significant at the .05 level. Those who are not familiar with concepts of statistical testing and probability should refer to Chapters 17 and 18 to clarify this discussion.

[‡]To calculate confidence intervals for relative risk, the formula is $CI = RR^{(1 \pm z/\sqrt{x^2})}$. For the 95% confidence interval, $z = 1.96$. For calculation of χ^2 see Chapter 25.

EVALUATING CAUSALITY IN OBSERVATIONAL STUDIES

The epidemiologist is ultimately concerned with identifying those factors, or exposures, that cause disease or disability. Because case-control and cohort studies do not involve direct experimentation or manipulation of variables, the validity of statistical association between exposure and disease with these observational designs must be made under conditions that are not strictly controlled. Therefore, the epidemiologist must first rule out influences of bias, confounding, and chance variation, and then must assess the strength of cause-and-effect criteria.

Perhaps most important is the establishment of a *time sequence* that documents the exposure preceding the disease. In addition, the researcher can look at the *strength of the association* using a measure of relative risk. The stronger the association, the more likely a causative relationship exists. The relationship should also have *biologic credibility*. The researcher should be able to postulate some mechanism by which the exposure might reasonably alter the risk of developing the disease. This may not be possible, depending on the state of knowledge, but it will make the conclusion more plausible if a realistic explanation can be offered. It is also helpful to show *consistency* with other studies. The more times a relationship can be documented by different researchers using different samples and conditions, the more likely it is true. Lastly, the presence of a **dose-response relationship** provides evidence for causality. This means that the severity of the disease can be associated with varying levels of the exposure. If the risk of developing the disease does not vary with increases or decreases in exposure, it is unlikely that the exposure is the true risk factor. These five criteria, taken together, can be used to provide evidence for a cause-and-effect relationship.

COMMENTARY

A New View of Outcomes

A traditional biomedical model defines health narrowly as the absence of disease. Based on this definition, epidemiologists collect data to determine frequency of occurrence of disease and risk factors for disease. Under this model, we open ourselves to looking at risk factors that have an effect at the biological level of the individual. Using a more complete model of health, epidemiology is able to focus on the occurrence of health-related states and risk factors related to physical, social, and psychological health status as well. The disablement model, described in Chapter 1, provides an excellent framework for this approach. We can begin to look at the concept of risk in terms of impairments that lead to physical disability, and use measures of risk to help us set priorities and evaluate outcomes.

This chapter has provided a broad view of epidemiology and has used the terms *condition, disorder, disease,* and *outcome* interchangeably. For example, in the study of risk factors and functional dependence, cited earlier, the outcome of functional dependence is in the realm of physical health status. Risk factors included impairments such as lower extremity mobility, upper extremity strength, vision, hearing, and depression. Many of the other examples in this chapter have also illustrated clinical applications of epidemiologic methods. Most clinicians, however, do not learn about epidemiologic approaches in basic research courses, and are not familiar with the use of measures of disease frequency, odds ratio, or relative risk. This is unfortunate, as there are many opportunities to answer important clinical questions using these techniques.

Questions that are appropriate for clinical epidemiologic study may deal with specific interventions, perhaps in a randomized clinical trial format, but may also be concerned with larger decision and policy issues that have direct application to practice. They can often be effectively answered using case-control methodology or analysis of cohort data. Decisions regarding choice of intervention, who gets intervention (including prevention), and the intensity and frequency of intervention may be aided by an understanding of the relative risks associated with specific patient characteristics, activities, or treatments. We may understand the physiological rationale for applying specific exercises for reducing pain or improving mobility, but do we know what factors may alter the success of our treatments, or which patients are more likely to improve? Such information can provide new insight into the rationales we use for making treatment decisions.

The information contained in this chapter is necessarily brief, and does not begin to cover the full scope of epidemiologic principles or analysis procedures. Readers are encouraged to refer to references listed at the end of this chapter and to consult with epidemiologists who can share their expertise and collaborate on relevant clinical studies.

KEY TERMS

epidemiology
exposure
risk factor
observational study
case report
correlational study
cross-sectional survey
prevalence
cumulative incidence (CI)
birth rate
mortality rate
cause-specific rate
case-fatality rate

age-specific rate
observational analytic
  designs
case-control study
case definition
population-based study
hospital-based study
selection bias
misclassification
observation bias
interviewer bias
recall bias
cohort study

randomized clinical trial
  (RCT)
relative risk (RR)
contingency table
odds ratio (OR)
attributable risk (AR)
confounding
effect modifier
Mantel-Haenszel pooled
  risk estimate
confidence interval (CI)
dose-response relationship

REFERENCES

1. World Health Organization. Constitution of the World Health Organization. *Basic Documents.* Geneva: World Health Organization, 1948.
2. Bajdik CD, Gallagher RP, Hill GB, Fincham S. Sunlight exposure, hat use, and squamous cell skin cancer on the head and neck. *J Cutan Med Surg* 1998;3:68–73.
3. Khuder SA, Dayal HH, Mutgi AB, Willey JC, Dayal G. Effect of cigarette smoking on major histological types of lung cancer in men. *Lung Cancer* 1998;22:15–21.

4. Klatsky AL, Armstrong MA, Friedman GD. Red wine, white wine, liquor, beer, and risk for coronary artery disease hospitalization. *Am J Cardiol* 1997;80:416–20.

5. Hennekens CH, Buring JE. *Epidemiology in Medicine.* Boston: Little, Brown, 1987.

6. Tobacman JK, Wenzel RP. Clinical epidemiology: further consideration. *J Clin Epidemiol* 1990;43:633–5.

7. Jordan WM. Pulmonary embolism. *Lancet* 1961;2:1146.

8. Davis JP, Chesney PJ, Wand PJ, LaVenture M. Toxic-shock syndrome: epidemiologic features, recurrence, risk factors, and prevention. *N Engl J Med* 1980;303:1429–35.

9. Centers for Disease Control. Pneumocystis pneumonia—Los Angeles. *MMWR* 1981;30:250.

10. Latham RH, Kehrberg MW, Jacobson JA, Smith CB. Toxic shock syndrome in Utah: a case-control and surveillance study. *Ann Intern Med* 1982;96:906–8.

11. Ammann AJ, Cowan MJ, Wara DW, et al. Acquired immunodeficiency in an infant: possible transmission by means of blood products. *Lancet* 1983;1:956–8.

12. US Department of Health and Human Services. *Health United States 1984.* DHHS Publication No. (PHS) 85-1232. Hyattsville, MD: National Center for Health Statistics, 1984.

13. Centers for Disease Control. Annual summary 1982. Reported morbidity & mortality in the United States. *MMWR* 1983;31:1–149.

14. Friedman GD. Cigarette smoking and geographic variation in coronary heart disease mortality in the United States. *J Chronic Dis* 1967;20:769–79.

15. Weissert WG. Estimating the long-term care population: prevalence rates and selected characteristics. *Health Care Financ Rev* 1985;6:83–91.

16. Bernard B, Sauter S, Fine L, Petersen M, Hales T. Job task and psychosocial risk factors for work-related musculoskeletal disorders among newspaper employees. *Scand J Work Environ Health* 1994;20:417–26.

17. Burdorf A, Van Der Steenhoven GA, Tromp-Klaren EG. A one-year prospective study on back pain among novice golfers. *Am J Sports Med* 1996;24:659–64.

18. Laden F, Spiegelman D, Neas LM, et al. Geographic variation in breast cancer incidence rates in a cohort of U.S. women. *J Natl Cancer Inst* 1997;89:1373–8.

19. Zaza C, Farewell VT. Musicians' playing-related musculoskeletal disorders: an examination of risk factors. *Am J Ind Med* 1997;32:292–300.

20. West DW, Schuman KL, Lyon JL, Robison LM, Allred R. Differences in risk estimations from a hospital and a population-based case-control study. *Int J Epidemiol* 1984;13:235–9.

21. McIntosh ID. Alcohol-related disabilities in general hospital patients: a critical assessment of the evidence. *Int J Addict* 1982;17:609–39.

22. Ray WA, Griffin MR, Schaffner W, Baugh DK, Melton LJD. Psychotropic drug use and the risk of hip fracture. *N Engl J Med* 1987;316:363–9.

23. Sorock GS. A case control study of falling incidents among the hospitalized elderly. *J Safety Res* 1983;14:47–52.

24. Dawber TR. *The Framingham Study: The Epidemiology of Atherosclerotic Disease.* Cambridge, MA: Harvard University Press, 1980.

25. Jette AM, Branch LG. The Framingham Disability Study: II. Physical disability among the aging. *Am J Public Health* 1981;71:1211–6.

26. Kelly-Hayes M, Jette AM, Wolf PA, D'Agostino RB, Odell PM. Functional limitations and disability among elders in the Framingham study. *Am J Public Health* 1992;82:841–5.

27. Guccione AA, Felson DT, Anderson JJ, et al. The effects of specific medical conditions on the functional limitations of elders in the Framingham study. *Am J Public Health* 1994;84:351–8.

28. Jette AM, Pinsky JL, Branch LG, Wolf PA, Feinleib M. The Framingham Disability Study: physical disability among community-dwelling survivors of stroke. *J Clin Epidemiol* 1988;41:719–26.

29. Benjamin EJ, D'Agostino RB, Belanger AJ, Wolf PA, Levy D. Left atrial size and the risk of stroke and death. The Framingham Heart Study. *Circulation* 1995;92:835–41.

30. Kannel WB, Shurtleff D. The Framingham study. Cigarettes and the development of intermittent claudication. *Geriatrics* 1973;28:61–8.
31. Jones BH, Cowan DN, Tomlinson JP, Robinson JR, Polly DW, Frykman PN. Epidemiology of injuries associated with physical training among young men in the army. *Med Sci Sports Exerc* 1993;25:197–203.
32. Kelsen DP, Ginsberg R, Pajak TF, et al. Chemotherapy followed by surgery compared with surgery alone for localized esophageal cancer. *N Engl J Med* 1998;339:1979–84.
33. Sacks H, Chalmers TC, Smith Jr H. Randomized versus historical controls for clinical trials. *Am J Med* 1982;72:233–40.
34. Fisher B, Redmond C, Fisher ER, et al. Ten-year results of a randomized clinical trial comparing radical mastectomy and total mastectomy with or without radiation. *N Engl J Med* 1985;312:674–81.
35. Fisher B, Bauer M, Margolese R, et al. Five-year results of a randomized clinical trial comparing total mastectomy and segmental mastectomy with or without radiation in the treatment of breast cancer. *N Engl J Med* 1985;312:665–73.
36. Francis T, Korns FT, Voight RB, et al. An evaluation of the 1954 poliomyelitis vaccine trials: summary report. *Am J Public Health* 1955;45:1.
37. Hennekens CH, Eberlein K. A randomized trial of aspirin and beta-carotene among U.S. physicians. *Prev Med* 1985;14:165–8.
38. Vickery DM, Kalmer H, Lowry D, Constantine M, Wright E, Loren W. Effect of a self-care education program on medical visits. *JAMA* 1983;250:2952–6.
39. Friedman LM, Furberg CD, DeMets DL. *Fundamentals of Clinical Trials.* 2d ed. Littleton, MA: PSG, 1985.
40. Wilhelmsen L, Ljungberg S, Wedel H, Werko L. A comparison between participants and nonparticipants in a primary preventive trial. *J Chronic Dis* 1976;29:331–9.
41. Stroke Prevention in Atrial Fibrillation Study Group. Preliminary report of the Stroke Prevention in Atrial Fibrillation Study. *N Engl J Med* 1990;322:863–8.
42. Tinetti ME, Inouye SK, Gill TM, Doucette JT. Shared risk factors for falls, incontinence, and functional dependence. Unifying the approach to geriatric syndromes. *JAMA* 1995;273:1348–53.
43. Buskin SE, Gale JL, Weiss NS, Nolan CM. Tuberculosis risk factors in adults in King County, Washington, 1988 through 1990. *Am J Public Health* 1994;84:1750–6.
44. Cole P, MacMahon B. Attributable risk percent in case-control studies. *Br J Prev Soc Med* 1971;25:242–4.
45. Mann JI, Inman WH, Thorogood M. Oral contraceptive use in older women and fatal myocardial infarction. *Br Med J* 1976;2:445–7.
46. Rothman KJ. *Modern Epidemiology.* Boston: Little, Brown, 1986.
47. Mantel N, Haenszel W. Statistical aspects of the analysis of data from retrospective studies of disease. *JNCI* 1959;22:719–748.

16

Other Research Approaches

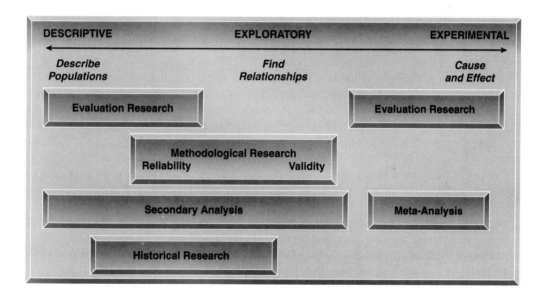

Because of the wide variety of research approaches available to the clinical scientist, it is often difficult to create appropriate classifications for all of them. Some research approaches incorporate elements of other designs, and some involve both experimental and nonexperimental elements. In this chapter, we present five additional research approaches: evaluation research, methodological research, secondary analysis, meta-analysis, and historical research. Each provides important and useful alternatives to approaches discussed in previous chapters.

EVALUATION RESEARCH

Health professionals are faced with many issues of practical concern related to the quality, effectiveness, efficiency, and impact of clinical and educational programs and policies. Rossi and Freeman define **evaluation research** as "the systematic application of social research procedures for assessing the conceptualization, design, implementation, and utility of social intervention programs."[1] Results of program evaluations provide practitioners, administrators, educators, legislators, and the public with important information about how well programs are meeting their goals and the needs of the community they serve. This information can then be used to support decisions about funding, resource allocation, and whether programs should be continued or modified. For example, program evaluation has been used to determine if an HIV/AIDS continuing education program increased the availability of HIV/AIDS services in rural communities,[2] to assess the success of a multidisciplinary day care program for patients with rheumatoid arthritis on overall disease activity and patients' perception of disease,[3] and to evaluate the effectiveness of an educational program designed to prevent work-related back injury in postal workers.[4]

Formative and Summative Evaluations

Evaluation research can be classified according to its focus on either process or outcomes. **Formative evaluation** studies are done as part of program planning or during early implementation.[1] These studies provide information to assist in the process of program development to meet specified needs or to monitor a program's achievements as service is delivered. Formative evaluation is generally a continuous process, designed to provide ongoing information for regular decision making and for "fine-tuning" the program.[1]

Summative evaluation addresses the outcomes or consequences of a program or policy after it has been implemented. It does not seek to change current practice, but provides information as a basis for deciding if a program should be continued, modified, or abandoned or for choosing among alternative strategies. The success of a program can be evaluated according to how effective it has been in achieving its goals. This requires operational definitions of success, which may be perceived differently by participants, administrators, and program personnel. For instance, participants may find an exercise program successful because they enjoy it and they feel better. Administrators may base success on numbers of patients treated and income generated. Clinicians may base success on how functional patients have become following participation. For summative evaluation to be useful, these definitions must be incorporated in the evaluation plan.

Summative evaluation is more limited in scope than formative evaluation in that it provides only an analysis of the consequences of program implementation. With summative data, the researcher can determine if a program is effective, but not why, thereby limiting the decision maker's ability to determine what changes would be necessary. Summative evaluation is most useful in a stable and efficient environment, where outcomes are of major importance. It is reasonable to consider both evaluative approaches, depending on administrative needs, the question of interest, and the program environment.

To illustrate the elements of formative and summative evaluations, consider a program to provide group treatment to patients who have had a stroke, as part of a department's effort to accommodate larger numbers of patients with fewer personnel.[5] A clinician might use formative evaluation to examine direct program implementation: Is the program being carried out as planned? Are patients being recruited in sufficient numbers? Are all patients who need the service being reached? Is there adequate access to resources? Are clinicians performing their tasks satisfactorily? What are program costs? On the basis of these evaluative data, an administrator might make changes while the program is ongoing, in scheduling personnel, seeking referrals, or providing financial or facility resources. It is also not unusual for this process to take different directions over time to meet changing interests.[6] A department administrator might become interested in evaluating the clinicians' satisfaction with the program or how the program is affecting participants' behavior in other departments. These are all formative elements of evaluation. In contrast, summative evaluation would be concerned with program outcomes, such as length of stay, discharge placement, functional level of patients at discharge, and effect on overall quality of care. The ultimate success of the program will often be determined based on these measurable factors. Clearly, both formative and summative data are of use to decision making.

Stages in Evaluation Research

Clarifying the Problem

Evaluation research begins by delineating specific questions or hypotheses concerning the program's effectiveness. Once these issues are determined, the researcher must gather relevant information to put the question in perspective. This may involve such tasks as studying records, analyzing organization and communication structures, examining space and resources, and looking at job descriptions, personnel ratios, and budgets. Evaluators will often interview individuals who can provide background information, and to whom the results of the evaluation will be important, such as program directors, professional personnel, sponsors, and clients. Specific goals and objectives should be stated, to put the program in an environmental context and to determine why the evaluation is wanted and what type of evaluation would be appropriate.

This first stage forces the evaluator to consider which variables will be indicative of success and which will affect outcomes. Variables should be sensitive to the types of changes that will be facilitated by the program. For some program components these measures will be straightforward. For example, a policy that is designed to reduce the costs of patient care can be easily evaluated according to budgetary criteria. It is more common, however, that program goals and processes are more complex and require consideration of a variety of related variables. Consider a program to treat workers with work-related back injuries.[7] The expressed goal of the program is to efficiently return the employee to the work setting. To evaluate the success of such a program, a researcher could simply look at the number of patients who returned to work; however, many other variables, such as gender, age, educational level, whether the patient was receiving workers' compensation, and the physical demands of employment, have potential impact on the outcomes. The researcher is forced to consider the interdependence of these factors and how they would influence the patient's reports of pain. As the researcher develops a conceptual framework for how these variables are related, a model is formulated that will provide a structure for interpreting the program's success.

Designs for Evaluation

The next step in evaluation research is to design the methodology. As in any other type of project, the researcher should first go to the literature to determine if evaluations have been done on this type of project before, what variables have been studied, and what designs or measurement tools were used. On the basis of this information and an understanding of the present environment, the researcher must structure a process of sampling, operationalizing measures, collecting data, and analyzing and interpreting outcomes.[8]

Designs for evaluation studies may be experimental, quasi-experimental, or descriptive, depending on the nature of the program and the desired outcomes, as well as the time frame and available resources. It is most desirable to attain maximal internal validity, so that observed outcomes can be reasonably attributed to the program. External validity will be more or less of an issue, depending on the context within which the evaluation is performed. Some evaluations are intended to demonstrate a program's effectiveness within a given setting only. Others attempt to provide some form of generalization to other settings, requiring more attention to external validity issues.

Whenever possible, evaluators should try to use the experimental model within the confines of the program situation. Some programs will permit randomization into experimental and control groups. When this is not possible, a comparison group can be chosen, necessitating the use of quasi-experimental models. Windsor et al. suggest that the following experimental or quasi-experimental designs are most useful for program evaluators: one-group pretest–posttest design, nonequivalent control group designs, time-series designs, and randomized pretest–posttest control group design.[9] The strengths and weaknesses of each design in internal and external validity should be examined in terms of the specific interpretation outcomes desired. Some evaluation studies will be more amenable to analysis using descriptive techniques, such as surveys, interviews, and behavioral observation, to describe attitudes, perceived outcomes, or changes that have occurred following program implementation.

There may also be situations when group comparisons will not be warranted, when an absolute standard of performance is set as a goal, and quality of performance can be measured against that standard.[10] For example, a department administrator may introduce a new scheduling system to increase the number of patients seen per day by 10%. If an increase of at least 10% is found, a comparison group would provide no additional useful information. In this situation, however, the researcher should take pre- and post-measures to determine the change observed after the program was implemented. The danger of this approach, of course, is the potential for other factors to have influenced the change.

Data Collection and Analysis

Evaluation data typically include a variety of behavioral and descriptive variables, such as demographic data; information about attitudes, motivations, knowledge, values, and personality characteristics; performance outcomes; utilization of services; and physiological measures of health. Evaluators use four major sources to obtain these data: program records, program staff, program participants, and relatives and friends of program participants.

Ultimately, the usefulness of an evaluative study depends on which variables have been measured. Choosing the appropriate variables to measure depends on how the program and its goals are conceptualized. For instance, if we were interested in demonstrating the effectiveness of an exercise education program for reducing sports-related injuries, it would be necessary to examine the interaction of the educational environment and the clients' social environment, and to evaluate outcomes relative to participation in sports activities, training and coaching, use of protective gear, and general physical fitness. It may also be important to monitor the knowledge, attitudes, and level of skill of participants, to determine how these influence their behaviors on and off the playing field.

It is also important to consider which variables have not been measured. For instance, to evaluate a group program for patients who have had a stroke, therapists might assess patients' capabilities for activities of daily living. If the patients varied in the side of their stroke, their responses might be different depending on how instructions were given and what types of perceptual motor activities were included. Therefore, the evaluator should probably record cognitive and speech functions as well as physical function to effectively estimate the program's success. If the impact of these confounding variables is ignored, the outcomes may be interpreted differently.

The researcher analyzes and interprets changes in these variables to determine if goals are indeed being met. Some studies will be enhanced by statistical handling of data, using a variety of procedures such as t-tests and analysis of variance; however, many forms of evaluation data will be best interpreted using descriptive data. In many cases, evaluation research does not adequately fit the experimental model, making it difficult to generate causal inferences. Therefore, evaluation data are often reported in terms of relationships rather than cause and effect, using correlation and regression statistics.

Evaluation of Program Objectives

In the traditional model of evaluation research, success of a program is based on how well its objectives are met. Unfortunately, programs often have multiple objectives, which may be stated in vague language, if they are stated at all. For instance, objectives may be phrased in broad terms, such as "improving competence in practice" or "improving attitudes toward patients." Such goals are conceptually clear, but they provide no direction for determining how success would be measured or documented.

Program objectives should be clarified in *quantitative* or *behavioral* terms whenever possible; that is, outcomes must be defined according to specific measurable change or the expected behaviors of those who are serviced by the program. For instance, a program might be developed to improve early targeting of geriatric patients who are at risk for developing cardiopulmonary complications following surgery. A goal of such a program could be to "reduce the number of patients who require therapy with an assistive breathing device" or "to demonstrate that the length of hospital stay is decreased." These statements delineate the specific criteria that can be used to determine if the program fulfilled its goals. The job of the evaluator is made so much easier when goals can be spelled out this way. There may, however, be a series of such objectives, creating a complex analysis.

Goal-Free Evaluation

There is some disagreement on the importance of specific objectives for evaluation research. Criticism is based on the tendency for evaluations to be narrow and unable to look at the full range of outcomes that might be observed. For example, one department designed a program specifically to increase the number of appropriate referrals to their service. The program involved the participation of personnel in several departments in the hospital in the effort to recruit patients who would benefit from treatment. The intended outcome of this program could be easily measured, of course, by counting the number of referrals; however, in addition to differences in referral patterns, therapists observed that the process had also enhanced communication among health care providers in the hospital. This outcome would not have been monitored in a strict goal-oriented evaluation. Therefore, some researchers prefer to use a **goal-free evaluation** approach, which does not focus the evaluation on predetermined goals, but instead examines the overall effect of the program.[11] This method allows the researcher to explore a program's general effects on the target population, without restricting interpretation to original objectives only. This method can be quite complex and requires extensive data collection. Its success will ultimately rest with the intuitive creativity of the evaluator. It is advantageous, however, in that initial goals are often modified or eliminated as a program progresses, and useful insights into a program's true significance can often be obtained.

Limitations of Evaluation Research

The nature of evaluation research presents several limitations to the interpretation of data. First, the researcher should realize that evaluation research has to be viewed within the political, administrative, financial, and social frameworks to which it contributes. Much of the decision making that formulates policy is directed by political value systems and vested interests,[8] and the results of evaluation research represent only a part of the rationale for the policy-making process. For this reason, researchers often find that personnel have too great a personal investment in a program to provide open or unbiased information that might jeopardize its existence. Evaluation research can also be significantly affected by biases in the researcher's choice of which variables are relevant to the program's goals.

It is not uncommon for a program or policy to address more than one goal. When this occurs the evaluation of a program's success can be very complex. Which goals should be evaluated? If some are met, but not others, is the program still considered successful? How are goals prioritized, if at all? Is a program successful if goals are only partially met? When many goals are addressed by different components of a single program, how does one evaluate the causes of change?

We also find that many program or policy goals are future directed, and their outcomes are not expected to be achieved within a short interval. Researchers and policy makers will often view outcomes relative to immediate, intermediate, and ultimate goals. Usually immediate goals are the only measurable ones within the time frame of a single project, unless a long-range study is undertaken; but this can be frustrating for a decision maker who needs information to make ongoing plans.

One frustration often experienced by evaluators is that even though research findings are objective, valid, and significant, they may go unused or unheeded by those to whom the data were presented. This possibility is mentioned here not to discourage working in evaluation research, but to make clear the considerations that should be addressed at the start to facilitate successful utilization of findings. First, the evaluator can involve decision makers in the process early, using them as guides to setting up the evaluation project. Evaluations are more likely to have an impact if given credibility by those who will use them. By focusing on issues of importance to administrators, evaluators will be better able to meet their information needs. In other words, an evaluation project must have face validity for those to whom results will be reported. Without this broad view, evaluations will not contribute significantly to change. In the long run, we can think of evaluation research as providing information that affects how decision makers think about programs and policies, helping to reduce uncertainty, and influencing them to move in progressive and supportive directions.[12]

METHODOLOGICAL RESEARCH

Methodological research involves the development and testing of measuring instruments for use in research or clinical practice. This approach is used extensively in health care research, as clinicians work toward establishing the reliability and validity of clinical measurement tools. In a research context, this approach does not involve the evaluation of treatment effectiveness, but rather, makes contributions to establishing the methods used to carry out that research. Methodological studies serve many purposes, all relating to the reliability and validity of a measurement tool. For many years, clinicians have realized the importance of documenting reliability, allowing us to have greater confidence in the accuracy of our measurements. More recently, the outcomes movement has provided the impetus for comprehensive methodological study of health status and functional assessment tools. These studies emphasize the use of outcome instruments as a way of indicating the success and quality of care. The implications of the results of these studies are far reaching, as we decide which tools will serve us best to demonstrate the effectiveness of our services. It is essential, therefore, that we understand the designs and analyses of methodological study, so we can make the most appropriate choices and be able to defend them.

Perhaps the most comprehensive approach to methodological study is in the development of a new tool. Although many clinicians have been motivated to find effective ways of measuring things within their practice environment, creating a new tool is truly an extensive process. It starts with a clear description of a problem for which a good measurement is not available. If the measurement is a physical property, it may be necessary to build a prototype to test the feasibility of building an instrument that will serve the desired purpose. This can be both time consuming and expensive. If the variable is a construct, such as pain or function, the researcher must be able to delineate the theoretical foundation for the phenomenon to be measured. For example, Williams and Myers approached the study of acute low back pain with the premise that it is important to understand factors that influence return to work in patients with low back injury.[13] They found that existing outcome measures failed to account for the patient's "normal" or "usual" state prior to low back injury, and they proposed that these were necessary considerations for assessing the extent of recovery. Therefore, they designed a new instrument called the Resumption of Activities of Daily Living (RADL) Scale, and studied its test–retest reliability, internal consistency, convergent and discriminant validity, and responsiveness to change.

Establishing reliability and validity of instruments is a painstaking process that requires multiple approaches and trials. If we look for studies that have examined these characteristics in tools such as the Functional Independence Measure (FIM), we find dozens of studies addressing the whole spectrum of measurement issues, from reliability,[14] to its application to various patient populations,[15, 16] to use of test scores for predicting function and discharge status.[17]

Methodological research can be used to compare the utility of different measuring tools for the same purpose. For example, Hsieh et al. compared three different instruments for measuring straight leg raising: a goniometer, a tape measure, and an inclinometer.[18] They determined that values obtained for the same joint measurement were different for the three instruments, with the tape measure consistently yielding the lowest values. In another context, Liang and coworkers were interested in finding the optimal technique for evaluating outcomes in patients who have undergone total joint arthroplasty.[19] They studied five health status instruments: the Arthritis Impact Measurement Scales (AIMS), Functional Status Index (FSI), Health Assessment Questionnaire (HAQ), Index of Well Being (IWB), and the Sickness Impact Profile (SIP). They compared the ability of these instruments to measure change in function and pain in a sample of 38 patients with arthritis. Their findings showed that these scales were not equivalent in all aspects of measurement. For instance, the HAQ was not sensitive to changes in mobility; the AIMS and IWB were least sensitive to changes in social function; the FSI and HAQ were less sensitive to changes in overall health status. All had similar sensitivity to measuring pain, however. This type of study addresses the issue of validity with the use of varied instruments, and provides important information for choosing an appropriate outcome measure, depending on the focus of intervention.

As new devices are developed for clinical measurement, clinicians are confronted with the need to validate them. For example, Fike and Rousseau compared the Jamar Dynamometer, which is widely used to test hand strength, with a less well-known instrument called the Vigorimeter.[20] The newer instrument had certain design advantages for reducing joint and skin pressure during testing, and so the researchers wanted to compare its performance with that of an established instrument for which norms had been developed. Using correlation procedures, they determined that both instruments were comparable in their measurements of hand strength. This information on concurrent validity now provides a basis for other researchers to use either instrument in their testing of treatment effectiveness.

Methodological studies are also used to find ways to improve the use of existing instruments. For example, investigators have looked at the effect of reducing the length of questionnaires on the validity of the instrument, with generally good results.[21] Researchers also consider the application of measurements under different conditions. For instance, Lynch and coworkers looked at reliability of the functional reach test, originally designed to test balance in the standing position, for assessing sitting balance in subjects with spinal cord injury.[22]

Sometimes it is important to evaluate instruments to determine their scope of applicability. Many health status and functional assessments have been designed as generic tools, as opposed to those that are geared toward a particular patient population or clinical condition. Therefore, some researchers have examined functional rating scales specifically for patients with amyotrophic lateral sclerosis (ALS),[23] asthma,[24] total knee replacement,[25] or shoulder disability,[26, 27] while others have tested the effectiveness of instruments across diverse patient groups.[28] Another significant consideration is the validity of an instrument as a measure of individual versus group characteristics. Many health status tools, for instance, have been validated as measures of group performance, but may not be useful for following individuals over time.[29] Or they may be validated as a measure of disability, but need to be examined for responsiveness to change over time.[30–32] These properties of instruments must be evaluated if we are to use these tools effectively.

Methodological studies make major contributions to research efforts, as it is virtually impossible to conduct meaningful research or clinical examinations without adequate measurement tools. These types of studies are of special importance to scientific disciplines that are engaged in human behavior research, for which objective and direct measuring tools are often unavailable. Reliability and validity studies are reported with increasing frequency in medical and rehabilitation journals, as clinicians continue to realize their importance for establishing measurement standards. We must stress, however, that methodological research is not intended as an end in itself; that is, the purpose of a methodological study is to develop instruments that can be used in practice or for further testing, not to establish reliability or validity for its own sake. The measurement properties of a test must be relevant to specific patient conditions and treatment choices. Published methodological studies on healthy subjects represent the beginning of this process. We must move forward, however, to examine reliability and validity within a context that will serve as a guide for clinical decisions. We must test measurement methods on appropriate patients under clinical conditions, so that our findings will be meaningful to practice. The concepts of reliability and validity are discussed in detail in Chapters 5 and 6.

SECONDARY ANALYSIS

Much of the research in health and social science involves the collection of large amounts of data, often more than the researcher actually analyzes. In **secondary analysis** a researcher uses an existing database to reexamine variables and answer questions other than those for which the data were collected. Investigators may analyze subsets of variables or subjects different from those analyzed in the initial study, or they may be interested in exploring new relationships among the variables. Sometimes the unit of analysis can be changed, so that one study might look at overall hospital characteristics, whereas another might look at individual responses of health care personnel. Researchers can also explore outcomes using different statistical techniques, either because initial findings were based on inappropriate statistical procedures or to test different hypotheses. When two or more comparable data sets can be combined for secondary analysis, researchers can expand the generalizability of outcomes. In this way secondary analysis can be especially useful for supporting theoretical hypotheses.

The major advantages of secondary analysis are the minimal expense involved, the ability to study large samples, and the elimination of the most time-consuming part of the research process—data collection. Researchers can formulate hypotheses and proceed to test them immediately. For new researchers, secondary analysis may provide a useful way to start the research process, especially when funds are limited. For experienced researchers, existing data sets may provide unexpected but important findings at little or no cost.[33]

The disadvantage of this approach relates to the researcher's lack of control over the data collection process. There is no way to ensure the quality of the data that are included in the data set. Questions may not have been asked in the appropriate format, or variables important to the analysis may not have been tested. Data may be missing or incorrectly entered. It is important to verify as much as possible how data were collected, what instruments were used, and how the sample was selected; however, even with this information, testing large samples creates great potential for error and makes specification of reliability difficult. The researcher interested in secondary analysis must consider the possible sources of error and judge their effect according to the documentation available on the data and the necessary rigor of the research hypothesis.

Finding a Question to Fit the Data—or Finding Data to Fit the Question

Secondary data analysis can proceed in two directions. Perhaps the more direct approach is to look carefully at existing data, to determine what types of questions would fit them. This requires a strong familiarity with the data and the variables that were measured. The researcher can then start to consider the possible relationships that might be of interest. Many studies involve the collection of large amounts of information that never get analyzed. Often the effect of demographic factors, such as age, gender, race, income level, and so on, can generate questions about their influence on physiological or performance variables. As a question begins to evolve, the researcher must proceed to the literature, so that a theoretical framework can be developed and hypotheses can be proposed.

The alternative process involves searching for a database that will provide the needed information to answer a given research question. The researcher must first develop a list of variables that are germane to the question, so that the viability of a particular database can be determined. For this process to work, the researcher must have some familiarity with databases that are available. It may be necessary to contact other individuals who have access to data, such as people in industry or hospital administration, who would know what kinds of information were accessible. Computerized databases from medical records may provide a rich source of information for clinical research.[34] The researcher may also explore collaborative relationships with other investigators.

Sources of Data

Secondary analysis has become increasingly common in recent years because of the availability of large data sets through data libraries and the widespread use of computers. Smaller-scale studies do not necessarily provide the same wealth of data, and data will not be available through data libraries, but researchers are often quite willing to share data or collaborate on secondary analyses. Information about these data sets may be obtained through journal articles or conference presentations. A variety of large databases are supported by data libraries such as the International Data Library and Reference Service at the University of California at Berkeley, the Council of Social Science Data Archives in New York City, the Roper Public Opinion Research Center at Williams College, and the Archive of the Inter-University Consortium for Political and Social Research at the University of Michigan. The U.S. government sponsors continued collection of health-related data through the National Center for Health Statistics (NCHS) and the U.S. Bureau of the Census, among others. Access to these databases can usually be obtained at minimal or no cost, often with direct online computer connections.

Databases such as the National Health Interview Survey, the National Hospital Discharge Survey, and the National Nursing Home Survey, all through NCHS, are continually used by researchers in public health, allied health, medicine, and social science to document health care utilization, health status of various age groups, and related personal and lifestyle characteristics. Data collected since 1950 as part of the Framingham Heart Study were originally intended to study risk factors for coronary heart disease, and have been used to study longitudinal changes in other factors, such as physical function,[35, 36] stroke,[37] and cognition.[38] Started in 1973, the Multiple Risk Factor Intervention Trial (MRFIT) was a randomized primary prevention trial to test the effect of a multifactor intervention program on mortality from coronary heart disease (CHD) in 12,866 high-risk men.[39] This data set has been used extensively, however, to answer other questions such as risk factors affecting the wives of participants,[40, 41] mortality from pulmonary disease,[42] risk associated with ethnicity,[43, 44] risk factors for stroke,[45] and alcohol use.[46] As these examples illustrate, with the availability of data through computer access, secondary analysis is an important research option, providing a rich source of information for clinicians to investigate important clinical questions.

META-ANALYSIS

As we explore literature on a particular topic, it is not unusual to find that many studies have approached the same research question but obtained different outcomes. The challenge for the clinician is to decide which studies are best, and which ones provide information that will be useful to practice. How do we take these varied results, from studies with different designs, and make sense of them?

We can think of these various studies as many trials, each one examining the same variables on different samples. Each trial gives us an estimate of the effect of the intervention. It would be helpful, then, if we could assume that all these studies provide estimates of the same thing, and that the samples are all part of one larger target population. If these assumptions are true, then we should be able to combine the studies to develop a single estimate of the intervention effect. This process should provide a convincing result that can then be used for clinical decision making, perhaps one that is more representative than any one small study could produce. We do this using a procedure called **meta-analysis,** a special case of secondary analysis, which is a statistical method of combining the results of a series of independent, previously published studies carried out for the same general purpose.

The idea of combining information from many studies is not new. Review articles are written frequently to provide a summary of findings from the literature. Meta-analysis does more than just summarize, however, by using statistical means to combine results. The major advantages of meta-analysis are to (1) increase power by increasing sample size, (2) improve estimates of effect size, (3) resolve uncertainty when conflicting results occur, and (4) improve the generalizability of findings.[47] Often, individual studies will result in nonsignificant findings, which may be a function of Type II error because of small sample size. Combining samples from several studies has the effect of increasing the power to detect important differences. Conflicts may be resolved because of this increased power. Improved generalizability occurs because each study will have been done under somewhat different conditions and with different sample sources.

Selecting Studies

The first step in a meta-analysis is to set a clear definition of the problem to be studied. Only then can we decide which studies should be included. Criteria must be established for using a study, including the specific purpose of each study, the description of subjects, the type of dependent variable, the study design, and the method of analysis. The researcher must look at each potential study critically to examine its design flaws, to determine if it should be included. How one chooses the studies for a meta-analysis will obviously have a considerable effect on the outcome. Researchers should state reasons for including or excluding specific studies in their research reports.

The potential problems in conducting and interpreting meta-analyses rest both with the realities of research publication and with the researcher. During the retrieval process, the researcher may fail to identify all of the relevant studies or the definition of inclusion criteria may not be definitive enough, making the combination of results impossible. A typical method of gathering research reports is through a MEDLINE search, but this should not be the only method. Unfortunately, data may exist that never come to publication because the results of the study were not statistically significant. In fact, research has shown that studies that do not produce significant differences are less likely to have been published than those that do show differences,[48, 49] or they take longer to reach publication.[50] This *publication bias* creates a situation where researchers must seek out unpublished works, perhaps from conference proceedings or other research contacts. These unpublished works can be included in the meta-analysis if they meet the established criteria.

Sample Size and Effect Size

A meta-analysis is not simply a compilation of group means to calculate an average. Although there are many different methods for analyzing this type of data, they are all based on utilization of estimates from individual studies to obtain a combined value that reflects the size of the effect of the independent variable, or the **effect size.** The concept of effect size is central to meta-analysis. It is an index of the degree of difference between groups.[51] The larger the difference, the greater the "effect" of the intervention. An effect size index is based on variance in the data as well as means for quantitative variables, proportions for categorical data, or correlations for measures of association. It is also directly influenced by sample size. For the comparison of two groups, the effect size index (given the symbol *d*) would be the difference between group means divided by the average standard deviation of the two groups (see Appendix C). Cohen has provided levels of interpretation for this index.[51] A large effect is defined as 0.8 or higher. This means that the groups are separated by 0.8 of a standard deviation. A medium effect size is 0.5, and a small effect size is 0.2.

The process of meta-analysis requires that the individual effect sizes for each study are combined to form a common estimate. In essence, we assume that each study that is included provides several observations of the same population value. The combined effect size and a confidence interval are then calculated. The statistical methods of combining effect sizes are beyond the scope of this book, but these methods are included in many advanced biostatistics texts.

Example

A meta-analysis was conducted by Ottenbacher and Jannell to examine the effectiveness of stroke rehabilitation on functional outcome.[52] They identified 124 reports through their literature search. They then established the inclusion criteria for which studies to include: (1) It had to be an investigation of stroke rehabilitation. (2) The primary diagnosis of the subjects had to be stroke with resultant hemiplegia. Studies that included patients with head trauma or brain tumor were excluded. (3) The dependent variables had to include motor function, cognitive skill, language ability, visual-perceptual function, and/or activities of daily living. (4) Studies had to include a comparison of at least two groups and analysis had to include means, standard deviations, t or F ratios, and p levels.

Of the 124 initially identified reports, 36 met the inclusion criteria, yielding a total of 3,717 subjects! Their analysis was based on the d-index, computed from 173 statistical tests included in the 36 reviewed trials. The combined effect size index showed a moderate difference between those who received a program of focused stroke rehabilitation and those in comparison groups. The results also showed an interaction between the type of research design and method of recording study outcomes. Blinding in the design was an important element in being able to establish treatment effectiveness. The researchers concluded that stroke rehabilitation may improve function, and that research design should be considered an important element in planning and interpreting clinical trials.

The number of meta-analyses appearing in the medical literature continues to grow each year, demonstrating an increased acceptance of this model for contributing to an understanding of clinical phenomena.* Meta-analysis offers an important approach given the real-world limitation that many individual researchers face in conducting studies of appropriately large scale to obtain convincing answers to practical research questions.

---

*An example of the international effort to conduct systematic reviews is the *Cochrane Collaboration*, which prepares and makes available meta-analyses. The collaboration consists of review groups representing many medical specialties and subspecialties. More information on the Cochrane Collaboration can be found on their website at <http://www.cochrane.org>.

HISTORICAL RESEARCH

Historical research involves the critical review of events, documents, literature, and other sources of data to reconstruct the past in an effort to understand how and why past events occurred. This approach has its foundations in the discipline of history, where past world events are examined and analyzed to determine how present conditions evolved and, ultimately, to anticipate future events. In similar fashion, historical research can build a foundation for interpreting current clinical theory and practice, providing a context within which we can evaluate professional trends. Historical research has received little attention in allied health, which is unfortunate, considering its potential for contributing to perspectives on professional issues, directions of professional growth and change, and effects of professional and societal trends on modes of practice. Historical research efforts in nursing are extensive. Lusk has presented a primer on historical research methodology that, although written in the context of nursing, provides comprehensive guidelines for all health professionals.[53]

The process of historical research starts with the determination of a research question appropriate for historical study. For example, clinicians might be interested in the influence of changes in entry-level education on practitioner roles or in how new technology and advanced basic research have affected the development of therapeutic programs. These types of questions can only be answered retrospectively within the historical perspective of events that precipitated change. Realistically, historical studies begin with general questions, as the scope of the topic may not be realized until after most of the relevant materials are identified.

Once a problem area is identified, a working hypothesis is developed, usually expressed in terms of the expected relationships among variables. This hypothesis is the element that distinguishes historical research from a critical review of literature or a chronological presentation of a series of events (although these will be major components of the historical research process). Historical research is not a collection of facts or dates, but is meant to incorporate judgments, analyses, and inferences in the search for relationships, by organizing and synthesizing data from the past, not just summarizing them.[53] Historical hypotheses are not tested in the traditional statistical sense, but they can be supported through study of historical sources. For example, one might hypothesize that surgical field units during World War II contributed to the present-day operating room staffing practices. Breakiron tested this hypothesis analyzing perioperative nursing practices during that war and relating them to current trends using nurses as first assistants in the operating room, including the evolution of core curricula and certification of these nurses.[54]

Sources of Historical Data

Historians use a variety of sources to accumulate data. The researcher must be critical in the acceptance of all that is read, recognizing that those who wrote in the past may have been selective in their presentation of facts or creative in their representation of the truth. For this reason, especially, the historical researcher should distinguish between firsthand and secondhand sources of information. For the historian, *primary sources* include original documents, such as letters, videotapes, photographs, or minutes of a meeting, eyewitness accounts, and direct recordings of events. This does not guarantee the truth or accuracy of the report, only that no intervening account has colored the information. *Secondary sources* may include biographies, textbooks, encyclopedias, literature reviews, newspaper accounts, and any summary of primary materials. As with all research, the historian should use primary sources whenever possible. The transmission of information from original to secondary accounts will invariably present some distortion or slant that could affect the validity of subsequent interpretations.[55]

Reliability and Validity

Historical data must also be evaluated for reliability and validity. Because historical information is subject to contamination, researchers will find that not all sources are of equal value.[56] The historian must be able to establish the authenticity of data, by subjecting the material to **external criticism.** This may involve determination that papers were indeed written by the ascribed author (not ghostwritten) or that documents have not been altered. The data must also be subjected to **internal criticism,** which questions the truth or worth of the material's content within the context of the research question. Although it is not a scientifically rigorous procedure, to some extent internal validity of information can be examined on the basis of corroboration from other sources or by finding no substantial contrary evidence.[56] It is also important to understand the relevant definitions and concepts used during the historical period and to recognize that standards and terminology change over time.

Synthesis of Historical Data

After the validity of historical data is established, the data must be synthesized and analyzed within an objective frame of reference that relates to the research hypothesis. The researcher must determine how much information is needed to draw valid conclusions. Some elements of data will be given more weight than others in their application to the hypothesis. The historian attempts to incorporate a scientific logic into this process, so that interpretations are made as objectively as possible. Because sources, measurements, and organization of data are not controlled, cause-and-effect statements cannot be made in historical research. One can only synthesize what is already known into systematized accounts of the past, and discuss potential relationships between variables based on sequencing of events and associated underlying characteristics of variables.

A useful example of historical research was presented by Levine, who examined the role of arts and crafts modalities in occupational therapy by tracing societal trends of industrialization and professionalization, along with the development of occupational therapy theory in the early 20th century.[57] She examined the concept of work as it reflected shifting values and social reforms in America, to document the important role of patient participation in occupational therapy practice. In another example, Gutman examined the evolution of the relationship between occupational therapists and othopedists that began during World War I, drawing conclusions about the development of models of care.[58]

COMMENTARY

Moving Forward

The second phase of the research process is the design of the study. On the basis of this and preceding chapters, it may seem a bit overwhelming to consider the full range of research approaches that are available to clinical researchers. Choosing one approach over the others is an important part of the planning process. This choice should be based on the nature of the research question, what it is that the researcher really wants to know, the availability of subjects, and what types of data can be collected.

The third and fourth phases of the research process involve the collection and analysis of data. In the next section of the book, we address methods of data description and analysis using statistical methods. Although this seems to be a separate phase in the evolution of a research study, the procedures for data analysis should be determined within the context of the chosen research approach. In fact, data analysis usually appears as the final section in a research proposal. Because the design of the study dictates how the data can be interpreted, the researcher must be able to see the intrinsic connection between design and analysis. As we begin to explore different data analysis procedures, we should keep in mind how these procedures can be applied to the various designs we have described.

KEY TERMS

evaluation research
formative evaluation
summative evaluation
goal-free evaluation

methodological research
secondary analysis
meta-analysis
effect size

historical research
external criticism
internal criticism

REFERENCES

1. Rossi PH, Freeman HE. *Evaluation: A Systematic Approach.* 5th ed. Newbury Park, CA: Sage Publications, 1993.
2. Sowell R, Seals G, Wilson B, et al. Evaluation of an HIV/AIDS continuing education program. *J Contin Educ Nurs* 1998;29:85–95.
3. Jacobsson LT, Frithiof M, Olofsson Y, Runesson I, Strombeck B, Wikstrom I. Evaluation of a structured multidisciplinary day care program in rheumatoid arthritis. A similar effect in newly diagnosed and long-standing disease. *Scand J Rheumatol* 1998;27:117–24.
4. Daltroy LH, Iversen MD, Larson MG, et al. A controlled trial of an educational program to prevent low back injuries *N Engl J Med* 1997;337:322–8.
5. Vickery DM, Kalmer H, Lowry D, Constantine M, Wright E, Loren W. Effect of a self-care education program on medical visits. *JAMA* 1983;250:2952–6.
6. Rocheleau B, MacKesey T. Utilization-focused evaluation: A case study from the human-services area. In: Palumbo DJ, Fawcett SB, Wright P, eds. *Evaluating and Optimizing Public Policy.* Lexington, MA: Lexington Books, 1981, 187–98.

7. Caruso LA, Chan DE, Chan A. The management of work-related back pain. *Am J Occup Ther* 1987;41:112–7.
8. Nachmias D. *Public Policy Evaluation: Approaches and Methods.* New York: Martin's Press, 1979.
9. Windsor RA, Baranowski T, Clark N, et al. *Evaluation of Health Promotion and Education Programs.* Mountain View, CA: Mayfield, 1984.
10. Posavac EJ, Carey RG. *Program Evaluation: Methods and Case Studies.* Englewood Cliffs, NJ: Prentice-Hall, 1980.
11. Scriven M. The methodology of evaluation. In: Tyler RW, Gagne RM, Scriven M, eds. *Perspectives of Curriculum Evaluation.* Chicago: Rand-McNally, 1967.
12. Palumbo DJ, Fawcett SB, Wright P. *Evaluating and Optimizing Public Policy.* Lexington, MA: Lexington Books, 1981.
13. Williams RM, Myers AM. A new approach to measuring recovery in injured workers with acute low back pain: Resumption of Activities of Daily Living Scale. *Phys Ther* 1998;78:613–23.
14. Dodds TA, Martin DP, Stolov WC, Deyo RA. A validation of the Functional Independence Measurement and its performance among rehabilitation inpatients. *Arch Phys Med Rehabil* 1993;74:531–6.
15. Oczkowski WJ, Barreca S. The Functional Independence Measure: its use to identify rehabilitation needs in stroke survivors. *Arch Phys Med Rehabil* 1993;74:1291–4.
16. DiScala C, Grant CC, Brooke MM, Gans BM. Functional outcome in children with traumatic brain injury: agreement between clinical judgment and the Functional Independence Measure. *Am J Phys Med Rehabil* 1992;71:145–8.
17. Mauthe RW, Haaf DC, Hayn P, Krall JM. Predicting discharge destination of stroke patients using a mathematical model based on six items from the Functional Independence Measure. *Arch Phys Med Rehabil* 1996;77:10–13.
18. Hsieh CY, Walker JM, Gillis K. Straight-leg-raising test. Comparison of three instruments. *Phys Ther* 1983;63:1429–33.
19. Liang MH, Fossel AH, Larson MG. Comparisons of five health status instruments for orthopedic evaluation. *Med Care* 1990;28:632–42.
20. Fike ML, Rousseau E. Measurement of adult hand strength: a comparison of two instruments. *Occup Ther J Res* 1982;2:43.
21. Shrout PE, Yager TJ. Reliability and validity of screening scales: effect of reducing scale length. *J Clin Epidemiol* 1989;42:69–78.
22. Lynch SM, Leahy P, Barker SP. Reliability of measurements obtained with a modified functional reach test in subjects with spinal cord injury. *Phys Ther* 1998;78:128–33.
23. The ALS CNTF Treatment Study (ACTS) Phase I-II Study Group. The Amyotrophic Lateral Sclerosis Functional Rating Scale. Assessment of activities of daily living in patients with amyotrophic lateral sclerosis. *Arch Neurol* 1996;53:141–7.
24. Steen N, Hutchinson A, McColl E, et al. Development of a symptom based outcome measure for asthma. *BMJ* 1994;309:1065–8.
25. Kantz ME, Harris WJ, Levitsky K, Ware Jr., JE, Davies AR. Methods for assessing condition-specific and generic functional status outcomes after total knee replacement. *Med Care* 1992;30:MS240–MS252.
26. Beaton DE, Richards RR. Measuring function of the shoulder. A cross-sectional comparison of five questionnaires. *J Bone Joint Surg [Am]* 1996;78:882–90.
27. Heald SL, Riddle DL, Lamb RL. The shoulder pain and disability index: the construct validity and responsiveness of a region-specific disability measure. *Phys Ther* 1997;77:1079–89.
28. McHorney CA, Ware Jr. JE, Lu JF, Sherbourne CD. The MOS 36-item Short-Form Health Survey (SF-36): III. Tests of data quality, scaling assumptions, and reliability across diverse patient groups. *Med Care* 1994;32:40–66.

29. MacKenzie CR, Charlson ME, DiGioia D, Kelley K. Can the Sickness Impact Profile measure change? An example of scale assessment. *J Chronic Dis* 1986;39:429–38.

30. Martin DP, Engelberg R, Agel J, Swiontkowski MF. Comparison of the Musculoskeletal Function Assessment questionnaire with the Short Form-36, the Western Ontario and McMaster Universities Osteoarthritis Index, and the Sickness Impact Profile health-status measures. *J Bone Joint Surg [Am]* 1997;79:1323–35.

31. Chambers LW, Haight M, Norman G, MacDonald L. Sensitivity to change and the effect of mode of administration on health status measurement. *Med Care* 1987;25:470–80.

32. Deyo RA, Centor RM. Assessing the responsiveness of functional scales to clinical change: an analogy to diagnostic test performance. *J Chronic Dis* 1986;39:897–906.

33. Hearst N, Hulley SB. Using secondary data. In: Hulley SB, Cummings SR, eds. *Designing Clinical Research: An Epidemiologic Approach.* Baltimore: Williams & Wilkins, 1988, p. 53–62.

34. Goldman L, Mushlin AI, Lee KL. Using medical databases for clinical research. *J Gen Intern Med* 1986;1:S25 – S30.

35. Guccione AA, Felson DT, Anderson JJ, et al. The effects of specific medical conditions on the functional limitations of elders in the Framingham Study. *Am J Public Health* 1994;84:351–8.

36. Visser M, Harris TB, Langlois J, et al. Body fat and skeletal muscle mass in relation to physical disability in very old men and women of the Framingham Heart Study. *J Gerontol* 1998;53A:M214–M221.

37. Benjamin EJ, D'Agostino RB, Belanger AJ, Wolf PA, Levy D. Left atrial size and the risk of stroke and death. The Framingham Heart Study. *Circulation* 1995;92:835–41.

38. Elias MF, Elias PK, D'Agostino RB, Silbershatz H, Wolf PA. Role of age, education, and gender on cognitive performance in the Framingham Heart Study: community-based norms. *Exp Aging Res* 1997;23:201–35.

39. Multiple Risk Factor Intervention Trial Research Group. Multiple risk factor intervention trial. Risk factor changes and mortality results. *JAMA* 1982;248:1465–77.

40. Sexton M, Bross D, Hebel JR, et al. Risk-factor changes in wives with husbands at high risk of coronary heart disease (CHD): the spin-off effect. *J Behav Med* 1987;10:251–61.

41. Svendsen KH, Kuller LH, Martin MJ, Ockene JK. Effects of passive smoking in the Multiple Risk Factor Intervention Trial. *Am J Epidemiol* 1987;126:783–95.

42. Kuller LH, Ockene JK, Townsend M, Browner W, Meilahn E, Wentworth DN. The epidemiology of pulmonary function and COPD mortality in the multiple risk factor intervention trial. *Am Rev Respir Dis* 1989;140:S76–S81.

43. Flack JM, Neaton JD, Daniels B, Esunge P. Ethnicity and renal disease: lessons from the Multiple Risk Factor Intervention Trial and the Treatment of Mild Hypertension Study. *Am J Kidney Dis* 1993;21:31–40.

44. Connett JE, Stamler J. Responses of black and white males to the special intervention program of the Multiple Risk Factor Intervention Trial. *Am Heart J* 1984;108:839–48.

45. Neaton JD, Wentworth DN, Cutler J, Stamler J, Kuller L. Risk factors for death from different types of stroke. Multiple Risk Factor Intervention Trial Research Group. *Ann Epidemiol* 1993;3:493–9.

46. Folsom AR, Hughes JR, Buehler JF, Mittelmark MB, Jacobs Jr. DR, Grimm Jr. RH. Do type A men drink more frequently than type B men? Findings in the Multiple Risk Factor Intervention Trial (MRFIT). *J Behav Med* 1985;8:227–35.

47. Sacks HS, Berrier J, Reitman D, Ancona-Berk VA, Chalmers TC. Meta-analyses of randomized controlled trials. *N Engl J Med* 1987;316:450–5.

48. Easterbrook PJ, Berlin JA, Gopalan R, Matthews DR. Publication bias in clinical research. *Lancet* 1991;337:867–72.

49. Dickersin K, Min YI. Publication bias: the problem that won't go away. *Ann NY Acad Sci* 1993;703:135–46.

50. Ioannidis JP. Effect of the statistical significance of results on the time to completion and publication of randomized efficacy trials. *JAMA* 1998;279:281–6.
51. Cohen J. *Statistical Power Analysis for the Behavioral Sciences.* 2d ed. Hillsdale, NJ: Lawrence Erlbaum, 1988.
52. Ottenbacher KJ, Jannell S. The results of clinical trials in stroke rehabilitation research. *Arch Neurol* 1993;50:37–44.
53. Lusk B. Historical methodology for nursing research. *Image J Nurs Sch* 1997;29:355–9.
54. Breakiron M. A salute to the nurses of World War II. *AORN J* 1995;62:710–22.
55. Kerlinger FN. *Foundations of Behavioral Research.* New York: Holt, Rinehart & Winston, 1973.
56. Christy TE. The methodology of historical research: a brief introduction. *Nurs Res* 1975;24:189–92.
57. Levine RE. Historical research: ordering the past to chart our future. *Occup Ther J Res* 1986;6:259.
58. Gutman SA. Influence of the U.S. military and occupational therapy reconstruction aides in World War I on the development of occupational therapy. *Am J Occup Ther* 1995;49:256–62.

PART IV

Data Analysis

CHAPTER

17

Descriptive Statistics and Measures of Variability

In the investigation of most clinical research questions, some form of quantitative data will be collected. Initially these data exist in *raw form*, which means that they are nothing more than a compilation of numbers representing empirical observations from a group of individuals. For these data to be useful as measures of group performance, they must be organized, summarized and analyzed, so that their meaning can be communicated. These are the functions of the branch of mathematics called statistics. **Descriptive statistics** are used to characterize the shape, central tendency, and variability within a set of data, often with the intent to describe a population. Measures of population characteristics are called **parameters.** A descriptive index computed from sample data is called a **statistic.** When researchers generalize sample data to populations, they use statistics to estimate population parameters. In this chapter we introduce the basic elements of statistical analysis for describing quantitative data.

FREQUENCY DISTRIBUTIONS

Because the numerical data collected during a study exist in unanalyzed, unsorted form, a structure is needed that allows us to recognize trends or averages. Table 17.1 presents a set of hypothetical scores of 48 physical therapists on a test of attitudes toward the disabled. For this example, a maximum score of 20 indicates an overall positive attitude; zero indicates a strong negative bias. The total set of scores for a particular variable is called a **distribution.** An arrangement of rank-ordered scores, such as this one, is called an **array.** The total number of scores in the distribution is given the symbol n.* In this sample, $n = 48$.

---

*The lowercase n is generally used to indicate the size of a sample; an uppercase N is used to represent the size of a population.

TABLE 17.1. RANK-ORDER DISTRIBUTION OF ATTITUDE SCORES ($n = 48$)

9	12	13	15	15	16	17	19
10	12	14	15	15	16	17	19
10	12	14	15	15	16	17	19
11	12	14	15	16	16	18	19
11	13	14	15	16	17	18	20
11	13	14	15	16	17	18	20

Although visual inspection of an array allows us to see the lowest and highest scores, this list is long and unwieldy, and inadequate for describing this group of therapists or comparing them with any other group. We can begin to summarize the data by presenting them in a **frequency distribution.** A frequency distribution is a table of rank-ordered scores that shows the number of times each value occurred, or its *frequency* (f). The first two columns in Table 17.2 show the frequency distribution for the raw scores presented in Table 17.1. Now we can tell more readily how the scores are distributed. We can determine the lowest and highest scores, where the scores tend to cluster, and which scores occurred most often. The sum of the numbers in the frequency column (f) equals n, the number of subjects or scores in the distribution. We can express this relationship using the symbol Σ (the capital Greek letter sigma) to denote "the sum of," so that $\Sigma f = n$ is read, "the sum of f equals n."

Sometimes frequencies are more meaningfully expressed as percentages of the total distribution. We can look at the percentage represented by each score in the distribution, or at the *cumulative percentage* obtained by adding the percentage value for each score to all percentages that fall below that score. For example, it may be useful to know that 18.7% of the sample had a score of 15 or that 56.2% of the sample had scores between 9

TABLE 17.2. FREQUENCY DISTRIBUTION OF ATTITUDE SCORES

Score (X)	Frequency (f)	%	Cumulative %
9	1	2.0	2.0
10	2	4.2	6.2
11	3	6.3	12.5
12	4	8.3	20.8
13	3	6.3	27.1
14	5	10.4	37.5
15	9	18.7	56.2
16	7	14.6	70.8
17	5	10.4	81.2
18	3	6.3	87.5
19	4	8.3	95.8
20	2	4.2	100.0
	$\Sigma f = n = 48$	100.0	

and 15. Percentages are useful for describing distributions because they are independent of sample size. For example, suppose in another sample of 150 therapists, 84 individuals obtained a score of 15 or less. Although there are more people in this second sample within this score range than in the first sample, they both represent the same percentage of the total sample (56.2%). Therefore, the samples may be more similar than frequencies would indicate.

Grouped Frequency Distributions

When clinical data are collected, researchers will often find that very few subjects, if any, obtain the exact same score. Consider a hypothetical sample of 30 patients for whom we obtained measurements of shoulder abduction range of motion, shown in the top of Table 17.3. Obviously, creating a frequency distribution is a useless process if every score has a frequency of one. In this situation, a *grouped frequency distribution* can be constructed by grouping the scores into *classes,* or intervals, where each class represents a unique range of scores within the distribution. Frequencies are then assigned to each interval.

The bottom of Table 17.3 shows a grouped frequency distribution for the range of motion data. The classes represent ranges of 10 degrees. The classes are *mutually exclusive* (no overlap) and *exhaustive* within the range of scores obtained. The choice of the number of classes to be used and the range within each class is an arbitrary decision. It depends on the overall range of scores, the number of observations, and how much detail is relevant for the intended audience. Although information is inherently lost in grouped data, this approach is often the only feasible way to present comprehensible data when large amounts of information are collected for continuous data. The groupings should be

TABLE 17.3. RAW SCORES AND GROUPED FREQUENCY DISTRIBUTION FOR SHOULDER ABDUCTION RANGE OF MOTION (n = 30)

84	98	94	115	90	85
68	96	132	93	86	112
125	60	105	80	108	91
72	102	77	95	77	130
95	92	94	110	100	82

Class	Frequency (*f*)
60–69	2
70–79	3
80–89	5
90–99	10
100–109	4
110–119	3
120–129	1
130–139	2
	$\Sigma f = n = 30$

clustered to reveal the important features of the data. The researcher must recognize that the choice of the number of classes and the range within each class can influence the interpretation of how a variable is distributed.

Graphing Frequency Distributions

Graphic representation of data often communicates information about trends and general characteristics of distributions more clearly than a tabular frequency distribution. The most common methods of graphing frequency distributions are the histogram, the frequency polygon, and the stem-and-leaf plot.

A **histogram** is a bar graph, composed of a series of columns, each representing one score or class interval. Figure 17.1 is a histogram showing the distribution of attitude scores given in Table 17.2. The frequency for each score is plotted on the Y-axis (vertical), and the measured variable, in this case attitude score, is on the X-axis (horizontal). The bars are centered over the scores.

A **frequency polygon** is a line plot, where each point on the line represents frequency or percentage. Figure 17.2 illustrates a frequency polygon for the attitude data. When grouped data are used, the dots in the graph are located at the midpoint of each class interval to represent the frequency in that class.

The **stem-and-leaf plot** is a refined grouped frequency distribution that is most useful for presenting the pattern of distribution of a continuous variable. The pattern is derived by separating each score into two parts. The *leaf* consists of the last or rightmost single digit of each score, and the *stem* consists of the remaining leftmost digits. Table 17.4 illustrates a stem-and-leaf plot for the shoulder range of motion data. These scores have leftmost digits of 6 through 13. These values become the stem. The last digit in each score becomes the leaf. To read the stem-and-leaf plot, we look across each row, attaching each single leaf digit to the stem. Therefore, the first row repre-

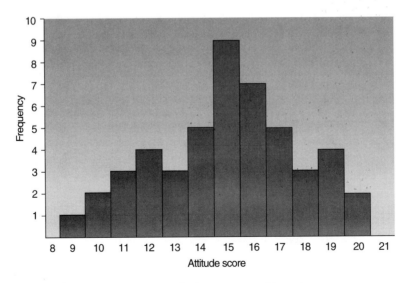

FIGURE 17.1   Histogram for attitude data given in Table 17.2.

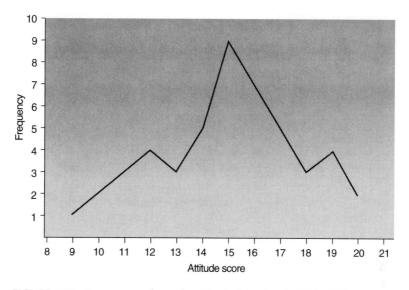

FIGURE 17.2 Frequency polygon for attitude data given in Table 17.2.

sents the scores 60 and 68; the second row 72, 77, and 77; the third row 80, 82, 84, 85, and 86; and so on. This display provides a concise summary of the data, while maintaining the integrity of the original data. If we compare this plot with the grouped frequency distribution in Table 17.3, it is clear how much more information is provided by the stem-and-leaf plot in a small space, and how it provides both tabular and graphic displays.

Shapes of Distributions

When graphs of frequency distributions are drawn, the distributions can be characterized by their shape. Although real data seldom achieve smooth curves, minor discrepancies are often ignored in an effort to describe overall the shape of a distribution.

TABLE 17.4. SHOULDER RANGE OF MOTION DATA PRESENTED IN RANK-ORDER DISTRIBUTION AND STEM-AND-LEAF PLOT

						Stem	Leaf
60	80	90	94	100	112	6	08
68	82	91	95	102	115	7	277
72	84	92	95	105	125	8	02456
77	85	93	96	108	130	9	0123445568
77	86	94	98	110	132	10	0258
						11	025
						12	5
						13	02

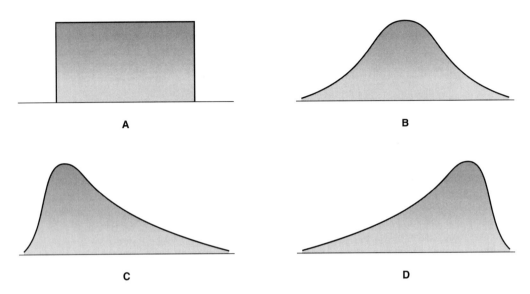

FIGURE 17.3   Common shapes of frequency distributions: **(A)** symmetrical rectangular; **(B)** normal curve; **(C)** skewed to the right; **(D)** skewed to the left.

Some distributions are symmetrical; that is, each half is a mirror image of the other. Curves A and B in Figure 17.3 are symmetrical. When scores are equal throughout the distribution, the shape is described as *uniform*, or rectangular, as shown in curve A. Curve B represents a special case of the symmetrical distribution called the **normal distribution.** In statistical terminology, "normal" refers to a specific type of bell-shaped distribution where most of the scores fall in the middle of the scale and progressively fewer fall at the extremes. The unique characteristics of this distribution curve are discussed in greater detail later in this chapter.

A **skewed distribution** is asymmetrical. The degree to which the distribution deviates from symmetry is its *skewness*. Curve C in Figure 17.3 is *positively skewed*, or skewed to the right, because most of the scores cluster at the low end and only a few scores at the high end have caused the tail of the curve to point toward the right. If we were to plot a distribution for annual family income in the United States, for example, it would be positively skewed, because most families have low to moderate incomes. When the curve "tails off" to the left, the distribution is *negatively skewed*, or skewed to the left, as in curve D. We might see a negatively skewed distribution if we plotted exam scores for an easy test, on which relatively few students achieved a low score.

MEASURES OF CENTRAL TENDENCY

Although frequency distributions enable us to order data and identify group patterns, they do not provide a practical quantitative summary of a group's characteristics. Numerical indices are needed to describe the "typical" nature of the data and to reflect different concepts of the "center" of a distribution. These indices are called measures of **central tendency,** or averages. The term *average* can denote three different measures of central tendency: the mode, the median, and the mean.

The Mode

The **mode** is the score that occurs most frequently in a distribution. It is most easily determined by inspection of a frequency distribution. Table 17.2 reveals that the mode for the attitude data is 15 because it occurs nine times, more than any other score. When class intervals are used, the mode is taken as the midpoint of the interval with the largest frequency. When more than one score occurs with the highest frequency, a distribution is considered *bimodal* (with two modes) or *multimodal* (with more than two modes). Many distributions of continuous variables do not have a mode.

The mode has only limited application as a measure of central tendency for continuous data, but can be useful in the assessment of categorical variables. For example, it may be of interest to determine the diagnostic category seen most often in a clinic.

The Median

The **median** of a series of observations is that value above which there are as many scores as below it; that is, it divides a rank-ordered distribution into two equal halves. When a distribution contains an odd number of scores, such as 4, 5, 6, 7, 8, the middle score, 6, is the median. With an even number of scores, the midpoint between the two middle scores is the median, so that for the series 4, 5, 6, 7, 8, 9, the median lies halfway between 6 and 7. Therefore, the median equals 6.5. For the distribution of attitude scores given in Table 17.2, with $n = 48$, the median will lie midway between the 24th and 25th scores. As both of these are 15, the median is 15.

The advantage of the median as a measure of central tendency is that it is unaffected by the value of extreme scores. It is an index of average *position* in a distribution, not amount. It is therefore a useful measure in describing skewed distributions. For instance, the average cost of a house is usually cited in terms of the median, because the distribution is skewed to the right.

The Mean

The **mean** is the sum of a set of scores divided by the number of scores, n. This value is what most people refer to as the "average." The symbol used to represent the mean of a population is the Greek letter mu, μ, and the mean of a sample is represented by $\overline{X}$. The bar above the X indicates that the value is an average score. The formula for calculation of the sample mean from raw data is

$$\overline{X} = \frac{\Sigma X}{n} \tag{17.1}$$

This is read, "the mean equals the sum of X divided by n," where X represents each individual score in the distribution. For example, we can apply this formula to the two sets of test scores shown in Table 17.5. In each distribution of eight students, the sum of scores is 669. Therefore, $\overline{X} = 669/8 = 83.6$.

Comparing Measures of Central Tendency

Determining which measure of central tendency is most appropriate for describing a distribution depends on several factors. Foremost is the intended application of the data.

TABLE 17.5. TEST SCORES OBTAINED FROM TWO GROUPS OF STUDENTS

	X_A	X_B	
	78	65	
	80	69	
$\overline{X}_A = 83.6$	82	78	$\overline{X}_B = 83.6$
Median = 85	85	85	Median = 85
Mode = 85	85	85	Mode = 85
$n = 8$	85	93	$n = 8$
	86	96	
	88	98	
	$\Sigma X_A = 669$	$\Sigma X_B = 669$	

The scale of measurement of the variable is another important consideration. All three measures of central tendency can be applied to variables on the interval or ratio scales, although the mean is most useful. For data on the nominal scale, only the mode is meaningful. If data are ordinal, both the median and mode can be applied.

It is necessary to consider how the summary measure will be used statistically. Of the three measures of central tendency, the mean is considered the most stable; that is, if we were to repeatedly draw random samples from a population, the means of those samples would fluctuate less than the mode or median. Only the mean can be subjected to arithmetic manipulations, making it the most reasonable estimate of population characteristics. For this reason, the mean is used more often than the median or mode for statistical analysis of ratio or interval data.

We can also consider the utility of the three measures of central tendency for describing distributions of different shapes. With uniform and normal distributions, any of the three averages can be applied with validity. With skewed distributions, however, the mean is limited as a descriptive measure because, unlike the median and mode, it is affected by the quantitative value of every score in a distribution and can be biased by extreme scores. For instance, in the previous example of test scores (Table 17.5), if the first subject obtained a score of 50 instead of 78, the mean would decrease from 83.6 to 80.1. The median and mode would be unaffected by this change.

The curves in Figure 17.4 illustrate how measures of central tendency are affected by skewness. The median will always fall between the mode and the mean in a skewed curve, and the mean will be pulled toward the tail. Because of these properties, the choice of which index to report with skewed distributions depends on what facet of information is appropriate to the analysis. It is often reasonable to report all three values, to present a complete picture of a distribution's characteristics.

MEASURES OF VARIABILITY

The shape and central tendency of a distribution are useful but incomplete descriptors of a sample. To illustrate this point, consider the following dilemma: You are responsible for planning the musical entertainment for a party of seven individuals, but you

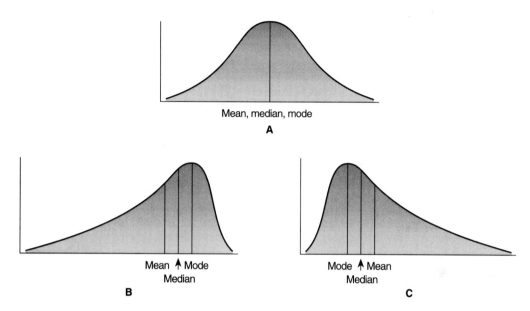

FIGURE 17.4   Relationship of mean, median, and mode in unimodal symmetrical **(A)** and skewed **(B)** and **(C)** distributions. The mean is pulled toward the tail of skewed curves.

don't know what kind of music to choose—so you decide to use their average age as a guide. The guests' ages are 3, 3, 13, 14, 59, 70, and 78 years. Based on the mode of 3 years, you would bring in characters from Sesame Street. Using the median of 14 years, you might hire a heavy metal band. And according to the mean age of 34.3 years, you might decide to play soft rock, although nobody in the group is actually in that age range. And the Tommy Dorsey fans are completely overlooked! What we are ignoring is the spread of ages within this group.

Consider now a more serious example, using the hypothetical exam scores reported in Table 17.5, obtained from two different groups of students. If we were to describe these two distributions using measures of central tendency only, then they would appear identical; however, a careful glance reveals that the scores for Group B are more widely scattered than those for Group A. This difference in **variability,** or dispersion of scores, is an essential element in data analysis. The description of a sample is not complete unless we can characterize the differences that exist *among* the scores as well as the central tendency of the data. In this section we describe five commonly used statistical measures of variability: range, percentiles, variance, standard deviation, and coefficient of variation.

Range

The simplest measure of variability is the **range,** which is the difference between the highest and lowest values in a distribution. For the test scores reported in Table 17.5, the range for Group A is 88 − 78 = 10, and that for Group B, 98 − 65 = 33.[†] These values

---

[†]Research reports will usually give ranges by providing the actual minimum and maximum scores, rather than their difference.

suggest that the first group was more homogeneous. Although the range is a relatively simple statistical measure, its applicability is limited because it is determined using only the two extreme scores in the distribution. It reflects nothing about the dispersion of scores between the two extremes. One aberrant extreme score can greatly increase the range, even though the variability within the rest of the data set is unchanged. In addition, the range of scores tends to increase with larger samples, making it an ineffective value for comparing distributions with different numbers of scores. Therefore, although it is easily computed, the range is usually employed only as a rough descriptive measure, and is typically reported in conjunction with other indices of variability.

Percentiles and Quartiles

Percentiles are used to describe a score's position within a distribution. Percentiles divide data into 100 equal portions. A particular score is located in one of these portions, which represents its position relative to all other scores. For example, if a student taking a college entrance examination scores in the 92nd percentile (P_{92}), that individual's score was higher than 92% of those who took the test. Percentiles are helpful for converting actual scores into comparative scores or for providing a reference point for interpreting a particular score. For instance, a child who scores in the 20th percentile for weight in his age group can be evaluated relative to his peer group, rather than considering only the absolute value of his weight.

Quartiles divide a distribution into four equal parts, or quarters. Therefore, three quartiles exist for any data set. Quartiles Q_1, Q_2, and Q_3 correspond to percentiles at 25%, 50%, and 75% of the distribution (P_{25}, P_{50}, P_{75}). The score at the 50th percentile or Q_2 is the median. The distance between the first and third quartiles, $Q_3 - Q_1$, is called the **interquartile range,** which represents the boundaries of the middle 50% of the distribution.

Quartiles are often used in clinical research as a basis for differentiating subgroups within a sample. For example, Hornsby and coworkers wanted to study the relationship between muscle length and plantar flexor torque by comparing subjects with "tight" and "loose" muscles.[1] Rather than specify range of motion criteria for tight and loose muscles and then seek out subjects to fit these criteria, the researchers evaluated their available subject pool and chose individuals whose scores fell below the first quartile (tight) and above the third quartile (loose). Subjects whose scores fell within the interquartile range were eliminated from the study. In this way, the researchers were able to create two groups with distinctly different inherent muscle lengths. In another example, researchers studied the relationship between bone density and walking habits in 239 postmenopausal women.[2] The sample was grouped into quartiles based on year-round distance walked, and these four groups were compared on bone density and several anthropometric variables. Quartiles provided the structure for creating comparison groups where no obvious criteria were available.

Variance

Measures of range have limited application as indices of variability because they are not influenced by every score in a distribution. To more completely describe a distribution we need an index that reflects the variation within a full set of scores. This value should

TABLE 17.6. RESTING PULSE RATE ($n = 10$) AND DEVIATION SCORES USED TO COMPUTE VARIANCE AND STANDARD DEVIATION

X	$(X - \overline{X})$	$(X - \overline{X})^2$	X^2
56	−9	81	3,136
58	−7	49	3,364
60	−5	25	3,600
62	−3	9	3,844
64	−1	1	4,096
66	1	1	4,356
68	3	9	4,624
70	5	25	4,900
72	7	49	5,184
74	9	81	5,476
$\Sigma X = 650$	0	$\Sigma(X - \overline{X})^2 = 330$	$\Sigma X^2 = 42{,}580$
$\overline{X} = 65$			

be small if scores are close together and large if they are spread out. It should also be objective so that we can compare samples of different sizes and determine if one is more variable than another.

We can begin to examine variability by looking at the deviation of each score from the mean; that is, we subtract the mean from each score in the distribution to obtain a *deviation score*, $X - \overline{X}$. Obviously, samples with larger deviation scores will be more variable around the mean. For instance, consider the distribution of pulse rate scores and deviation scores shown in Table 17.6. The mean of the distribution is 65 beats/minute. Note that the first five deviation scores are negative values because these scores are smaller than the mean.

As a measure of variability, the deviation score has intuitive appeal, as these scores will obviously be larger as scores become more heterogeneous and farther from the mean. It might seem reasonable, then, to take the average of these values, or the mean deviation, as an index of dispersion within the sample. This is a useless exercise, however, because the sum of the deviation scores will always equal zero, $\Sigma(X - \overline{X}) = 0$, as illustrated in the second column in Table 17.6. If we think of the mean as a central balance point for a distribution, then it makes sense that the scores will be equally dispersed about that central point.

This dilemma is solved by squaring each deviation score to get rid of the minus signs, as shown in the third column of Table 17.6. The sum of the squared deviation scores, $\Sigma(X - \overline{X})^2$, is called the **sum of squares** (SS). As variability increases, the sum of squares will be larger.

We now have a number we can use to describe the sample's variability. In this case, $\Sigma(X - \overline{X})^2 = 330$. As an index of relative variability, however, the sum of squares is limited because it can be influenced by the sample size; that is, as n increases, the sum will also tend to increase simply because there are more scores. To eliminate this problem, the sum of squares is divided by n, to obtain the mean of the squared deviation scores (shortened to **mean square,** MS). This value is a true measure of variability and is called the **variance.**

For population data, the variance is symbolized by σ^2 (lowercase Greek sigma). When the population mean is known, deviation scores are obtained by $X - \mu$. Therefore, the population variance is defined by

$$\sigma^2 = \frac{SS}{N} = \frac{\Sigma(X - \mu)^2}{N} \tag{17.2}$$

With sample data, deviation scores are obtained using $\overline{X}$, not μ. Because sample data do not include all the observations in a population, this substitution results in a sample variance slightly smaller than the true population variance. To compensate for this bias, the sum of squares is divided by $n - 1$ to calculate the sample variance, given the symbol s^2:

$$s^2 = \frac{SS}{n-1} = \frac{\Sigma(X - \overline{X})^2}{n - 1} \tag{17.3}$$

This corrected statistic is considered an *unbiased estimate* of the parameter σ^2. For the data in Table 17.6, SS = 330 and n = 10. Therefore,

$$s^2 = \frac{330}{10 - 1} = 36.67$$

Computational Formulas

Equation 17.3 defines variance on the basis of deviation scores; however, when the mean is not a whole number or when large samples are used, computation of deviation scores can be quite tedious and tends to be less reliable because of rounding off. Therefore, a computational formula for variance that uses raw scores is preferred:[‡]

$$s^2 = \frac{\Sigma X^2 - \dfrac{(\Sigma X)^2}{n}}{n - 1} \tag{17.4}$$

where ΣX^2 is the sum of the squared raw scores. The numerator in this formula is the computational expression for sum of squares.

[‡]The corresponding computational formula for population variance is $\sigma^2 = \dfrac{\Sigma X^2 - \dfrac{(\Sigma X)^2}{N}}{N}$

Using the computational formula for data shown in Table 17.6,

$$s^2 = \frac{(42{,}580) - \frac{(650)^2}{10}}{10 - 1} = \frac{330}{9} = 36.67$$

Standard Deviation

The drawback of variance as a descriptive measure of a sample's variability is that it was calculated using the squares of the deviation scores. It is generally not useful to describe sample variability in terms of squared units, such as degrees squared or pounds squared. Therefore, to bring the index back into the original units of measurement, we take the square root of the variance. This value is called the **standard deviation,** symbolized by s.[§] The formula for standard deviation is

$$s = \sqrt{s^2} = \sqrt{\frac{SS}{n-1}} = \sqrt{\frac{\Sigma(X - \overline{X})^2}{n-1}} \tag{17.5}$$

The corresponding computational formula is

$$s = \sqrt{\frac{\Sigma X^2 - \frac{(\Sigma X)^2}{n}}{n-1}} \tag{17.6}$$

For the preceding example,

$$s^2 = \sqrt{\frac{(42{,}580) - \frac{(650)^2}{10}}{10 - 1}} = \sqrt{36.67} = 6.06$$

The standard deviation of sample data is usually reported with the mean so that the data are characterized according to both central tendency and variability. A mean may be expressed as $\overline{X} = 65 \pm 6.06$, which tells us that the average of the deviations on either side of the mean is 6.06. Graphs will often show an *error bar* to indicate the mean and standard deviation (see Figure 17.5).

The standard deviation can be used as a basis for comparing samples. Suppose that pulse rate measures were taken for another group of subjects with a mean of 65 ± 20, as in Figure 17.5B. Because this second standard deviation is larger, we know that the second group's scores were more spread out around the mean. In clinical studies it may be relevant to describe the degree of variability among subjects as a way of estimating the generalizability of responses. Variance and standard deviation are fundamental components

---

[§]The corresponding formulas for the population standard deviation are

$$\sigma = \sqrt{\sigma^2} = \sqrt{\frac{SS}{N}} = \sqrt{\frac{\Sigma(X - \mu)^2}{N}} = \sqrt{\frac{\Sigma X^2 - \frac{(\Sigma X)^2}{N}}{N}}$$

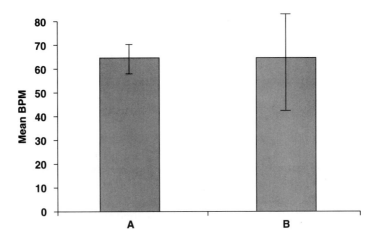

FIGURE 17.5 Example of a bar graph showing the mean and error bar indicating the standard deviation. Some authors will only show the error bar in one direction. The error bars indicate that the distribution in **(A)** is less variable than the distribution in **(B)**, even though they have the same mean.

of any analysis of data. We explore the application of these concepts to many statistical procedures throughout the coming chapters.

Coefficient of Variation

The **coefficient of variation (***CV***)** is another measure of variability that can be used to describe data measured on the interval or ratio scale. It is the ratio of the standard deviation to the mean, expressed as a percentage:

$$CV = \frac{s}{\overline{X}} \times 100 \tag{17.7}$$

There are two major advantages to this index. First, it is independent of units of measurement because units will mathematically cancel out. Therefore, it is a practical statistic for comparing distributions recorded in different units. Second, the coefficient of variation expresses the standard deviation as a proportion of the mean, thereby accounting for differences in the magnitude of the mean. The coefficient of variation is, therefore, a measure of *relative variation,* most meaningful when comparing two distributions.[11]

These advantages can be illustrated using data from a study of normal values of lumbar spine range of motion, in which data were recorded in both degrees and inches of excursion.[3] The mean ranges for 21- to 29-year-olds were $\overline{X} = 41.2 \pm 9.6$ degrees, and $\overline{X} = 3.7 \pm 0.72$ inches, respectively. The absolute values of the standard deviations for these two measurements suggest that the measure of inches, using a tape measure, was much less variable; however, because the means are substantially different and because

---

[11]The coefficient of variation cannot be used when a variable mean is a negative number. Because *CV* is expressed as a percentage, it cannot be interpreted as a negative value.

the units are different, we would expect the standard deviations to be different as well. By calculating the coefficient of variation, we get a better idea of the relative variation of these two measurements:

$$\text{Degrees:} \quad CV = \frac{9.6}{41.2} \times 100 = 23.3\%$$

$$\text{Inches:} \quad CV = \frac{0.72}{3.7} \times 100 = 19.5\%$$

Now we can see that the variability within these two distributions is actually quite comparable. As this example illustrates, the coefficient of variation is a useful measure for making comparisons among patient groups or different clinical assessments to determine if some are more stable than others.

THE NORMAL DISTRIBUTION

Earlier in this chapter we discussed the symmetrical distribution known as the *normal distribution*. This distribution represents an important statistical concept because so many biological, psychological, and social phenomena manifest themselves in populations according to this shape. If we were to graph the population frequency distribution of variables such as height or intelligence, the graph would resemble the bell-shaped curve. Unfortunately, in the real world we can only estimate such data from samples and, therefore, cannot expect data to fit the normal curve exactly. For practical purposes, then, the normal curve represents a theoretical concept only, with well-defined properties that allow us to make statistical estimates about populations using sample data.

The fact that the normal curve is important to statistical theory should not imply, however, that data are not useful or valid if they are not normally distributed. Many sociological variables such as socioeconomic class, income, ethnic background, and age are skewed. Such data can be handled using statistics appropriate to non-normal distributions (see Chapter 22).

Proportions of the Normal Curve

The statistical appeal of the normal distribution is that its characteristics are constant and, therefore, predictable. As shown in Figure 17.6, the curve is smooth, symmetrical, and bell shaped, with most of the scores clustered around the mean. The mean, median, and mode have the same value. The frequency of scores decreases steadily as scores move in a negative or positive direction away from the mean, with relatively rare observations at the extremes. Theoretically, there are no boundaries to the curve; that is, scores potentially exist with infinite magnitude above and below the mean. Therefore, the tails of the curve approach but never quite touch the baseline.

Because of these standard properties, we can also determine the proportional areas under the curve represented by the standard deviations in a normal distribution. Statisticians have shown that 34.13% of the area under the normal curve is bounded by the mean and the score one standard deviation above or below the mean. Therefore, 68.26%

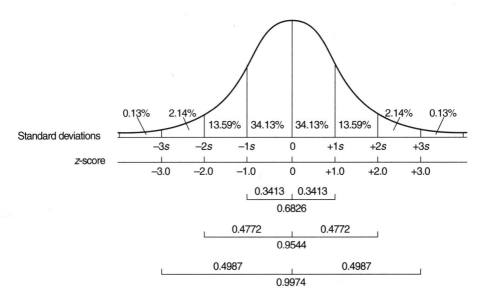

FIGURE 17.6   Areas under the normal curve, showing standard deviations and corresponding z-scores.

of the total distribution (the majority) will have scores within ±1 standard deviation (±1s) from the mean. Similarly, ±2s from the mean will encompass 95.45%, and ±3s will cover 99.73% of the total area under the curve. At ±3s we have accounted for virtually the entire distribution. Because we can never discount extreme values at either end, we never account for the full 100%. This information can be used as a basis for interpreting standard deviations. For example, if we are given $\overline{X} = 65 \pm 6.06$, we can estimate that approximately 68% of the individuals in the sample have scores between 58.94 and 71.06.

Standardized Scores   *S = Std. Dev. of a sample*

Statistical data are meaningful only when they are applied in some quantitative context. For example, if a patient has a pulse rate of 58 beats/min, the implication of that value is evident only if we know where that score falls in relation to a distribution of normal pulse rates. If we know that $\overline{X} = 68$ and $s = 10$ for a given sample, then we know that a score of 58 is one standard deviation below the mean. This gives us a clearer interpretation of the score. When we express scores in terms of standard deviation units, we are using **standardized scores,** also called **z-scores.** For this example, a score of 58 can be expressed as a z-score of −1.0, the minus sign indicating that it is one standard deviation unit below the mean. A score of 88 is similarly transformed to a z-score of +2.0, or two standard deviations above the mean.

A z-score is computed by dividing the deviation of an individual score from the mean by the standard deviation:

$$z = \frac{X - \overline{X}}{s} \tag{17.8}$$

Using the example of pulse rates, for an individual score of 85 beats/min, with $\overline{X} = 68$ and $s = 10$,

$$z = \frac{85 - 68}{10} = \frac{17}{10} = 1.7$$

Thus, 85 beats/min is 1.7 standard deviations above the mean.

The Standardized Normal Curve

The normal distribution can also be described in terms of standardized scores. The mean of a distribution of z-scores will always equal zero (no deviation from the mean), and the standard deviation will always be 1.0. As shown in Figure 17.6, the area under the standardized normal curve between $z = 0$ and $z = +1.0$ is approximately 34%, the same as that defined by the area between the mean ($z = 0$) and one standard deviation. The total area within $z = \pm 1.00$ is 68.26%. Similarly, the total area within $z = \pm 2.00$ is 95.45%. Using this model, we can determine the proportional area under the curve bounded by any two points in a normal distribution. These values are given in Appendix Table A.1.

Determining Areas under the Normal Curve

We can illustrate this process using hypothetical values for pulse rates, with $\overline{X} = 68$ and $s = 10$. Suppose we want to determine what percentage of our sample has a pulse rate above 50 beats/min. First, we determine the z-score for 50 beats/min:

$$z = \frac{50 - 68}{10} = \frac{-18}{10} = -1.8$$

Therefore, 50 beats/min is slightly less than two standard deviations below the mean.

Now we want to determine the proportion of our total sample that is represented by all scores above 50, or above $z = -1.8$. We already know that the scores above the mean (above $z = 0$) represent 50% of the curve, as shown by the dark gray area in Figure 17.7. Therefore, we are now concerned with the light gray area between 68 and 50, which is equal to the area from $z = 0$ to $z = -1.8$. Together these two shaded areas represent the total area above 50.

We can now refer to Table A.1. This table is arranged in three columns, one containing z-scores and the other two representing areas either from 0 to z or above z (in one tail of the curve). For this example, we are interested in the area from 0 to z, or from 0 to -1.8. This table uses only absolute values of z. Because it includes standardized units for a symmetrical curve, the proportional area from 0 to $z = +1.8$ is the same as the area from 0 to $z = -1.8$.

If we look to the right of $z = 1.80$ in Table A.1, we find that the area from 0 to z equals .4641, or 46.41% of the curve. Therefore, the total area under the curve for all scores above 50 beats/min will be $.50 + .4641 = .9641$, or 96.41%.

We might also be interested in determining the area above 80 beats/min, as shown by the gray area in Figure 17.8. For this example, we are interested in the area above z.

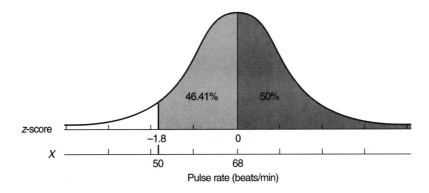

FIGURE 17.7   Distribution of pulse rates with $\overline{X} = 68$ and $s = 10$, showing the area under the normal curve above 50 beats/minute, or $z = -1.8$. The light gray area represents $z = 0$ to $-1.8 = .4641$ (from Table A.1). Together, the gray areas represent 96.41% of the total area under the curve.

First we find the z-score for 80 beats/min:

$$z = \frac{80 - 68}{10} = \frac{12}{10} = 1.2$$

This score is slightly more than one standard deviation above the mean. From Table A.1 we find that for $z = 1.20$, the tail of the curve represents .1151, or 11.51% of the curve.

   Standardized scores are very useful for interpreting an individual's standing relative to a normalized group. For example, many standardized tests, such as psychological, developmental, and intelligence tests, use z-scores to demonstrate that an individual's score is above or below the "norm" (the standardized mean) or to show what proportion of the subjects in a distribution fall within a certain range of scores.

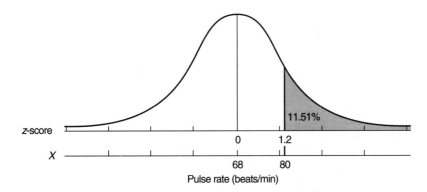

FIGURE 17.8   Distribution of pulse rates with $\overline{X} = 68$ and $s = 10$, showing the area under the normal curve above 80 beats/minute, or $z = 1.2$. The gray area in the tail of the curve represents 11.51% of the curve (from Table A.1).

The validity of estimates using the standard normal curve depends on the closeness with which a sample approximates the normal distribution. Many clinical samples are too small to provide an adequate approximation and are more accurately described as skewed. Unfortunately, many researchers do not test for skewness as part of their analysis; however, because many statistical procedures are based on assumptions of normality in the underlying distribution, results of analyses may be suspect if the researcher has not examined data for "goodness-of-fit" to the normal distribution (see Chapter 25). Many computer programs for descriptive statistics will compute measures of skewness. Skewness should be reported to help readers understand the shape of a distribution and to evaluate the appropriate use of statistical procedures.

COMMENTARY

Description Only Goes So Far

Descriptive statistics are the building blocks for data analysis. They serve an obvious function in that they summarize important features of numerical data. Descriptive measures are limited in their application because they do not attempt to infer anything that goes beyond the data themselves. Therefore, if we collect information about the average performance of a group of patients, we are using a descriptive process; however, if we use this information to predict future performance of these patients or to make generalizations about the effectiveness of the treatment they received, we are going beyond the scope of descriptive data. Consider the elusive cure for the common cold:

> Each of a dozen different independent studies showed that a considerable percentage of colds cleared up after treatment with antihistamines. A great fuss ensued, at least in the advertisements, and a medical product boom was on. It was based on an eternally springing hope and also on a curious refusal to look at a fact that has been known for a long time. Henry G. Felsen, a humorist and no medical authority, pointed out some time ago, proper treatment will cure a cold in 7 days, but left to itself a cold will hang on for a week.[4]

It is important to remain cognizant of the limitations of descriptive information for generalization. Interpretations that go beyond sample data are based on inferential statistics.

Measures of central tendency and variance form the foundation for most inferential procedures, but they cannot be used alone to support generalizations. For instance, suppose we calculate means and standard deviations for outcomes under two different treatment conditions, and these values turn out to be different from each other. These descriptive measures tell us only how each group performed, but cannot tell us anything about the true experimental differences that exist between them. The application of inferential statistics is discussed in the next chapter.

KEY TERMS

descriptive statistics
parameter
statistic
distribution
array
frequency distribution
histogram
frequency polygon
stem-and-leaf plot

normal distribution
skewed distribution
central tendency
mode
median
mean ($\overline{X}$)
variability
range
percentiles

quartiles
interquartile range
sum of squares (SS)
mean square (MS)
variance (s^2)
standard deviation (s)
coefficient of variation (CV)
standardized score
(z-score)

REFERENCES

1. Hornsby TM, Nicholson GG, Gossman MR, Culpepper M. Effect of inherent muscle length on isometric plantar flexion torque in healthy women. *Phys Ther* 1987;67:1191–7.
2. Krall EA, Dawson-Hughes B. Walking is related to bone density and rates of bone loss. *Am J Med* 1994;96:20–6.
3. Fitzgerald GK, Wynveen KJ, Rheault W, Rothschild B. Objective assessment with establishment of normal values for lumbar spinal range of motion. *Phys Ther* 1983;63:1776–81.
4. Huff D. *How to Lie with Statistics*. New York: Norton, 1954, p. 8.

18

Statistical Inference

In the previous chapter we presented statistics that can be used to summarize and describe data. Descriptive procedures are not sufficient, however, for testing theories about the effects of experimental treatments or for generalizing the behavior of samples to a population. For these purposes, researchers use a process of statistical *inference*. The process of drawing inferences from samples is familiar to everybody. When an individual decides to read a book by a certain author after having enjoyed other books by that same author, that person is inferring something about the probable quality of the new book. When a specific treatment approach produces beneficial effects for a particular patient, a clinician might decide to use that approach for other patients with similar conditions. The difference between these subjective inferences and statistical inference is that the researcher uses objective criteria to make such decisions.

Inferential statistics involve a decision-making process that allows us to estimate population characteristics from sample data. The success of this process requires that we make certain assumptions about how well the sample represents the larger population. These assumptions are based on two important concepts of statistical reasoning: **probability** and **sampling error.** The purpose of this chapter is to introduce these fundamental concepts and to demonstrate the principles of their application for drawing valid conclusions from research data.

PROBABILITY

Probability is a complex but essential concept for understanding inferential statistics. We all have some notion of what probability means, as evidenced by the use of terms such as "likely," "probably," or "a good chance." We use probability as a means of prediction: "There is a 50% chance of rain tomorrow," or "This operation has a 75% chance of success." Statistically, we can view probability as a system of rules for analyzing a complete set of possible outcomes, or a *sample space*. For instance, a sample space could represent the two sides of a coin or the six faces on a die. An event is a single observable happening or outcome, such as the appearance of tails on the flip of a coin or a 3 on the toss of a die. A sample space could be a set of IQ scores for all students in a given school system. An event might be the random selection of one student's IQ score of 110. In other words, each score in the sample space is a potential event.

Probability is the likelihood that any one event will occur, given all the possible outcomes. We use a lowercase *p* to signify probability, expressed as a ratio or decimal. For example, given the two possible outcomes for the flip of a coin, the likelihood of getting tails on any single flip will be 1 of 2, or 1/2, or .5. Therefore, we say that the probability of getting tails is 50%, or $p = .5$. Suppose we want to know the probability of getting a 3 when a die is thrown. The sample space is the set of six faces of the die, or six possible outcomes. Therefore, the probability that we will roll a 3 is 1 of 6, or 1/6, or $p = .167$. Conversely, the probability that we will not roll a 3 is 5 of 6, or 5/6, or $p = .833$. What is the probability that we will roll a 3 or higher? There are now four possible events—3, 4, 5, and 6—that meet this criterion. Therefore, the probability is 4 of 6, 2/3, or $p = .667$, that we will roll a 3 or higher on any single roll of one die.

For an event that is certain to occur, $p = 1.00$. For instance, if we toss a die, the probability of rolling a 3 or not rolling a 3 is 1.00 ($p = .167 + .833$). These two events are *mutually exclusive* and *complementary* events because they cannot occur together and because they represent all possible outcomes. Therefore, the sum of their probabilities will always equal 1.00. We can also establish that the probability of an impossible event is zero. For instance, the probability of rolling a 7 with one die is 0 of 6, or $p = 0.00$. In the real world, the probability for most events falls somewhere between 0 and 1. Scientists will generally admit that nothing is a "sure bet" and nothing is impossible!

This concept can now be applied to a distribution of scores. Suppose we had access to the population of scores for height of all adult men alive today. This distribution of millions of scores would approximate the normal curve. Suppose, too, that the mean height was 69 in., with a standard deviation of 3 in. What is the probability that any one man selected at random from this population will be between 66 and 72 in. tall, or within ±1 standard deviation? We know this range represents 68.26% of the population as shown by the center gray area in Figure 18.1. This means that approximately 68 of 100 men can be expected to be between 66 and 72 in. tall, or that there is a 68% probability ($p = .68$) that any one man we select will fall within this range. Similarly, the probability of selecting a man 78 in. or taller (scores beyond +3 standard deviations) is .0013, as this area represents 0.13% of the total distribution, as shown by the gray area in the tail of Figure 18.1.

It is important to understand that probability is predictive in that it reflects what *should* happen over the long run, not necessarily what *will* happen for any given trial or event. When a surgeon advises that an operation has a 75% probability of success, it means that in the long run, for all such cases, 75% can be expected to be successful. For any single patient the surgery will not be 75% successful; it will either be a success or not. Therefore, once an event occurs, it is no longer "probable." It either happened as predicted or not. Probability applies to the proportion of time we can *expect* a given outcome to occur in the idealized "long run."

We use probability in research as a guideline for making decisions about how well sample data estimate the characteristics of a population. We also use probabilities to determine if observed treatment differences are likely to be representative of population differences or if they could have occurred *by chance.* We try to determine if we can estimate what would happen to others in the population on the basis of our limited sample.

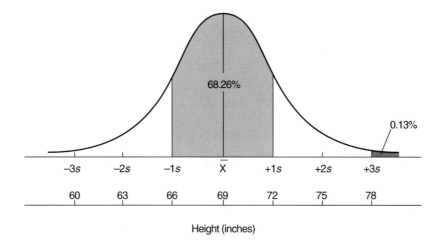

FIGURE 18.1   Hypothetical distribution of heights for adult males, with $\bar{X} = 69$ and $s = 3$. Center area represents $\pm 1s$, or 68.26% of the population. Gray area to the right represents $\geq 3s$, or 0.13% of the population.

To understand these applications of probability, we must first understand the statistical relationship between samples and populations.

SAMPLING ERROR

The estimation of population characteristics from sample data is based on the assumption that samples are random and valid representatives of the population. Even when truly random samples are used, however, we cannot be sure that one sample's characteristics will be identical to those of the population, simply because fewer cases are included in the sample. For example, if we had access to birth records for all liveborn babies in the United States for the past year, we might find that the population parameters for birth weight were $\mu = 120$ ounces and $\sigma = 5$. Now suppose we randomly select a sample of 10 babies, and find that $\bar{X} = 115$ ounces and $s = 30$. Because selection was unbiased, this sample should be a good representative of the population; however, the sample mean and standard deviation are somewhat different from the population values and, therefore, do not provide accurate estimates. What would account for this difference? Random selection implies that all members of a population have an equal opportunity of being chosen, but, obviously, this does not guarantee proportional representation of all parts of the population. We could obtain a sample with many lighter babies just by chance. It is highly unlikely that a sample of 10 would match the overall distribution of population characteristics.

    If we choose a second sample of 10 babies, the odds are that we will obtain yet a different mean and standard deviation. The laws of chance tell us that through a process of infinitely repeated random sampling, we should expect to see such differences among the sample means. The tendency for sample values to differ from population values is called **sampling error.** Sampling error of the mean for any single sample is equal to the difference between the sample mean and the population mean ($\bar{X}-\mu$). The greater the sampling error, the less accurate $\overline{X}$ is as an estimate of μ. In practice, sampling error is unpredictable because it occurs strictly by chance—by virtue of who happens to get picked for any one sample.

Theoretically, if we were to randomly draw an infinite number of samples from a population, each with $n = 10$, the means of these samples would exhibit varying degrees of sampling error. We would expect, by chance, that most of the sample means would be close to the population mean. If we plotted the sample means, we would find that the distribution would take the shape of a normal curve, and that the mean of all the sample means would be equal to the population mean. This distribution of sample means is called a **sampling distribution of means.** A sampling distribution will consistently take the shape of the normal curve.*

Obviously, a sampling distribution is a theoretical concept only, because one does not go through such a sampling process in practice. Clinical researchers work with only one sample from which inferences are made about a population; however, because of the predictable properties of the normal curve, we can use the concept of the sampling distribution to formulate a basis for making inferences from sample data.

Standard Error of the Mean

The standard deviation of a theoretical sampling distribution of means is called the **standard error of the mean ($\sigma_{\overline{X}}$).** This value is considered an estimate of the population standard deviation, σ. The curve in Figure 18.2A represents a hypothetical sampling distribution formed by repeated sampling of birth weights, with samples of $n = 10$. The means of such small samples tend to vary, and in fact, we see a wide curve with great variability. The sampling distribution in the curve in Figure 18.2B was constructed from the same population, but with samples of $n = 50$. These sample means form a narrower distribution curve with less variability and, therefore, a smaller standard deviation. As sample size increases, samples become more representative of the population, and their means are more likely to be closer to the population mean; that is, their sampling error will be smaller. Therefore, the standard deviation of the sampling distribution is an indicator of the degree of sampling error, reflecting how accurately the various sample means estimate the population mean.

Because we do not actually construct a sampling distribution, we need some useful way to estimate the standard error of the mean from sample data. This estimate, $s_{\overline{X}}$, is based on the standard deviation and size of the sample:

$$s_{\overline{X}} = \frac{s}{\sqrt{n}} \tag{18.1}$$

Using our example of birth weights, for a single sample of 10 babies, we found a mean of 115 with a standard deviation of 30 (Figure 18.2A). Therefore, $s_{\overline{X}} = 30/\sqrt{10} = 9.5$. With a sample of $n = 50$, $s_{\overline{X}} = 30/\sqrt{50} = 4.2$. As illustrated in Figure 18.2, as n increases, the stan-

---

*This phenomenon is explained by the *central limit theorem,* which demonstrates that even for skewed distributions, the sampling distribution of means will approach the normal curve as n increases. Therefore, we can use sampling distributions and the probabilities associated with the normal curve to predict population characteristics for any distribution.

dard error of the mean decreases. With larger samples the sampling distribution is expected to be less variable, and therefore, a statistic based on a large sample is considered a better estimate of a population parameter than one based on a smaller sample.

A sample mean, together with its standard error, helps us imagine what the sampling distribution curve would look like. For example, for a sample of $n = 50$, with $\overline{X} = 115$ and $s_{\overline{X}} = 4.2$, the theoretical sampling distribution might look like the curve shown in Figure 18.2B. If we use this curve as an estimate of the population distribution, we can determine the probability of drawing a single sample with a certain mean. Based on our knowledge of the normal curve, the chances are 95.45 of 100 that any single random sample we might draw from this population would have a mean between 106.6 and 123.4 ($\pm 2 s_{\overline{X}}$). Therefore, the probability is 95.45% that a sample mean will lie within this range,

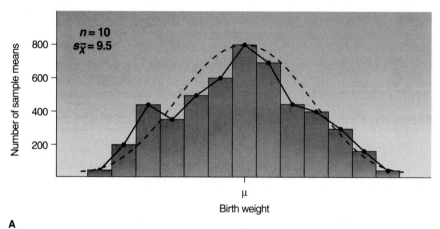

A

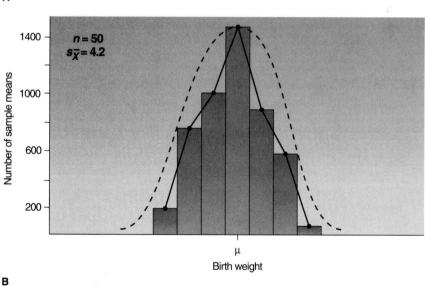

B

FIGURE 18.2   Hypothetical sampling distributions for birth weight. Curve A is drawn for samples with $n = 10$. Curve B is drawn for samples with $n = 50$.

or there is less than a 5% chance that any sample mean drawn from this population will be less than 106.6 or above 123.4. We should note that the standard error cannot be a direct measure of variance in the population, because it is a function of sample size.

CONFIDENCE INTERVALS

For many research applications, sample data are used to estimate unknown population parameters. For example, we can sample medical records to determine length of hospital stay for patients with certain diagnoses or we could study normative values for tests of motor function. The purpose of these types of analyses is to estimate how the population behaves and to use this information for decision making or as a foundation for further research.

We can use our knowledge of sampling distributions to estimate population parameters in two ways. A **point estimate** is a single value obtained by direct calculation from sample data, such as using $\overline{X}$ to estimate μ. We know, however, that any single sample value will most likely contain some degree of error as a population estimate. Therefore, it is often more meaningful to use an **interval estimate,** by which we specify an interval within which we believe the population parameter will lie. Such an estimate takes into consideration not only the value of a single sample statistic, but also the relative accuracy of that statistic.

For example, Fitzgerald et al. estimated the population mean for lumbar spinal extension for 30- to 39-year-olds.[1] Based on a random sample of 42 individuals, they determined that $\overline{X} = 40.0$ degrees and $s = 8.8$ degrees. Therefore, the point estimate of μ is the sample mean, 40.0 degrees. How can we tell how accurate this estimate is? Perhaps we would be more comfortable giving a range of values within which we are fairly sure the population mean will fall. For instance, we might guess that the population mean is likely to be within 5 degrees of the sample mean, to fall within the interval 35 to 45 degrees. We must be more precise than guessing allows, however, in proposing such an interval, so that we can be "confident" that the interval is an accurate estimate.

A **confidence interval (CI)** is a range of scores with specific boundaries, or *confidence limits,* that should contain the population mean. The boundaries of the confidence interval are based on the sample mean and its standard error. The wider the interval we propose, the more confident we will be that the true population mean will fall within it. This degree of confidence is expressed as a probability percentage, such as 95% confidence.

To illustrate the procedure for constructing a 95% confidence interval, consider the earlier example of lumbar spine extension, with $\overline{X} = 40.0$, $s = 8.8$, $n = 42$, and $s_{\overline{X}} = 8.8/\sqrt{42} = 1.36$. The sampling distribution estimated from this sample is shown in Figure 18.3. We know that 95.45% of the total distribution will fall within $\pm 2s_{\overline{X}}$ from the mean, or within the boundaries of $z = \pm 2$. Therefore, to determine the proportion of the curve within 95%, we need to determine points just slightly less than $z = \pm 2$. By referring to Table A.1 in the Appendix, we can determine that 0.95 of the total curve (0.475 on either side of the mean) is bounded by a z-score of ± 1.96, just less than 2 standard error units above and below the mean. Therefore, as shown in Figure 18.3, 95% of the total sampling distribution will fall between $-1.96s_{\overline{X}}$ and $+1.96s_{\overline{X}}$. We are 95% sure that the population mean will fall within this interval. This is called the *95% confidence interval.*

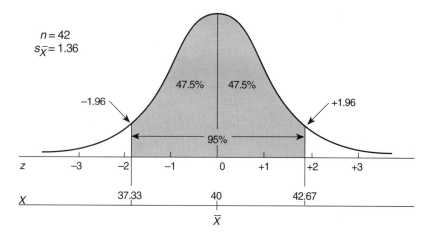

FIGURE 18.3   95% confidence interval for sampling distribution of lumbar extension range of motion for 30- to 39-year-olds.

We obtain the boundaries of a confidence interval using the formula

$$CI = \bar{X} \pm (z)s_{\bar{X}} \qquad\qquad (18.2)$$

For 95% confidence intervals, $z = \pm1.96$.
For our data, therefore,

$$95\% \ CI = 40.0 \pm (1.96)(1.36)$$

$$= 40.0 \pm 2.67$$

$$95\% \ CI = 37.33 \ to \ 42.67$$

We are 95% confident that the population mean of lumbar extension for 30- to 39-year-olds will fall between 37.33 and 42.67 degrees.

How can we interpret this statement? Because of sampling error, one sample we select may have a mean of 50 degrees, with 95% confidence limits between 47.3 and 52.7 degrees. Another sample could have a mean of 52 degrees, with 95% confidence limits between 49.3 and 54.7 degrees. The 95% confidence limits indicate that if we were to draw 100 random samples, each with $n = 42$, we could construct 100 confidence intervals around the sample means, 95 of which could be expected to contain the true population mean. Five of the 100 intervals would not contain the population mean. This would occur just by chance, because the scores chosen for those five samples would be too extreme and not good representatives of the population. In reality, however, we construct only one confidence interval based on the data from only one sample. Theoretically, then, we cannot know if that one sample would produce one of the 95 correct intervals or one of the 5 incorrect ones. Therefore, there is a 5% chance that the population mean is not included in the obtained interval, that is, a 5% chance the interval is one of the incorrect ones.

To be more confident of the accuracy of an interval, we can construct a 99% confidence interval, allowing only a 1% risk that the interval we propose will not contain the true population mean. Using Table A.1, we can determine that 99% of the area under the

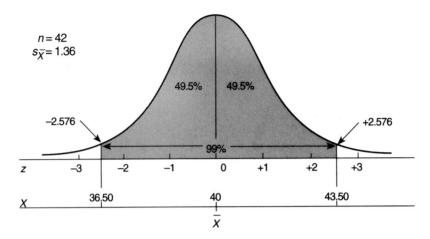

FIGURE 18.4 99% confidence interval for sampling distribution of lumbar extension range of motion for 30- to 39-year-olds.

curve (0.495 on either side of the mean) is bounded by $z = \pm2.576$, as shown in Figure 18.4. Therefore,

$$99\% \text{ CI} = \bar{X} \pm (2.576)s_{\bar{X}} \qquad (18.3)$$

For our data,

$$99\% \text{ CI} = 40 \pm (2.576)(1.36)$$

$$= 40 \pm 3.50$$

$$99\% \text{ CI} = 36.5 \text{ to } 43.5$$

We are 99% confident that the population mean falls between 36.5 and 43.5 degrees.

Note that the confidence limits get wider as our confidence level increases. We reduce the risk of being wrong by sacrificing precision. The choice of confidence interval depends on the nature of the variables being studied and the researcher's desired level of accuracy. By convention, the 95% and 99% confidence intervals are used most often.

Confidence Intervals with Small Samples

The process we have just described is appropriate for calculating confidence intervals for large samples. With smaller samples, however, sampling distributions tend to be more spread out than the normal distribution, and, therefore, the standard normal curve is not considered an adequate representation with samples of n less than 30. Thus, an alternate theoretical sampling distribution, called the **t-distribution,** is used to evaluate smaller samples.

The major statistical contrast between the t-distribution and the standard normal distribution is the difference in their configuration. The t-distribution is flatter and wider at the tails than the normal curve. This shape changes with different sample sizes, so that there are actually many t-distributions, one for each sample size. As sample size increases, the sampling distribution becomes narrower and approaches the shape of the normal curve.

The spread of the *t*-distribution changes the proportions under the curve; that is, we cannot estimate the percentages within standard deviation units in the same proportions as in the normal curve. For example, we know that 95% of the normal sampling distribution falls within $z = \pm 1.96$, slightly less than 2 standard deviation units. To find this area with smaller samples, we use values of *t* instead of *z*. These values are given in Table A.2 in the Appendix, and summarized here in Table 18.1 for 90%, 95%, and 99% confidence intervals. For reasons we will explain later in this chapter, statisticians use **degrees of freedom (*df*)** to identify the various *t*-distributions, rather than *n*. For the creation of confidence intervals, degrees of freedom will equal $n - 1$. Therefore, for a sample of $n = 6$, $df = 5$; with $n = 10$, $df = 9$; and so on.

By referring to Table 18.1, we find that for $n = 6$ ($df = 5$), 95% of the total area falls within $t = \pm 2.571$. With a sample of $n = 10$ ($df = 9$), 95% of the area falls within $t = \pm 2.262$. With $n = 30$, this area is bounded by $t = \pm 2.042$. As *n* increases, the value of *t* approaches $z = 1.96$.

We use these values to create confidence intervals using the formula

$$\text{CI} = \bar{X} \pm (t)s_{\bar{X}} \tag{18.4}$$

TABLE 18.1. VALUES OF *t* FOR 90%, 95%, AND 99% CONFIDENCE INTERVALS

df	90%	95%	99%
5	2.015	2.571	4.032
6	1.943	2.447	3.707
7	1.895	2.365	3.499
8	1.860	2.306	3.355
9	1.833	2.262	3.250
10	1.812	2.228	3.169
11	1.796	2.201	3.106
12	1.782	2.179	3.055
13	1.771	2.160	3.012
14	1.761	2.145	2.977
15	1.753	2.131	2.947
16	1.746	2.120	2.921
17	1.740	2.110	2.898
18	1.734	2.101	2.878
19	1.729	2.093	2.861
20	1.725	2.086	2.845
30	1.697	2.042	2.750
40	1.684	2.021	2.704
60	1.671	2.000	2.660
120	1.658	1.980	2.617
∞	1.645	1.960	2.576

Therefore, to create a 95% confidence interval for a sample with $n = 18$, $\bar{X} = 5.0$, and $s_{\bar{X}} = 2.0$, we locate $t = 2.110$ for 17 df. Thus,

$$95\% \text{ CI} = 5.0 \pm (2.110)(2.0)$$

$$= 5.0 \pm 4.22$$

$$95\% \text{ CI} = 0.78 \text{ to } 9.22$$

This means that we are 95% confident that the population mean falls between 0.78 and 9.22. If our sample size increases to $n = 31$ ($df = 30$, $t = 2.042$), our confidence interval changes:

$$95\% \text{ CI} = 5.0 \pm (2.042)(2.0)$$

$$= 5.0 \pm 4.084$$

$$95\% \text{ CI} = .916 \text{ to } 9.084$$

Note that the interval is narrower when more scores are used. We have become more precise in our estimate by using a larger sample.

Application of Confidence Intervals

The process of estimating population values is useful only if we can apply those values to practice. In fact, many clinical judgments are based on some value that has been established as the "norm." We can use confidence intervals to estimate normative population values as a basis for clinical evaluation. For example, Fitzgerald and coworkers established the 95% confidence intervals for lumbar extension range of motion for several age groups, as shown in Table 18.2.[1] These intervals were calculated using the appropriate t-distributions.

We can interpret these intervals in several ways. First, they show us that extension range of motion decreases as one ages. The variability in lumbar range, indicated by the standard error of the mean, is small for younger subjects but increases with age. We also see that a great deal of overlap exists in confidence intervals across age groups, demonstrating that a single mean value alone would be a misleading criterion for assessing if

TABLE 18.2.   MEANS, STANDARD DEVIATIONS, AND 95% CONFIDENCE INTERVALS IN 10-YEAR AGE GROUPS FOR LUMBAR EXTENSION RANGE OF MOTION (IN DEGREES)

Age	n	$\bar{X}$	s	$s_{\bar{X}}$	95% CI
20–29	31	41.2	9.6	1.7	37.7 to 44.7
30–39	44	40.0	8.8	1.3	37.3 to 42.7
40–49	16	31.1	8.9	2.2	26.4 to 35.8
50–59	43	27.4	8.0	1.2	24.9 to 29.9
60–69	27	17.4	7.5	1.4	14.4 to 20.4
70–79	10	16.6	8.8	2.8	10.3 to 22.9

Source: Fitzgerald GK, Wynveen KJ, Rheault W, Rothschild B: Objective assessment with establishment of normal values for lumbar spinal range of motion. *Phys Ther* 1983;63:1776–81. Reprinted with permission of the American Physical Therapy Association.

a patient's performance was "within normal limits." In this case, it is also clear that the limits within an age group encompass a narrow range, generally less than 10 degrees. The samples in this study are actually relatively small for establishing normative values. In practice, both the validity and reliability of normative studies depend on the use of large samples and repeated testing; however, these interpretations illustrate how confidence intervals can provide a guide for establishing normal limits of performance and for deciding if a patient's condition should be considered pathological.

HYPOTHESIS TESTING

The estimation of population parameters is only one part of statistical inference. More often inference is used to answer questions concerning comparisons or relationships, such as, "Is one treatment more effective than another?" or "Is there a relationship between the length of time a treatment is applied and the degree of improvement observed?" These types of questions usually involve the comparison of means, proportions, correlations, or some other statistic.

According to the concept of sampling error, we would expect to see some differences between groups even when a treatment is not at all effective, because of chance differences in subject characteristics. Therefore, we need some mechanism for deciding if an observed effect reflects chance only or if we can argue with confidence that the differences represent "real" effects. We do this through a process of *hypothesis testing.*

Statistical Hypotheses

To illustrate this process, consider a study in which a hypothesis was proposed that short leg casting will improve gait characteristics of children with cerebral palsy.[2] Experimental and control groups were formed through random assignment. Measurements were taken for stride length, among several other gait variables, and the percentage of improvement from pretest to posttest was calculated for each subject. The researcher found that the mean improvement in stride length was 27.0 cm for the casted group and -13.0 cm for the control group. On the basis of the large difference between these means, should the researcher conclude that the research hypothesis has been supported?

The Null Hypothesis

Before we can interpret observed differences, we must consider two possible explanations for this outcome. The first supposes that the research hypothesis is correct and that the observed difference in stride length is due to the effect of casting. The second possible explanation is that the observed difference between the groups occurred by chance, as a result of sampling error. This second explanation is the **statistical hypothesis,** called the **null hypothesis,** H_0, which states that any observed differences between means are due to chance. No matter how the research hypothesis is stated, the researcher's goal will always be to statistically test the null hypothesis, usually with the intention of rejecting it. This concept is analogous to the legal assumption that a person is innocent until proven guilty. It suggests that we assume no relationship exists between variables until reasonable evidence is accumulated to convince us otherwise. Statistical tests, which are described in detail in subsequent chapters, are used to make this judgment as objective as possible.

We can never actually "prove" the null hypothesis. The purpose of an experiment is to give the data a chance of *disproving* it.[3] In essence, we are using a decision-making process based on the concept of negative inference. No one experiment can establish that a null hypothesis is true; that is, it would take an infinite number of unsuccessful experiments to prove that casting has no effect on stride length. We can, however, discredit the null hypothesis by any one trial that shows that casting is effective. Therefore, the purpose of testing the statistical hypothesis is to decide whether H_0 is *false*. We can only legitimately say that we *reject* or *do not reject* the null hypothesis. It is not appropriate to "accept" the null hypothesis, because this implies proof of its validity. This is analogous to the use of *guilty* and *not guilty* in a court of law. A jury can reach a guilty verdict if evidence does not support innocence. Otherwise, the verdict is not guilty. The jury cannot find the defendant innocent. A not guilty verdict, however, is expected if the evidence is not sufficient for guilt (beyond a reasonable doubt). Using a similar logic, the null hypothesis can be rejected if the evidence is strong enough. If the evidence is not sufficient, we do not reject the null hypothesis, but that does not necessarily mean it is true.

By rejecting the null hypothesis, the researcher concludes that it is unlikely that chance is operating to produce observed differences. This is called a **significant effect,** that is, one that is *probably not due to chance.* When the null hypothesis is not rejected, the researcher concludes that the observed difference may be due to chance and is not significant. This does not necessarily mean that there is no true effect, however. It only means that the evidence is too weak to substantiate the effect. We will discuss the importance of this concept shortly.

The null hypothesis can be stated formally as

$$H_0: \mu_A = \mu_B \quad \text{or} \quad H_0: \mu_A - \mu_B = 0$$

which predicts that the mean of Population A is not different from the mean of Population B. In this example, under H_0, the stride lengths for the population with casting and the population without casting would not be significantly different; that is, any observed difference between groups would probably be the result of chance.

The Alternative Hypothesis

Researchers usually propose two statistical hypotheses, one to be rejected and another to be accepted. In addition to the null hypothesis, an **alternative hypothesis (H_1)** is stated as

$$H_1: \mu_A \neq \mu_B \quad \text{or} \quad H_1: \mu_A - \mu_B \neq 0$$

These statements predict that the observed difference between the two population means is not due to chance. We say, then, that the observed difference is "real," or that the likelihood that the difference is due to chance is very small. In most cases, the researcher hopes that the data will support the alternative hypothesis, and that H_0 will be rejected; that is, the alternative hypothesis represents the research hypothesis. There may be situations, however, when the researcher does not expect a difference, such as trying to show that a standard treatment is as effective as an experimental one. In such a case, the research hypothesis will be the same as the null hypothesis, and the researcher will want to reject the alternative hypothesis.

The preceding alternative hypotheses state that a difference will exist between Populations A and B. These are considered **nondirectional hypotheses,** because they do not specify which group mean is expected to be larger. Alternative hypotheses can also be expressed in **directional** form, indicating the expected direction of difference between sample means. We could state

$$H_1: \mu_A > \mu_B \qquad (H_1: \mu_A - \mu_B > 0)$$

or

$$H_1: \mu_A < \mu_B \qquad (H_1: \mu_A - \mu_B < 0)$$

These hypotheses predict that the mean of Population A is either greater or smaller than the mean of Population B. For instance, we might predict that the experimental group receiving casting will show a greater improvement than the control group.

Statistical hypotheses are formally stated in terms of the population parameter, μ, even though the actual statistical tests will be based on sample data. For instance, for this example, the hypotheses predict either that the casted group is from a different population than the control group (H_1) or that they are from the same population (H_0).

ERRORS IN HYPOTHESIS TESTING

The decision to reject or not reject the null hypothesis is based on the results of objective statistical procedures; however, this objectivity does not guarantee that a correct decision will be made. Because such decisions are based on sample data only, it is always possible that the true relationship between experimental populations is not accurately reflected in the statistical outcome.

Hypothesis testing will always result in one of two decisions: either reject or do not reject the null hypothesis. Any one decision can be either correct or incorrect. Therefore, we can classify four possible decision outcomes, shown in Figure 18.5. If we do not reject H_0 when it is in fact true (observed differences are really due to chance), we have made a correct decision. If we reject H_0 when it is false (differences are real), we have also made a correct decision. If, however, we decide to reject H_0 when it is true, we have made an error, called a **Type I error.** In this case, we have concluded that a real difference exists, when in fact, the differences are due to chance. Having committed this type of statistical error, we might decide to use a treatment that is not really effective. Conversely, if we do not reject H_0 when it is false, we have committed a **Type II error.** Here we would conclude that differences are due to chance, when, in fact, the samples represent different populations. In this situation, we might ignore an effective treatment or abandon a potentially fruitful line of research.

	Truth	
	H_0 is true	H_0 is false
Reject H_0	Type I error (α)	Correct
Accept H_0	Correct	Type II error (β)

FIGURE 18.5 Potential errors in hypothesis testing.

In any statistical analysis we may draw a correct conclusion, or we may commit one of these two types of errors. If we reject the null hypothesis, and decide that treatment groups are different, we may be correct or we may be making a Type I error (but not Type II). If we do not reject the null hypothesis, and decide that no differences exist, we may be correct or we may be making a Type II error (but not Type I). The seriousness of one type of error over the other is relative. Historically, statisticians and researchers have focused attention on Type I error as the primary basis of hypothesis testing; however, the consequences of failing to recognize an effective treatment may be equally important. Although we never know for sure if we are committing one or the other type of error, we can take steps to decrease the probability of committing one or both.

TYPE I ERROR: LEVEL OF SIGNIFICANCE

If we want to determine the probability of committing a Type I error, we must set some standard for rejecting the null hypothesis. This standard is called the **level of significance,** denoted as **alpha (α).** The level of significance represents a criterion for judging if an observed difference can be considered sampling error or real. The larger an observed difference is, the less likely it occurred by chance. The probability that an observed difference did occur by chance is determined by statistical tests (which are covered in the coming chapters). This probability is denoted as p. For example, we might find that an analysis comparing two means yields $p = .18$. This means that there is an 18% probability that the difference between the means occurred by chance. Therefore, if we decide to reject H_0, and conclude that the tested groups are different from each other, we have an 18% chance of being wrong, that is, an 18% chance of committing a Type I error.

The question facing the researcher is how to decide if this probability is acceptable. We know there is some chance that any observed difference will be the result of sampling error. But how much of a chance is small enough that we would be willing to accept the risk of being wrong? Is an 18% chance of being wrong acceptable?

The selected alpha level defines the *maximal acceptable risk* of making a Type I error if we reject H_0. Typically, researchers set this standard at 5%, which is considered a small risk. This means that we would be willing to accept a 5% chance of *incorrectly rejecting* H_0, but no more. Therefore, for a given analysis, if p is less than .05 we would be willing to reject the null hypothesis; that is, the difference would be considered significant. If p is greater than .05, then we would not reject the null hypothesis. For the earlier example with $p = .18$, if we set $\alpha = .05$, then we would not reject the null hypothesis. At $p = .18$, the probability that the observed difference is due to chance is too great. If a statistical test demonstrates that two means are different at $p = .04$, we could reject H_0, with only a small acceptable risk (4%) of committing a Type I error.

Choosing a Level of Significance

How does a researcher decide on a level of significance as the criterion for statistical testing? The traditional designation of .05 is really an arbitrary standard. A researcher may choose other criterion levels depending on how critical a Type I error would be. For example, suppose we were involved in the study of a drug to reduce spasticity, comparing control and experimental groups. This drug could be very beneficial to patients with upper motor neuron involvement; however, the drug has potentially serious side effects and is very expensive to produce. In such a situation we would want to be very confident that observed results were real, and not due to chance. If we reject the null hypothesis and recommend the drug, we would want the probability of our committing a Type I error to be very small. We do not want to encourage the use of the drug unless it is clearly and markedly beneficial. We can minimize the risk of statistical error by lowering the level of significance to .025 or .01. If we use $\alpha = .01$ as our criterion for rejecting H_0, we would have only 1 of 100 chances of making a Type I error. This would mean that we could have greater confidence in our decision to reject the null hypothesis.

Although researchers usually choose .05 as a convenient standard, there are situations, as just described, when lower levels of significance are appropriate. In the absence of compelling justification, however, it is not necessary to make the level of significance more rigorous than $\alpha = .05$. It is generally considered unacceptable to designate values of alpha higher than .05.

Researchers should specify the minimal level of significance required for rejecting the null hypothesis prior to data collection. The decision to use .05 or .01, or any other value, should be based on the concern for Type I error, not on what the data look like. If a researcher chooses $\alpha = .01$ as the criterion, and statistical testing shows significance at $p = .04$, the researcher would not reject H_0. If $\alpha = .05$ had been chosen as the criterion, the opposite conclusion would be reached. It is not appropriate to decide on the criterion level after the statistical probabilities have been determined. Because data are influenced by sampling error, it is important that the determination of the level of significance remains an unbiased process.

Interpreting *p* Values

Researchers must be aware of the appropriate interpretation of p values: The p value is the probability of finding an effect as big as the one observed when the null hypothesis is true. Therefore, with $p = .02$, even if there is no true difference, you would expect to observe this size effect 2% of the time. Said another way, if we performed 100 similar experiments, 2 of them would result in a difference this large, even though no true difference exists.

It is tempting, then, to reverse this definition, to assume that there is a 98% probability that a real difference exists. This is not the case, however. The p value is based on the assumption that the null hypothesis is true, although it cannot be used to prove it. The p value will only tell us how rarely we would expect a difference this large in the population. It is the researcher's responsibility to determine if this result is sufficiently unlikely that the null hypothesis should be rejected.

We must also be careful to avoid using the magnitude of p as an indication of the degree of validity of the research hypothesis. It is inadvisable to use terms such as "highly significant" and "more significant" because they imply that the value of p is a measure of experimental effect, which it is not. The level of significance can be considered a point along a continuum that demarcates the line between chance and reality. Once the level of significance is chosen, it represents a decision rule. The decision is dichotomous: either yes or no, significant or not significant. Once the decision is made, the magnitude of p reflects only the relative degree of confidence that can be placed in that decision. That said, researchers will still caution that a nonsignificant p value is not necessarily the end of the story, especially if it is close to α. The pragmatic difference in clinical effect with $p = .04$ or $p = .06$ may truly be negligible. We must, therefore, also consider the possibility of Type II error.

TYPE II ERROR: STATISTICAL POWER

We have thus far established the logic behind classical statistical inference, based on the probability associated with rejecting a true null hypothesis, or Type I error. What happens when we find no significant difference between groups and we do not reject the null hypothesis? Does this necessarily mean that there is no real effect?

If we do not reject the null hypothesis when it is indeed false, we have committed a Type II error; that is, we have found no significant difference when a difference really does exist. Unfortunately when results are not significant, researchers may assume that the experimental treatment was not effective. Researchers are often unable or unwilling to publish reports that end in nonsignificant outcomes.[4] A nonsignificant outcome may, however, simply mean that the available evidence is not strong enough to reject the null hypothesis. The implications of this issue can be far-reaching. For instance, the literature may demonstrate conflicting results, with some studies showing that a treatment is effective and others failing to do so. Researchers may try to explain these apparent discrepancies by unknowingly proposing flawed theoretical models, or abandoning important research directions prematurely. We may be losing a great deal of valuable information or moving critically off course by ignoring the possibilities of Type II error.[5]

The probability of making a Type II error is denoted by **beta (β),** which is the *probability of failing to reject a false null hypothesis.* If $\beta = .20$, there is a 20% chance that we will make a Type II error, or that we will not reject H_0 when it is really false. The fact that samples are really different does not guarantee that a statistically significant finding will result. The value of β represents the likelihood that we will be unable to statistically identify real differences.

The complement of β error, $1 - \beta$, is the statistical **power** of a test. *Power is the probability that a test will lead to rejection of the null hypothesis,* or the probability of attaining statistical significance. If $\beta = .20$, $1 - \beta$ or power $= .80$. Therefore, for a statistical test at 80% power, the probability is 80% that we would correctly demonstrate a statistical difference and reject H_0 if actual differences exist. The more powerful a test, the less likely one is to make a Type II error. Power can be thought of as sensitivity. The more sensitive a test, the more likely it will detect important clinical differences that truly exist. Where $\alpha = .05$ has become the conventional standard for Type I error, it has been suggested that $\beta = .20$, with corresponding power of 80%, represents a reasonable protection against Type II error.[6,7]

The Determinants of Statistical Power

The statistical power of a test is a function of four factors: the significance criterion (α), the variance in the data (s^2), sample size (n), and a factor that reflects the magnitude of the observed differences, called the **effect size (ES).**

The Significance Criterion

Although no direct mathematical relationship exists between α and β, there is trade-off between them. Lowering the level of significance reduces the chance of Type I error by requiring stronger evidence for a statistical test to demonstrate significant differences. This also means that the chance of missing a true effect is increased. As the probability of committing a Type I error decreases, the probability of committing a Type II error increases. By making the standard for rejecting H_0 more rigorous (lowering α), we make it harder for sample results to meet this standard.

Variance

The power of a statistical test is increased as the variance within a set of data is reduced. The ability to detect differences between groups is enhanced when the groups are distinctly different. When the variability within groups is large, differences between groups will be less obvious. Variance can be reduced, and power increased, by experimental design, such as using repeated measures or homogeneous blocks of subjects, by controlling for sources of random measurement error, or by increasing the size of the sample.

Sample Size

The influence of sample size on the power of a test is critical. The larger the sample, the greater the statistical power. Smaller samples are less likely to be good representations of population characteristics, and, therefore, true differences between groups are less likely to be recognized. When very small samples are used ($n < 30$), as is often the case in clinical research, power is substantially reduced.

Effect Size

Power is also influenced by the size of the "effect" of the experimental variable. When comparing groups, this effect will be the difference between sample means, or an estimate of the effect of the independent variable. In studies where relationships are of interest, this effect will be the degree of correlation or association between variables. This is the essence of most research questions: "How large an effect will my treatment have?" or "How strong is the relationship between two variables?" Treatments that result in large changes or correlations are more likely to produce significant outcomes than those with small or negligible effects.

Therefore, effect size is a measure of the *degree to which the null hypothesis is false.*[6] For instance, if we hypothesize that no difference exists between strength scores for two groups, we are hypothesizing that the effect size is zero. If we find an actual difference of 20 foot-pounds, the effect size is 20. The larger the effect size, the greater the effective difference between the groups.

Power Analysis

We can use power analysis in two ways. One purpose is to estimate the sample size needed to obtain a desired level of power before data collection and to use this estimate in recruiting a sample. One of the first questions researchers ask when planning a study is, "How many subjects are needed?" An easy answer is as many subjects as possible;

however, this is not helpful when one is trying to place realistic limits on time and resources for data collection. Researchers may arbitrarily suggest that a sample size of 30 or 50 is "reasonable." Unfortunately, these estimates may be inadequate for many research designs or for studies with small effect sizes. By specifying a level of significance and desired power in the planning stages of a study, a researcher can estimate how many subjects would be needed to detect a significant difference for an expected effect size. The larger the effect size, the smaller the required sample. When the sample size estimate is beyond realistic limits, a researcher may try to redesign the study by controlling variability in the sample, choosing a different dependent variable or increasing effect size, or the researcher may decide not to conduct the study, given that significant results are so unlikely. Many clinical variables will produce small to medium effect sizes because of the inherent variability among patients and the lack of standardization and sensitivity in clinical measures.[5] Therefore, sample size becomes extremely important in designing a study that has a reasonable chance of success.

It should also be noted that this type of power analysis may provide a basis for limiting sample size when a researcher is fortunate enough to have access to large numbers of subjects. There will come a point when additional subjects provide no additional power, and the extra effort and expense are not warranted. Although most researchers say, "The more subjects, the better," this is only true up to a point.

The second purpose of power analysis is to determine the probability that a Type II error was committed when a study results in a nonsignificant finding. By knowing the observed effect size, the level of significance, and the sample size, the researcher can determine the degree of power that was achieved in the analysis. If power is low, the researcher might draw only tentative conclusions about the lack of significant treatment effect, and consider replicating the study with a larger sample to increase the power of the test.

Power analysis should be incorporated into the planning stages of every experimental or correlational study. The lack of such planning often results in a high probability of Type II error and needlessly wasted efforts.[8] It is also useful to evaluate the power of nonsignificant tests reported in the literature. In some cases, the clinical significance of a study will be greater than suggested by the statistical outcome because of the lack of power.[9] For example, many meta-analyses have demonstrated important treatment effects even when individual clinical trials did not produce significant outcomes because they used small samples.[10]

Procedures for power analysis are described in Appendix C for t-tests, analysis of variance, correlation, regression, and chi-square tests. Some computer programs include analyses of effect size and power for various tests.[11]

CONCEPTS OF STATISTICAL TESTING

Statistical procedures are used to test hypotheses through the calculation of a test statistic, or test ratio. Different statistics are used to test differences between means, correlations, and proportions. The test statistic is used to determine if a significant difference is attained, by establishing the probability that such a difference would occur if H_0 were true.

To illustrate this concept, let us assume we want to determine whether the mean IQ of 3-year-old children who were born prematurely is different from the mean IQ of the general population of 3-year-old children, which is known to be 100. The null hypothesis, H_0: μ = 100, states that the mean of the population of premature children is 100; that is, the premature children are from the general population. The alternative hypothesis, H_1: $\mu \neq$ 100, states that the premature children come from a population with a mean IQ different from 100, that is, different from the overall population. This is a nondirectional hypothesis. We draw a random sample of n = 30 premature children, with mean $\bar{X}$ = 105 and standard deviation s = 16. The difference between this sample mean and the hypothesized population mean may be the result of chance, or it may indicate that premature children should not be considered part of the overall population. The researcher must determine the probability that one would observe a difference as large as 5 points by chance if the population mean for premature children is truly 100.

We begin by assuming that the null hypothesis is true; that is, the observed difference of 5 points is due to chance. We then ask, "How often would we expect to see a difference of 5 points or more if H_0 were true?" The answer is based on the defined properties of the normal sampling distribution and our desired level of significance, α = .05.

The z-Ratio

Recall from Chapter 17 that we can determine the area beyond any point in a normal distribution using values of z, or standard deviation units. For an individual sample score, X, a z-score represents the distance between that score and the sample mean, $\bar{X}$, divided by the standard deviation of the distribution (see Equation 17.8). When z is applied to a sampling distribution of means, the ratio reflects the distance between an individual sample mean, $\bar{X}$, and the population mean, μ, divided by the standard error of the mean:

$$z = \frac{\bar{X} - \mu}{s_{\bar{X}}} \tag{18.5}$$

For our example, $\bar{X}$ with = 105, s = 16, n = 30, and μ = 100, we calculate $s_{\bar{X}}$ = $16/\sqrt{30}$ = 2.9. Therefore,

$$z = \frac{105 - 100}{2.9} = \frac{5.0}{2.9} = 1.72$$

Therefore, the sample mean for premature children is 1.72 standard error units above the hypothesized mean of 100. The question we must ask is, "Does this difference represent a significant difference?" That is, is the difference large enough that we would consider the mean IQ of premature children to be different from 100?

Let us assume we could plot the sampling distribution of means of IQ for the general population, which takes the form of the normal curve. We know that 95% of the area under the curve is bounded by z = ±1.96, as shown in Figure 18.6. Therefore, there is a 95% chance that any one sample chosen from this population would have a mean within those boundaries. Said another way, it is *highly likely* that any one sample chosen from this general population would have a mean IQ within this range. Conversely, there is

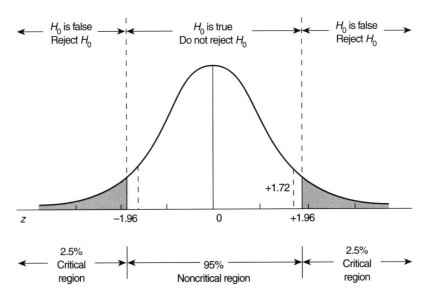

FIGURE 18.6 Standard normal distribution of z-scores showing critical values for a two-tailed test (nondirectional) at α_2 = .05 and the calculated z-score for IQ.

only a 5% chance that any sample mean would fall above or below those points. This means that it is *unlikely* that a sample mean from this general population would have a z-score greater than ±1.96. Any value that has only a 5% chance of occurring is considered unlikely, based on a .05 level of significance. In other words, if our sample yields a mean with a z-ratio beyond ±1.96, it is unlikely that that sample is from the general population (H_1). If the sample mean of IQ for premature children falls within z = ±1.96, then there is a 95% chance that the sample comes from a population with μ = 100 (H_0).

The Critical Region

The tails of the curve depicted in Figure 18.6, representing the area above and below z = ±1.96, encompass the **critical region,** or the *region of rejection.* The value of z that defines these areas is the **critical value.** When we calculate z for our study sample, it must be *equal to or greater than* the absolute critical value if H_0 is to be rejected. If a calculated z-ratio falls within the critical region (z ≥ ±1.96), the ratio is *significant.* If the ratio is less than the critical value (z < ±1.96), it represents a difference that is likely due to chance.

In our example, z = 1.72 for the mean IQ of premature children. This value is less than the critical value of 1.96 and falls within the central *noncritical region* of the curve. Therefore, it is likely that this sample comes from a population with μ = 100, or the general population. In other words, the observed difference between the means of the general population and the sample of premature children is not large enough to be considered significant at α = .05. The difference between the sample mean and population mean is probably due to chance. We do not reject the null hypothesis.

Directional versus Nondirectional Tests

The process we have just described is considered *nondirectional* because we did not predict the direction of the difference between the sample means. Consequently, the critical region was established in both tails, so that a large enough positive or negative z-ratio would lead to rejection of the null hypothesis. This is considered a **two-tailed test.** For convenience, we can designate our level of significance as $\alpha_2 = .05$, to indicate a two-tailed probability with $\alpha/2$ in each tail.

The critical value, against which the calculated z-ratio is compared, is determined according to the specified level of significance. If $\alpha_2 = .05$, then a total of 5% of the curve must be in the two tails of the curve. Therefore, using Appendix Table A.1, we see that for $\alpha_2 = .01$ (.005 in each tail), the critical value of $z = \pm 2.576$. Similarly, for $\alpha_2 = .10$ (.05 in each tail), $z = \pm 1.645$.

When a researcher has sufficient reason to propose an alternative hypothesis that specifies which mean will be larger, a *directional* test can be performed. For example, we could hypothesize that the mean IQ of premature children is greater than 100, which is a directional hypothesis. In this case, it is not necessary to locate the critical region in both tails, because we do not expect a negative ratio. We are only interested in the positive tail of the curve. Therefore, we would perform a **one-tailed test.** We can specify the level of significance as $\alpha_1 = .05$ because the full 5% will be located in one tail of the curve. The critical value will now represent that point at which the area in the positive tail equals 5% of the total curve. Using Table A.1, we find that this area starts at $z = 1.645$, as shown in Figure 18.7. We are hypothesizing that there is only a 5% chance that any sample chosen from the general population would have a mean IQ above $z = 1.645$. The value of the calculated z-ratio must be greater than or equal to 1.645 to be considered significant. Based on our example, $z = 1.72$ would now fall in the critical region,

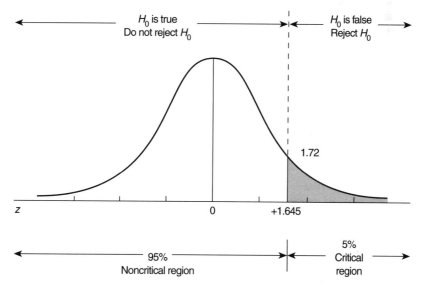

FIGURE 18.7 Standard normal distribution of z-scores showing critical values for a one-tailed test (directional) at $\alpha_1 = .05$ and the calculated z-score for IQ.

and, therefore, be considered significant. With a one-tailed test, we would reject the null hypothesis.

One-Tailed or Two-Tailed?

Note that the z-ratio in this example is considered significant with a one-tailed test, but not with a two-tailed test, because the critical value for the one-tailed test is lower. Therefore, the one-tailed test is more powerful; that is, one is less likely to commit a Type II error using the one-tailed test. One would think, then, that researchers would routinely use one-tailed tests, making it easier to attain significance. This situation has sparked many debates about the appropriate use of directional and nondirectional alternative hypotheses. Some statisticians favor exclusive use of two-tailed (nondirectional) tests, based on a conservative and traditional approach to data analysis.[12] With this argument, one-tailed tests should only be used when it is impossible for the difference to go in the opposite direction. A test of IQ, for instance, would not fit this criterion. Others have argued that the rationale behind most research questions supports one-sided tests, especially in studies where a control or placebo group is involved.[13] These proponents argue that the ethics of research would demand that a study be based on a sound theoretical rationale that would identify an expected direction of difference.

We think the middle ground on this issue is most reasonable: Researchers are obliged to justify whether the research hypothesis is directional or nondirectional, and use the appropriate statistical approach.[14] This means that the decision to use a one- or two-tailed test is a reasoned one, not an arbitrary one, and certainly not made after data are collected and analyzed. With sufficient manipulation of statistics, almost any result can be given statistical significance. The interpretation of statistical outcomes is, however, based on the search for truth about clinical phenomena, not contrived outcomes. Therefore, if a researcher decides on the directionality of a test after the experimental results are known, the theoretical probabilities associated with the test cannot be considered an accurate representation of the data. It is also important to realize that if a directional hypothesis is proposed, and results go in the direction opposite to that expected, H_0 cannot be rejected because it is not possible to accept the alternative. Therefore, a one-tailed test should be applied only when a sound rationale can be provided. The choice of a one- or two-tailed test should always be specified prior to data analysis and should be reported with published data.

Degrees of Freedom

The last concept we introduce here is that of degrees of freedom (df). We can think of degrees of freedom geometrically, indicating the available directions of movement within a given space. A point on a line is free to move in one dimension only, and has one degree of freedom. A point in a three-dimensional space, such as a cube, has three degrees of freedom. Therefore, degrees of freedom refer to those components that are *free to vary* within a defined system.

In statistical terminology, degrees of freedom refer to the number of components that are free to vary within a set of data. For example, suppose we took five measurements with a sum of 30 and a mean of 6. Theoretically, any set of five numbers could be specified to equal a sum of 30; however, once four of the scores are known, the fifth is automatically determined. If we measured 8, 9, 10, and 11, then the fifth score would have to be -8 to get a total of 30. Therefore, this set of data has four degrees of freedom. Four values are free to vary, given the restrictions imposed on the data, in this case a sum of 30 with a mean of 6. In this situation, the degrees of freedom will equal one less than the number of scores, or $n - 1$. As we present statistical tests in the coming chapters, we will describe the rules for determining the degrees of freedom associated with specific procedures.

PARAMETRIC VERSUS NONPARAMETRIC STATISTICS

Statistics that are used to estimate population parameters are called **parametric statistics.** The validity of parametric tests is dependent on certain assumptions about the nature of data. The primary assumption is that samples are randomly drawn from parent populations with normal distributions. Therefore, the sample should be a useful representation of population "parameters." With small samples, or with distributions that have not been previously described, it may be unreasonable to accept this assumption. Tests of "goodness of fit" can be performed to determine how well data match the normal distribution (see Chapter 25). A second assumption is that variances in the samples being compared are roughly equal, or homogeneous. A test for *homogeneity of variance* can substantiate this assumption. A third assumption is that data are measured on the interval or ratio scales. Therefore, scores can be subjected to arithmetic manipulations to calculate means and standard deviations.

When statistical conditions do not meet these requirements, **nonparametric tests** can be used. Nonparametric tests make fewer assumptions about population data, and can be used when normality and homogeneity of variance criteria are not satisfied. They can be used effectively, therefore, with very small samples. In addition, they have been specifically developed to operate on data at the nominal and ordinal scales. Alternatively, data can be transformed to another scale of measurement, such as a logarithmic scale, to create distributions that more closely satisfy the necessary assumptions for parametric tests (see Appendix D).

Statisticians do not agree on absolute rules for using parametric or nonparametric procedures. The classical school insists that if all the assumptions behind parametric tests are not met, nonparametric tests should be used; however, parametric tests are generally considered robust enough to withstand even major violations of these assumptions without seriously affecting the validity of statistical outcomes,[15,16] including their use with ordinal data.[17] Many researchers prefer to use parametric procedures because they are generally considered more powerful. As this is not the appropriate forum to settle this debate, we take a moderate position and suggest that nonparametric tests are most useful when ordinal or nominal data are collected and when samples are small and normality cannot be assumed. When their application is justified, parametric tests are preferred because they are more powerful and more versatile with complex research designs. This issue is discussed further in Chapter 22.

A summary of parametric and nonparametric statistical tests can be found in Appendix B.

COMMENTARY

Statistical versus Clinical Significance

The emphasis placed on significance testing in clinical research must be tempered with an understanding that statistical tests are tools for analyzing data and should never be used as a substitute for knowledgeable interpretation of outcomes. A big difference exists between **statistical significance** and **clinical significance.** Statistical tests are not sensitive to units of measurement, nor can they be responsive to the practical or clinical implications of the data. Suppose we did a study that resulted in a significant difference between groups with means of 90 and 95 degrees shoulder range of motion. Knowing the inherent error in range of motion testing, could we reasonably conclude that 5 degrees represents a clinically important difference? A mean difference that is small can be statistically significant just because enough subjects were used in the experiment to make the test powerful; but the difference may be very unimportant. The word *significant* should not be used in research literature to mean important, conclusive, distinctive, or marked. Its use should be reserved for the reporting of statistical results. Confidence intervals offer one solution to this interpretation problem, as the values that define the confidence interval can be interpreted according to their clinical relevance. The researcher must determine when the observed difference is large enough to warrant corrective action or a change in practice. This concept is of great importance to clinical researchers, who should use statistics as a form of input to, but not the sole criterion for, clinical decisions. The researcher must have a thorough knowledge of the phenomenon being studied.

The converse of this reasoning is also important. When a test does not result in a statistically significant outcome, but the effect size is clinically meaningful, we should be aware of the possibility of Type II error, and not automatically assume that the treatment is not effective. The effect size can be an important benchmark to understand responses obtained with various instruments, such as health status measures, and for interpreting change in responses over time.[18] With new treatment approaches, we must consider the effect size over statistical significance to avoid discarding potentially important discoveries.[10]

As we search for the answers to research questions, we are constantly aware of the need to consider the validity of our design, measurements, and theoretical constructs. In addition to these elements, however, we must also consider the validity of analysis procedures, or **statistical conclusion validity** (see Chapter 9). We can start with a well-designed study, but our outcomes will not be meaningful unless we choose appropriate statistical tests and interpret them accurately. For example, we would want to know that we had sufficient power, that we have not violated the assumptions of the statistical procedure, and that our measurements are reliable.

This is an issue that must be addressed in the planning stages of a study. All too often statistical consultants are handed the results of a study and asked to help analyze the data. This requires retrospective definition of assumptions, often a frustrating task. It is impossible to correct deficiencies in design or data collection after the fact. A statistician should be consulted in the design phase of a study, to set the proper operational definitions, to determine appropriate procedures, and to ensure that the research question can be answered. There is no greater disappointment than the realization that months of hard work are fruitless because the data cannot be analyzed to generate the desired interpretation.

Because statistics are essential for interpreting clinical research, we must be educated consumers as we read reports of research and as participants in a study. We do not have to be statisticians to have a working knowledge that will allow us to be critical in the use of statistical information for clinical decision making. Read on!

KEY TERMS

inferential statistics
probability
sampling error
sampling distribution
standard error of the mean
    $(s_{\overline{X}})$
point estimate
interval estimate
confidence interval (CI)
t-distribution
degrees of freedom (df)
statistical hypothesis

null hypothesis (H_0)
significant effect
alternative hypothesis (H_1)
directional hypothesis
nondirectional hypothesis
Type I error
Type II error
level of significance
alpha (α)
beta (β)
power ($1-\beta$)
effect size (ES)

critical region
critical value
two-tailed test (α_2)
one-tailed test (α_1)
parametric statistics
nonparametric statistics
statistical significance
clinical significance
statistical conclusion
    validity

REFERENCES

1. Fitzgerald GK, Wynveen KJ, Rheault W, Rothschild B. Objective assessment with establishment of normal values for lumbar spinal range of motion. *Phys Ther* 1983;63:1776–81.
2. Bertoti DB. Effect of short leg casting on ambulation in children with cerebral palsy. *Phys Ther* 1986;66:1522–9.
3. Fisher RA. *The Design of Experiments.* 6th ed. New York: Hafner, 1951.
4. Ioannidis JP. Effect of the statistical significance of results on the time to completion and publication of randomized efficacy trials. *JAMA* 1998;279:281–6.
5. Matyas TA, Ottenbacher KJ. Confounds of insensitivity and blind luck: statistical conclusion validity in stroke rehabilitation clinical trials. *Arch Phys Med Rehabil* 1993;74:559–65.
6. Cohen J. *Statistical Power Analysis for the Behavioral Sciences.* 2d ed. Hillsdale, NJ: Lawrence Erlbaum, 1988.
7. Young MJ, Bresnitz EA, Strom BL. Sample size nomograms for interpreting negative clinical studies. *Ann Intern Med* 1983;99:248–51.
8. Freiman JA, Chalmers C, Smith H, Kuebler RR. The importance of beta, the type II error and sample size in the design and interpretation of the randomized control trial. *New Engl J Med* 1978;299:690.
9. Ottenbacher KJ. Statistical power and research in occupational therapy. *Occup Ther J Res* 1982;2:13.

10. Altman DG, Bland JM. Absence of evidence is not evidence of absence. *BMJ* 1995;311:485.

11. Green SB, Salkind NJ, Akey TM. *Using SPSS for Windows: Analyzing and Understanding Data.* Upper Saddle River, NJ: Prentice-Hall, 1997.

12. Fleiss JL. Some thoughts on two-sided tests. *J Controlled Clin Trials* 1987;8:394.

13. Peace KE. The alternative hypothesis: one-sided or two-sided? *J Clin Epidemiol* 1989;42:473–6.

14. Feinstein AR. Clinical biostatistics. XXXII. Biological dependency, hypothesis testing, unilateral probabilities and other issues in scientific direction vs statistical duplexity. *Clin Pharmacol Ther* 1975;17:498–513.

15. Kerlinger FN. *Foundations of Behavioral Research.* New York: Holt, Rinehart & Winston, 1973.

16. Nunally JC. *Psychometric Theory.* 2d ed. New York: McGraw-Hill, 1978.

17. Gaito J. Measurement scales and statistics: resurgence of an old misconception. *Psychol Bull* 1980;87:564–7.

18. Kazis LE, Anderson JJ, Meenan RF. Effect sizes for interpreting changes in health status. *Med Care* 1989;27:S178–S189.

19

The t-Test

The simplest experimental comparison involves the use of two independent groups created by random assignment. This design allows the researcher to assume that all individual differences are evenly distributed among the groups, so that the groups are equivalent at the start of the experiment. Statistically, the groups are considered random samples of the same population, and therefore, any observed differences among them should be the result of sampling error or chance. After the application of a treatment variable, the researcher wants to determine if the groups are still from the same population, or if their means can be considered significantly different. This determination is made through a test of statistical significance.

The purpose of this chapter is to introduce procedures for evaluating the comparison between two means using the *t*-test and confidence intervals. These procedures can be applied to differences between two independent samples or between scores obtained with repeated measures. These procedures are based on parametric operations and, therefore, are subject to all assumptions underlying parametric statistics. Recall from our discussion in Chapter 18 that the *t*-distribution is an analogue of the standard normal distribution, developed to represent smaller sampling distributions. The *t*-distribution was originally developed by W. S. Gossett in 1908, who wrote under the pseudonym of "Student."[1] Therefore, the *t*-test is often referred to as Student's *t*-test.

THE CONCEPTUAL BASIS FOR COMPARING GROUP MEANS

The concept of statistical significance for comparing means is based on the relationship between two sample characteristics: the mean and the variance. The difference between group means indicates the degree of separation *between* groups (the effect size). Variance measures tell us how variable the scores are *within* each group. Both of these characteristics represent sources of variability that are used to describe the extent of treatment effects.

Suppose we wanted to compare two randomly assigned groups, one experimental and one control, to determine if their performances were different. Theoretically, if the experimental treatment was effective, and all other factors were equal and constant, all subjects within a group would achieve the same score, but scores would be different between groups, as illustrated in Figure 19.1A. In this scenario, all the observed differences are due to the group assignment. There is a difference *between the groups,* but no variance *within the groups.* All differences among scores can be *explained* by the effect of treatment.

Now let us consider the more realistic situation when subjects within a group do not all respond the same way. As shown in Figure 19.1B, the scores in the treatment and control groups are variable, but we tend to see higher scores among those who received treatment. If we try to account for the observed differences among these scores, a portion of the differences can be *explained* by the treatment. However, the scores are also influenced by personal characteristics, inconsistencies in measurement, and a host of unknown behavioral and environmental factors. This variance within the groups is *unexplained,* due to all the other factors influencing the response. This unexplained portion is called **error variance.** The concept of statistical "error" does not mean mistakes or miscalculation. It refers to all sources of variability within a set of data that cannot be explained by the independent variable.

The distribution in Figure 19.1B is represented by a pair of curves. This graph shows means that are far apart, with few overlapping scores (the gray area) at one extreme of each curve. The curves show that the individuals in the treatment and control groups behaved very differently, whereas subjects within each group performed within a narrow range. In such a comparison, the null hypothesis would probably be rejected. These groups would be seen as different.

Contrast this with the distribution in Figure 19.1C, which shows the same means, but greater variability within the groups, as evidenced by the wider spread of the curves. Factors other than the treatment variable are causing subjects to respond very differently from each other. Here we find a great deal of overlap, indicating that many subjects from both groups had the same score, regardless of whether they received the experimental treatment. These curves reflect a greater degree of error variance. In this case, it is less likely that the treatment is differentiating the groups, and the null hypothesis would probably not be rejected. Any differences observed here are probably due to chance.

These subjective judgments are not adequate, however, for making research decisions. How do we objectively determine if observed differences between groups are true population differences or only chance differences? In other words, how do we decide if we should reject the null hypothesis? We make this decision on the basis of its *probability of being true.* This is what a test of statistical significance is designed to do.

The Statistical Ratio

The significance of the difference between group means is judged by a ratio derived as follows:

$$\text{Ratio} = \frac{\text{difference } between \text{ group means}}{\text{variability } within \text{ groups}}$$

The numerator represents the separation between the groups, which is a function of all sources of variance, including treatment effects and error. The denominator reflects the variability within groups as a result of error alone. Therefore, when H_0 is false, that is, when a treatment effect exists ($\mu_1 \neq \mu_2$), the ratio is conceptually represented as

$$\frac{\text{treatment effect} + \text{error}}{\text{error}}$$

When H_0 is true, that is, when no real treatment effect exists ($\mu_1 = \mu_2$), the ratio reduces to

$$\frac{\text{error}}{\text{error}}$$

As the treatment effect increases, the absolute value of this ratio gets larger. As the error variance increases, the ratio gets smaller, approaching 1.0. If we want to demonstrate that two groups are significantly different, this ratio should be as large as possible. Thus, we would want the separation between the group means to be large and the variability within groups to be small. We emphasize the **variance between** and **within** groups as essential elements of significance testing which will be used repeatedly as we continue our discussion. Most statistical tests are based on this relationship. We now examine how this ratio is applied to the *t*-test to determine the significance of the difference between two means.

Statistical Hypotheses

The null hypothesis for a two-level design states that the two population means are equal:

$$H_0: \mu_1 = \mu_2$$

The alternative hypothesis can be stated in a nondirectional format, $H_1: \mu_1 \neq \mu_2$, or a directional format, $H_1: \mu_1 > \mu_2$ or $H_1: \mu_1 < \mu_2$. Nondirectional hypotheses are tested using a two-tailed test of significance. Directional hypotheses are tested using a one-tailed test.

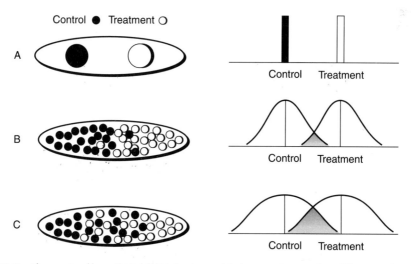

FIGURE 19.1 Three sets of hypothetical distributions with the same means, but different variances. In **(A)** all subjects in each group received the same score, but the groups were different from each other. In **(B)** the subjects' scores were more spread out, but the control and treatment conditions are still clearly different. In **(C)** the subjects are much more variable, and the groups are not distinctly different.

THE *t*-TEST FOR INDEPENDENT SAMPLES

The **independent** or **unpaired t-test** is used when two independent groups of subjects are compared. Such groups are usually created through random assignment, although samples of convenience or intact groups may be used.* Groups are considered independent because each is composed of an independent set of subjects, with no inherent relationship derived from repeated measures or matching.

Equality of Variance Assumption

The unpaired *t*-test is based on the assumption that the variances of the two groups are not different. This is called the assumption of **equality of variance** or **homogeneity of variance.** This assumption is routinely tested as part of the *t*-test in a computer analysis (see Tables 19.1 and 19.2). The two tests used most often for this purpose are *Levene's test* and *Bartlett's test*, both based on the *F* statistic. If variances are *not significantly different* ($p > .05$), then they are considered *equal.* When variances are unequal, an alternative formula for *t* is applied.

The *t* Statistic: Equal Variances

The test statistic for the unpaired *t*-test is calculated using the formula

$$t = \frac{\overline{X}_1 - \overline{X}_2}{s_{\overline{X}_1 - \overline{X}_2}} \tag{19.1}$$

The numerator of this ratio represents the difference between the independent group means, or the effect size. The term in the denominator is called the **standard error of the difference between the means,**[†] representing the variability within the two samples. Equation 19.1 can be used in situations when $n_1 = n_2$, or when $n_1 \neq n_2$ if variances are equal. An alternative formula for *t*, to be described shortly, is used when the assumption of equality of variance is not met.

We estimate $s_{\overline{X}_1 - \overline{X}_2}$ using a **pooled variance estimate,** given the symbol s_p^2:

$$s_p^2 = \frac{s_1^2(n_1 - 1) + s_2^2(n_2 - 1)}{n_1 + n_2 - 2} \tag{19.2}$$

where s_1^2 and s_2^2 are the group variances, and n_1 and n_2 are the respective sample sizes. This estimate provides a *weighted average* of s_1^2 and s_2^2.[‡] The pooled variance estimate is based on the assumption that both samples come from the same population and that

---

*When intact groups are used, regression procedures may be the more appropriate form of analysis because groups cannot be randomly assigned to treatment conditions. See Chapters 24 and 27 for a discussion of regression procedures.

[†]In Chapter 18 we introduced the concept of standard error as an estimate of population variability based on a sampling distribution of means. In this case we are estimating the variability in a sampling distribution of *differences between means*.

[‡]With two samples of equal size, this equation reduced to $s_p^2 = \dfrac{s_1^2 + s_2^2}{2}$

they have equal variances (any difference between variances is due to chance). Therefore, the pooled variance should estimate the population variance.

The standard error of the difference between the means is then given by[§]

$$s_{\overline{X}_1 - \overline{X}_2} = \sqrt{\frac{s_p^2}{n_1} + \frac{s_p^2}{n_2}} = \sqrt{s_p^2 \left(\frac{1}{n_1} + \frac{1}{n_2} \right)} \tag{19.3}$$

Degrees of Freedom

The number of degrees of freedom associated with the independent t-test is the total of the degrees of freedom for both groups. Therefore, $df = (n_1 - 1) + (n_2 - 1) = (n_1 + n_2 - 2)$. This can also be written $df = N - 2$, where N is the combined sample size.

Example

Suppose we are interested in testing the hypothesis that a newly designed splint will improve hand function of patients with rheumatoid arthritis, as measured by pinch strength in pounds. We propose a directional hypothesis (H_1: $\mu_1 > \mu_2$) because we are interested only in documenting an improvement in function. Results that show no change or a negative change would not be significant.

We assemble a random sample of 20 subjects with rheumatoid arthritis, with similar degrees of deformity in the hand and wrist. The subjects are randomly assigned to an experimental group ($n_1 = 10$) or a control group ($n_2 = 10$). The experimental subjects wear the splint for 1 week, in addition to participating in their regularly scheduled activities. The control subjects engage in similar activities, with no splint. Pinch strength is measured on day 1 and day 8 for both groups, and the change between the pretest and posttest measurements is used for analysis. Therefore, this study is structured as a pretest–posttest control group design, testing H_0: $\mu_1 = \mu_2$ against H_1: $\mu_1 > \mu_2$.

Hypothetical data are reported in Table 19.1A. The mean improvement in strength was 10.11 pounds for the splinted group and 5.45 pounds for the control group. The variances associated with these means are not significantly different (Levene's test, $p = .419$, Table 19.1D❷).

To calculate the t-ratio for this comparison, we first determine the value of the denominator, $s_{\overline{X}_1 - \overline{X}_2} = 1.714$, as shown in Table 19.1B. We substitute this value in Equation 19.1, and arrive at a *calculated* t-ratio of 2.718. Now we must determine if this calculated ratio is sufficiently large to be considered significant. We do this by comparing the calculated value with a **critical value** at a specified level of significance. The larger the ratio, the more likely the difference is *not* due to chance.

Critical Values of t

Table A.2 in the Appendix is a table of critical values associated with t-distributions for samples of various sizes. At the top of the table, levels of significance are identified for one-tailed (α_1) and two-tailed (α_2) tests. Because we proposed a directional alternative hypothesis in this example, we will perform a one-tailed test at $\alpha_1 = .05$.

[§]With equal sample sizes $s_{\overline{X}_1 - \overline{X}_2} = \sqrt{\dfrac{2s_p^2}{n}}$, where n is the number of subjects in each group.

TABLE 19.1. COMPUTATION OF THE UNPAIRED t-TEST (EQUAL VARIANCES): CHANGE IN PINCH STRENGTH FOLLOWING HAND SPLINTING

A. DATA	Group 1 (Splint)	Group 2 (Control)
	$\overline{X}_1 = 10.11$	$\overline{X}_2 = 5.45$
	$n_1 = 10$	$n_2 = 10$
	$s_1^2 = 13.81$	$s_2^2 = 15.58$

B. COMPUTATIONS

$$s_p^2 = \frac{s_1^2(n_1 - 1) + s_2^2(n_2 - 1)}{n_1 + n_2 - 2} = \frac{13.81(10 - 1) + 15.58(10 - 1)}{10 + 10 - 2} = 14.695$$

$$s_{\overline{X}_1 - \overline{X}_2} = \sqrt{\frac{s_p^2}{n_1} + \frac{s_p^2}{n_2}} = \sqrt{\frac{14.695}{10} + \frac{14.695}{10}} = 1.714 \qquad t = \frac{\overline{X}_1 - \overline{X}_2}{s_{\overline{X}_1 - \overline{X}_2}} = \frac{10.11 - 5.45}{1.7143} = 2.718$$

C. HYPOTHESIS TEST

$$H_0: \mu_1 = \mu_2 \quad H_1: \mu_1 > \mu_2 \qquad _{(\alpha_1 = .05}t_{(18)} = 1.734 \text{ (Table A.2)}$$
Reject H_0

D. OUTPUT

```
                        Independent t-test

  Group         n of cases       mean      std.dev.      std.err.

  SPLINT            10           10.110      3.716         1.175
  CONTROL           10            5.450      3.947         1.248

      ❶ mean difference 4.660       std.err. difference 1.714

  ❷ Levene's test for equality of variance    F = 0.685   p = .419

       t-test            t         df       2-tailed sig       CI

  Equal variances      2.718       18         .014❸       1.058, 8.262❹
  Unequal variances    2.718      17.935       .014       1.058, 8.263
```

❶ The difference between the means of group 1 and 2 (the numerator of the t-test). The standard error of the difference between the means (denominator of the t-test).

❷ Levene's test is not significant ($p = .419$). Therefore, we will use the t-test for equal variances.

❸ The two-tailed significance is .014. Because this analysis was based on a one-tailed test (directional alternative hypothesis), we use half of the two-tailed value. Therefore, $p = .007$. This is a significant test, and we reject H_0.

❹ 95% confidence interval does not contain zero. Therefore, the difference between the means is significant.

The column along the left side of the table, labeled *df*, identifies the degrees of freedom associated with different size samples. In this study there are $10 + 10 - 2 = 18$ *df*. We look across the row for 18 *df* to the column labeled $\alpha_1 = .05$ and find the critical value 1.734. We use the summary form

$$_{(\alpha_1 = .05)}t_{(18)} = 1.734$$

to indicate the critical value of *t* associated with $\alpha_1 = .05$ and 18 *df*.

For a *t*-ratio to represent a significant difference, the absolute value of the calculated ratio must be *greater than or equal to* the critical value. In a one-tailed test, the calculated ratio must also be of the appropriate sign; that is, the predicted direction of difference must be supported. In this example, the calculated value $t = 2.718$ is greater than the critical value 1.734. The ratio is positive, because $\overline{X}_1$ was larger than $\overline{X}_2$, as predicted. Therefore, the group means are considered significantly different at $\alpha_1 = .05$ (see Table 19.1C). We reject H_0 and accept H_1, and conclude that patients wearing the hand splint improved more than those in the control group.

One- versus Two-Tailed Tests

Note that each column in Table A.2 represents both a one- and a two-tailed probability. Note, too, that each two-tailed probability is twice its corresponding one-tailed probability. For instance, the critical value of *t* at $\alpha_1 = .05$ for 18 *df* is 1.734. This is also the critical value for *t* at $\alpha_2 = .10$. The critical value for $\alpha_1 = .01$ is the same as that for $\alpha_2 = .02$. Some statistical tables and computer packages provide values for only a one- or two-tailed test. If this occurs, it is a simple matter to convert the probability values. The probability reported for a one-tailed test is doubled to get a two-tailed test. Conversely, the probability reported for a two-tailed test is halved to get a one-tailed test. For instance, for the data in Table 19.1, we performed a one-tailed test. The computer output reports only a two-tailed significance (Table 19.1D❸). Therefore, to get the one-tailed significance we divide .014 by 2, and $p = .007$. Please be clear that it is the probabilities that are doubled or halved, not the critical values.

The astute reader will also note that the same calculated value of *t* may be significant for a one-tailed test but not for a two-tailed test; that is, critical values are lower for one-tailed tests at a given alpha level. In other words, the one-tailed test is more powerful. This occurs because one-tailed tests require proof in only one direction, and the full 5% probability can fall in one tail of the curve rather than being split between both sides. This concept is clarified in Chapter 18 (see Figures 18.6 and 18.7). Because of the different critical values associated with one- or two-tailed tests at the same probability level, the type of *t*-test used should always be specified in advance of data analysis and should be stated in a research report.

The Sign of t

Critical values of *t* are absolute values, so that negative or positive ratios are tested against the same criteria. The sign of *t* can be ignored when a nondirectional hypothesis has been proposed. The critical region for a two-tailed test is located in both tails of the *t*-distribution, and therefore a positive or negative value can be considered significant. The sign will be an artifact of which group happened to be designated group 1. If the groups were arbitrarily reversed, the ratio would carry the opposite sign, with no change in outcome.

The sign is of concern, however, when a directional hypothesis is proposed. In a one-tailed test, the researcher is predicting that one specific mean will be larger than the other, and the sign must be in the predicted direction for the alternative hypothesis to be accepted. If the difference is in the opposite direction to that predicted, the researcher cannot reverse the alternative hypothesis, and H_0 cannot be rejected. It is important, therefore, to be sure of direction when performing a one-tailed test.

The *t* Statistic: Unequal Variances

Studies have shown that the validity of the unpaired *t*-test is not seriously compromised by violation of the assumption of equality of variance when $n_1 = n_2$;[2] however, when sample sizes are unequal, differences in variance can affect the accuracy of the *t*-ratio. If a test for equality of variance shows that variances are significantly different, the *t*-ratio must be adjusted.

Consider the previous example, in which we examined the effect of a hand splint on pinch strength. Table 19.2 shows alternative data for this comparison, with unequal sample sizes ($n_1 = 15$, $n_2 = 10$). The variances in this analysis are significantly different (Levene's test, $p = .038$, Table 19.2D❷).

When the larger sample also has the larger variance, as in this example ($n_1 > n_2$ and $s_1^2 > s_2^2$), the *t*-test becomes less powerful; that is, fewer significant differences will be found. Therefore, this issue is moot if significant differences are obtained, but is of concern in cases where H_0 is not rejected.

This problem is of a different import when the smaller sample has the larger variance ($n_1 < n_2$ and $s_1^2 > s_2^2$), especially when one variance is more than twice the other. In this case, the probability of a Type I error is increased. A test that is significant at $p = .05$ may actually be significant at a higher probability, such as .09 or .12. This discrepancy increases as the relative sample sizes and variance differences become more disparate.[3] Obviously, this issue is of concern only when a significant difference is obtained.

When sample size and variances are unequal, the *t*-ratio is modified so that it is no longer based on a pooled variance estimate, but instead uses the *separate variances* of the two groups (see Table 19.2B):

$$t = \frac{\overline{X}_1 - \overline{X}_2}{\sqrt{\dfrac{s_1^2}{n_1} + \dfrac{s_2^2}{n_2}}} \tag{19.4}$$

The degrees of freedom associated with the *t*-test for unequal variances are also adjusted downward,[4] so that the critical value for *t* is also modified. In this example, 20.6 degrees of freedom are used to determine the critical value of *t* (see Table 19.2D❸).[||]

Computer packages will automatically run the *t*-test with both pooled and separate variance estimates, and will print out the *t*-values, degrees of freedom, and probabilities

---

[||]The adjusted degrees of freedom are determined according to: $df = \dfrac{(s_1^2/n_1 + s_2^2/n_2)^2}{(s_1^2/n_1)^2\left(\dfrac{1}{n_1 - 1}\right) + (s_2^2/n_2)^2\left(\dfrac{1}{n_2 - 1}\right)}$

TABLE 19.2. COMPUTATION OF THE UNPAIRED *t*-TEST (UNEQUAL VARIANCES): CHANGE IN PINCH STRENGTH FOLLOWING HAND SPLINTING

A. DATA	Group 1 (Splint)	Group 2 (Control)
	$\bar{X}_1 = 10.80$	$\bar{X}_2 = 5.65$
	$n_1 = 15$	$n_2 = 10$
	$s_1^2 = 25.17$	$s_2^2 = 4.89$

B. COMPUTATIONS

$$t = \frac{\bar{X}_1 - \bar{X}_2}{\sqrt{\dfrac{s_1^2}{n_1} + \dfrac{s_2^2}{n_2}}} = \frac{10.80 - 5.65}{\sqrt{\dfrac{25.17}{15} + \dfrac{4.89}{10}}} = \frac{5.15}{1.472} = 3.498 \qquad (19.4)$$

C. HYPOTHESIS TEST

$H_0: \mu_1 = \mu_2 \qquad H_1: \mu_1 > \mu_2 \qquad {}_{(\alpha_1 = .05)}t_{(20.6)} \cong 1.723$ (Table A.2)

Reject H_0

D. OUTPUT

```
                        Independent t-test

Group        n of cases        mean      std.dev.     std.err.

SPLINT           15           10.800       5.017        1.295
CONTROL          10            5.650       2.212        0.699

     ❶ mean difference 5.415      std.err. difference 1.472

❷ Levene's test for equality of variance   F = 4.866   p = .038

    t-test              t        df      2-tailed sig      95% CI

Equal variances      3.039      23           .006        1.644, 8.656
Unequal variances    3.498    20.625❸        .002❹       2.085, 8.215❺
```

❶ Difference between the means of group 1 and 2 (numerator of the *t*-test). Standard error of the difference (denominator of the *t*-test).

❷ Levene's test is significant ($p = .038$). Therefore, we will use the *t*-test for unequal variances.

❸ With 25 subjects, the adjusted total degrees of freedom for the test of unequal variances is 20.625.

❹ The two-tailed significance for the *t*-test is .002. This analysis was based on a one-tailed test (directional alternative hypothesis). The one-tailed significance level is half of the two-tailed value. Therefore, $p = .001$. This is significant, and we reject H_0.

❺ 95% confidence interval does not contain zero. Therefore, the difference between means is significant.

associated with a test for equal and unequal variances (see Table 19.1D). The programs will also show the results of the test for equality of variance. On the basis of these results, it is the researcher's task to choose which t values will be used for the analysis. In this instance, we will use the second line of data in the output, for unequal variances.

THE t-TEST FOR PAIRED SAMPLES

Researchers often use repeated measures or matched designs to improve the degree of control over extraneous variables in a study. In these designs subjects may be matched on relevant variables, such as age and intelligence, or any other variable that is potentially correlated with the dependent variable. Sometimes twins or siblings are used as matched pairs. More commonly, however, clinical researchers will use subjects as their own controls, exposing each subject to both experimental conditions and then comparing their responses across these conditions.

In these types of studies, data are considered *paired* or correlated, because each measurement has a matched value for each subject. To determine if these values are significantly different from each other, a **paired t-test** is performed. This test analyzes **difference scores (d)** within each pair, so that subjects are compared only with themselves or with their match. Statistically, this has the effect of reducing the total error variance in the data because most of the extraneous factors that influence data will be the same across both treatment conditions. Therefore, tests of significance involving paired comparisons tend to be more powerful than unpaired tests.

The t Statistic: Paired Data

The test statistic for paired data is based on the ratio

$$t = \frac{\bar{d}}{s_{\bar{d}}} \tag{19.5}$$

where $\bar{d}$ is the mean of the difference scores, and $s_{\bar{d}}$ represents the **standard error of the difference scores.**[#] This ratio also reflects the relationship of *between-* and *within-group* variance components. The numerator is a measure of the differences between pairs of scores, and the denominator is a measure of the variability within the difference scores.

The paired t-test is also based on the assumption that samples are randomly drawn from normally distributed populations with equal variances; however, because the number of scores in both treatment conditions must be the same, it is unnecessary to test this assumption with correlated samples.

Degrees of Freedom

The total df associated with a paired t-test are $n - 1$, where n is the number of pairs of scores.

Example

Suppose we set up a study to test the effect of using a lumbar support pillow on angular position of the pelvis in relaxed sitting. We hypothesize that pelvic tilt will change

---

[#] $s_{\bar{d}} = \dfrac{s_d}{\sqrt{n}}$, where s_d is the standard deviation of the difference scores.

with use of a support pillow (a nondirectional hypothesis). We test eight subjects, each one sitting relaxed in a straight-back chair with and without the pillow (in random order). The angle of the pelvic tilt is measured using a flexible ruler, with measurements transformed to degrees.

Because each subject is measured under both experimental conditions, this is a repeated measures design, testing the hypothesis H_0: $\mu_1 = \mu_2$ against H_1: $\mu_1 \neq \mu_2$, where means represent repeated conditions. These hypotheses may also be expressed in terms of difference scores: H_0: $\bar{d} = 0$ and H_0: $\bar{d} \neq 0$.

Hypothetical data are reported in Table 19.3A. A difference score, d, is calculated for each pair of scores. The standard deviation of these difference scores, s_d, is 4.62. Therefore, the standard error of the differences, $s_{\bar{d}} = 4.62 \sqrt{8} = 1.63$. By substituting values in Equation 19.5, we obtain $t = 8.74$ (see Table 19.3B and D).

The absolute value of the calculated ratio is compared with a critical value obtained from Table A.2, in this case for a two-tailed test with $N - 1 = 7$ df: $_{(\alpha_2 = .05)} t_{(7)} = 2.365$. Because the calculated value is greater than the critical value, these conditions are considered significantly different. Therefore, H_0 is rejected and H_1 is accepted (see Table 19.3C). Even though we have proposed a nondirectional hypothesis, we are justified in concluding that the pillow produces a decrease in pelvic tilt, based on the observed magnitude of the means for each treatment condition.

INAPPROPRIATE USE OF MULTIPLE *t*-TESTS

The *t*-test is one of the most commonly applied statistical tests. Unfortunately, it is also one of the most misused.[5] The sole purpose of the *t*-test is to compare two means. Therefore, when more than two means are analyzed within a single sample, the *t*-test is inappropriate. For instance, if we wanted to compare three types of exercise, it would be incorrect to use the *t*-test because the analysis involves three comparisons within one sample.

The problem with using multiple *t*-tests within one set of data is that the more comparisons one makes, the more likely one is to commit a Type I error, that is, to find a significant difference when none exists. Remember that α is the probability of committing a Type I error for any single comparison. At $\alpha = .05$, there is a 5% chance we will be in error if we say that group means are different. Although it is true that $\alpha = .05$ for each individual comparison, the potential *cumulative error* in a set of comparisons is actually greater than .05. Consider the interpretation that, for $\alpha = .05$, if we were to repeat a study 100 times when no difference really existed, we could expect to find a significant difference five times, just by chance. Five percent of our conclusions could be in error. For any one comparison, however, we cannot know if a significant finding represents one of the potentially correct or incorrect decisions. Theoretically, any one test could be in error. A logical argument can then be postulated—the more we repeat comparisons within a sample, the greater are our chances that one or more of those comparisons will fall into that 5% category.

This problem can be avoided by using the more appropriate *analysis of variance (ANOVA)*, which is a logical extension of the *t*-test specifically designed to compare more than two means. As an adjunct to the analysis of variance, *multiple comparison procedures* have been developed that control the Type I error rate, allowing valid interpretations of several comparisons at the desired α level. These procedures are discussed in Chapters 20 and 21.

TABLE 19.3. COMPUTATION OF THE PAIRED t-TEST: ANGLE OF PELVIS WITH AND WITHOUT A LUMBAR SUPPORT PILLOW

A. DATA

Subject	X_1 (without pillow)	X_2 (with pillow)	d
1	120	108	12
2	110	96	14
3	115	98	17
4	130	110	20
5	110	100	10
6	105	85	20
7	106	92	14
8	102	95	7
	$\Sigma X_1 = 898$	$\Sigma X_2 = 784$	$\Sigma d = 114$
	$\bar{X}_1 = 112.25$	$\bar{X}_2 = 98.00$	$\bar{d} = 14.25$
			$s_a = 4.62$

B. COMPUTATIONS

$$s_{\bar{d}} = \frac{s_d}{\sqrt{n}} = \frac{4.62}{\sqrt{8}} = 1.633 \qquad t = \frac{\bar{d}}{s_{\bar{d}}} = \frac{14.25}{1.63} = 8.742$$

C. HYPOTHESIS TEST

$H_0: \mu_1 = \mu_2 \qquad H_0: \mu_1 \neq \mu_2 \qquad _{(\alpha_2 = .05)}t_{(7)} = 2.365$ (Table A.2)

Reject H_0

D. OUTPUT

```
                          Paired t-test

Variable   n of cases   corr   sig      mean     std.dev.   std.err.

PILLOW                                  112.250    9.176      3.244
                8       .864❶  .006
NONE                                     98.000    8.159      2.884


   t-test none - pillow                          2-tailed
mean diff   std.dev.   std.err   t       df       sig       95% CI

14.250❷     4.621      1.633❸  8.742     7       .000❹   9.947, 18.553❺
```

❶ The analysis includes the correlation of pillow and non-pillow scores and significance of that correlation.

❷ Mean of the difference scores, $\bar{d}$ (numerator of the t-test).

❸ Standard error of the difference scores, $s_{\bar{d}}$ (denominator of the t-test).

❹ The computer generates a probability value with a precision of three places. This does not indicate a zero probability. The probability is some value less than .0001.

❺ 95% confidence interval of the difference scores does not contain zero, indicating a significant difference.

USE OF CONFIDENCE INTERVALS TO TEST DIFFERENCES BETWEEN MEANS

We can also use the *t*-distribution to construct confidence intervals around mean differences. Recall that a confidence interval specifies an interval or range of scores within which the population mean is likely to fall. For small samples, the 95% confidence interval is given by $\overline{X} \pm (t)s_{\overline{x}}$, where *t* is the critical value at $n - 1$ degrees of freedom at the desired level of α. Using a similar approach, we can set a confidence interval to estimate the *difference between group means* that exists in the population as follows:

$$95\% \text{ CI} = (\overline{X}_1 - \overline{X}_2) \pm (t)s_{\overline{X}_1 - \overline{X}_2} \tag{19.6}$$

where $s_{\overline{X}_1 - \overline{X}_2}$ is calculated using Equation 19.3. We will be 95% confident that the true *difference between population means* will fall within this interval.

Consider again the data shown in Table 19.1 for changes in pinch strength, with a difference between means of 4.66. The unpaired *t*-test is significant at $\alpha_1 = .05$, and H_0 is rejected. Now let us examine how we can use a confidence interval to arrive at the same conclusion.

We create the 95% confidence interval using $_{(a_2 = .05)} t_{(18)} = 2.101$ (from Table A.2). By definition, confidence intervals only look at two-tailed test values. The standard error of the difference between means is 1.714, calculated using the pooled variance estimate as shown in Table 19.1B. We substitute these values in Equation 19.6 to determine the 95% confidence limits:

$$95\% \text{ CI} = (10.11 - 5.45) \pm 2.101\,(1.714)$$

$$= 4.66 \pm 3.60$$

$$= 1.06 \text{ to } 8.26$$

We are 95% confident that the true mean difference, $\mu_1 - \mu_2$, lies between 1.06 and 8.26 (see Table 19.1D❹).

The null hypothesis states that the difference between two means will be zero. If we look carefully at the 95% confidence interval for these data, we see that the null value, zero, is not contained within it. As we are 95% confident that the true mean difference lies somewhere within this interval, it is unlikely that the true mean difference is zero. Therefore, we can reasonably reject H_0. This confirms the results of the *t*-test for these same data. If the confidence interval did contain zero (with confidence limits ranging from a negative to a positive value), then we would not reject the null hypothesis.

For the paired *t*-test, the same process will yield a confidence interval for the paired difference. The results, shown in Table 19.3, are obtained using the formula:

$$95\% \text{ CI} = \overline{d} \pm t(s_{\overline{d}})$$

Therefore,

$$95\% \text{ CI} = 14.25 \pm 2.635\,(1.633)$$

$$= 14.25 \pm 4.30$$

$$= 9.95 \text{ to } 18.55$$

We are 95% confident that the true difference in pelvic angle between the pillow and non-pillow conditions is between 9.95 and 18.55 degrees (see Table 19.3D❺).

COMMENTARY

The Significance of Significance

Researchers in many disciplines, epidemiologists and biostatisticians foremost among them, have become disenchanted with the overemphasis placed on reporting p values in research literature.[5] In an effort to make hypothesis testing more meaningful, investigators in these disciplines have relied on the confidence interval as a more practical estimate of a population's characteristics. The outcomes of hypothesis testing using either confidence intervals or t-tests will be the same; however, the confidence interval gives the researcher information not provided by the t-test. Rather than just indicating if two means are significantly different, the confidence interval essentially estimates true effect size; that is, it estimates how large a difference can be expected in the population. This information can then be used for evaluating the results of assessments and for framing practice decisions. Confidence intervals may be more clinically useful than relying on probability values when the magnitude of differences is relevant to clinical decision making and prediction of normal or abnormal responses.

KEY TERMS

error variance
between-groups variance
within-groups variance
unpaired t-test
  (independent t-test)
homogeneity (or equality)
  of variance

standard error of the
  difference between
  means ($s_{\overline{X}_1 - \overline{X}_2}$)
pooled variance estimate (s_p^2)
critical value
paired t-test

difference score (d)
standard error of the
  difference scores ($s_{\overline{d}}$)

REFERENCES

1. "Student." The probable error of a mean. *Biometrika* 1908;6:1.
2. Glass GV, Peckham PD, Sanders JR. Consequences of failure to meet assumptions underlying the fixed effects analysis of variance and covariance. *Rev Educ Res* 1972;42:237.
3. Scheffe H. *The Analysis of Variance.* New York: Wiley, 1959.
4. Cochran WG, Cox GM. *Experimental Designs.* 2d ed. New York: Wiley, 1957.
5. Ottenbacher K. A "tempest" over t-tests. *Am J Occup Ther* 1983;37:700–2.

20

Analysis of Variance

As knowledge and clinical theory have developed, clinical researchers have proposed more complex research questions, necessitating the use of elaborate multilevel and multi-factor experimental designs. The **analysis of variance** (ANOVA) is a powerful analytic tool for analyzing such designs, where three or more conditions or groups are compared. The analysis of variance is used to determine if the observed differences among a set of means are greater than would be expected by chance alone. The ANOVA is based on the F statistic, which is similar to t in that it is a ratio of between-groups treatment effects to within-group variability. The test can be applied to independent groups or repeated measures designs.*

The purpose of this chapter is to describe the application of the analysis of variance for a variety of experimental research designs. An introduction to the basic concepts underlying analysis of variance is most easily addressed in the context of a single-factor experiment (one independent variable) with independent groups. We then follow with discussions of more complex models, including factorial designs and repeated measures designs.

ANALYSIS OF VARIANCE FOR INDEPENDENT SAMPLES: ONE-WAY CLASSIFICATION

In a single-factor experiment, the one-way analysis of variance is applied when three or more independent group means are compared. The descriptor "one-way" indicates that the design involves one independent variable, or factor, with three or more levels.

---

*As with all parametric tests, the ANOVA is based on the assumption that samples are randomly drawn from normally distributed populations with equal variances. Tests for homogeneity of variance can be performed to validate the latter assumption. With samples of equal size, the analysis of variance is considered "robust" in that reasonable departures from the assumptions of normality and homogeneity will not seriously affect the validity of inferences drawn from the data.[1] With unequal sample sizes, gross violations of homogeneity of variance can increase the chance of Type I error. In such cases, a nonparametric analysis of variance can be applied (see Chapter 22), or data can be transformed to a different scale that improves homogeneity of variance within the sample distribution (see Appendix D).

Although the ANOVA can be applied to two-group comparisons, the t-test is generally considered more efficient for that purpose.[†]

Statistical Hypothesis

The null hypothesis for a one-way multilevel study is stated in the form

$$H_0: \mu_1 = \mu_2 = \mu_3 = \ldots = \mu_k$$

where k is the number of groups or levels of the independent variable. Usually a general alternative hypothesis is proposed that states that *at least two means* will differ. A set of specific alternative hypotheses can be proposed to indicate expected differences among subsets of means. For example, $H_1: (\mu_1 = \mu_2) \neq (\mu_3 = \mu_4)$.

Sums of Squares

In the last chapter we established that mean differences can be evaluated using a statistical ratio that relates the treatment effect to experimental error. The analysis of variance uses the same process, except that the ratio must now account for the relationships among several means. The F-test (named for Sir Ronald Fisher who developed the test) is used to determine how much of the total observed variability in scores can be explained by differences among several treatment means and how much is attributable to unexplained differences among subjects. To analyze this variability with several groups, we must refer back to the concept of **sum of squares (SS),** introduced in Chapter 17. The sum of squares is calculated by subtracting the sample mean from each score ($X-\bar{X}$), squaring those values, and taking their sum ($SS = \Sigma(X-\bar{X})^2$). The larger the sum of squares, the greater the variability of scores within a sample.

Example

To illustrate how this concept is applied to analysis of variance, consider a hypothetical study on the effect of using different types of assistive devices on step length in a population of above-knee amputees. Through random assignment, we create three independent groups: one using a cane, a second using crutches, and a third group to serve as a control, using no assistive device. We use a lowercase n to indicate the number of subjects in each group ($n = 5$) and an uppercase N to represent the total number of subjects in the study ($N = 15$). The independent variable, type of assistive device, has three levels ($k = 3$). Therefore, this is a single-factor, multilevel design. The dependent variable is stride length, measured in inches. Hypothetical data for this study are reported in Table 20.1A.

Total Sum of Squares

To estimate the total variability in these data, consider the set of 15 scores as one total sample, ignoring group assignment. We can calculate a mean for this total sample, called the **grand mean,** $\bar{X}_G$, around which all 15 scores will vary. For the data in Table 20.1, the

---

[†]The results of a t-test and analysis of variance with two groups will be the same. The t-test is actually a special case of the analysis of variance, with the relationship $F = t^2$.

TABLE 20.1. COMPUTATION OF ONE-WAY ANALYSIS OF VARIANCE FOR INDEPENDENT SAMPLES: STEP LENGTH (IN INCHES) WITH DIFFERENT ASSISTIVE DEVICES ($k = 3$, $N = 15$)

A. DATA	Group 1: Cane		Group 2: Crutches		Groups 3: Control	
	X_1	X_1^2	X_2	X_2^2	X_3	X_3^2
	9	81	8	64	6	36
	15	225	17	289	7	49
	16	256	9	81	8	64
	13	169	11	121	4	16
ΣX_i	65		55		30	
ΣX_i^2		875		655		190
$\bar{X}_i$	13		11		6	

B. COMPUTATIONS $\Sigma X = 65 + 55 + 30 = 150$ $\Sigma X^2 = 875 + 655 + 190 = 1720$

C. COMPUTATIONS

$$SS_t = \Sigma X^2 - \frac{(\Sigma X)^2}{N} = 1720 - \frac{(150)^2}{15} = 220 \tag{20.1}$$

$$SS_b = \sum \frac{(\Sigma X_i)^2}{n} - \frac{(\Sigma X)^2}{N} = \left[\frac{(65)^2}{5} + \frac{(55)^2}{5} + \frac{(30)^2}{5}\right] - \frac{(150)^2}{15} = 130 \tag{20.2}^a$$

$$SS_e = \Sigma X^2 - \sum \frac{(\Sigma X_i)^2}{n} = 1720 - \left[\frac{(65)^2}{5} + \frac{(55)^2}{5} + \frac{(30)^2}{5}\right] = 90 \tag{20.3}$$

D. COMPUTATIONS

$$df_b = k - 1 = 3 - 1 = 2 \qquad df_e = N - k = 15 - 3 = 12$$

$$MS_b = \frac{SS_b}{df_b} = \frac{130}{2} = 65 \qquad MS_e = \frac{SS_e}{df_e} = \frac{90}{12} = 7.5$$

$$F = \frac{MS_b}{MS_e} = \frac{65}{7.5} = 8.67$$

E. HYPOTHESIS TEST

$H_0: \mu_1 = \mu_2 = \mu_3$ $H_1: \mu_1 \neq \mu_2 \neq \mu_3$ $_{(\alpha=.05)}F_{(2,12)} = 3.89$

Reject H_0

F. OUTPUT: SUMMARY TABLE

Source of Variation	df	Sum of Squares	Mean Square	F	Sig.
Between Groups	2	130.00	65.00	8.67	.005
Within Groups (Error)	12	90.00	7.50		
Total	14	220.00			

---

[a] Note that the term $(\Sigma X_i)^2/n$ in equation 20.2 represents the square of the sum of scores within each individual group divided by the number of subjects in that group.

sum of all 15 scores is 150, and $\bar{X}_G = 10$. The sum of squares for this total sample repre-sents the square of the deviations of each individual score from the grand mean, $(X - \bar{X}_G)^2$. This *total sum of squares* (SS_t) reflects the *total variability* that exists within this set of data ($SS_t = \Sigma [X - \bar{X}_G]^2$).

Partitioning Sum of Squares

As we have described before, some of this total variability can be attributed to a treat-ment effect (*between* the groups), and the rest can be attributed to unexplained sources of variance, or **error variance,** among the subjects (*within* the groups). The analysis of variance partitions the total variance within a set of data (SS_t) into these two compo-nents. The *between-groups effect* reflects the spread of group means around the grand mean ($\bar{X} - \bar{X}_G$). The larger this effect, the greater the separation between the groups. The *within-groups effect* reflects the spread of scores within each group around the group mean, or the differences between subjects ($X - \bar{X}$).

Calculating Sums of Squares

To facilitate calculations, and to avoid rounding errors introduced by using the mean, we use computational formulas that have been developed for sum of squares. The val-ues needed for these computations are the individual scores (X) and their squares (X^2), as shown in Table 20.1A. In Table 20.1B we have calculated the sum of all scores, ΣX, and the sum of all squared scores, ΣX^2.

In Table 20.1C, the total sum of squares (Equation 20.1) is calculated, where N is the total number of subjects for all groups combined.[‡] We then calculate separate sums of squares for the between-groups effect (SS_b) and the within-groups error effect (SS_e) (Equations 20.2 and 20.3). The within-groups error sum of squares can be calculated us-ing Equation 20.3, or by subtraction using $SS_e = SS_t - SS_b$.

The *F* Statistic

Degrees of Freedom

The total degrees of freedom (df_t) within a set of data will always be one less than the to-tal number of observations, in this case $N-1$. In our example, $N = 15$ and $df_t = 14$. The number of degrees of freedom associated with the between-groups variability (df_b) is one less than the number of groups ($k - 1$), in this case $df_b = 2$. There are $n - 1$ degrees of freedom within each group, so that the number of degrees of freedom for the within-groups error variance (df_e) for all groups combined will be $(n_1 - 1) + (n_2 - 1) + \ldots + (n_k - 1)$, or $N - k$. For the data in Table 20.1, $df_e = 15 - 3 = 12$. The degrees of freedom for the separate variance components are additive, so that $(k - 1) + (N - k) = (N - 1)$.

[‡]Note that this is the same term used in the numerator for the computational formula of variance and standard deviation, which were defined in Chapter 17 (Equation 17.4).

Mean Squares

The concepts of between-groups and within-groups variability are once again used to define a statistical ratio. These sources of variability are defined as between-groups and error sums of squares. We convert the sums of squares to a variance estimate, or **mean square (*MS*),** by dividing each sum of squares by its respective degrees of freedom. A mean square can be calculated for the between- and within-variance components as follows:

$$MS_b = \frac{SS_b}{df_b} \qquad (20.4a)$$

$$MS_e = \frac{SS_e}{df_e} \qquad (20.4b)$$

The F-Ratio

Mean square values are used to calculate the **F statistic** as a ratio of the between-groups variance to the error variance:

$$F = \frac{MS_b}{MS_e} \qquad (20.5)$$

When H_0 is true and no treatment effect exists, the total variance in a sample is due to error, and MS_e is equal to or larger than MS_b, yielding an F-ratio of approximately 1.0 or less. When H_0 is false and the treatment effect is significant, the between-groups variance is large, yielding an F-ratio greater than 1.0. The larger the F-ratio, the greater the difference between the group means relative to the variability within the groups. In our example, $F = 8.67$, as shown in Table 20.1D.

Critical Values of F

Like t, the calculated F-ratio is compared with a critical value to determine its significance. Table A.3 in the Appendix contains critical values of F at $\alpha = .05$ and .01 (each in a separate subtable). Because mean squares are based on squared values, the F-ratio cannot be a negative number, and the F distribution will be skewed to the right. Therefore, we do not distinguish tails for an F-test.

The critical value of F for the desired α is located in the table by the degrees of freedom associated with the between-groups and error variances, with df_b across the top of the table and df_e along the side. For our example, $df_b = 2$ and $df_e = 12$ (always given in that order). Therefore, from Table A.3,

$$_{(.05)}F_{(2,12)} = 3.89$$

We compare this critical value with our calculated value, $F = 8.67$. The calculated value must be *greater than or equal to* the critical value to achieve statistical significance. In this case, we can reject H_0 and accept H_1. There is less than a 5% chance that the observed differences within the overall set of means are due to chance or experimental error alone.

A significant F-ratio does not indicate that each group is different from all other groups. Actually, it only tells us that there is a significant difference between at least two of the means (largest versus smallest). At this point, a separate test must be done to determine exactly where the significant differences lie. Various **multiple comparison tests** are described for this purpose in the next chapter. When the F-ratio is smaller than the critical value, H_0 is not rejected and no further analyses are appropriate.

The ANOVA Summary Table

Computer-generated output will present the results of an analysis of variance in a summary table that provides sums of squares and mean square data for determination of the F-ratio. The table presents data for the between-groups and error sources of variance, as shown in Table 20.1F. This table will often be included in the results section of a research report. Terminology used in the table will vary among computer programs and research reports. Rather than listing "between groups" as a source of variance, some researchers list the name of the independent variable. The error variance may be called the within-groups variance, residual, or between-subjects variance, or may be given the symbol S/A, which is read "subjects (S) within A," where A is the independent variable.

The probability level associated with the F-ratio is given in the last column of the summary table (as in Table 20.1F). Some researchers may simply indicate if the ratio has achieved significance, indicating $p < .05$, although most reports will include the exact probability obtained by computer analysis, as shown.

Some authors do not include summary tables in their research reports, choosing instead to report F-ratios in the body of the text. When this is done, the calculated value of F is given, along with the associated degrees of freedom and probability. For example, for the data in Table 20.1, we could say that there was a significant difference among the three experimental groups ($F = 8.67$, $df = 2,12$, $p = .005$). This practice is not problematic with single-factor analyses. Basically all relevant information is included in the parentheses. It does become somewhat cumbersome when multifactor analyses are reported.

ANALYSIS OF VARIANCE: TWO-WAY CLASSIFICATION

Because of the complexity of human behavior and physiological function, many clinical investigations are designed to study the simultaneous effects of two or more independent variables. This approach is often more economical than testing each variable separately and provides a stronger basis for generalization of results to clinical practice.

Example

As an example, let us assume we wanted to compare the effect of prolonged versus quick stretch for improving ankle range of motion against a control (Factor A). At the same time, we are interested in determining if the position of the knee during stretch (flexed or extended) will affect the outcome (Factor B). Instead of looking at each of these factors separately, we can examine their combined influence using a two-way factorial design. This design involves two independent variables: type of stretch

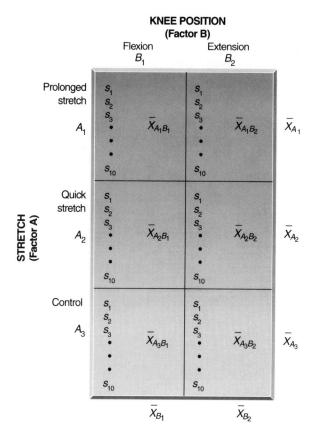

**KNEE POSITION
(Factor B)**

Flexion B_1 Extension B_2

FIGURE 20.1 Two-way (3×2) factorial design testing the effects of **(A)** stretch ($k = 3$) and **(B)** knee position ($k = 2$) on ankle range of motion. Sixty subjects are randomly assigned to each of six experimental conditions ($n = 10$). The marginal means for each independent variable are obtained by pooling data across the second variable.

(with three levels) and knee position (with two levels). Within the 3×2 framework are six treatment combinations. As shown in Figure 20.1, we can arrange the design in a table with six cells, so that rows correspond to type of stretch and columns to positions. Each cell represents a unique combination of levels for A and B. We could allocate 10 subjects per cell, for a total of 60 subjects. The design of factorial experiments was discussed in Chapter 10.

The appropriate statistical analysis for this design is a **two-way analysis of variance.** The descriptor "two-way" indicates a two-dimensional analysis, involving two independent variables. In this example, each variable is an independent factor (not repeated). The two-way ANOVA is an extension of the one-way analysis. It, too, partitions the total variance in the set of scores into between-groups and error components. The between-groups variance explains the independent variable effects, and the error variance accounts for all sources of variation unexplained by treatment; however, because the design incorporates two independent variables, the between-groups component must be further partitioned to account for the separate and combined effect of each independent variable. Therefore, we can ask three questions of these data:

1. What is the effect of variable A, independent of variable B?
2. What is the effect of variable B, independent of variable A?
3. What is the joint effect or interaction of variables A and B?

These components are called main effects and interaction effects, each explaining part of the total treatment effect.

Main Effects

In a two-way design, the effect of each independent variable can be examined separately, essentially creating two single-factor experiments. These effects are called **main effects,** illustrated in Figure 20.2. For instance, using the preceding example, we can study the main effect of stretch (Factor A) by collapsing or pooling data for the two knee positions. With 10 subjects in each of the original cells, we would now obtain a mean for 20 scores at each level of stretch ($\bar{X}_{A_1}, \bar{X}_{A_2}$, and $\bar{X}_{A_3}$ in Figure 20.2A). These three means represent the average between-groups effect of stretch, independent of the effect of knee position.

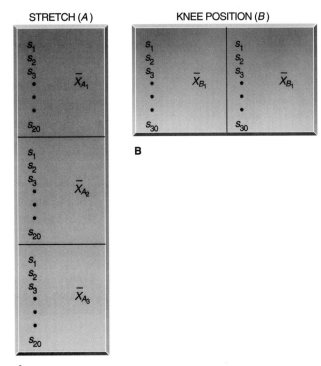

FIGURE 20.2 Diagrams of main effects for stretch treatment and knee position in a two-way factorial design.

The sum of squares associated with this main effect accounts for the separation among groups that received different forms of stretch.

Similarly, we can collapse the levels of stretch to obtain two means for the main effect of knee position (Factor B). There will be 30 scores per cell ($\overline{X}_{B_1}$ and $\overline{X}_{B_2}$), as shown in Figure 20.2B. These two means reflect the average between-groups effect of knee position, independent of type of stretch. A second sum of squares will be calculated to account for the separation between these two groups.

The means for levels of the main effects are called **marginal means.** They represent the average separate effect of each independent variable in the analysis. Comparison of the marginal means within each factor indicates how much of the variability in all 60 scores can be attributed to the overall effect of stretch alone or knee position alone.

Interaction Effects

In addition to the analysis of main effects, the factorial experiment has the added advantage of being able to look at combinations of levels of each independent variable. Statistically, these are referred to as **interaction effects.** Interaction is present when the effects of one variable are not constant across different levels of the second variable, that is, when various combinations of levels cause differential effects.

To illustrate this concept, consider the hypothetical means for dorsiflexion given for the six groups in Figure 20.3. Each mean represents a unique treatment combination of stretch

| | | Knee position *(B)* | |
| | | Flexion | Extension |
Stretch *(A)*		B_1	B_2
Prolonged	A_1	20	25
Quick	A_2	10	15
Control	A_3	3	8

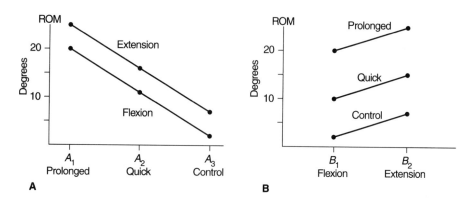

FIGURE 20.3 Plots of data showing no interaction between stretch treatment and knee position. Parallel lines indicate that responses on one variable are constant across the second variable.

and knee position. We can plot these means to more clearly illustrate these relationships. In Figure 20.3A, we have represented range of motion, the dependent variable, along the Y-axis. The three stretch groups are represented along the X-axis. The means for range of motion for each knee position are plotted at each level of stretch, with lines connecting the means. Note that in this example, the lines are parallel, which means that the pattern of response at each knee position is consistent across all levels of stretch. We can reverse the plot, as shown in Figure 20.3B, with knee position on the X-axis, demonstrating a constant pattern for each level of stretch across both knee positions. These graphs demonstrate a situation where there is no interaction; that is, prolonged stretch (A_1) will generate the greatest ankle response under both knee conditions and scores with knee extension are higher across all levels of stretch.

Now consider a different set of results for the same study, given in Figure 20.4. The plots for these data show lines that are not parallel; that is, the pattern of the baseline variable across all levels of the second variable is not constant. For example, in Figure 20.4A, the plot for knee flexion indicates little difference across levels of stretch. On the other hand, the line for knee extension shows a distinct difference for prolonged stretch. In Figure 20.4B, we see that the three flexion measures are fairly close (between 8 and 10 degrees), and two of the extension measures are also close (between 3 and 4 degrees), but the effect of prolonged stretch with knee extension is quite different. When lines are not parallel or when they cross, interaction is present. In this example, it is not the use of prolonged stretch alone that makes the treatment more effective. It is the combination of prolonged stretch with knee extension. Therefore, there is an interaction between the two in-

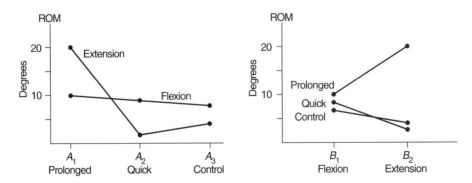

| Stretch (A) | | Knee position (B) | |
		Flexion B_1	Extension B_2
Prolonged	A_1	10.3	19.6
Quick	A_2	9.1	3.1
Control	A_3	8.0	3.6

FIGURE 20.4   Plots of data showing interaction between stretch treatment and knee position. Lines that are not parallel or that cross indicate that responses on one variable will vary depending on the level of the second variable. In this example, prolonged stretch with knee extension consistently produces a greater response than other combinations of the two variables.

dependent variables. The analysis of variance will account for this difference among the interaction means as a third component of the between-groups sum of squares.

The graphs shown in Figures 20.3 and 20.4 are called interaction plots, often used to visually clarify data from a two-factor analysis of variance. Although either factor can be plotted along the X-axis there will usually be one more informative way to present the graph, depending on how the relationship between variables will be interpreted. For example, we might be interested primarily in the effect of different types of stretching exercises, with knee position included as a variation of that exercise. Figure 20.4A is probably more useful for this interpretation, because it allows us to see how the ankle responses differ across the three levels of stretch at each separate knee position. If knee position were of primary interest, Figure 20.4B would be more meaningful.

Statistical Hypotheses

When two independent variables are examined in a single experiment, three statistical hypotheses are usually proposed, one for each main effect and one for the interaction effect. For example, for a 3×2 factorial design, the following hypotheses would be proposed:

1. $H_0: \mu_{A_1} = \mu_{A_2} = \mu_{A_3}$
2. $H_0: \mu_{B_1} = \mu_{B_2}$
3. $H_0: \mu_{A_1B_1} = \mu_{A_1B_2} = \mu_{A_2B_1} = \mu_{A_2B_2} = \mu_{A_3B_1} = \mu_{A_3B_2}$

An alternative hypothesis can be proposed for each null hypothesis. These hypotheses may be general statements of difference, or they may specify differences between specific means. An F-ratio is calculated to test each null hypothesis.

Presentation of Data for a Two-Way ANOVA

We have chosen not to include a mathematical example for a two-way analysis of variance, as we expect that all such analyses will be done by a computer. Those interested in details of the computations should refer to advanced statistical texts, such as those references given at the end of this chapter.[1-3] We will examine the format for presentation of results of a two-way ANOVA, as shown in Table 20.2.

TABLE 20.2. SUMMARY TABLE FOR A TWO-WAY ANALYSIS OF VARIANCE: EFFECT OF STRETCH AND KNEE POSITION ON ANKLE RANGE OF MOTION ($N = 60$) (DATA TAKEN FROM FIGURE 20.4)

Source	df	SS	MS	F	Sig.
Stretch(A)	2	1080.73	540.37	41.843	.000[a]
Position(B)	1	2.02	2.02	.156	.694
Stretch × Position (A × B)	2	707.72	353.86	27.401	.000
Error	54	697.36	12.91		
Total	59	2487.83			

[a]Computer programs will generate *p* values with a specified level of precision, that is, to a set number of decimal places. Therefore, a *p* value of .000 does not indicate zero probability. It simply means that the probability is <.0001, but the precision of the output does not allow the exact value to be printed.

Note that there are three between-groups sources of variance listed—two main effects and the interaction effect. These are often listed in the summary table according to the name of the independent variable. Alternatively, each variable may be given a letter designation, such as A and B, or the first letter of the variable name can be used. Thus, for our example, type of "stretch" (A) and "knee position" (B) are listed as main effects. The interaction between two variables is signified by an $\times$, such as Stretch $\times$ Knee Position ($A \times B$), read "stretch by knee position." The error term represents the unexplained variability between subjects within all combinations of A and B.[§]

Degrees of Freedom

The number of degrees of freedom associated with each main effect is one less than the number of levels of that independent variable ($k - 1$). To clarify this notation, we use ($A - 1$) degrees of freedom for Factor A, and $B - 1$ for Factor B, where the letters A and B represent the number of levels of each factor. Therefore, for stretch with three levels, $df = 2$. For knee position with two levels, $df = 1$. The number of degrees of freedom for the interaction between these variables is the product of their respective degrees of freedom, ($A - 1$)($B - 1$). Therefore, the interaction effect in this example has $2 \times 1 = 2$ degrees of freedom.

The total degrees of freedom associated with an experiment will always be one less than the total number of observations, $N - 1$. In this study, with $n = 10$ per group ($N = 60$), $df_t = 59$. The error degrees of freedom can be determined by using (A)(B)($n - 1$) with equal size groups or by subtracting the combined between-groups degrees of freedom from the total degrees of freedom. For this example, $df_e = (3)(2)(9) = 59 - 2 - 1 - 2 = 54$.

The F Statistic and Critical Values

Calculation of F is based on the ratio of between-groups to error mean squares. Mean square values are determined by dividing the sum of squares for each effect by its associated degrees of freedom. Each between-groups effect generates an F-ratio, based on its own mean square divided by the mean square for the common error term, MS_e. For example, for the data shown in Table 20.2, the F-ratios for the main effects of stretch (A) and knee position (B)[||] are obtained by

$$F_A = \frac{MS_A}{MS_e} = \frac{540.37}{12.91} = 41.86 \qquad F_B = \frac{MS_B}{MS_e} = \frac{2.02}{12.91} = .156$$

Similarly, the F-ratio for the interaction term, $A \times B$, is calculated according to

$$F_{AB} = \frac{MS_{AB}}{MS_e} = \frac{353.86}{12.91} = 27.41$$

where the subscript AB is used to denote the interaction between A and B.

[§]The error variance is sometimes given the abbreviation S/AB, which is read, "subjects within AB."
[||]The use of the subscript B to denote Factor B should not be confused with the use of subscript b to denote "between-groups" in previous examples. In this example, both A and B represent between-groups sources of variance for the two independent variables.

Each *F*-ratio is compared with a critical value from Appendix Table A.3. The degrees of freedom associated with the specific between-groups effect (main effect or interaction) are located across the top and the degrees of freedom associated with the error term are listed along the side. The critical values ($\alpha = .05$) for each effect shown in Table 20.2 are

$$\text{Stretch } (A) \qquad _{(.05)}F_{(2,54)} = 3.17$$

$$\text{Knee Position } (B) \qquad _{(.05)}F_{(1,54)} = 4.02$$

$$A \times B \qquad _{(.05)}F_{(2,54)} = 3.17$$

Therefore, this hypothetical ANOVA demonstrates a significant main effect for type of stretch and a significant interaction effect between stretch and knee position.

The ANOVA Summary Table

The information contained in an ANOVA table provides a convenient summary of a study's design and results. For example, from Table 20.2 we can tell that there are two independent variables, stretch and knee position, with three and two levels, respectively (by looking at degrees of freedom); that there are 60 subjects in the study ($df_t = N - 1 = 59$); and that the outcome was dependent on which type of stretch was used in a particular knee position.

Interpreting Interaction and Main Effects

Simple Effects

In most cases, researchers develop factorial designs with the expectation of specific patterns of interaction between the independent variables; that is, they hypothesize that certain combinations of treatments will be most effective. If this were not the case, the researcher could just as easily design separate one-way studies. Clinical interpretation of interaction is often facilitated by dividing the factorial design into several smaller "single-factor" experiments, each represented by the rows and columns in the design, as shown in Figure 20.5. These separate effects are called **simple effects.** Interaction is defined as a significant difference between simple effects.[2] Each line in an interaction plot (see Figures 20.3 and 20.4) represents a simple effect. Simple effects are distinguished from main effects which are based on averaged values across a second variable. An analysis of simple effects will reveal differential patterns within each of the independent variables. Such an analysis can be carried out on row effects, column effects, or both. With simple effects, the researcher can inspect the data to determine which levels of either variable contribute most to the observed differences. The analysis of simple effects is similar to carrying out several single-factor analyses of variance, with between-groups effects extracted from the larger factorial design.[#]

[#]See Keppel[2] and Green et al.[3] for detailed discussion of statistical procedures for analyzing simple effects.

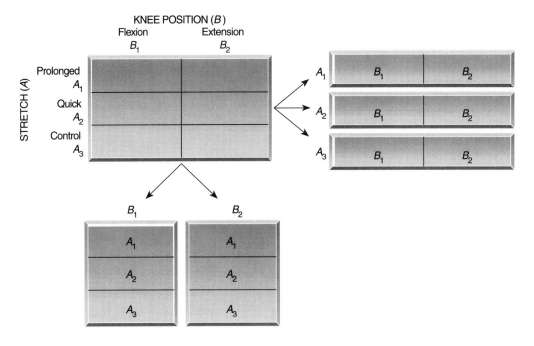

FIGURE 20.5   Simple effects for a 3 × 2 factorial design.

Main Effects

When there is no interaction effect in an experiment, the main effects are easily interpreted by referring to the outcome of the *F*-test for each independent variable. In that case, the analysis is essentially reduced to a one-way design, and combinations of treatments are ignored. If an interaction effect is present and main effects are not significant, interpretation is also straightforward; however, when an interaction effect is present, significant main effects are more difficult to interpret. For example, look again at the interaction plots in Figure 20.3. With no interaction present, it is easy to see that range of motion was consistently higher with the knee in extension and with prolonged stretch.

In Figure 20.4, where there is a significant interaction, the separate effects of knee position and type of stretch must be examined more carefully. In Figure 20.4A, with type of stretch (Factor A) along the baseline, we can see that the level of response at different knee positions changes at different levels of stretch. Therefore, we cannot draw any general conclusions about the main effect of knee position. This is called a *disordinal interaction* and the main effect of knee position is ignored in the interpretation of results. In Figure 20.4B, however, where knee position is plotted on the baseline, we can see that although prolonged stretch with knee extension shows the largest difference, it is also true that prolonged stretch is consistently above all other levels of stretch. This illustrates an *ordinal interaction,* where the relative ranking of the levels of Factor A does not change at different levels of Factor B. Therefore, it would be appropriate to conclude that, in general, treatment with prolonged stretch consistently results in greater range of motion than treatment with quick stretch or no stretch.

Multiple Comparisons

Multiple comparison tests are also used to compare means for each significant effect following an analysis of variance. For significant main effects, the marginal means are compared. For example, we would compare $\overline{X}_{A_1}, \overline{X}_{A_2}$, and $\overline{X}_{A_3}$ (Figure 20.2) to examine the main effect of stretch. When a main effect has only two levels, as with knee position in this example, a multiple comparison is unnecessary. The F-test functions like a t-test. Therefore, if F is significant, one need only look at the two main effect means to determine which is greater.

For significant interaction effects, the individual group means are compared. For example, we could determine which of the six combinations of stretch and knee position would produce the greatest changes in ankle range of motion. Based on the data shown in Figure 20.4, we might expect to find that prolonged stretch with knee extension (A_1B_2) elicits a more effective response than the other five combinations.**

ANALYSIS OF VARIANCE: THREE-WAY CLASSIFICATION

A multifactor analysis of variance can be performed with any number of independent variables, although we rarely see analyses beyond three dimensions. For example, we could expand the preceding study to look at the effects of stretch, knee position, and three forms of exercise for increasing ankle range of motion.

The analysis of a three-way design is a direct extension of the two-way ANOVA. With three independent variables, *A, B,* and *C,* the total variability in the data is divided into seven parts: three main effects (one for each independent variable), three double interactions testing each pair of independent variables in combination ($A \times B$, $A \times C$, and $B \times C$), and a triple interaction ($A \times B \times C$) testing all possible combinations of the three variables.[††] A sum of squares is calculated for each of these effects, to account for their contribution to the total variance in the sample. As in other analyses, each main effect has k–1 degrees of freedom, and degrees of freedom for the interaction terms are the product of the degrees of freedom for each effect in the interaction. The total degrees of freedom will be $N - 1$, and the error term will have $(A)(B)(C)(n - 1)$ degrees of freedom. An F-ratio is calculated for each main effect and each interaction effect, using the mean square for the error term in the denominator.

The advantage of higher-order factorial designs is the ability to examine how combinations of several variables influence behavior. Because treatment variables rarely exist in isolation, this approach can greatly enhance the construct validity and generalization of research results to practice. Unfortunately, such designs can also become overly complex, requiring large numbers of treatment groups and subjects. In addition, because the statistical analysis breaks down the total variance into so many components, interaction tests for the ANOVA will generally have lower power.

One way to overcome this problem is to use a repeated measures design, where subjects are tested under all treatment conditions. This approach serves to decrease the overall sample size and to increase statistical power. This design is discussed in the following section. Of course, some phenomena cannot be studied with repeated

---

*See Tables 21.5 and 21.6 for results of multiple comparison tests for the analysis of variance shown in Table 20.2.
[††]These interactions are illustrated in Design 3b in Chapter 10.

measurements, such as the study we have described for increasing ankle range of motion. It would not make sense to test one subject in more than one treatment combination because of the potential carryover effects. Researchers will usually try to limit the number of variables within a single study because of these difficulties inherent in multifactor analysis.

REPEATED MEASURES ANALYSIS OF VARIANCE

Up to now we have discussed the analysis of variance only as it is applied to completely randomized designs. These designs, where subjects are randomly assigned to treatment groups, are also called *between-subjects designs* because all sources of variance represent differences between subjects (within a group and between groups). Clinical investigators, however, often use repeated factors to evaluate the performance of each subject under several experimental conditions. The repeated measures design is logically applied to study variables when practice or carryover effects are minimal and when differences in an individual's performance across treatment levels are of interest. This type of study can involve one or more independent variables.

In a repeated measures design, all subjects are tested under k treatment conditions. The analysis of variance is modified to account for the correlation among successive measurements on the same individual. For this reason, such designs are also called *within-subjects designs.* The statistical hypotheses proposed for repeated measures designs are the same as those for independent samples, except that the means represent treatment conditions rather than groups.

The statistical advantage of using repeated measures is that individual differences are controlled. When independent groups are compared, it is likely that groups will differ on extraneous variables and that these differences will be superimposed on treatment effects; that is, both treatment differences and error variance will account for observed differences between groups. With repeated measures designs, however, we have only one group, and differences between treatment conditions should primarily reflect treatment effects. Therefore, error variance in a repeated measures analysis will be smaller than in a randomized experiment. Statistically, this has the effect of reducing the size of the error term in the analysis of variance, which means that the F-ratio will be larger. Therefore, the test is more powerful than when independent samples are used.

Single-Factor Repeated Measures Designs

Example

The simplest repeated measures design involves one independent variable, where all levels of treatment are administered to all subjects. To illustrate this approach, let us consider a single-factor experiment designed to look at differences in isometric elbow flexor strength with the forearm in three positions: pronation, neutral, and supination. The independent variable, forearm position, has three levels ($k = 3$). Logically, this question warrants a repeated measures design, where each subject's strength is tested in each position.

In a repeated measures design, we are interested in a comparison across treatment conditions *within each subject.* It is not of interest to look at averaged group performance

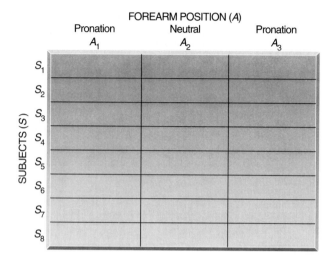

FIGURE 20.6 Diagram for a single-factor repeated measures design.

at each condition. Therefore, statistically, each subject is considered a unique block in the design. We can represent the design diagrammatically as shown in Figure 20.6, with rows corresponding to subjects ($n = 9$), and columns representing experimental conditions. Note that this diagram resembles a two-way factorial design, with forearm position as one independent variable and subjects as the other. Using this interpretation, each cell in the design has a sample size of $n = 1$. Each individual subject is considered a separate level of the independent variable *subjects.*

Using the format of a two-way analysis, the **repeated measures analysis of variance** will look at the main effect of forearm position (Factor A), the main effect of subjects (Factor S), and the interaction between these two factors. Because each cell in the design has only one score, there can be no variability within a cell. Therefore, the error term for this analysis is actually the interaction between subjects and treatment; that is, interaction reflects the inconsistency of subjects across the levels of treatment. This interaction represents the variance that is unexplained by the treatment variable and will serve as the denominator for the F-ratio. Calculations for a single-factor repeated measures analysis of variance are similar to those performed in a one-way ANOVA, except that an additional sum of squares is calculated for the effect of subjects (SS_s). These calculations are shown in Table 20.3.

Degrees of Freedom

The total degrees of freedom associated with a repeated measures design will equal one less than the total number of observations made, or $nk - 1$. In our example, $df_t = (9)(3) - 1 = 26$.

As in other analyses, the number of degrees of freedom associated with the main effects will be $k - 1$ for the independent variable, and $n - 1$ for subjects. The degrees of freedom for the error term are determined as they are for an interaction, so that $df_e = (k - 1)(n - 1)$. Table 20.4 shows these values for the current example in a summary table.

TABLE 20.3.   COMPUTATION OF A SINGLE-FACTOR REPEATED MEASURES ANALYSIS OF VARIANCE: ELBOW FLEXOR STRENGTH TESTED IN THREE FOREARM POSITIONS ($N = 9$)

A. DATA Subject	Pronation X_1	Neutral X_2	Supination X_3	ΣX_s	$(\Sigma X_s)^2/k$
1	10	18	20	48	768
2	12	20	19	51	867
3	38	51	52	141	6,627
4	14	22	27	63	1,323
5	28	37	43	108	3,888
6	9	25	26	60	1,200
7	21	29	31	81	2,187
8	7	23	24	54	972
9	17	23	20	60	1,200
ΣX_1	156	248	262		
ΣX_i^2	3,528	7,702	8,656		
$\bar{X}$	17.3	27.56	29.11		$\Sigma(\Sigma X_s)^2/k = 19{,}032$

B. COMPUTATIONS

$$\Sigma X = 156 + 248 + 262 = 666 \qquad \Sigma X^2 = 3{,}528 + 7{,}702 + 8{,}656 = 19{,}886$$

$$\frac{(\Sigma X)^2}{nk} = \frac{(666)^2}{27} = 16{,}428 \qquad \Sigma \frac{(\Sigma X_i)^2}{n} = \frac{(156)^2}{9} + \frac{(248)^2}{9} + \frac{(262)^2}{9} = 17{,}164.89$$

C. COMPUTATIONS

$$SS_t = \Sigma X^2 - \frac{(\Sigma X)^2}{nk} = 19{,}886 - 16{,}428 = 3{,}458 \tag{20.7}$$

$$SS_b = \Sigma \frac{(\Sigma X_i)^2}{n} - \frac{(\Sigma X)^2}{nk} = 17{,}164.89 - 16{,}428 = 736.89 \tag{20.8}$$

$$SS_s = \Sigma \frac{(\Sigma X_s)^2}{k} - \frac{(\Sigma X)^2}{nk} = 19{,}032 - 16{,}428 = 2{,}604 \tag{20.9}^a$$

$$SS_e = \Sigma X^2 - \Sigma \frac{(\Sigma X_i)^2}{n} - \Sigma \frac{(\Sigma X_s)^2}{k} + \frac{(\Sigma X)^2}{nk} = 19{,}886 - 17{,}164.89 + 16{,}428 = 117.11 \tag{20.10}$$

D. COMPUTATIONS

$$df_b = k - 1 = 3 - 1 = 2 \qquad df_e = (n-1)(k-1) = (8)(2) = 16$$

$$MS_b = \frac{SS_b}{df_b} = \frac{739.89}{2} = 368.44 \qquad MS_e = \frac{SS_e}{df_e} = \frac{117.11}{16} = 7.32$$

$$F = \frac{MS_b}{MS_e} = \frac{368.44}{7.32} = 50.34$$

E. HYPOTHESIS TEST $H_0: = \mu_1 = \mu_2 = \mu_3$ $H_1: \neq \mu_1 \neq \mu_2 \neq \mu_3$ $(\alpha = .05) F_{(2,16)} = 3.63$
Reject H_0

---

[a] The term ΣX_s in Equation 20.9 is the sum of scores across treatment conditions for each subject.

TABLE 20.4. RESULTS OF A REPEATED MEASURES ANALYSIS OF VARIANCE: ELBOW FLEXOR STRENGTH TESTED IN THREE FOREARM POSITIONS (DATA FROM TABLE 20.3)

Source	df ❶	SS	MS	F	Sig
Subjects	8	2604.00	325.50	❷	
Forearm Position	2	736.89	368.44	50.341	.000 ❸
Error	16	117.11	7.32		
Total	26	3458.00			

Mauchly's Test of Sphericity

				Epsilon ❺	
Mauchly's W ❹	Chi-Square	df	Sig	Greenhouse-Geisser	Huynh-Feldt
.664	2.861	2	.239	.749	.883

❶ Degrees of freedom associated with repeated measures effects.
❷ The program does not generate an *F*-ratio for the between-subjects effect.
❸ The repeated measure of forearm position is significant.
❹ Mauchly's Test of Sphericity is used to determine if adjustments to degrees of freedom are needed for the repeated measure. Many statistics are converted to familiar values to determine their associated probabilities. In this case, Mauchly's *W* is converted to chi-square for this purpose.
❺ Two versions of epsilon are used for the adjustment of *p*.

The F *Statistic*

The sums of squares for the treatment effect and the error effect are divided by their associated degrees of freedom to obtain the mean squares. These mean square values are then used to calculate the *F*-ratio for treatment according to

$$F_A = \frac{MS_A}{MS_{AS}} \tag{20.6}$$

where MS_A is the mean square for the treatment variable, and MS_{AS} is the mean square for the interaction of treatment and subjects, or the error term. As shown in Table 20.3D, the *F*-ratio for the treatment (*A*) effect is 50.34.

We can calculate an *F*-ratio for the effect of subjects, using $F_S = MS_S/MS_{AS}$; however, this is not a meaningful test. We expect subjects to differ from each other, and it is generally of no experimental interest to establish that they are different. The *F*-ratio for subjects is not given in most computer printouts (Table 20.4 ❷), and this effect is generally ignored in the interpretation of data.[‡‡]

The critical value for the *F*-ratio for treatment is located in Appendix Table A.3, using the degrees of freedom for treatment (df_b) and the degrees of freedom for the error

---

[‡‡]The one-way repeated measures ANOVA is used to generate MS values for calculation of models 2 and 3 of the ICC reliability coefficient (see Chapter 26). For interpretation of the ICC, it is useful to determine that the between-subjects effect is significant. These computations are easily done by hand if they are not generated in the computer analysis.

term (df_e). Therefore, the critical value for this effect will be $_{(.05)}F_{A(2,16)} = 3.63$. The calculated F-ratio exceeds this critical value and, therefore, is significant. The null hypothesis for treatment effects is rejected. The summary table shows that this difference is significant at $p < .0001$ (Table 20.4 ❸). We conclude that elbow flexor strength is related to forearm position. It will be appropriate at this point to perform a multiple comparison test on the three treatment means to determine which forearm positions are significantly different from the others.[§§]

Variance Assumptions with Repeated Measures Designs

We have previously discussed the fact that the analysis of variance is based on an assumption about the homogeneity of variances among treatment groups. This assumption is also made with repeated measures designs; however, with repeated measures we cannot examine variances of different groups because only one group is involved. Instead, the variances of interest reflect difference scores across treatment conditions within a subject. For example, with three repeated treatment conditions, A_1, A_2, A_3, we will have three difference scores: $A_1 - A_2$, $A_1 - A_3$, and $A_2 - A_3$. When used in this way with repeated measures, the homogeneity of variance assumption is called the **assumption of sphericity,** which states that the variances within each of these sets of difference scores will be relatively equal and correlated with each other.

We have also established that reasonable departures from the variance assumption would not seriously affect the validity of the analysis of variance, except in situations where sample sizes were grossly unequal. One might think, then, that violations of the variance assumption would be unimportant for repeated measures, where treatment conditions must have equal sample sizes, but this is not the case. Because the repeated measures test examines correlated scores across treatment conditions, it is especially sensitive to variance differences, biasing the test in the direction of Type I error. In other words, the repeated measures test is considered too liberal when variances are not correlated, increasing the chances of finding significant differences above the selected α level.

To address this concern, most computer programs will run a repeated measures ANOVA in two different ways, using multivariate and univariate statistics. Multivariate tests are preferable in that they do not require the assumption of sphericity. Several multivariate tests are usually run simultaneously, with unfamiliar names such as Pillai's Trace, Wilks' Lambda, Hotelling's Trace, and Roy's Largest Root. Because these tests are all based on different procedures, they are usually converted to a common reference, an F-ratio. These tests examine all possible sets of difference scores to determine if there is a significant difference among them. If they are significant, multiple comparison tests should follow. Because researchers are generally less familiar with these multivariate tests, they do not tend to be reported, but they appear prominently in computer output.

The second approach, used more often in clinical research, involves the standard repeated measures F-test, but with an adjustment to the value of p to account for possible

---

[§§]See Table 21.7 for an example of a multiple comparison for the repeated measures analysis of variance shown in Table 20.3.

violations of sphericity. A test called *Mauchly's Test of Sphericity* (Table 20.4❹) is performed first to determine if the adjustment is needed.[†] If the sphericity test is significant, correction is achieved by decreasing the degrees of freedom used to determine the critical value of *F*, thereby making the critical value larger. If the critical value is larger, then the calculated value of *F* must be larger to achieve significance. This compensates for bias toward Type I error by making it harder to demonstrate significant differences. Note that there is no difference in how the ANOVA is run, and the generated *F*-ratio with its associated degrees of freedom for the ANOVA remains unchanged. Only the probability associated with that *F* will change. This adjustment is only relevant, however, when the *F*-ratio is significant.

The degrees of freedom for the *F*-ratio are adjusted by multiplying them by a correction factor given the symbol **epsilon** (Table 20.4❺). Two different versions of epsilon are used: the **Greenhouse-Geisser (G-G) correction**[4] and the **Huynh-Feldt (H-F) correction.**[5] The Greenhouse-Geisser correction is usually considered first. If it results in a significant *F*, agreeing with the original analysis, then the probability associated with the Greenhouse-Geisser correction is used. When it does not result in a significant outcome, disagreeing with the original analysis, then the Huynh-Feldt correction is applied. These correction factors are shown in Table 20.4❺ for the one-way repeated measures analysis originally shown in Table 20.3, for the comparison of elbow flexor strength across three forearm positions. Because the test for sphericity is not significant ($p = .239$), we are not concerned about this adjustment. If the test for sphericity had been significant, however, the probabilities generated in the computer analysis for the ANOVA table would be the corrected ones.

Multifactor Repeated Measures Designs

The concepts of repeated measures analysis can also be applied to multifactor experiments. Such designs can include all repeated factors or a combination of repeated and independent factors. When all factors are repeated, the design is referred to as a repeated measures or within-subjects design. When a single experiment involves at least one independent factor and one repeated factor, the design is called a **mixed design.** We present the general concepts behind these types of analyses and describe the format for presentation of results. We base our examples on a two-factor design, although these concepts can be easily expanded to accommodate more complicated designs. Those interested in calculations for multifactor repeated measures designs should consult references given at the end of this chapter.[1,2,6]

Within-Subjects Designs

With two repeated factors, the design is an extension of the single-factor repeated measures design. Suppose we redesigned our previous example to study isometric elbow flexor strength with the forearm in three positions and with the elbow at two

---

[†]The power of Mauchly's test will vary with sample size.[3] With small samples it loses power. With large samples it may be significant even though the impact of violating the sphericity assumption is minor.

different angles. We would then be able to see if the position of the elbow had any influence on strength when combined with different forearm positions. In this 3×2 repeated measures design, if $n = 8$, each subject would be tested six times, for a total of 48 measurements.

With two repeated factors, variance is partitioned to include a main effect for subjects and for each treatment variable, as well as for subject by treatment interactions (forearm × subjects, elbow × subjects, and forearm × elbow × subjects). These interactions represent the random or chance variations among subjects for each treatment effect. The mean squares for these interaction terms are used to calculate an error term for each repeated main effect, as shown in Table 20.5. The assignment of degrees of freedom for each of these variance components follows the rules used for the regular two-way analysis of variance: for each main effect $df = k - 1$; for each interaction effect $df = (A - 1)(B - 1)$.

Each treatment effect in this study (forearm, elbow, and forearm × elbow) is tested by the ratio $F = MS/MS_e$, where the error term is the interaction of that particular treatment effect with subjects. As shown in Table 20.5❷, each repeated factor is essentially being tested as it would be in a single-factor experiment, with its own error term. By separating out an error component for each treatment effect, we have created a more powerful test than we would have with one common error term; that is, the error component is smaller for each separate treatment effect than it would be with a combined error term. Therefore, F-ratios tend to be larger. In this example, only the main effect of forearm position is significant ($p = .013$).

Once again, researchers will generally ignore ratios for the effect of subjects (Table 20.5❶). The effect of subjects is only important insofar as it is used to determine the error terms for the treatment effects. This effect will often be omitted from the summary table.

TABLE 20.5. SUMMARY TABLE FOR A TWO-FACTOR REPEATED MEASURES ANALYSIS OF VARIANCE: ELBOW FLEXOR STRENGTH WITH VARIATIONS IN THREE FOREARM POSITION AND TWO ELBOW POSITIONS ($N = 8$)

Source	df	SS	MS	F	Sig.
Subjects (S)❶	7	982.48	140.35		
Forearm (A)	2	1145.17	572.27	6.07	.013
Error (A × S) ❷	14	1319.83	94.27		
Elbow (B)	1	368.52	368.52	1.11	.327
Error (B × S)	7	22319.98	331.43		
Forearm × Elbow (A × B)	2	27.17	13.58	.12	.888
Error (A × B × S)	14	1587.83	113.42		

❶ The between-subjects effect is often eliminated from the summary table in a research report. It does not provide important information to the interpretation of the main or interaction effects, but is used in the determination of the error term for each effect.

❷ Each repeated measures effect is tested against its own error term, which is the interaction between that effect and the effect of subjects.

Mixed Designs

In a two-factor analysis, where only one factor is repeated, the overall format for the analysis of variance is a combination of between-subjects (independent factors) and within-subjects (repeated factors) analyses. In a mixed design, the independent factor is analyzed as it would be in a regular one-way analysis of variance, pooling all data for the repeated factor. The repeated factor is analyzed using techniques for a repeated measures analysis.

For example, suppose we wanted to look at the effect of ice applied to the biceps brachii on elbow flexor strength in three forearm positions. Ice (A) is an independent factor, and forearm position (B) is a repeated factor. Assume we have three levels of ice (ice pack, placebo, and control), and three levels of forearm position, as before. We randomly assign eight subjects ($n = 8$) to each ice group, for a total of 24 subjects ($N = 24$), each tested in three forearm positions.

The first part of the ANOVA for this type of study is an analysis of the independent factor, ice. Each level of this factor is assigned to eight different subjects. Comparison across these three groups is a *between-subjects* analysis, shown in Table 20.6 ❶. This is actually a one-way analysis of variance for the effect of ice, with two sources of variance: the between-groups effect (ice) and the within-groups variance, or error term. In this example, there is no significant difference among the three levels of ice ($p = .352$).

The table also shows the *within-subjects* analysis, or the analysis of all factors that include the repeated factor (Table 20.6 ❷). This section lists the main effect for forearm position (B), the interaction between forearm position and ice ($A \times B$), and a common error term to test these two effects. In this example, the main effect of forearm position is significant ($p < .0001$), as is the interaction effect ($p = .035$).

TABLE 20.6.   SUMMARY TABLE FOR TWO-WAY ANALYSIS OF VARIANCE WITH ONE REPEATED FACTOR (MIXED DESIGN): ELBOW FLEXOR STRENGTH WITH VARIATIONS OF ICE AND FOREARM POSITION (N :EQ 24)

Source of Variance	df	SS	MS	F	Sig.
Between subjects ❶					
Ice (A)	2	377.08	188.54	1.09	.352
Error	21	3606.18	171.72		
Total	32	3983.21			
Within subjects ❷					
Forearm (B)	2	1870.58	935.29	17.018	.000
Ice × Forearm (A × B)	4	629.83	157.46	2.865	.035
Error	42	2308.25	54.96		

❶ The between-groups effect is computed for the independent measure, ice. This section is a one-way analysis of variance.

❷ The within-subjects effect includes the repeated measure and the interaction of the repeated measure with the independent measure.

COMMENTARY

Beyond Analysis of Variance

The analysis of variance provides researchers with a statistical tool that can adapt to a wide variety of design situations. We have covered only the most common applications in this chapter. Many other designs, such as nested designs, randomized blocks, and studies with unequal samples, require mathematical adjustments in the analysis that are too complex for us to cover here. Fortunately, computer packages are readily available for performing analyses of variance, and are generally flexible enough to accommodate all the design variations that researchers might require in clinical research. The **general linear model (GLM)** is usually used to accommodate the variety of design options for the ANOVA.

The *t*-test and analysis of variance are based on several assumptions about the nature of data. We have reviewed these assumptions in several places in this and previous chapters. In general, these tests are robust to violations of these assumptions (with the exception of repeated measures designs), so that they can be used with confidence in most research situations; however, when clinical experiments are performed with very small samples, the data may violate these assumptions sufficiently to warrant transforming the data to a different scale of measurement that better reflects the appropriate characteristics for statistical analysis (see Appendix D), or it may be appropriate to use nonparametric statistics that do not make the same demands on the data. In Chapter 22 we describe several nonparametric tests that can be used in place of the *t*-test and the single-factor analysis of variance.

When the analysis of variance results in a significant finding, researchers are usually interested in pursuing the analysis to determine which specific levels of the independent variables are different from each other. Multiple comparison tests, designed specifically for this purpose, are described in the next chapter. At that time we look at some of the data presented here, and show how those data can be analyzed further using multiple comparison techniques.

As we continue to discuss statistical tests in subsequent chapters, many readers will find it helpful to refer to the chart provided in Appendix B, which presents an overview of statistical tests and criteria for choosing a particular test for analyzing different types of data and designs.

KEY TERMS

analysis of variance (ANOVA)
sum of squares (SS)
grand mean ($\bar{X}_G$)
error variance
mean square (MS)
F statistic
multiple comparison tests

two-way analysis of variance
main effects
marginal means
interaction effects
simple effects
repeated measures analysis of variance

assumption of sphericity
epsilon
Greenhouse-Geisser (G-G) correction
Huynh-Feldt (H-F) correction
mixed design
general linear model (GLM)

REFERENCES

1. Ferguson GA. *Statistical Analysis in Psychology and Education.* 5th ed. New York: McGraw-Hill, 1981.
2. Keppel G. *Design and Analysis: A Researcher's Handbook.* 2d ed. Englewood Cliffs, NJ: Prentice-Hall, 1982.
3. Green SB, Salkind NJ, Akey TM. *Using SPSS for Windows: Analyzing and Understanding Data.* Upper Saddle River, NJ: Prentice-Hall, 1997.
4. Geisser S, Greenhouse SW. An extension of Box's results on the use of the F distribution in multivariate analysis. *Ann Math Statist* 1958;29:885.
5. Huynh H, Feldt LS. Estimation of the Box correction for degrees of freedom from sample data in the randomized block and split-plot designs. *J Educ Statist* 1976;1:69.
6. Kirk RE. *Experimental Design: Procedures for the Behavioral Sciences.* 2d ed. Belmont, CA: Brooks/Cole, 1982.

21

Multiple Comparison Tests

When an analysis of variance results in a significant *F*-ratio, the researcher is justified in rejecting the null hypothesis and concluding that not all *k* population means are equal; however, this outcome tells us nothing about which means are significantly different from which other means. In this chapter we describe the most commonly used statistical procedures for deciding which population means are significantly different. These procedures are called **multiple comparison tests.**

Several multiple comparison procedures are available, most given names for the individuals who developed them. Each test involves the rank ordering of means and successive contrasts of pairs of means. The pairwise differences between means are tested against a critical value to determine if the difference is large enough to be significant. The major difference between the various tests lies in the degree of protection offered against Type I and Type II error. A conservative test will protect against Type I error, requiring that means be far apart to establish significance. A more liberal test will find a significant difference with means that are closer together, thereby offering greater protection against Type II error.

Most multiple comparison procedures are classified as **post hoc** because specific comparisons of interest are decided *after* the analysis of variance is completed. These are considered **unplanned comparisons,** in that they are based on exploration of the outcome. Therefore, these tests are most useful when a general alternative hypothesis has been proposed. We will describe the three most commonly reported post hoc multiple comparison procedures: Tukey's honestly significant difference method, the Newman-Keuls test, and Scheffé's comparison.*

Other multiple comparison tests are classified as **a priori,** or **planned comparisons,** because specific contrasts are planned *prior to* data collection based on the research rationale. Technically, these comparisons are appropriate even when an *F*-test is not significant, as they are planned before data are collected, and therefore, the

---

*Other post hoc tests used less often include *Duncan's Multiple Range Test*[2] and *Fisher's Least Significant Difference*.[3] These tests are generally considered too liberal, resulting in too great a risk of Type I error.[4, 5]

overall null hypothesis is not of interest. Although several planned comparison tests are available, we describe one commonly used method called the Bonferroni t-test.[†]

As many statistical computer packages do not include multiple comparison tests for the analysis of variance, it is useful to be able to perform these tests by hand. Fortunately, most multiple comparison procedures are simple enough to be carried out efficiently with a hand calculator once the analysis of variance data are obtained.

THE TYPE I ERROR RATE: PER COMPARISON VERSUS FAMILY

At the end of Chapter 19 we discussed the inappropriate use of multiple t-tests when more than two comparisons are made within a single set of data. This issue is based on the desired protection against Type I error, which is specified by α. At $\alpha = .05$, we limit ourselves to a 5% chance that we will be in error if we say that group means are different for any single comparison. We must differentiate this **per comparison error rate (α_{PC})** from the situation where α is set at .05 for each of several comparisons in one experiment. Although it is true that $\alpha = .05$ for each individual comparison, the potential cumulative error for the set of comparisons is actually greater than .05. This cumulative probability has been called the **familywise error rate (α_{FW})** and represents the probability of making at least one Type I error in a set or "family" of statistical comparisons.[‡]

The Type I error rate for a family of comparisons, where each individual comparison is tested at $\alpha = .05$, is equal to

$$\alpha_{FW} = 1 - (1 - \alpha)^c \tag{21.1}$$

where c represents the total number of comparisons. The maximum number of pairwise contrasts for any set of data will be $k(k-1)/2$. If we want to compare three means, testing each comparison at $\alpha = .05$, we will perform $c = 3(3-1)/2 = 3$ comparisons. Therefore,

$$\alpha_{FW} = 1 - (1 - .05)^3 = 1 - (.95)^3 = .143$$

This means that if we perform three t-tests and find three significant differences, there is a greater than 14% chance that at least one of these significant differences occurred by chance. This exceeds the generally accepted standard of 5% risk for Type I error.

As the number of comparisons increases, so does the probability that at least one significant difference will occur by chance. For example, with α_{PC} set at .05, tests involving four, five, and six means will result in the following familywise probabilities of Type I error:

(Four means: 6 comparisons) $\alpha_{FW} = 1 - (1 - .05)^6 = .26$

(Five means: 10 comparisons) $\alpha_{FW} = 1 - (1 - .05)^{10} = .40$

(Six means: 15 comparisons) $\alpha_{FW} = 1 - (1 - .05)^{15} = .54$

[†]Other types of planned comparisons include *orthogonal contrasts*, which allow for comparison of specific combinations of means, and *Dunnett's test*[6] which focuses on comparison of a control group with each of several experimental groups. See references for fuller discussions of these procedures.[1, 7, 8]

[‡]Some statistical references use the term *experimentwise error rate* to indicate the error for all effects within an experiment, whereas *familywise error rate* is used to indicate specific sets of effects, such as main effects and interaction effects in an analysis of variance.[7]

Clearly, the likelihood of finding significant differences among a set of means, even when H_0 is true for all comparisons, will be extremely high as the number of comparisons increases.

Several of the multiple comparison procedures we describe base their critical values on per comparison error rates; others base their Type I error rate on the entire family of comparisons. There is no consensus about preferences for one approach over the other. Use of a per comparison error rate will result in greater statistical power, but with the potential for more Type I errors. Conversely, use of the familywise error rate will produce fewer Type I errors, but will result in fewer significant differences. Researchers must determine if Type I or Type II error is of greater concern in a particular study and apply statistical tests accordingly. In most cases, one hopes to strike a balance between the two types of statistical error.

One-Tailed versus Two-Tailed Tests

Post hoc comparisons are usually tested using two-tailed probabilities. When specific contrasts are not specified in advance, it follows that directions of difference cannot be predicted. One-tailed tests can be performed for planned comparisons; however, unless evidence in favor of directional hypotheses is quite strong, it is generally statistically safer to perform two-tailed tests. Contrasts involving two-tailed tests will always be based on the absolute difference between means. One-tailed tests must result in a statistical ratio that supports the directional hypothesis.

STATISTICAL RATIOS FOR MULTIPLE COMPARISON TESTS

To illustrate the concept of multiple comparison tests, we will use a hypothetical study comparing the effects of ultrasound (US), ice, and friction massage for relieving pain in 44 patients with elbow tendonitis. The four group means, shown in Table 21.1A, represent the change in pain-free range of motion for three treatment groups and a control group. Eleven subjects were tested in each group. The null hypothesis for this study states that no differences exist among the four group means:

$$H_0: \mu_A = \mu_B = \mu_C = \mu_D$$

The analysis of variance for these data, shown in Table 21.1B, is significant, and it is now of interest to examine individual differences among means.

The process of testing differences among several means is fairly consistent for all multiple comparison procedures. In each test, means are first arranged in *order of size*, and differences between pairs of means are obtained, as shown in Table 21.1C. This table shows the absolute differences between all pairs of means, using a triangular format. With $k = 4$, there will be a total of $4(4 - 1)/2 = 6$ comparisons. The entries in the body of the table are the pairwise mean differences. Values are not entered below the diagonal to avoid redundancies. Each pairwise comparison, or contrast, is tested against a **minimum significant difference (MSD):**

$$| \bar{X}_1 - \bar{X}_2 | \geq \text{minimum significant difference}$$

If the absolute difference between a pair of means is *equal to or greater than* the minimum significant difference, then the contrast is considered significant. If the pairwise difference is smaller than the minimum significant difference, the means are not significantly different from each other.

TABLE 21.1.   DATA FOR MULTIPLE COMPARISON TESTS: CHANGE IN PAIN-FREE ELBOW ROM FOLLOWING TREATMENT FOR TENDONITIS ($N = 44$)

A. GROUP MEANS ($k = 4$)

(A) Ultrasound	$\bar{X}_A = 44.18$	$n_A = 11$
(B) Ice	$\bar{X}_B = 45.27$	$n_B = 11$
(C) Massage	$\bar{X}_C = 35.39$	$n_C = 11$
(D) Control	$\bar{X}_D = 24.18$	$n_D = 11$

B. ANALYSIS OF VARIANCE

Source	df	SS	MS	F	p
Between groups	3	3153.12	1051.04	11.83	.000
Within groups (Error)	40	3554.86	88.87		

C. TABLE OF MEAN DIFFERENCES

	Means	Control D 24.18	Massage C 35.39	Ultrasound A 44.18	Ice B 45.27
D	24.26	—	11.13	19.92	21.01
C	35.76		—	8.42	9.51
A	44.18			—	1.09

Calculation of the minimum significant difference is based on the error mean square, MS_e, taken from the analysis of variance, and a critical value taken from a statistical table. The MS_e reflects the degree of variance within groups (between subjects). Logically, the greater the variance within groups, the less likely we will see a significant difference between means. Critical values for the MSD are used differently, depending on the number of means being compared and the type of error rate used (per comparison or familywise). The relevant critical values are located according to the degrees of freedom associated with the error term, df_e, in the analysis of variance.[§] For the example we are using, the error mean square is 88.87, with 40 degrees of freedom (see Table 21.1B).

TUKEY'S HONESTLY SIGNIFICANT DIFFERENCE

Tukey developed one of the simplest multiple comparison procedures, which he called the **honestly significant difference (HSD)** method.[9] Tukey's procedure sets a familywise error rate, so that α identifies the probability that one or more of the pairwise com-

---

[§]It is not uncommon to find that the exact value for the error degrees of freedom is not listed in these tables. In that case, it is usually sufficient to refer to the closest value for degrees of freedom for an approximate critical value. To be conservative, the next lowest value for degrees of freedom should be used.

parisons will be falsely declared significant. Therefore, this test offers generous protection against Type I error.

Tukey's HSD test is calculated using the **studentized range statistic,** given the symbol q. Critical values of q are found in Appendix Table A.6. The q statistic is influenced by the overall number of means that are being compared. At the top of Table A.6, the number of means being compared is given the symbol r.[||] Logically, as the number of sample means increases, the size of the difference between the largest and smallest means will also increase, even when H_0 is true. The q statistic provides a mechanism for adjusting critical values to account for the effect of larger numbers of means.

Minimum Significant Difference

The minimum significant difference for Tukey's procedure is given by

$$\text{MSD} = q\sqrt{\frac{MS_e}{n}} \tag{21.2}$$

where MS_e is the mean square error, n is the number of subjects *in each group* (assuming equal sample sizes[#]), and q is taken from Appendix Table A.6, for the desired level of α, df_e, and the number of means, r. For the example we are using, $q = 3.79$ for $\alpha = .05$, $r = 4$, and $df_e = 40$. Therefore,

$$\text{MSD} = 3.79\sqrt{\frac{88.07}{11}} = 10.76$$

This minimum significant difference is compared with each pairwise mean difference in Table 21.2. Absolute differences that are equal to or greater than this value are significant. For example, the difference between the largest and smallest means ($\bar{X}_B - \bar{X}_D$) is equal to 21.01. This value exceeds the minimum significant difference and is, therefore, significant. To present these results in a clear format, an asterisk denotes those differences that are significant in Table 21.2. According to these results, the three experimental groups are different from the control, but the three treatment groups are not different from each other.

NEWMAN-KEULS METHOD

The **Newman-Keuls (NK) test** (sometimes called Student-Newman-Keuls test) is similar to the Tukey method, except that it uses a per comparison error rate.[4] Therefore, α specifies the Type I error rate for each pairwise contrast, rather than for the entire set of

---

[||]In this case, r stands for *range*. This symbol should not be confused with the use of the r for correlation coefficient.

[#]When samples are not of equal size, the *harmonic mean* of the sample size is used in calculations of the minimum significant difference. The harmonic mean, n', is equal to $\dfrac{k}{\Sigma\left(\frac{1}{n}\right)}$ where k is the number of groups, and n is the sample size for each group. Therefore, if there are two groups, with $n_1 = 10$ and $n_2 = 5$, $n' = \dfrac{2}{\left(\frac{1}{10} + \frac{1}{5}\right)} =$ 6.67. This procedure can be used with all multiple comparison tests.

TABLE 21.2. SIGNIFICANT DIFFERENCES (*) FOR TUKEY'S HSD TEST (α = .05)

A. MINIMUM SIGNIFICANT DIFFERENCE: 10.76

B. TABLE OF MEAN DIFFERENCES

	Control D	Massage C	Ultrasound A	Ice B
Means	**24.18**	**35.39**	**44.18**	**45.27**
D 24.18	—	11.13*	19.92*	21.01*
C 35.39		—	8.42	9.51
A 44.18			—	1.09

comparisons. Overall, then, as the number of comparisons increases, the chances of committing a Type I error are greater using this procedure than using Tukey's test.

The Newman-Keuls method is also based on the studentized range q; however, values of q are used differently for each contrast, depending on the number of *adjacent* means, r, within an ordered **comparison interval.** To illustrate how this is applied, consider the four sample means for the tendonitis study, ranked in ascending size order: D, C, A, B (see Figure 21.1). If we compare the two smaller means, the comparison interval D → C includes two adjacent means. Therefore, r = 2 for that comparison. If we compare the largest and smallest means, the interval D → B contains four adjacent means, D, C, A, and B (r = 4). Similarly, if we compare means C and B, the comparison interval C → B contains three adjacent means, C, A, and B (r = 3). Therefore, a comparison interval represents the steps between ordered means for a given comparison. As shown in Figure 21.1, with four means we will have intervals of two, three, and four means. In contrast to Tukey's approach which uses one critical difference for all comparisons, the Newman-Keuls test will use a larger critical difference as r increases. This adjusts for the fact that larger differences are expected with a greater range of means, even when H_0 is true.

Minimum Significant Difference

The minimum significant difference for the Newman-Keuls comparison is

$$\text{MSD} = q_{(r)}\sqrt{\frac{MS_e}{n}} \tag{21.3}$$

where values of $q_{(r)}$ are obtained from Table A.6 for each comparison interval. For the example we are using, we find q for α = .05 and df_e = 40 for comparison intervals of r = 2, 3, and 4:

$$q_{(r = 2)} = 2.86$$

$$q_{(r = 3)} = 3.44$$

$$q_{(r = 4)} = 3.79$$

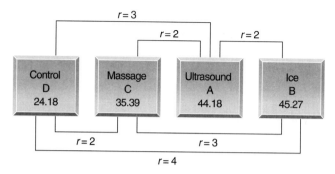

FIGURE 21.1 Comparison intervals for a set of four group means, arranged in size order. Based on data from Table 21.1.

With $MS_e = 88.87$ and $n = 11$, we find the corresponding minimum significant differences:

$$MSD\ (r = 2) = 2.86\sqrt{\frac{88.87}{11}} = 8.12$$

$$MSD\ (r = 3) = 3.44\sqrt{\frac{88.87}{11}} = 9.77$$

$$MSD\ (r = 4) = 3.79\sqrt{\frac{88.87}{11}} = 10.76$$

These minimum significant differences are compared with the appropriate mean differences in Table 21.3. Significant differences are noted with an asterisk. For example, the difference between means D and B is 21.01, which exceeds the critical difference 10.76 for $r = 4$. Therefore, these two means are significantly different. The difference between means C and B is 9.51, which does not exceed the critical difference 9.77 for $r = 3$. These two means are not significantly different from each other. Of the six comparisons, four are significant. This test demonstrates that the three experimental groups are different from the control, and ultrasound is different from massage.

The reader may note that the minimum difference for the Newman-Keuls test with $r = 4$ is the same as the minimum difference used for Tukey's test (in this case 10.76). The Tukey procedure uses this one minimum difference for all comparisons, whereas the Newman-Keuls test adjusts the minimum differences for smaller comparison intervals. Therefore, the minimum differences will be lower for some contrasts using the Newman-Keuls method. Consequently, the Newman-Keuls test results in a greater number of significant differences, and is the more powerful of the two comparisons; however, because the Newman-Keuls procedure does not control for the familywise error rate, it will produce a greater number of Type I errors than the Tukey method over the long run.

TABLE 21.3.   SIGNIFICANT DIFFERENCES (*) FOR NEWMAN-KEULS TEST ($\alpha = .05$)

A. MINIMUM SIGNIFICANT DIFFERENCES (MSD):

Comparison Intervals:	$r = 2$	MSD = 8.12
	$r = 3$	MSD = 9.77
	$r = 4$	MSD = 10.76

B. TABLE OF MEAN DIFFERENCES

	Control D	Massage C	Ultrasound A	Ice B
Means	**24.18**	**35.39**	**44.18**	**45.27**
D 24.18	—	11.13* ($r = 2$)	19.92* ($r = 3$)	21.01* ($r = 4$)
C 35.39		—	8.42* ($r = 2$)	9.51 ($r = 3$)
A 44.18			—	1.09 ($r = 2$)

SCHEFFÉ'S COMPARISON

The **Scheffé comparison** is the most flexible and most rigorous of the post hoc multiple comparison tests.[10] It is also popular with many researchers because it is based on the familiar F distribution. It is a conservative test because it adopts a familywise error rate that applies to all contrasts. This provides strong protection against Type I error, but it also makes the procedure much less powerful than the other tests we have described. Scheffé has recommended that a less stringent level of significance be used, such as $\alpha = .10$, to avoid excess Type II error.[11]

Minimum Significant Difference

The minimum significant difference for the Scheffé comparison is given by

$$\text{MSD} = \sqrt{(k-1)F}\sqrt{\frac{2MS_e}{n}} \tag{21.4}$$

where k is the total number of means involved in the set of comparisons, and F is the critical value for df_b and df_e obtained from Appendix Table A.3 (not the calculated value of F from the ANOVA). For the example we are using, $k = 4$ and $F = 2.84$ for 3 and 40 degrees of freedom at $\alpha = .05$. Therefore,

$$\text{MSD} = \sqrt{(4-1)\,(2.84)}\sqrt{\frac{2(88.87)}{11}} = 11.73$$

All differences between means must meet or exceed this value to be significant. Therefore, as denoted by asterisks in Table 21.4, this analysis results in two significant com-

TABLE 21.4.   SIGNIFICANT DIFFERENCES (*) FOR SCHEFFÉ'S COMPARISON

A. MINIMUM SIGNIFICANT DIFFERENCE: 11.73

B. TABLE OF MEAN DIFFERENCES

Means	Control D 24.18	Massage C 35.39	Ultrasound A 44.18	Ice B 45.27
D 24.18	—	11.13	19.92*	21.01*
C 35.39		—	8.42	9.51
A 44.18			—	1.09

parisons (less than with the Newman-Keuls or Tukey method), demonstrating the lower power associated with the Scheffé comparison. According to this test, the control and massage groups (D and C) are not significantly different from each other, where they were considered significantly different with the other tests.

BONFERRONI *t*-TEST

Researchers often designate specific contrasts of interest prior to data collection. These contrasts usually relate to theoretical expectations of the data. When comparisons are planned in advance and when they are relatively limited in number,** a priori tests can be used. The rationale for valid application of planned comparisons must be established before data are collected, so that the choice of specific hypotheses cannot be influenced by the data. Because the researcher is not necessarily interested in all possible contrasts, it is actually unnecessary to test the overall null hypothesis with the analysis of variance. Regardless of whether the ANOVA demonstrates a significant *F*-ratio, planned comparisons can be made.

The **Bonferroni *t*-test** (also called *Dunn's multiple comparison procedure*) is a planned comparison, using a familywise error rate that is the sum of the per comparison significance levels. Therefore, α_{FW} is dependent on the number of planned comparisons, *c*:

$$\alpha_{FW} \le \alpha_1 + \alpha_2 + \ldots + \alpha_c \tag{21.5}$$

For example, with four planned comparisons, each tested at $\alpha = .01$, the probability of one or more Type I errors for the entire family of contrasts is not greater than $\alpha = .04$. Essentially, the procedure splits α evenly among the set of planned contrasts, so that each contrast is tested at α_{FW}/c. Therefore, if a researcher wants an overall probability of .05 for a set of four contrasts, each individual comparison will have to achieve significance at .05/4, or $p = .013$. This process of adjusting α, called **Bonferroni's correction,** is used extensively as a protection against Type I error.

The Bonferroni test is based on Student's *t* distribution, with adjustments made for the number of contrasts being performed within a set of data. To facilitate these adjustments, a special table of critical values has been developed for Bonferroni's *t* [given the symbol *t*(B)].[12]

**Glass and Hopkins define a small number of comparisons as less than $k(k-1)/4$.[4]

Minimum Significant Difference

The minimum significant difference for the Bonferroni test can be computed using

$$MSD = t(B)\sqrt{\frac{2MS_e}{n}} \tag{21.6}$$

where $t(B)$ is taken from Appendix Table A.7 for α_{FW}, df_e, and c, where c is the total number of comparisons in the experiment. Continuing with the example we have been using, for six comparisons performed at $\alpha_{FW} = .05$, with $df_e = 40$, we find $t(B) = 2.77$. Therefore,

$$MSD = 2.77\sqrt{\frac{2(88.87)}{11}} = 11.13$$

All pairwise differences are compared with this one minimum significant difference, as shown in Table 21.5B by asterisks. In this case, three of the six comparisons are significant. According to these results, the three intervention groups are different from the control.

SIMPLE AND COMPLEX CONTRASTS

The contrasts we have described so far in this chapter are considered **simple contrasts** because they involve the comparison of pairs of means. We can also specify contrasts in terms of differences between subsets of means. For example, in the study of treatment for elbow tendonitis, we might want to compare the group that receives ultrasound with

TABLE 21.5.   SIGNIFICANT DIFFERENCES (*) FOR THE BONFERRONI *t*-TEST (α = .05)

A. MINIMUM SIGNIFICANT DIFFERENCE: 11.13

B. TABLE OF MEAN DIFFERENCES

	Control D 24.18	Massage C 35.39	Ultrasound A 44.18	Ice B 45.27
Means	24.18	35.39	44.18	45.27
D 24.18	—	11.13*	19.92*	21.01*
C 35.39		—	8.42	9.51
A 44.18			—	1.09

C. OUTPUT: Homogeneous Subsets of Means

			Subset for alpha = .05	
Bonferroni	Group	N	1	2
	D	11	24.18	
	C	11		35.39
	A	11		44.18
	B	11		45.27

both groups that do not receive thermal intervention (massage and control). The hypothesis for this comparison would be

$$H_0 : \mu_A = \frac{\mu_C + \mu_D}{2}$$

This is a **complex contrast** because it involves more than two means. The multiple comparison test will respond to the question, "Is the mean of Group A significantly different from the average of means of Groups C and D?" As the number of means in a study increases, the number of potential complex contrasts also increases. Complex contrasts are designed to answer specific questions in a research study that offer different theoretical explanations of the data. By looking at subsets of data, investigators can often clarify relationships that may not be evident with simple contrasts. Both the Scheffé and Bonferroni comparison procedures will handle complex contrasts.[4, 7, 8] See Kirk[1] and Keppel[7] for calculations of complex contrasts.

PRESENTATION OF RESULTS OF MULTIPLE COMPARISONS

The results of multiple comparison tests can be presented in several ways. The triangular matrix of mean differences has been illustrated throughout this chapter. Mean differences that are significant are usually starred within the body of the table. Many computer programs will generate output for multiple comparisons by listing *homogeneous subsets* of means. For example, the results of the Bonferroni *t*-test for the elbow tendonitis study could be reported as shown in Table 21.5C. The means that are listed together as a subset are considered homogeneous; that is, they are not significantly different. This output shows that means for C, A, and B are not different from each other, and that mean D is different from all other means.

A corresponding method uses underscoring to identify homogeneous subsets. Some authors choose to display the set of means arranged in ascending order, with a line drawn beneath means that are *not significantly different* from each other. Any means that are not underscored by the same line are significantly different. For example, the results of the Bonferroni *t*-test for the elbow tendonitis study, reported in Table 21.5C, could be given as follows:

Group	Control	Massage	Ultrasound	Ice
Mean	24.26	35.76	44.18	45.44

This presentation provides the same information in a concise space.

Many authors do not use tables, but choose to present the results of a multiple comparison within the narrative portion of a paper. With a limited number of comparisons this is often sufficient; however, when several measures are compared, a tabulated presentation may facilitate interpretation.

MULTIPLE COMPARISON PROCEDURES FOR FACTORIAL DESIGNS

Multiple comparison procedures are applicable to all analysis of variance designs. So far, we have described their use following an analysis with only one independent variable. When multifactor experiments are analyzed, the multiple comparison procedures can be used to compare means for main effects and interaction effects.

To illustrate this application, let us refer back to a study presented in Chapter 20, involving the comparison of stretch and knee position for increasing ankle range of motion. Factor A (stretch) had three levels: prolonged, quick, and control. Factor B (knee position) had two levels: flexion and extension. This design is shown in Figure 21.2. Ten subjects were tested in each of the six treatment combinations. Recall that the marginal means, $\bar{X}_A$ and $\bar{X}_B$, represent main effects for each independent variable separately. The six cells of the design (A_1B_1 through A_3B_2) represent all combinations of the two independent variables, or the interaction means.

The outcome of the analysis of variance for this study is shown in Table 20.2. The main effect of stretch is significant, as is the interaction effect. In practice, we would usually ignore the main effects because of the significant interaction, and proceed to analyze the six individual cell means. For purposes of illustration, however, we look at the main effect of stretch using a multiple comparison procedure. Had it been significant, we would not have to perform a multiple comparison for the variable of knee position because it has only two levels. Therefore, a significant effect could be interpreted by simply looking at the marginal means, as with a t-test.

Main Effects

The analysis of a significant main effect requires examination of differences among marginal means. For the main effect of stretch, we compare $\bar{X}_{A1}, \bar{X}_{A2}$, and $\bar{X}_{A3}$. The application of multiple comparison tests to marginal means is the same as in previous examples, except that n must reflect the total number of subjects contributing to each mean in a contrast. Therefore, if $n = 10$ for each cell in the design, then $n = 20$ for each marginal

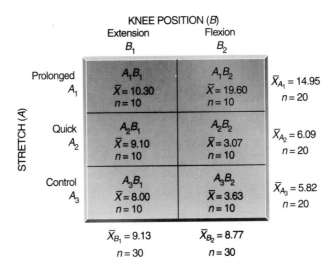

FIGURE 21.2   Two-way design (3 × 2) for a study comparing effect of type of stretch (Factor A) and knee position (Factor B) on ankle range of motion ($N = 60$). Six individual cell means are shown, as are marginal means for each independent variable.

mean for Factor A (see Figure 21.2). The values of MS_e and df_e used for calculations are taken from the analysis of variance summary table. In this case, $MS_e = 12.91$ and $df_e = 54$ (we will use $df_e = 60$ for locating tabled values).

To apply Tukey's HSD to these data, we calculate the minimum significant difference:

$$\text{MSD} = q\sqrt{\frac{MS_e}{n}} = 3.40\sqrt{\frac{12.91}{20}} = 2.73$$

with q taken from Table A.6 for $\alpha = .05$, $df_e = 60$, and $r = 3$. Note that $n = 20$ represents the pooled sample size for each marginal mean. The pairwise differences between the marginal means are shown in Table 21.6B. Differences that exceed 2.73 are significant. Results in Table 21.6C show that prolonged stretch ($\overline{X}_{A1}$) is significantly different from quick stretch ($\overline{X}_{A2}$) and the control ($\overline{X}_{A3}$), but that the latter two means are not significantly different from each other.

Interaction Effects

When an interaction effect is significant, multiple comparison tests are usually performed on pairwise contrasts of individual cell means. Formulas are used exactly as they were for the one-way design. In this example, we would be comparing six means.

TABLE 21.6. SIGNIFICANT DIFFERENCES (*) AMONG MARGINAL MEANS FOR MAIN EFFECT OF STRETCH USING TUKEY'S HSD TEST ($\alpha = .05$)

A. MINIMUM SIGNIFICANT DIFFERENCE: 2.73

B. TABLE OF MEAN DIFFERENCES

	A_1 Prolonged	A_2 Quick	A_3 Control
Means	14.95	6.09	5.82
A_1 14.95	—	8.86*	9.13*
A_2 6.09		—	0.27

C. OUTPUT: Homogeneous Subsets of Means

			Subsets	
Tukey's HSD	Group	N	1	2
	A3	20	5.82	
	A2	20	6.09	
	A1	20		14.95

If we choose to analyze all pairwise differences with $k = 6$, we will obtain $6(6-1)/2 = 15$ comparisons. To use Tukey's HSD as an example, we calculate the minimum significant difference:

$$\text{MSD} = q\sqrt{\frac{MS_e}{n}} = 4.16\sqrt{\frac{12.91}{10}} = 6.16$$

with q obtained from Table A.6 for $\alpha = .05$, $df_e = 60$, and $r = 6$. Note that $n = 10$ reflects the sample size for each of the six individual cell means.

The mean differences, shown in Table 21.7, must exceed this minimum significant difference to be considered significant. Results demonstrate that range of motion achieved with prolonged stretch with knee extension (A_1B_2) is significantly greater than with all other treatment combinations. In addition, prolonged stretch with knee flexion (A_1B_1) is greater than quick stretch and control with knee extension.

Interpretation of pairwise differences for interactions will often be more meaningful by limiting contrasts to row or column effects, eliminating comparisons that move diagonally within the design. In other words, we would probably not be interested in the contrast of prolonged stretch in flexion with the other forms of stretch in extension, which are diagonal comparisons (see Figure 21.2). This type of comparison is actually confounded, because it involves different levels of both variables. We are more interested in the contrasts across A_1, across A_2, and across A_3, and three contrasts within B_1 and within B_2. This would result in a total of 9 contrasts, rather than 15. When using tests such as Bonferroni's t, where the number of comparisons is the basis for adjusting critical values, this process can significantly improve statistical power as well as clarify explanations.

MULTIPLE COMPARISON PROCEDURES FOR REPEATED MEASURES

The standard post hoc multiple comparison procedures just described are not generally run for repeated measures analyses. Because repeated measures involve within-subject comparisons, the multiple comparison procedures do not logically fit, as they are based on over-

TABLE 21.7. SIGNIFICANT DIFFERENCES (*) AMONG INTERACTION MEANS FOR TYPE OF STRETCH AND KNEE POSITION USING TUKEY'S HSD TEST ($\alpha = .05$)

A. MINIMUM SIGNIFICANT DIFFERENCE: 6.16

B. TABLE OF MEAN DIFFERENCES

Stretch Knee Means	A_2B_2 Quick Ext 3.07	A_3B_2 Control Ext 3.63	A_3B_1 Control Flex 8.00	A_2B_1 Quick Flex 9.10	A_1B_1 Prolonged Flex 10.30	A_1B_2 Prolonged Ext 19.60
3.07	—	0.56	4.93	6.03	7.23*	16.53*
3.63		—	4.37	5.47	6.67*	15.97*
8.00			—	1.10	2.30	11.60*
9.10				—	1.20	10.50*
10.30					—	9.30*

all group differences. Therefore, the paired *t*-test has been used as a reasonable approach for looking at differences between pairs of means within a repeated measures design.[13, 14] Each pairwise comparison is entered as a difference score, and the analysis will determine which means are significantly different. For example, let us reconsider the hypothetical study described in Chapter 20 that looked at elbow flexor strength in three forearm position for nine subjects. The mean for pronation was 17.33, for neutral 27.56, and for supination 29.11 pounds. The results of the repeated measures analysis of variance showed that a significant difference existed among the three forearm positions (see Table 20.3). Therefore, a post hoc multiple comparison test is warranted to compare the three means.

Table 21.8 presents a summary of results of the paired *t*-test for three pairwise comparisons in this example. The differences for neutral-pronation and pronation-supination are significant ($p = .000$), but the difference for neutral-supination is not ($p = .127$). This analysis presents a problem, however, in terms of familywise error rate. Because several analyses are being run on the same sample, we risk inflating the value of α if each test is performed at the same .05 criterion. Therefore, this approach requires the use of a **Bonferroni correction,** whereby the overall value for α is divided by the number of comparisons. For instance, with three comparisons $\alpha_{FW} = .05/3 = .017$. This means that the p value for each individual comparison must be .017 or less to be considered significant. In our current example, with the two significant effects at $p = .000$, we have clearly achieved this criterion. However, if we had found a difference for any one comparison at .02, for example, where it would typically be considered significant at $\alpha = .05$, we would not consider it significant for this multiple comparison.

TREND ANALYSIS

Multiple comparison tests are most often used in studies where the independent variable is qualitative, or nominal, and where the researcher's interest focuses on determining which categories are significantly different from the others. When an independent variable is quantitative, the treatment levels no longer represent categories, but differing amounts of something, such as age, duration or intensity of a modality, dosage of a drug,

TABLE 21.8. PAIRED *t*-TEST FOR MULTIPLE COMPARISON OF THREE PAIRWISE CONTRASTS FOLLOWING REPEATED MEASURES ANOVA: ELBOW FLEXOR STRENGTH IN THREE FOREARM POSITIONS (DATA FROM TABLE 20.3)

A. PAIRED *t*-TESTS

Pair	Mean Diff	Std. Dev.	Std. Error	*t*	*df*	*Sig.*
Neutral-Pronation	10.22	3.77	1.26	8.140	8	.000
Supination-Neutral	1.56	2.74	.91	1.701	8	.127
Supination-Pronation	11.78	4.71	1.57	7.500	8	.000

B. TABLE OF MEAN DIFFERENCES

		Pronation	Neutral	Supination
	Means	17.33	27.56	29.11
	17.33	—	10.22*	11.78*
	27.56		—	1.56

or time intervals for repeated testing. When the levels of an independent variable are ordered along a continuum, the researcher is often interested in examining the shape of the response rather than differences between levels. This approach is called a **trend analysis.**

The purpose of a trend analysis is to find the most reasonable description of continuous data based on the number of turns, or "ups and downs" seen across the levels of the independent variable. For example, if we wanted to study the changes that occur in strength as one ages, we might study 10 blocks of subjects, each representing a different age category from 8 to 80 years old. A hypothetical plot of such data is shown in Figure 21.3. A multiple comparison of means will not tell us about the directions of change across age, but a trend analysis will.

Basically, trends are classified as either linear or nonlinear. In a **linear trend,** all data rise or fall at a constant rate as the value of the independent variable increases. This trend is characterized by a straight line, as shown in Figure 21.4A. For example, we might use this function to represent the relationship between height and age in children. As a child grows older, height tends to increase proportionally.

A *nonlinear trend* demonstrates "bends" or changes in direction. A **quadratic trend,** shown in Figure 21.4B, demonstrates a single turn upward or downward, creating a concave shape to the data. This means that following an initial increase or decrease in the dependent variable, scores vary in direction or rate of change. Learning curves can be characterized as quadratic. Performance generally increases at a sharp rate through early trials and then plateaus.

Higher-order nonlinear trends are more complex and are often difficult to interpret. As shown in Figure 21.4C and D, a *cubic trend* involves a second change of direction, and a *quartic trend* a third turn. As the number of levels of the independent variable increases, the number of potential trend components will also increase. There can be a maximum of $k - 1$ turns, or trend components, within any data set.

The curves in Figure 21.4 are examples of pure trends. Real data seldom conform to these patterns exactly. Even with data that represent true trends, chance factors will produce dips and variations that may distort the observed relationship. The purpose of a trend analysis is

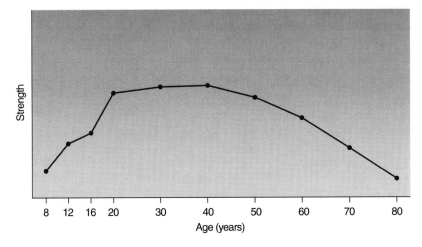

FIGURE 21.3   Hypothetical data for strength changes over 10 age ranges.

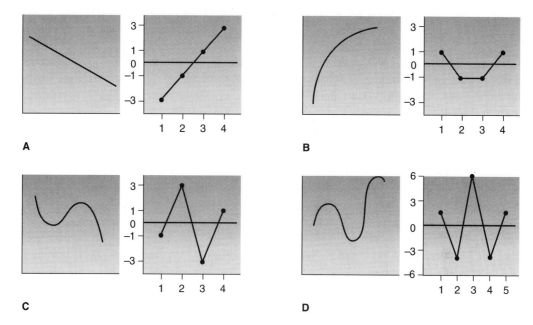

FIGURE 21.4 Examples of several types of trends: (**A**) linear trend, (**B**) quadratic trend, (**C**) cubic trend, (**D**) quartic trend.

to describe the overall tendency in the data using the least number of trend components possible. Some data can be characterized by a single trend; others demonstrate more than one pattern within a single data set. The hypothetical data for strength and age illustrate this possibility (Figure 21.3). The portion of the data from 8 to 20 years can probably be best described as linear, even though it is not perfectly straight. This indicates that individuals tend to get stronger as they grow within this age range. Many times slight dips, such as that seen at age 16, reflect random error in the sample studied, and are not indicative of true changes in direction. This would be hard to determine based on visual criteria alone, which is why a statistical trend analysis is needed. We can also see a quadratic component within this curve after age 20. Strength appears to plateau at age 30, after which a gradual dropoff is evident. One might even suspect that a second linear component exists after age 40.

Significance of Trend Components

Trends are tested for significance as part of an analysis of variance.[tt] The mathematical basis for analyzing trends is beyond the scope of the present discussion. Most statistical computer packages are able to run a trend analysis.[‡‡]

The results of trend analyses are listed as part of an ANOVA summary table. An example of this type of output for an independent samples test is given in Table 21.9, based

---

[tt]Those interested in mathematical computations of trends will find useful examples in Kirk,[1] Keppel,[7] and Ferguson.[8]

[‡‡]Some computer packages will refer to trend analyses as *orthogonal decomposition,*[15] or *orthogonal polynomial contrasts.*[16, 17]

TABLE 21.9. EXAMPLE OF AN ANALYSIS OF VARIANCE WITH A TREND ANALYSIS FOR INDEPENDENT SAMPLES: CHANGES IN STRENGTH ACROSS 10 AGE GROUPS (N = 100)

A. ANALYSIS OF VARIANCE

Source	df	SS	MS	F	Sig.
Age	9	750	83.33	5.40	.001
Error	90	1250	15.43		
Total	99	2000			

B. TREND ANALYSIS

Source	df	SS	MS	F	Sig.
Age	9	750	83.33	5.40	.001
Linear	1	230	230.00	14.91	.008
Quadratic	1	492	492.00	31.89	.000
Residual	7	28	4.00	0.26	.683
Error	90	1250	15.43		
Total	99	2000			

on the hypothetical age and strength data in Figure 21.3. The top portion of the table shows how the standard analysis of variance is presented. In the bottom portion, the trend analysis is added. Note that the between-groups sum of squares for the effect of age (SS_b = 750) has been partitioned into three parts: a linear trend (SS_{lin} = 230), a quadratic trend (SS_{quad} = 492), and a *residual* that represents all other possible trend components (SS_{res} = 28). Because there are 10 measurement intervals, we have the potential for 9 trend components; however, testing beyond the quadratic component usually yields uninterpretable results. Therefore, variance attributable to all higher-order trends is included in the residual variance. We can also see that the total degrees of freedom for these three trend components account for the possibility of 9 trend components.

Each specific trend component (linear, quadratic, and residual) is tested by an F-ratio, calculated using the mean square for that trend and the error term. In this example, both the linear and quadratic trends are significant. No higher-order trends are important to description of these data, based on the low residual variance. When a trend component is statistically significant, subjective examination of graphic patterns of the data is usually sufficient for further interpretation.

Limitations of Trend Analysis

Two important limitations should be considered when interpreting trend analyses. First, the number and spacing of intervals between levels of the independent variable can make a difference to the visual interpretation of the curve. Obviously, with only two levels of an independent variable no trend can be established. A linear trend requires a minimum of three points, a quadratic trend a minimum of four points, and so on. With larger spans in the quantitative variable, more intervals may be necessary.

Most investigators try to use equally spaced intervals to achieve consistency in the interpretation. Others will purposefully create unequal intervals to best represent the samples of interest. For instance, trends that are established over time may involve some intervals of hours and others of days. Most computer packages that perform trend analyses will accommodate equal or unequal intervals, but distances between unequal intervals must be specified.

The second caution for interpreting trend analysis is to avoid extrapolating beyond the upper and lower limits of the selected intervals. For example, based on Figure 21.3, if we had tested only individuals between 20 and 80, we might conclude that strength declines linearly with age. Conversely, if we looked only at ages 8 through 20, we might conclude that strength increases linearly with age. By limiting the range of intervals we would have missed the quadratic function that more accurately describes the relationship between strength and age across the life span. Therefore, the nature of the relationship between the independent and dependent variables should be examined within and across the ranges that will allow the most complete interpretation.

COMMENTARY

Choices, Choices, Choices

There are no widely accepted criteria for choosing one multiple comparison test over another, and the selection of a particular procedure is often made either arbitrarily or on the basis of available software; however, two basic issues should guide the choice of a multiple comparison procedure.

The first issue relates to the decision to conduct either planned or unplanned contrasts. This decision rests with the researcher during the planning stages of the study, in response to theoretical expectations. With planned comparisons, the researcher asks, "Is *this* difference significant?" With post hoc tests the question shifts to, "*Which* differences are significant?" When the researcher is interested in exploring all possible combinations of variables, unplanned contrasts should be used.

The second issue concerns the importance of Type I or Type II error. Each multiple comparison test will control for these errors differently, depending on the use of per comparison or familywise error rates. Of the three post hoc comparisons described here, the Newman-Keuls test is the most powerful. Scheffé's comparison gives the greatest control over Type I error, but at the expense of power. Researchers often prefer Tukey's HSD because it offers both reasonable power and protection against Type I error. The power of the Newman-Keuls procedure is increased by using different comparison intervals, but use of the per comparison error rate increases the risk of Type I error.

Researchers must examine the research question to determine which multiple comparison test is most appropriate in terms of the research design. These decisions should be based on the research question, not on which test is most likely to find significant differences. The decision to run planned or unplanned comparisons and simple or complex contrasts should be made before the data are analyzed. Other than these rather straightforward criteria, when there is no overriding concern for either Type I or Type II error, there may be no obvious choice for a specific test. The researcher is obliged to consider the rationale for comparing treatment conditions or groups and to justify the basis for making these comparisons.

KEY TERMS

multiple comparison tests
post hoc (unplanned)
  comparisons
a priori (planned)
  comparisons
per comparison error rate
  (α_{PC})
familywise error rate (α_{FW})

minimum significant
  difference (MSD)
Tukey's honestly significant
  difference (HSD)
studentized range statistic
  (q)
Newman-Keuls (NK) test
comparison interval (r)

Scheffé's comparison
Bonferroni t-test
Bonferroni's correction
simple contrast
complex contrast
trend analysis
linear trend
quadratic trend

REFERENCES

1. Kirk RE. *Experimental Design: Procedures for the Behavioral Sciences*. 2d ed. Belmont, CA: Brooks/Cole, 1982.
2. Duncan DB. Multiple range and multiple F tests. *Biometrics* 1955;11:1.
3. Fisher RA. *The Design of Experiments*. 6th ed. New York: Hafner, 1951.
4. Glass GV, Hopkins KD. *Statistical Methods in Education and Psychology*. 2d ed. Englewood Cliffs, NJ: Prentice-Hall, 1984.
5. Miller RG. *Simultaneous Statistical Inference*. New York: McGraw-Hill, 1966.
6. Dunnett CW. A multiple comparison procedure for comparing several treatments with a control. *J Am Statist Assoc* 1955;50:1096.
7. Keppel G. *Design and Analysis: A Researcher's Handbook*. 2d ed. Englewood Cliffs, NJ: Prentice-Hall, 1982.
8. Ferguson GA. *Statistical Analysis in Psychology and Education*. 5th ed. New York: McGraw-Hill, 1981.
9. Tukey JW. *The Problem of Multiple Comparisons*. Ditto: Princeton University, 1953.
10. Scheffé HA. A method for judging all contrasts in the analysis of variance. *Biometrika* 1953;40:87.
11. Scheffé HA. *The Analysis of Variance*. New York: Wiley, 1959.
12. Dunn OJ. Multiple comparison among means. *J Am Statist Assoc* 1961;56:52.
13. Green SB, Salkind NJ, Akey TM. *Using SPSS for Windows: Analyzing and Understanding Data*. Upper Saddle River, NJ: Prentice-Hall, 1997.
14. Maxwell SE. Pairwise multiple comparisons in repeated measures designs. *J Educ Stat* 1980;5:269–87.
15. Dixon WJ. BMDP Statistical Software. Berkeley: University of California Press, 1988.
16. SAS Institute Inc. *SAS/STAT User's Guide*. Cary, NC: SAS Institute, Inc., 1988.
17. SPSS Inc. *SPSS Base 7.0 for Windows, User's Guide*. Chicago: SPSS Inc., 1996.

22

Nonparametric Tests for Group Comparisons

In previous chapters we have presented several statistical tests that are based on certain assumptions about the parameters of the population from which the samples were drawn. These **parametric tests** require that the assumptions of normality and homogeneity of variance are met to a reasonable degree for validity of analysis. In this chapter, we present a set of statistical procedures classified as **nonparametric,** which test hypotheses for group comparisons without normality or variance assumptions. For this reason, these methods are sometimes referred to as *distribution-free tests.*

Nonparametric methods are similar to parametric methods in that both test hypotheses and both involve the use of a statistical ratio or test statistic, with an associated probability. Similarly, the outcomes of these tests are evaluated according to a predetermined alpha level of significance. In this chapter we describe five nonparametric procedures that are the most commonly used analogues of the parametric *t*-test and *F*-test: the **Mann–Whitney *U*-test, sign test, Wilcoxon signed-ranks test, Kruskal-Wallis one-way analysis of variance by ranks,** and the **Friedman two-way analysis of variance by ranks.** Although these tests are easily computed with a handheld calculator, they are also included in most statistical packages for computer analysis.

CRITERIA FOR CHOOSING NONPARAMETRIC TESTS

Two major criteria are generally adopted for choosing a nonparametric test over a parametric procedure. The first is that assumptions of population normality and homogeneity of variance cannot be satisfied. Many clinical investigations involve variables that have not been studied sufficiently to support these assumptions. In all likelihood, most pathological conditions are represented by skewed distributions rather than symmetrical ones. In addition, small clinical samples and samples of convenience cannot automatically be considered representative of larger normal distributions.

The second criterion for choosing a nonparametric test is that data are measured on the nominal or ordinal scale. Many assessment tools have been developed around these scales. Nonparametric tests provide an objective mechanism for supporting statistical hypotheses when these levels of measurement are used.

Although nonparametric tests require fewer statistical assumptions than parametric procedures, they still put some restrictions on data. Some type of randomization procedure should be used in forming groups. This allows the researcher to make assumptions about the equality of groups before the independent variable is administered. In addition, the nonparametric tests described in this chapter apply to data that are at least at the ordinal level (see Chapter 25 for tests appropriate to nominal level data); that is, the variable of interest has an underlying continuous distribution that can be ranked, even if it cannot be measured quantitatively. For instance, strength can be measured using discrete manual muscle test grades on an ordinal scale, even though strength truly exists along a continuum. Ordinal scales are used often to measure relative changes in clinical variables such as sitting balance, function, or sensation. Analysis of these types of variables represents the most appropriate use of nonparametric statistics. The major disadvantage of nonparametric tests is that they generally cannot be adapted to complex clinical designs, such as factorial designs and tests of interactions.

Power-Efficiency in Nonparametric Tests

Many researchers prefer to use parametric tests because they are generally more powerful. Nonparametric tests are less sensitive than parametric tests because most of them involve ranking scores rather than comparing precise metric changes. Nonparametric and parametric methods have been compared on the basis of their *power-efficiency*, which is a test's relative ability to identify significant differences for a given sample size. Generally, an increase in sample size is needed to make a nonparametric test as powerful as a parametric test. For instance, a nonparametric test may require a sample size of 50 to achieve the same degree of power as a parametric test with 30 subjects. This relationship can be expressed as a percentage that indicates the relative power-efficiency of the nonparametric test. For example, if power-efficiency is 60%, then with equal sample sizes, the nonparametric test is 60% as powerful as the parametric test. In other words, to achieve equal power with the nonparametric test, we would need 10 subjects for every 6 used with the parametric procedure.

With equal sample sizes, nonparametric tests will generally be less powerful than their parametric counterparts; however, with larger samples this discrepancy is minimized. Most of the nonparametric tests described here can achieve approximately 65% to 95% power-efficiency in comparison to their most powerful parametric analogues.[1] These figures apply to calculations based on comparisons of normal populations. With very small samples, as with six subjects or less, many nonparametric tests will be as powerful as their parametric counterparts. With larger nonnormal populations, the nonparametric statistics may actually be more powerful.[2] As power is an issue only when significant results are not obtained, a researcher need not be concerned with the relative power of nonparametric tests when the null hypothesis is rejected.

TABLE 22.1. EXAMPLE OF RANKED SCORES WITHOUT TIES (A) AND WITH TIES (B)

Sample A (n = 8)	Rank	Sample B (n = 8)	Rank
6	4	8	3
2	3	11	5
8	5	3	1.5
9	6	17	8
−3	1	11	5
0	2	3	1.5
16	8	11	5
12	7	12	7

PROCEDURE FOR RANKING SCORES

Most nonparametric tests are based on rank ordering of scores. The procedure for ranking will be illustrated using the two samples shown in Table 22.1. Scores are always ranked from smallest to largest, with the rank of 1 assigned to the smallest score. Algebraic values are taken into account, so that the lowest ranks are assigned to the largest negative values, if any. The highest rank will equal n. As shown in Sample A, the rank of 1 is assigned to the smallest score (−3), the rank of 2 goes to the next smallest (0), and so on, until the rank of 8 is assigned to the highest score (16).

When two or more scores in a distribution are tied, they are each given the same rank, which is the average of the ranks they occupy. For instance, in Sample B, there are two scores with the smallest value (3). They occupy ranks 1 and 2; therefore, they are each assigned the average of their ranks: $(1 + 2)/2 = 1.5$. The next highest value (8) receives the rank of 3, as the first two ranks are filled. The next highest value is 11, which appears three times. As we have already filled ranks 1, 2, and 3, we average the next three ranks: $(4 + 5 + 6)/3 = 5$. Each score of 11 is assigned the rank of 5. Having filled the first 6 rank positions, the last two values in the distribution are assigned ranks 7 and 8.

TEST FOR TWO INDEPENDENT SAMPLES: MANN-WHITNEY *U*-TEST

The **Mann-Whitney *U*-test** is one of the more powerful nonparametric procedures, designed to test the null hypothesis that two independent samples come from the same population.* This test is analogous to the parametric *t*-test for independent samples. Like the unpaired *t*-test, the *U*-test does not require that groups be of the same size. It is, therefore, an excellent alternative to the *t*-test when parametric assumptions are not met.

Example

A researcher is interested in the effect of body position on a person's ability to relax, as measured by EMG biofeedback from the frontalis muscle. To study this question, 11 subjects are randomly assigned to two groups in a pretest–posttest design, with one group

---

*Some statisticians prefer to use the Wilcoxon Rank Sum Test to test the difference between two independent samples. This test is equivalent to the Mann-Whitney *U*-test.

TABLE 22.2   MANN-WHITNEY U-TEST: CHANGE IN MICROVOLT ACTIVITY FOLLOWING RELAXATION IN TWO POSITIONS

A. DATA	Supine $(n_1 = 5)$	Rank	Sitting $n_2 = 6$	Rank
	20	5	10	3
	30	7	5	2
	50	11	35	8
	45	10	25	6
	40	9	0	1
			15	4
		$R_1 = 42$		$R_2 = 24$

B. COMPUTATIONS

$$U_1 = R_1 - \frac{n_1(n_1 + 1)}{2} = 42 - \frac{5(5 + 1)}{2} = 27$$

$$U_2 = R_2 - \frac{n_2(n_2 + 1)}{2} = 24 - \frac{6(6 + 1)}{2} = 3$$

$\boxed{U = 3}$

C. TEST FOR LARGE SAMPLES

$$z = \frac{U - \dfrac{n_1 n_2}{2}}{\sqrt{\dfrac{n_1 n_2(n_1 + n_2 + 1)}{12}}} = \frac{3 - \dfrac{(5)(6)}{2}}{\sqrt{\dfrac{(5)(6)(5 + 6 + 1)}{12}}} = \frac{-12}{\sqrt{30}} = -2.19$$

D. OUTPUT: HYPOTHESIS TEST

Critical Value of U: For $n_1 = 5$, $n_2 = 6$, at $\alpha_2 = .05$, $U = 3$
          (Table A.8)   Reject H_0

z test: $z = -2.19 > 1.96$ (two-tailed $p = .0286$)
          (Table A.1)   Reject H_0

```
Mann-Whitney U = 3.000
z = -2.191
Sig (2-tailed) = .028
```

positioned supine, the other sitting. Results are recorded as changes in microvolt activity. The researcher hypothesizes that the positions will facilitate different levels of relaxation (a nondirectional hypothesis).

Procedure

Hypothetical data for this example are given in Table 22.2A. The first step is to combine both groups and rank all the scores in order of increasing size. The sum of the ranks assigned to each group is designated R_1 or R_2. Under the null hypothesis, we would expect the groups to be equally distributed with regard to high and low ranks, and the mean of the ranks would be equal for both groups. Any differences between the ranks should be the result of chance. The test will determine if the difference between the sums of ranks is sufficiently large to be considered significant. An alternative hypothesis can be directional or nondirectional.

The U *Test Statistic*

The test statistic, U, is calculated using each group as a reference, as follows:

$$U_1 = R_1 - \frac{n_1(n_1 + 1)}{2} \tag{22.1a}$$

$$U_2 = R_2 - \frac{n_2(n_2 + 1)}{2} \tag{22.1b}$$

where n_1 is the smaller sample size, n_2 is the larger sample size, and R_1 and R_2 are the sums of the ranks for the groups. Designation of n_1 or n_2 is arbitrary if groups are of equal size. Obviously, these formulas will yield different values of U. For example, using calculations shown in Table 22.2B, we obtain $U_1 = 27$, with Group 1 as the reference group. Using Group 2 as the reference group, we obtain $U_2 = 3$. We can show that these values are mathematically related as

$$U_1 = n_1 n_2 - U_2 \tag{22.2}$$

and vice versa. For example, for the data in Table 22.2, we can demonstrate this relationship:

$$U_1 = (5)(6) - 3 = 27$$
$$U_2 = (5)(6) - 27 = 3$$

The smaller of these two values is assigned to the test statistic U. In this case, then, $U = 3$.

Critical Values of U

Critical values of U are given in Appendix Table A.8 for one- and two-tailed tests at several levels of significance. These values are compared with the *smaller value* of either U_1 or U_2. The appropriate critical values are located in the table for n_1 and n_2. The calculated value of U must be *equal to or less than* the tabled value to be significant. (*Note:* This is opposite to the way we have used critical values with parametric tests.)

For the current example, at $\alpha_2 = .05$, with $n_1 = 5$ and $n_2 = 6$, the critical value of U is 3. Because the calculated value, $U = 3$, is equal to this critical value, we can reject H_0. Our conclusion is then based on visual examination of the mean ranks, which shows that greater relaxation (higher mean rank) is attained in the supine position.

Large Samples

When sample size exceeds 25, Table A.8 cannot be used. In this situation, the value of U is converted to z and tested against the standard normal distribution:

$$z = \frac{U - \dfrac{n_1 n_2}{2}}{\sqrt{\dfrac{n_1 n_2 (n_1 + n_2 + 1)}{12}}} \tag{22.3}$$

Even though the present example does not warrant it, we have used the data to illustrate this application in Table 22.2C. In this formula it does not matter if U_1 or U_2 is used. The absolute value of z will be the same either way.

We can determine the exact probability associated with the test by finding the tail probability for z in Appendix Table A.1. For $z = 2.19$, the one-tailed probability is .0143. Because we have proposed a nondirectional hypothesis, we double this value for a two-tailed test. Therefore, $p = .0286$. Critical values of z (in Table A.1) can also be used to determine if this ratio is significant.[†] For a two-tailed test at .05 (we proposed a nondirectional hypothesis), $z = 1.96$. Our calculated value exceeds this critical value, and the null hypothesis is rejected. This outcome agrees with the results obtained using Table A.8.

TEST FOR THREE OR MORE INDEPENDENT SAMPLES: KRUSKAL-WALLIS ONE-WAY ANALYSIS OF VARIANCE BY RANKS

When three or more groups are compared ($k \geq 3$), a nonparametric analysis of variance is appropriate for the same reasons that an F-test is used with parametric data. The **Kruskal-Wallis one-way analysis of variance by ranks** is a nonparametric analogue of the one-way analysis of variance. It is a powerful alternative to the F-test when variance and normality assumptions for parametric tests are not met. It is also the most appropriate way to handle ordinal level data when more than two groups are compared. With $k = 2$, this test is equivalent to the Mann-Whitney U-test. Multiple comparison procedures can also be applied.

Example

We want to study the effect of three modalities for relieving chronic low back pain. We randomly assign 17 subjects ($N = 17$) to receive ice ($n = 6$), hot pack ($n = 6$), or ultrasound ($n = 5$). Pain is measured on a visual analogue scale from 0 mm (pain free) to 100 mm (severe pain). Scores are recorded as the change in level of pain from pretreatment to posttreatment levels.

Procedure

Hypothetical data are reported in Table 22.3A. The procedures for the Kruskal-Wallis ANOVA are similar to those used for the Mann–Whitney U-test. The first step is to combine data for all groups and rank scores from the smallest to the largest. The smallest score receives the rank of 1, and the largest score is assigned the rank of N. Ties are assigned average ranks.

The ranks are then summed for each group separately, as shown in Table 22.3A. If the null hypothesis is true, we would expect an equal distribution of ranks under the three conditions.

[†]For one-tailed tests at .05 and .01, the critical values are 1.645 and 2.326, respectively. For two-tailed tests, these critical values are 1.96 and 2.576, respectively. The calculated value of z must be *greater than or equal to* the critical value to be considered significant.

TABLE 22.3 KRUSKAL-WALLIS ONE-WAY ANALYSIS OF VARIANCE BY RANKS: CHANGES IN LEVEL OF PAIN ($N = 14$)

A. DATA	Group 1: Ice		Group 2: Hot Packs		Group 3: Ultrasound	
	Change score	Rank	Change score	Rank	Change score	Rank
	40	8	35	6	80	14
	60	11	25	2.5	50	10
	10	1	30	4.5	75	13
	25	2.5	40	8	70	12
	30	4.5	40	8		
R		27		29		49
n		5		5		4
$\bar{R}$		5.4		5.8		12.25

B. COMPUTATIONS

$$H = \frac{12}{N(N+1)} \sum \frac{R_2}{n} - 3(N+1)$$

$$= \frac{12}{14(14+1)} \left[\frac{(27)^2}{5} + \frac{(29)^2}{5} + \frac{(49)^2}{4} \right] - 3(14+1)$$

$$= \frac{12}{210} [914.25] - 45 = 7.243$$

C. OUTPUT: HYPOTHESIS TEST

For $df = 2$, $\chi^2 = 5.99$ (Table A.5)

Reject H_0

```
Chi-Square = 7.243
df = 2
Sig = .025
```

The H Statistic

The test statistic for the Kruskal-Wallis test is H, calculated according to

$$H = \frac{12}{N(N+1)} \sum \frac{R^2}{n} - 3(N+1) \tag{22.4}$$

where N is the number of cases in all samples combined, n is the number of cases in each individual sample, and R is the sum of ranks for each individual sample. This calculation is illustrated in Table 22.3B. For this example, $H = 7.243$.

Critical Values

The H statistic is tested using the chi-square distribution with $k - 1$ degrees of freedom (Table A.5).[‡] With three groups, $df = 2$. Therefore, we test H against the critical value of

---

[‡]When samples are very small, with five subjects or fewer per group, alternative tables can be used to obtain critical values of H (see Siegel and Castellan[3]).

5.99 at $\alpha = .05$. H must be greater than or equal to χ^2 to be considered significant: Our calculated value of $H = 7.243$ is significant, and we can reject H_0. We now need to perform a multiple comparison procedure to determine which groups are different. This will be described shortly.

Ties

A substantial number of ties can have a conservative effect on the value of H, making the test less powerful. This may be a concern when the test result is not significant and when greater than 25% of the scores are tied. A correction factor can be applied to increase the value of H under these conditions. Unless the number of ties is substantial, however, the effect of the correction will be minimal. Obviously, if H is significant without the correction, there is no point in making the adjustment. Procedures for this correction can be found in the text by Siegel and Castellan.[3]

Multiple Comparison for the Kruskal-Wallis ANOVA

When H is significant, it is usually of interest to determine which specific groups are different from each other. The Mann-Whitney U-test is often used as a multiple comparison procedure; however, a Bonferroni correction should be applied to control for the increased risk of Type I error, using the same rationale that applies to multiple t-tests. Siegel and Castellan present a multiple comparison procedure to protect against this increased error rate.[3]

A multiple comparison for the Kruskal-Wallis ANOVA tests the significance of pairwise differences between conditions, based on the *mean of the ranks* for each sample: $\bar{R} = R/n$. For the data in Table 22.3, $\bar{R}_1 = 5.4$, $\bar{R}_2 = 5.8$, and $\bar{R}_3 = 12.25$. The total number of pairwise comparisons associated with an analysis will be equal to $k(k - 1)/2$. With three mean rankings ($k = 3$), we will have $3(3 - 1)/2 = 3$ comparisons.

Minimum Significant Difference

Each pairwise comparison is tested against a minimum significant difference (MSD) based on the formula

$$|\bar{R}_1 - \bar{R}_2| \geq z \sqrt{\frac{N(N + 1)}{12}\left(\frac{1}{n_1} + \frac{1}{n_2}\right)} \tag{22.5}$$

where N is the total number of subjects in all samples combined, and n_1 and n_2 are the respective sample sizes for the two groups involved in the specific pairwise comparison. Any absolute difference between mean ranks that is *equal to or larger than* the minimum significant difference is considered significant.

The value of z in Equation 22.5 is based on the total number of comparisons to be made and the desired level of significance for the overall test. We obtain z from Table 22.4. The α level selected in the table is based on the desired *familywise error rate* (α_{FW}), that is, the overall probability associated with the entire set of comparisons. Researchers may choose to keep α_{FW} at .05, which is considered a conservative practice, or they may accept

TABLE 22.4. CRITICAL VALUES OF *z* TO BE USED IN CALCULATING MULTIPLE COMPARISONS WITH *H* AND X_r^2 STATISTICS

Number of comparisons	α_{FW}				
	.25	.20	.15	.10	.05
1	1.150	1.282	1.440	1.645	1.960
2	1.534	1.645	1.780	1.960	2.241
3	1.732	1.834	1.960	2.128	2.394
4	1.863	1.960	2.080	2.241	2.498
5	1.960	2.054	2.170	2.326	2.576
6	2.037	2.128	2.241	2.394	2.638
7	2.100	2.189	2.300	2.450	2.690
8	2.154	2.241	2.350	2.498	2.734
9	2.200	2.287	2.394	2.539	2.773
10	2.241	2.326	2.432	2.576	2.807

Adapted from Table A.II of Siegel S, Castellan NJ: *Nonparametric Statistics for the Behavioral Sciences*, ed 2. New York, McGraw-Hill, 1988, with permission.

higher probability levels, such as .15 or .20, when the risk of Type I error is not of great concern.[§] Typically, a larger α is chosen as *k* increases.[4]

Example

We can illustrate this procedure using the data in Table 22.3. To compare Groups 1 ($n_1 = 5$) and 2 ($n_2 = 5$), we first specify our desired familywise error rate, say $\alpha_{FW} = .15$. Next, we determine that there will be a total of three comparisons. According to Table 22.4, at $\alpha_{FW} = .15$, $z = 1.96$ for three comparisons. We can now compute the minimum significant difference for this comparison using Equation 22.7:

$$\text{MSD} = 1.96\sqrt{\frac{14(14 + 1)}{12}\left(\frac{1}{5} + \frac{1}{5}\right)} = 1.96\sqrt{7} = 5.19$$

We compare this minimum difference with the absolute difference between the mean ranks for Groups 1 and 2:

$$|\bar{R}_1 - \bar{R}_2| = |5.4 - 5.8| = 0.4$$

Because this difference is less than the minimum significant difference, it is not considered significant. There is no significant difference between ice and hot packs for relieving pain.

[§]The actual probability associated with each individual comparison is $\alpha_{FW}/k(k-1)$. Therefore, with $k = 3$, and $\alpha_{FW} = .05$, the per comparison error rate is $.05/3(3-1) = .008$. At $\alpha_{FW} = .20$, the per comparison error rate would be $.20/3(3-1) = .03$.

We compare Groups 1 and 3 ($n_1 = 5$, $n_3 = 4$) using

$$\text{MSD} = 1.96\sqrt{\frac{14(14 + 1)}{12}\left(\frac{1}{5} + \frac{1}{4}\right)} = 1.96\sqrt{7.875} = 5.50$$

The difference, $|\bar{R}_1 - \bar{R}_3| = |5.4 - 12.25| = 6.85$, is greater than this minimum significant difference, and, therefore, this represents a significant effect. Ultrasound ($\bar{R}_3$) is more effective than ice ($\bar{R}_1$).

Finally, we compare Groups 2 and 3 ($n_2 = 5$, $n_3 = 4$) using the minimum significant difference of 5.50 (obtained earlier for the same sample sizes):

$$|\bar{R}_2 - \bar{R}_3| = |5.8 - 12.25| = 6.45$$

This comparison is also significant. We can now conclude that ultrasound ($\bar{R}_3$) is more effective for reducing low back pain than either ice ($\bar{R}_1$) or hot packs ($\bar{R}_2$) in this hypothetical study.

When all k samples are of equal size, one minimum significant difference can be used for all comparisons, using the formula

$$\text{MSD} = z\sqrt{\frac{k(N - 1)}{6}} \tag{22.6}$$

TESTS FOR TWO CORRELATED SAMPLES: SIGN TEST AND WILCOXON SIGNED-RANKS TEST

Two procedures are commonly used for testing the difference between correlated samples: the sign test and the Wilcoxon signed-ranks test. These tests are used with two-level repeated measures designs. They are analogous to the parametric t-test for correlated or paired samples.

The Sign Test

The **sign test** is one of the simplest nonparametric tests because it requires no mathematical calculations. It is used with binomial data, and does not require that measurements be quantitative. As its name implies, the data are analyzed using plus and minus signs rather than numerical values. Therefore, this test provides a mechanism for testing relative differentiations such as more–less, higher–lower, or larger–smaller. It is particularly useful when quantification is impossible or unfeasible and when subjective ratings are necessary.

Example

We are interested in the effect of knee angle on knee extensor strength. Using a manual muscle test (MMT), we will study 10 patients, 6 months following total knee replacement. MMT grades are recorded from 0 (no muscle activity) to 11 (normal strength). Using $\alpha = .05$, we hypothesize that knee extensor strength will be different with the knee in 90 and 15 degrees of flexion.

TABLE 22.5.   SIGN TEST AND WILCOXON SIGNED-RANKS TEST: MMT GRADES FOR KNEE EXTENSION WITH KNEE AT TWO ANGLES

A. DATA

Subject	Angle 90°	Angle 15°	Sign	d	Rank of d	Ranks with less frequent sign
1	8	8	0	0		
2	10	11	–	−1	−1	−1
3	7	7	0	0		
4	9	7	+	+2	+3	
5	10	8	+	+2	+3	
6	11	7	+	+4	+7	
7	10	8	+	+2	+3	
8	10	7	+	+3	+5.5	
9	8	8	0	0		
10	10	7	+	+3	+5.5	

$T = -1$

**B. HYPOTHESIS TEST:
   OUTPUT FOR THE SIGN TEST**

6 plus signs, 1 minus sign, $x = 1$ (number of fewer signs)

For $x = 1$, $n = 7$, $p = .124$ (Table A.9)

$$z = \frac{|5| - 1}{\sqrt{7}} = 1.51$$

Do not reject H_0

```
SIGN TEST

Negative differences     1
Positive differences     6
Ties                     3
Total                    10
Sig (2-tailed) = .125
```

**C. HYPOTHESIS TEST:
   OUTPUT FOR THE SIGNED-RANKS TEST**

Sum ranks with less frequent sign $= -1$

For $n = 7$ at $\alpha_2 = .05$, $T = 2$ (Table A.10) Reject H_0

$$z = \frac{T - \dfrac{n(n + 1)}{4}}{\sqrt{\dfrac{n(n + 1)(2n + 1)}{24}}} = \frac{1 - \dfrac{7(7 + 1)}{4}}{\sqrt{\dfrac{7(7 + 1)(2(7) + 1))}{24}}} = \frac{-13}{\sqrt{35}} = -2.20$$

```
WILCOXON SIGNED-RANKS
                    N    Sum
Negative
  Ranks            1    1.00
Positive           6   27.00
  Ranks
Ties               3
Total              10
z = 2.217
Sig (2-tailed) = .027
```

Procedure

Hypothetical data are shown in Table 22.5A. The sign test is applied to the differences between each pair of scores, based on whether the direction of difference is positive or negative. In this example, we will use the grades measured at 15 degrees as the reference and record whether the grade at 90 degrees is greater (+), the same

(0), or less (–) than the reference grade, always maintaining the same direction of comparison. With a nondirectional hypothesis it does not matter which value is used as the reference, as long as the order is consistent. In the fourth column in Table 22.5A, the signs of the differences are listed. When no difference is obtained, a zero is recorded.

Under the null hypothesis, we would expect half the differences to be positive and the other half to be negative. We will reject H_0 if one sign occurs sufficiently less often. If we propose a directional alternative hypothesis, we must be sure that the direction of comparison supports the predicted direction of change. For this illustration, we have proposed a nondirectional hypothesis.

To proceed with the test, we count the number of plus signs and the number of minus signs. Ties, recorded as zeros, are discarded from the analysis, and n is reduced accordingly. In this example, 7 of the 10 subjects showed differences, with three ties. Therefore, $n = 7$. There are 6 plus signs and 1 minus sign (see Table 22.5A). We take the smaller of these two values, the *number of fewer signs,* and assign it the test statistic, x. In this case, $x = 1$, the number of minus signs.

Test Probabilities

To determine the probability of obtaining x under H_0, we refer to Appendix Table A.9. This table lists one-tailed probabilities associated with x for values up to $n = 30$, where n is the number of pairs whose differences showed direction. Two-tailed tests require doubling the probabilities given in the table.

For $x = 1$ and $n = 7$, the table shows $p = .062$. Because we have proposed a nondirectional hypothesis, we double this value for a two-tailed probability of $p = .124$. This is greater than the acceptable level of .05, and we cannot reject H_0. The probability that the difference in the number of plus and minus signs occurred by chance is too great. We conclude that there is no significant difference in knee extensor strength with the knee at 90 and 15 degrees.

The determination of the probability associated with x is based on a theoretical distribution called the *binomial probability distribution.* A binomial outcome is one that can take only two forms, in this case either positive or negative. The binomial test determines the likelihood of getting the smaller number of plus or minus signs out of the total number of differences just by chance.

Large Samples

With sample sizes greater than 30, x is converted to z and tested against the normal distribution according to the formula

$$z = \frac{|D| - 1}{\sqrt{n}} \tag{22.7}$$

where $|D|$ is the absolute difference between the number of plus and minus signs.

This calculation is illustrated in Table 22.5B for data with six plus signs and one minus sign, resulting in $z = 1.51$ [$p = .13$ (two-tailed) from Table A.1]. Using the critical value of $z = 1.96$ for $\alpha_2 = .05$, this outcome does not achieve significance.

The Wilcoxon Signed-Ranks Test

The sign test evaluates differences within paired scores based solely on whether one score is larger or smaller than the other. This is often the best approach with subjective clinical variables that offer no greater precision; however, if data are able to provide information on the relative magnitude of differences, the more powerful **Wilcoxon signed-ranks test** can be used. This test examines both the direction of difference and the relative amount of difference.

Example

Consider the example presented in the previous section. In Table 22.5A, we have listed the manual muscle test grades as ordinal values, based on a scale of 0 to 11 (Normal). We obtain a difference score for each subject, labeled d. When $d = 0$, the subject is dropped from the analysis, and n is reduced, as it was in the sign test.

Procedure

We proceed by ranking the difference scores, *without regard to sign*, and discarding any pairs with no difference. We then attach the sign of the difference to the obtained ranks. For instance, in our example, the rank of 1 is given to the smallest difference score (subject 2), and then assigned –1 because it reflects a negative difference. Tied difference scores are given the mean of their ranks. Therefore, ranks 2, 3, and 4 are taken by subjects 4, 5, and 7, who all have a difference score of 2. These scores are each assigned the average rank of 3. Subjects 8 and 10 are tied with difference scores of 3, filling ranks 5 and 6, which are averaged to rank 5.5. The final rank of 7 is assigned to subject 6.

If the null hypothesis is true, we would expect to find an equal representation of positive and negative signs among the larger and smaller ranks; that is, the sum of the positive ranks should be equal to the sum of the negative ranks. We reject H_0 if either of these sums is too small.

The T *Statistic*

We determine if there are fewer positive or negative ranks, and then sum the ranks for the *less frequent sign*. This sum is assigned the *test* statistic, T. In this example, there are fewer ranks with negative signs, with the sum of –1. Therefore, $T = -1$. Only the absolute value of T is used to determine significance. The sign of T is of concern only when performing a one-tailed test.

Critical Values

Critical values of T are given in Table A.12 for one- and two-tailed tests, where n is the number of pairs with nonzero differences. The absolute calculated value of T must be *less than or equal to* the critical value to achieve significance. Note once again that this is opposite to the way most critical values are used. For this analysis, at $\alpha_2 = .05$, with $n = 7$, the critical value of T is 2. Therefore, our calculated value of $T = 1$ is significant. We can reject H_0 and conclude that knee extensor strength is different with the knee at

90 and 15 degrees. Visual examination of the data tells us that strength is greater with the knee at 90 degrees.

It is interesting to note the difference between the outcome of this analysis and the outcome of the sign test on the same data. We were able to substantiate a significant difference using the Wilcoxon procedure, because it is sensitive to relative differences, not just direction. Therefore, if data achieve adequate precision, the Wilcoxon test is recommended over the sign test.

Large Samples

With sample sizes over 25, the absolute value of T can be converted to z according to

$$z = \frac{T - \dfrac{n(n + 1)}{4}}{\sqrt{\dfrac{n(n + 1)(2n + 1)}{24}}} \tag{22.8}$$

where n is the number of paired observations. For this analysis, $z = -2.20$ ($p = .028$ from Table A.1), as shown in Table 22.5C. The absolute value of z is greater than the critical value 1.96, which represents a significant difference at $\alpha_2 = .05$.

TEST FOR MORE THAN TWO CORRELATED SAMPLES: FRIEDMAN TWO-WAY ANALYSIS OF VARIANCE BY RANKS

In this section we present a nonparametric test to analyze data from a single-factor repeated measures design with three or more experimental conditions. The **Friedman two-way analysis of variance by ranks** is a powerful alternative to the parametric repeated measures ANOVA when ordinal data are used or when parametric assumptions are not tenable. The test is given the designation "two-way" based on the interpretation that "subjects" is treated as an independent variable with $n = 1$ per cell of the design. It is assumed that the number of measurements in each experimental condition will be the same.

Example

We are interested in measuring the effect of changing body position on blood pressure in six patients with chronic pulmonary disease. Each patient will be placed in three positions—level, head down, and head elevated—in random order. Blood pressure will be measured within 1 minute of assuming the position. We may choose to use a nonparametric form of analysis for this study because the sample is small, and because we do not have sufficient reason to assume that blood pressure for a population of patients with this disease will be normally distributed. In addition, although blood pressure measurements can be considered ratio level data, we can rationalize that the lack of reliability in the data warrants using a nonparametric test.

TABLE 22.6. FRIEDMAN TWO-WAY ANALYSIS OF VARIANCE BY RANKS: BLOOD PRESSURE IN THREE POSITIONS ($n = 6$)

A. DATA	(1) Level		(2) Elevated		(3) Down	
Subject	BP	Rank	BP	Rank	BP	Rank
1	110	1	150	2	175	3
2	100	1.5	100	1.5	110	3
3	120	1	140	3	135	2
4	110	1	130	2	155	3
5	120	1	130	2	145	3
6	130	1	155	2	170	3
R		6.5		12.5		17
R^2		42.25		156.25		289.0

B. COMPUTATIONS

$$X_r^2 = \frac{12}{nk(k+1)} \sum R^2 - 3n(k+1)$$

$$= \frac{12}{(6)(3)(3+1)} [42.25 + 156.25 + 289] - 3(6)(3+1)$$

$$= \frac{12}{72}[487.5] - 72 = 9.25$$

C. OUTPUT: HYPOTHESIS TEST

For $k = 3$ ($df = 2$)

$\chi^2 = 5.99$ at $\alpha = .05$ (Table A.5)

Reject H_0

```
FRIEDMAN TEST
                  Mean Rank              N = 6
Down                2.83        Chi-square = 9.652
Elevated            2.08               df = 2
Level               1.08              Sig = .008
```

Procedure

Hypothetical data for this study are reported in Table 22.6A. Data are arranged so that rows represent subjects (n) and columns represent experimental conditions (k). In this example, $n = 6$ and $k = 3$. We begin by converting all scores to ranks; however, the ranking process for this test is different from that used with the Kruskal-Wallis ANOVA. Here the ranks are assigned across each row (within a subject). Ties are assigned average ranks within a row. The highest rank within a row will equal k. This process is illustrated in Table 22.6A.

The next step is to sum the ranks within each column. If the null hypothesis is true, we would expect the distribution of ranks to be a matter of chance, and high and low ranks should be evenly distributed across all treatment conditions. Therefore, the rank sums within each column should be equal. If the alternative hypothesis is true, at least one pair of conditions will show a difference.

The χ_r^2 Statistic

The test statistic for the Friedman ANOVA is χ_r^2 (read "chi square r"). It is computed using the formula

$$X_r^2 = \frac{12}{nk(k+1)} \sum R^2 - 3n(k+1) \tag{22.9}$$

where n is the number of subjects (rows), k is the number of treatment conditions (columns), and ΣR^2 is the sum of the squared ranks across treatment conditions. Calculation of χ_r^2 is illustrated in Table 22.6B. For this analysis, $\chi_r^2 = 9.25$.

Critical Values

The distribution of χ_r^2 follows the standard χ^2 distribution with $k - 1$ degrees of freedom, where k is the number of experimental conditions (Table A.5).[1][1] With 2 df, we measure our calculated value of 9.25 against 5.99 (at $\alpha = .05$). The calculated value must be *equal to or larger than* the critical value to be significant. Therefore, our test is significant.

Multiple Comparison for the Friedman ANOVA

When χ_r^2 is significant, we can test all pairwise differences using a multiple comparison procedure.[3] We propose a familywise error rate as an overall level of significance for the combined set of contrasts in the experiment.

Minimum Significant Difference

The expression used to determine the minimum significant difference (MSD) for all pairwise contrasts is

$$|R_1 - R_2| \geq z \sqrt{\frac{nk(k+1)}{6}} \tag{22.10}$$

where R_1 and R_2 are the rank totals for each treatment condition, n is the number of subjects, and k is the number of treatment conditions. The value of z is taken from Table 22.5 for the appropriate number of comparisons ($k(k - 1)/2$) and the desired familywise α level for the combined set of comparisons. For the current example, we have a total of three comparisons, and we propose a familywise α level of .10. Therefore, $z = 2.128$.

We compute the minimum significant difference:

$$\text{MSD} = 2.128 \sqrt{\frac{6(3)(3+1)}{6}} = 2.128 \sqrt{12} = 7.37$$

---

[1][1]Alternative tables are available when three groups are tested with $n \leq 15$ (see Siegel and Castellan[3]).

For this analysis, contrasts are made between *rank totals* for each treatment condition, not mean ranks. The absolute value of differences between rank sums for each pair of treatment conditions must be *greater than or equal to* the obtained critical value. Because we are dealing with repeated measures, and all subjects are represented under each treatment, there is only one critical value for all contrasts. The three pairwise comparisons for this study are

$$|R_1 - R_2| = |6.5 - 12.5| = 6.0$$

$$|R_1 - R_3| = |6.5 - 17.0| = 10.5$$

$$|R_2 - R_3| = |12.5 - 17.0| = 4.5$$

The only difference score that exceeds the MSD of 7.37 is obtained from the second comparison between Conditions 1 and 3. Therefore, there is a significant difference in blood pressure when an individual is positioned level versus head down, with higher pressures obtained in the head-down position. No other contrasts are significant.

COMMENTARY

Decisions, Decisions, Decisions

Nonparametric procedures offer clinical researchers a powerful and easily understood statistical mechanism for analyzing changes measured with subjective tools. Because of the nature of many clinical assessments, the ability to analyze ordinal data is important. There is still some debate among statisticians and researchers concerning the appropriate application of parametric versus nonparametric statistics with ordinal data. The classical view is that only nonparametric procedures should be used with ordinal measurements; however, many researchers apply parametric tests to ordinal data, presumably because parametric tests have greater statistical power. This practice has been justified by assuming that the ordinal intervals are consistent, even though sensitivity of measurement may be unable to document this. Therefore, the analysis would not conceptually violate the assumptions of the parametric test.[5, 6] Although some assessment scales can be constructed in such a way as to define intervals as precisely as possible, it is probably unreasonable to assume that constructs such as manual resistance, sensation, and so on, typically measured as ranks, can be measured with sufficient reliability that intervals can be considered equal. It is also likely that many of these scales are nonlinear, so that intervals at extremes of the scale will be different from those toward the center. Those who use this approach or who interpret findings of others who have used it must consider the potential for jeopardizing the validity of statistical outcomes by treating ordinal data as interval data.[7] Therefore, we generally advocate the use of nonparametric methods with ordinal data.

Nonparametric methods are also appropriate for use with interval or ratio data when distributions are skewed or when sample sizes are too small to assume representation of a normal distribution; however, nonparametric procedures can be wasteful of information when used with data on the interval or ratio scales, because precise data are reduced to ranks. Therefore, when the criterion for using nonparametric tests is based on violations of normality only, it may be useful to transform data using a logarithmic transformation to achieve a normal distribution (see Appendix D) and to apply a parametric test.

The tests that have been included in this chapter are only a sampling of available nonparametric procedures. Statisticians continue to develop and refine these tests and to expand the capabilities of nonparametric methods into areas such as regression and factorial designs. Many tests have been developed with very specific purposes, such as comparing several treatment groups with a single control or looking at differences in variables that have an inherent order. Nonparametric statistics can also be used for correlation procedures and for testing nominal scale data. These procedures are presented in Chapters 23 and 25. We encourage the interested reader to explore these and other approaches further using the readings listed at the end of this chapter.

KEY TERMS

parametric tests
nonparametric tests
Mann-Whitney U-test (U)
sign test (x)
Wilcoxon signed-ranks
    test (T)

Kruskal-Wallis one-way
    analysis of variance by
    ranks (H)

Friedman two-way
    analysis of variance by
    ranks (χ^2_r)

REFERENCES

1. Winer BJ, Michels KM, Brown DR. *Statistical Principles in Experimental Design.* 3d ed. New York: McGraw-Hill, 1991.
2. Neave HR, Granger WJ. A Monte Carlo study comparing various two-sample tests for differences in means. *Technometrics* 1968;10:509.
3. Siegel S, Castellan NJ. *Nonparametric Statistics for the Behavioral Sciences.* 2d ed. New York: McGraw-Hill, 1988.
4. Daniel WW. *Applied Nonparametric Statistics.* Boston: Houghton Mifflin, 1978.
5. Gaito J. Measurement scales and statistics: Resurgence of an old misconception. *Psychol Bull* 1980;87:564–7.
6. Nunally J, Bernstein IH. *Psychometric Theory.* 3d ed. New York: McGraw-Hill, 1994.
7. Royeen CB, Seaver WL. Promise in nonparametrics. *Am J Occup Ther* 1986;40:191–3.

23

Correlation

The statistical procedures we have described thus far have all focused on the comparison of a measured dependent variable across categories of an independent variable. These procedures are generally applied to experimental and quasi-experimental designs for the purpose of group comparisons. We will now begin to examine procedures for exploratory analyses, where the purpose of the research question is to evaluate the relationship between two measured variables. Where statistical tests of group differences address the question, "Is group A different from group B?" or "Does this treatment cause this outcome?" measures of **correlation** ask, "What is the relationship between A and B?" or "Does variable A increase with variable B?"

The concept of correlation is, by and large, a familiar one. Pairs of observations, X and Y, are examined to see if they tend to "go together." For instance, we generally accept that taller people tend to weigh more than shorter people, that children resemble their parents in intelligence, and that heart rate increases with physical exertion. These variables are correlated, in that the value of one variable (X) is associated with the value of the other variable (Y). With a strong correlation, we can infer something about the second value by knowing the first. Correlation can be applied to paired observations on two different variables, such as heart rate and level of exertion, or to one variable measured on two occasions, such as intelligence of a parent and child.

Correlation coefficients are used to quantitatively describe the strength and direction of a relationship between two variables. The purpose of this chapter is to introduce several types of correlation coefficients that can be applied to a variety of exploratory research designs and types of data. The most commonly reported measure is the Pearson product–moment coefficient of correlation, for use when both X and Y are on the interval or ratio scales. We include procedures for correlating ranked data using the Spearman rho (r_s) and several correlation methods for use with data in the form of dichotomies.

SCATTER PLOTS

It is often useful to examine a statistical relationship by creating a **scatter diagram** or **scatter plot,** as shown in Figure 23.1. In a scatter plot each point (dot) represents the intersection of a pair of related observations. With a sufficient number of data points, a scatter plot can visually clarify the strength and shape of a relationship. For instance, the points in Figure 23.1A show a pattern in which the values of Y increase in exact proportion to the values of X. This is considered a perfect positive relationship, with data points falling on a straight line. In Figure 23.1B, the data demonstrate a negative slope in a perfect negative relationship, with lower values of Y associated with higher values of X.

Perfect relationships are truly rare, however. Generally the association between X and Y does not follow a perfect pattern, and values of X and Y will change in varying proportions. Figure 23.1C shows a strong positive correlation; this pattern might reflect the relationship between height and weight, for example. Figure 23.1D shows a strong negative correlation; this might represent the relationship between leg length and the number of steps needed to walk a given distance. These two patterns reveal data that are clustered in relatively linear patterns. Figure 23.1E shows a weaker positive relationship, one that is harder to visually interpret than the others. We might see such a pattern if we looked at lower extremity strength and overall physical function, where a relationship exists, but individuals respond differently for a variety of reasons. Scatter plots that oc-

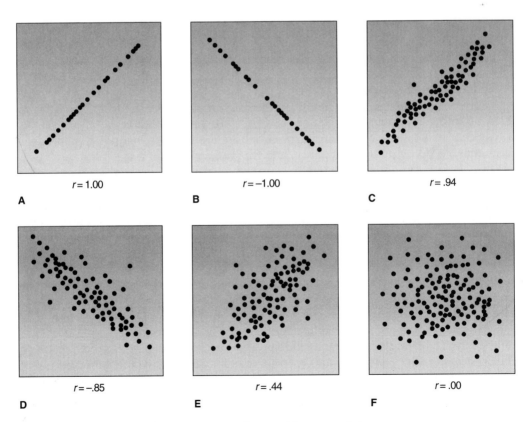

FIGURE 23.1 Scatter plots illustrating various degrees of linear correlation.

cur in random or circular patterns, as in Figure 23.1F, reflect no linear relationship between X and Y, or near-zero correlation. This might be the case if we studied the relationship between students' exam grades and height, for example. In this case, the value of Y is not associated with the value of X; that is, all observed variability is random.

CORRELATION COEFFICIENTS

Inspection of data in a scatter plot provides some idea about a relationship, but is not adequate for summarizing that relationship. The correlation coefficient is used to provide an index that reflects a quantitative measure of the relationship between two variables. For most applications, a lowercase r is used to represent a sample correlation coefficient. Correlation coefficients can take values ranging from –1.00 for a perfect negative relationship, to 0.00 for no correlation, to +1.00 for a perfect positive relationship. The *magnitude* of the correlation coefficient indicates the *strength* of the association between X and Y. The closer the value is to ±1.00, the stronger the association. The *sign* of the correlation coefficient indicates the *direction* of the relationship. In a positive relationship, X increases as Y increases, and X decreases as Y decreases. In a negative relationship, X increases as Y decreases, and vice versa.

In reality, because of random effects, we seldom see either perfect or zero correlation. We will typically encounter values of r that fall between 0.00 and ±1.00. These values are expressed as decimals, usually to two places, such as $r = .75$ or $r = -.62$. The plots in Figure 23.1 represent a variety of potential outcomes for a correlation analysis between variables X and Y, showing different values of correlation coefficients. Data that cluster closer to a straight line have higher correlation coefficients.

LINEAR VERSUS CURVILINEAR RELATIONSHIPS

The pattern of a relationship between two variables is often classified as linear or nonlinear. The plots in Figures 23.1A and B are perfectly linear because the points fall on a single straight line. The plots in Figures 23.1C through E can also be considered linear, although as they begin to deviate from a straight line, their correlation decreases. The closer the points are to a straight line, the higher the value of r.

The coefficient r is a measure of **linear relationship** only, which means that the value of r reflects the true nature of a relationship only when scores vary in a linear fashion. When a **curvilinear relationship** is present, the linear correlation coefficient will not be able to describe it accurately.* For instance, a curvilinear shape typically characterizes the relationship between strength and age. As age increases so does strength,

---

*The eta coefficient (η), also called the correlation ratio, is an index that does not assume a linear relationship between two variables.[1] To establish nonlinear correlation using eta, one variable must be nominal (i.e., categorical). If both variables are continuous, one must be converted to categories or groups. An ANOVA can be used to compare these groups on the continuous variable. The eta coefficient can then be computed as follows:

$$\eta = \sqrt{\frac{SS_b}{SS_t}},$$ where SS_b is the between-groups sum of squares, and SS_t is the total sum of squares from the ANOVA.

The interpretation of η is the same as r, although η can only range from 0.00 to +1.00 (it cannot be negative). The square of eta (η^2) is interpreted as r^2 (see Chapter 24). The value of η^2 is also an effect size index for the t-test and ANOVA (see Appendix C).[2,3]

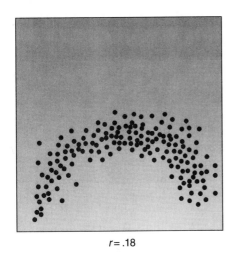

$r = .18$

FIGURE 23.2   Illustration of a strong curvilinear relationship, yielding a poor linear correlation.

reaching a plateau in adulthood, followed by a decline in elderly years. This type of relationship is illustrated in Figure 23.2.

Because r measures only linear functions, the correlation coefficient for a curvilinear relationship can be close to zero, even when X and Y are indeed related. For example, a systematic relationship is clearly evident between X and Y in Figure 23.2, although $r = .18$ suggests a very weak relationship. This should caution the researcher to be critical about the interpretation of correlation coefficients. It may not be reasonable to conclude that two variables are unrelated solely on the basis of a low correlation. By plotting a scatter diagram for all correlation analyses, researchers can observe whether the association in a set of data is linear or curvilinear, and thereby decide if r is an appropriate statistic for analysis.

CRITERIA FOR EVALUATING CORRELATION COEFFICIENTS

The value of the correlation coefficient is a measure of strength of association between two variables. There are no widely accepted criteria for defining a strong versus moderate versus weak association. As a general guideline we offer the following: Correlations ranging from 0.00 to .25 indicate little or no relationship; those from .25 to .50 suggest a fair degree of relationship; values of .50 to .75 are moderate to good; and values above .75 are considered good to excellent. We hasten to emphasize, however, that *these values should not be used as strict cutoff points,* as they are affected by sample size, measurement error, and the types of variables being studied. Sociological and behavioral scientists often use lower correlations as evidence of functionally useful relationships for the interpretation of complex abstract phenomena. Such interpretations must be based on the nature of the data, the purpose of the research, and the researcher's knowledge of the subject matter.

It is also important to understand that correlation coefficients cannot be interpreted as proportions. Therefore, a coefficient of .40 does not represent an association twice as

TABLE 23.1. INTERCORRELATIONS OF ROLE CHARACTERISTICS OF PARENTAL CAREGIVERS

Variable	1	2	3	4	5	6	7
1 Primary caregiver	1.000	.002	.019	.089*	.082*	.118***	.112**
2 Parent with dementia		1.000	.453***	.011	.117***	.064	.083*
3 Parent with behavioral problem			1.000	.165***	.423***	.156***	.252***
4 Hours of care				1.000	.225***	.159***	.144***
5 Increased stress					1.000	.209***	.342***
6 Poor physical health						1.000	.623***
7 Poor emotional health							1.000

*p<.05; **p<.01; ***p<.001

Adapted from: Penning MJ. In the middle: parental caregiving in the context of other roles. *J Gerontol* 1998;53B:S188–S197, Table 4, p. S193. Reprinted with permission of the Gerontological Society of America.

strong as a coefficient of .20. The difference in the degree of relationship between .50 and .60 is not necessarily the same as the difference between .80 and .90. Each coefficient must be interpreted relative to the context of the variables under study.

The Correlation Matrix

Studies using correlation analysis often examine several variables at one time, and may include a matrix of **intercorrelations,**[†] which presents the correlation coefficients for all pairs of variables. Table 23.1 shows such an arrangement for some of the data collected in a study of role characteristics of parental caregivers.[4]

Note that the table is triangular; that is, values below the diagonal would be redundant of those above the diagonal and, therefore, are not included. The values on the diagonal are all 1.00, representing the perfect correlation of each variable with itself. Some authors omit these values, as they are always understood. The values off the diagonal are the correlation coefficients for each pair of variables. For example, Table 23.1 shows that increased stress (variable 5) is associated with having a parent with behavioral problems (variable 3, $r = .42$), and dementia (variable 2, $r = .45$). The caregiver's perception of poor physical health (variable 6) is associated with poor emotional health (variable 7, $r = .62$). This correlation matrix provides the reader with a useful overview of data in a complete and concise format.

Significance of the Correlation Coefficient

Just like other sample statistics, the correlation coefficient is subject to sampling error; that is, the observed correlation is considered one of an infinite number of possible correlations that could be obtained from random samples of a population. A theoretical sampling distribution could be created by obtaining correlation coefficients from many random

---

[†]This terminology should not be confused with the *intraclass correlation coefficient (ICC),* which is used in reliability studies (see Chapter 26).

samples. Most of the samples would show correlations close to the actual population value, and fewer would be distributed at the extremes. We can subject the correlation coefficient to a test of significance based on this theoretical distribution, to determine if the observed value is a random effect or if it is a good estimate of the population correlation.

The null hypothesis states that there is no relationship between X and Y in the underlying population, and therefore, the value of the correlation coefficient is zero, $H_0: r = 0$. A test of significance will determine how likely it is that an observed correlation value would have occurred by chance. Although a nondirectional alternative hypothesis can be proposed ($H_1: r \neq 0$), it is usually stated with direction, predicting either a positive or a negative relationship ($H_1: r > 0$ or $H_1: r < 0$). We present specific methods for testing the significance of various correlation coefficients in the sections that follow.

The significance of a correlation coefficient does not mean that a correlation coefficient represents a strong relationship. Statistical significance only indicates that an observed value is unlikely to be the result of chance. Correlation coefficients are very sensitive to sample size, and statistical power can be relatively high even with smaller samples. Using the Pearson r, for example, with $n \geq 15$, a moderate correlation of $r = .45$ will be significant ($p < .05$). With larger samples, such as $n > 60$, even values as small as $r = .20$ will be significant. Therefore, a correlation coefficient should always be interpreted in relation to the size of the sample from which it was obtained. With a sufficient increase in sample size almost any observed correlation value will be statistically significant, even if it is so small as to be a meaningless indicator of association. For example, the data shown in Table 23.1 were obtained from a sample of over 3,000 subjects, resulting in high power. However, many of the correlations are quite small (less than .30), even though they are significant at $p < .001$. Although many authors report p values associated with correlation coefficients, significance is not as useful to interpretation of r as it is with t-tests or F-tests. Low correlations should not be discussed as clinically important just because they have achieved statistical significance. Such interpretations should be made only on the basis of the magnitude of the correlation coefficient.

PEARSON PRODUCT–MOMENT CORRELATION COEFFICIENT

The most commonly reported measure of correlation is the **Pearson product–moment coefficient of correlation,** developed by the English statistician Karl Pearson. The statistic is given the symbol r for sample data and ρ (rho) for a population parameter. This statistic is appropriate for use when X and Y are continuous variables with underlying normal distributions on the interval or ratio scales.

Product–moment correlation is based on the concept of **covariance.** With proportional consistency in two sets of scores, we expect that a large X is associated with a large Y, a small X with a small Y, and so on. Therefore, X and Y are said to covary; that is, they vary in similar patterns. With a strong positive relationship, then, an X score that is above the mean $\bar{X}$ should be associated with a Y score that is above the mean $\bar{Y}$. With a strong negative relationship a low X score (below $\bar{X}$) is associated with a high Y score (above $\bar{Y}$). Therefore, if we take the deviation of each score from its mean, called a *moment*, the moments for X and Y scores should be related. The product of the moments for X and Y is a reflection of the degree of consistency within the distributions, hence the name of the statistic.

Example

To illustrate the calculation of r, we use the data in Table 23.2, representing developmental scores on tests of proximal (reaching) and distal (prehensile skill) behaviors in 12 normal infants, 30 weeks of age.[5] The null hypothesis states that there is no relationship between these two behaviors and that the correlation coefficient will be equal to zero, H_0: $\rho = 0$. The alternative hypothesis states that there will be a positive relationship, H_1: $\rho > 0$.

The r Statistic

The computational formula for the Pearson r is

$$r = \frac{n\Sigma XY - (\Sigma X)(\Sigma Y)}{\sqrt{\left[n\Sigma X^2 - (\Sigma X)^2\right]\left[n\Sigma Y^2 - (\Sigma Y)^2\right]}} \quad (23.1)$$

where n is the number of pairs of scores.

To calculate r, we determine X^2, Y^2, and XY for each subject's scores and then substitute the sums of these terms into Equation 23.1 as shown in Table 23.2B. The calculations yield $r = .365$. This would be considered a relatively weak correlation, suggesting that there is little association between proximal and distal skills in this sample.

Test of Significance

The product–moment correlation coefficient can be subjected to a test of significance, to determine if the observed value could have occurred by chance (if it is significantly different from zero). Critical values of r are provided in Appendix Table A.4 for one- and two-tailed tests of significance with $n - 2$ degrees of freedom. The observed value of r must be *greater than or equal to* the tabled value to be significant. For this example, we locate the critical value $_{(a_1 = .05)}r_{(10)} = .497$. The observed value, $r = .365$, is less than this critical value, and H_0 is not rejected. Computer output shows that $p = .121$ (Table 12.2C). These data do not support a relationship between proximal and distal motor skills at 30 weeks of age.[‡]

CORRELATION OF RANKS: SPEARMAN RANK CORRELATION COEFFICIENT

The **Spearman rank correlation coefficient,** given the symbol r_s (sometimes called Spearman's rho), is a nonparametric analogue of the Pearson r, to be used with ordinal data.

Example

To illustrate this procedure, we examine the relationship between verbal and reading comprehension for a sample of 10 children with learning disability. The hypothetical scores are

---

[‡]See Appendix C for a power analysis for these data.

TABLE 23.2.   COMPUTATION OF THE PEARSON PRODUCT–MOMENT CORRELATION COEFFICIENT: PROXIMAL VERSUS DISTAL DEVELOPMENT SCORES ($n = 12$)

A. DATA

Subject	Proximal (X)	Distal (Y)	X^2	Y^2	XY
1	17	11	289	121	187
2	10	8	100	64	80
3	14	13	196	169	182
4	21	14	441	196	294
5	16	21	256	441	336
6	21	19	441	361	399
7	22	14	484	196	308
8	18	21	324	441	378
9	18	16	324	256	288
10	16	16	256	256	256
11	18	10	324	100	180
12	20	14	400	196	280
	$\Sigma X = 211$	$\Sigma Y = 177$	$\Sigma X^2 = 3835$	$\Sigma Y^2 = 2797$	$\Sigma XY = 3168$

B. COMPUTATIONS

$$r = \frac{n\Sigma XY - (\Sigma X)(\Sigma Y)}{\sqrt{\left[n\Sigma X^2 - (\Sigma X)^2\right]\left[n\Sigma Y^2 - (\Sigma Y)^2\right]}}$$

$$= \frac{12(3{,}168) - (211)(177)}{\sqrt{\left[12(3{,}835) - (211)^2\right]\left[12(2{,}797) - (177)^2\right]}} = .365$$

C. OUTPUT: HYPOTHESIS TEST

$_{(\alpha_1 = .05)}r_{(10)} = .497$ (Table A.4)

$H_0: \rho = 0;\ H_1: \rho > 0$

Do not reject H_0

Pearson		Distal	Proximal
Correlation	Distal	1.000	.365
	Proximal	.365	1.000
Sig (1-tailed)	Distal	—	.121
	Proximal	.121	—
N	Distal	12	12
	Proximal	12	12

based on an ordinal scale (1–100), as shown in Table 23.3. The null hypothesis states that there is no association between one's verbal and reading comprehension ability, $H_0: r_s = 0$. The alternative hypothesis states that a positive correlation is expected, $H_1: r_s > 0$.

Procedure

To calculate r_s we must first rank the observations within the X and Y distributions separately, with the rank of 1 assigned to the smallest values. Ties are given the average of

TABLE 23.3. COMPUTATION OF THE SPEARMAN RANK CORRELATION COEFFICIENT (r_S): VERBAL AND READING COMPREHENSION SCORES ($n = 10$)

A. DATA

Subject	Verbal X	Reading Y	R_X	R_Y	d	d^2
1	73	71	6	5	1	1
2	59	63	3	3	0	0
3	86	92	9	10	-1	1
4	81	64	8	4	4	16
5	76	73	7	7	0	0
6	90	80	10	9	1	1
7	55	45	2	1	1	1
8	61	72	4	6	-2	4
9	41	48	1	2	-1	1
10	69	75	5	8	-3	9
						$34 = \Sigma d^2$

B. COMPUTATIONS

$$r_s = 1 - \frac{6\Sigma d^2}{n(n^2 - 1)} = 1 - \frac{6(34)}{10(100 - 1)} = .79$$

C. OUTPUT: HYPOTHESIS TEST

$(\alpha_1 = .05)\, r_{s(10)} = .564$ (Table A.13)

$H_0: r_s = 0;\ H_1: r_s > 0$

Reject H_0

Spearman rho		Reading	Verbal
Correlation	Reading	1.000	.794
	Verbal	.794	1.000
Sig (1-tailed)	Reading	—	.003
	Verbal	.003	—
N	Reading	10	10
	Verbal	10	10

their ranks (the procedure for ranking scores was described at the beginning of Chapter 22). These rankings are listed under R_X and R_Y in Table 23.3A. If there is a strong positive relationship between X and Y, then we would expect these rankings to be consistent; that is, low ranks in X will correspond to low ranks in Y, and vice versa. The Spearman procedure examines the disparity between the two sets of rankings by looking at the difference between the ranks of X and Y assigned to each subject, given the value d. We then square values of d to eliminate minus signs. The sum of the squared differences, Σd^2, is an indicator of the strength of the observed relationship between X and Y, with higher sums reflecting greater disparity.

The r_s Statistic

The value of r_s is determined by the computational formula

$$r_s = 1 - \frac{6\Sigma d^2}{n(n^2 - 1)} \tag{23.2}$$

where Σd^2 is the sum of the squared rank differences, and n is the number of pairs. As shown in Table 23.3, $r_s = .79$ for this example. This would be considered a relatively strong relationship.

Test of Significance

We can test the significance of r_s using critical values in Appendix Table A.11. This table uses n rather than degrees of freedom to locate critical values. The observed value of r_s must be *greater than or equal to* the tabled value to achieve significance. For this example, we find the critical value $_{(\alpha_1 = .05)}r_{s(10)} = .564$. Therefore, our calculated value of $r_s = .79$ is significant.

Ties

When ranked data result in many ties, the value of r_s can be inflated. A correction factor can be introduced and an alternative formula used to calculate r_s. This correction is described by Siegel and Castellan[6] and Daniel.[7] The effect of the correction is generally negligible, unless there is a large proportion of ties in either X or Y.

CORRELATION OF DICHOTOMIES

Measures of association are also useful with dichotomous variables. A **dichotomy** is a nominal variable that can take only two values, such as male–female, diseased–nondiseased, and yes–no responses on surveys. The integers 0 and 1 are usually assigned to represent the levels of a dichotomous variable. When either X or Y (or both) is a dichotomy, specialized correlation coefficients are used to test associations.

Phi Coefficient

The **phi coefficient,** given the symbol Φ, is used when both X and Y are dichotomous variables. The phi coefficient is a special case of the product–moment correlation coefficient, given only two values of X and Y. For ease of analysis, data are arranged in a 2×2 table, called a **contingency table.**

Example

Suppose we studied the relationship between motor and verbal skills in a group of 60 adults with traumatic brain injury. We devise a set of test items for which scores are graded as Pass or Fail. We assign 1 to Pass and 0 to Fail, as shown in Table 23.4. We organize our findings in a contingency table that shows how many of the patients achieved passing or failing scores on both verbal and motor tests. The table is arranged so that we can identify cells using the letters A, B, C, and D in the order shown in Table 23.4A. For the sake of consistency, the order of this notation has become standard. We can also identify marginal totals for each type of test.

TABLE 23.4. COMPUTATION OF THE PHI COEFFICIENT: ASSOCIATION OF SUCCESS IN MOTOR AND VERBAL SKILLS ($n = 60$)

A. DATA

		Motor Skills			
		Fail 0	Pass 1		
Verbal skills	Fail 0	(A) 8	(B) 25	Total 33	(A+B)
	Pass 1	(C) 20	(D) 7	27	(C+D)
	Total	28 (A+C)	32 (B+D)	60	

B. COMPUTATIONS

$$\Phi = \frac{BC - AD}{\sqrt{(A + B)(C + D)(A + C)(B + D)}}$$

$$= \frac{(25)(20) - (8)(7)}{\sqrt{(33)(27)(28)(32)}} = .497$$

C. OUTPUT: HYPOTHESIS TEST

$z = \Phi \sqrt{n} = .497 \sqrt{60} = 3.85$ $p = .00007$ (Table A.1)

$H_0: \Phi = 0;\ H_1: \Phi > 0$ Reject H_0

```
Phi = .497
Sig = .000
N of valid cases = 60
```

The Φ Statistic

We use the phi coefficient to test $H_0: \Phi = 0$ against $H_1: \Phi > 0$, according to

$$\Phi = \frac{BC - AD}{\sqrt{(A + B)(C + D)(A + C)(B + D)}} \tag{23.3}$$

Note that the denominator is the square root of the product of the four marginal totals.[§]
As shown in Table 23.4B, $\Phi = .497$, representing a moderate relationship. We can interpret the strength of this association based on a range of –1.00 to +1.00, although, theoretically, Φ can achieve a perfect correlation only when the two variables are evenly divided.

Test of Significance

The significance of Φ can be determined using the standard normal distribution, based on the relationship

$$z = \Phi \sqrt{N} \tag{23.4}$$

[§]An alternative formula involves use of chi-square (see Chapter 25, Equation 25.8).

For this example, $z = 3.85$. This observed value exceeds the critical value $z = 1.645$ for $\alpha_1 = .05$. The exact probability associated with this value can be obtained from Appendix Table A.1 (see Table 23.4C). The significance of Φ can also be tested using chi-square, which is described in Chapter 25. The phi coefficient is most reliable with samples of $n > 8$.[8]

Point Biserial Correlation

When one dichotomous variable (X) is correlated with one continuous variable (Y), the **point biserial correlation coefficient, r_{pb},** is used. It, too, is a special case of the product–moment coefficient, given that scores on Y are classified into two series: those who scored 0 and those who scored 1 on X. The point biserial coefficient can be used as a measure of the degree to which the continuous variable can be used to discriminate between the two categories of the dichotomous variable. If the two categories are perfectly divided so that all high scores on Y belong to one category, and all low scores belong to the other, r_{pb} would assume its maximum value. This maximum value will never reach 1.00 or –1.00 because of the inexact nature of dichotomized data. With a random distribution (no relationship), the coefficient would equal 0.00.

Example

Table 23.5A shows a set of hypothetical data for ratings of elbow flexor spasticity (resistive force in kilograms) for patients who have had a stroke on the right (1) and left (0) sides. We can use the point biserial correlation to test $H_0: r_{pb} = 0$, against $H_1: r_{pb} \neq 0$, to determine if the degree of spasticity is related to side of involvement.

The r_{pb} Statistic

We calculate the point biserial coefficient according to

$$r_{pb} = \frac{\bar{Y}_1 - \bar{Y}_0}{s_Y} \sqrt{\frac{n_1 n_0}{N(N-1)}} \tag{23.5}$$

where $\bar{Y}_1$ = mean of Y scores for $X = 1$ (right-side involvement)
        $\bar{Y}_0$ = mean of Y scores for $X = 0$ (left-side involvement)
        s_Y = standard deviation for the entire distribution of Y scores
        n_1 and n_0 = number of subjects in each group
        N = total sample

For this example, $N = 10$, $n_1 = 5$ and $n_0 = 5$. According to the calculations shown in Table 23.5B, $r_{pb} = .781$, which is a relatively strong association. These hypothetical results would suggest that degree of spasticity is a distinguishing factor related to side of involvement.

This formula for r_{pb} (Equation 23.5) is actually derived from the Pearson correlation (Equation 23.1). The results using either equation will be identical. Therefore, the point biserial correlation can be run using computer programs for the Pearson r (see Table 23.5C).

TABLE 23.5. COMPUTATION OF THE POINT BISERIAL CORRELATION COEFFICIENT: SPASTICITY AND SIDE OF INVOLVEMENT ($N = 10$)

A. DATA

Subject	Side[a] X	Spasticity Y
1	0	20
2	1	35
3	0	16
4	0	22
5	1	28
6	1	34
7	0	18
8	1	25
9	0	20
10	1	22

[a]0 = Left; 1 = Right

B. COMPUTATIONS

$$\bar{Y}_0 = 19.20$$
$$\bar{Y}_1 = 28.80$$
$$s_x = 6.48$$
$$n_0 = 5$$
$$n_1 = 5$$

$$r_{pb} = \frac{\bar{Y}_1 - \bar{Y}_0}{s_Y} \sqrt{\frac{n_1 n_2}{N(N-1)}}$$

$$= \frac{28.80 - 19.20}{6.48} \sqrt{\frac{(5)(5)}{(10)(9)}} = .781$$

C. OUTPUT: HYPOTHESIS TEST

$_{(\alpha_2 = .05)}r_{(8)} = .632$ (Table A.4)

$H_0: r_{pb} = 0; \; H_1: r_{pb} \neq 0$

Reject H_0

Pearson		Spasticity	Side
Correlation	Spasticity	1.000	.781
	Side	.781	1.000
Sig	Spasticity	—	.008
(2-tailed)	Side	.008	—
N	Spasticity	10	10
	Side	10	10

Test of Significance

A test of significance can be applied to the point biserial coefficient using critical values for r (Appendix Table A.4) with $N - 2$ degrees of freedom (see Table 23.5C). The independent t-test can also be used, with side of involvement as the independent variable. According to these hypothetical data, side of involvement is significantly related to degree of spasticity ($p = .008$).

Rank Biserial Correlation

A variant of the point biserial procedure, called the **rank biserial correlation,** r_{rb}, is used when a dichotomy is correlated with a continuous variable on the ordinal scale.[9]

Example

Consider the situation when we are interested in exploring the relationship between sex (Y) and functional ability (X) in elderly patients. Function is graded on a 0 to 10 point scale, with 0 representing total independence. We test 10 individuals, 5 males (coded 0) and 5 females (coded 1). Hypothetical data are shown in Table 23.6A.

TABLE 23.6. COMPUTATION OF THE RANK BISERIAL CORRELATION COEFFICIENT: ASSOCIATION OF FUNCTION AND SEX ($n = 10$)

A. DATA	Function	Sex $\left(\begin{array}{l}1 = \text{Female} \\ 0 = \text{Male}\end{array}\right)$			R_X for	
Subject	X	Y	R_X	Y_1	Y_0	
1	9	1	10	10	
2	8	0	8.5		8.5
3	7	1	6.5	6.5	
4	3	1	4	4	
5	4	1	5	5	
6	7	0	6.5		6.5
7	2	1	3	3	
8	8	0	8.5		8.5
9	1	0	2		2
10	0	0	1		1
				$\Sigma R_{X_1} = 28.5$	$\Sigma R_{X_0} = 26.5$
				$\bar{R}_1 = 5.7$	$\bar{R}_0 = 5.3$

B. COMPUTATIONS

$$r_{rb} = \frac{2}{n}(\bar{R}_1 - \bar{R}) = \frac{2}{10}(5.7 - 5.3) = .08$$

We compute r_{rb} by ranking the ordinal responses on the X variable (R_X) for all subjects, and then listing these ranks separately for the two values of Y, as shown in the last two columns of Table 23.6A. The ranks assigned to each female subject are listed under Y_1, and the ranks assigned to each male subject are listed under Y_0. We add the ranks for X associated with each group, and then calculate the average rank for each group ($\bar{R}_1$ and $\bar{R}_0$).

The r_{rb} Statistic

The average ranks are substituted in the formula

$$r_{rb} = \frac{2}{n}(\bar{R}_1 - \bar{R}_0) \tag{23.6}$$

As shown in Table 23.6B, $r_{rb} = .08$, which suggests that there is no association between sex and functional ability in this hypothetical sample. No test of significance is available for this procedure.

Other Correlation Procedures for Dichotomies

Two other procedures can be used in situations when a variable with an underlying continuous distribution is treated as a dichotomy. For instance, attitudes can be scored as approve–disapprove, although these scores are based on an underlying continuum. We could grade a patient's gait as normal–abnormal, even though a continuum of quality in gait is present. Such dichotomies are considered artificial in that they are artifacts of a measurement method. When one continuous variable is correlated with an artificial dichotomy, the **biserial correlation coefficient** is used. When both X and Y are artificial dichotomies, the **tetrachoric correlation coefficient** is used. Both of these correlation procedures are uncommon, but will occasionally be seen in the literature. Procedures for calculating these coefficients can be found in the text by Glass and Hopkins.[10]

INTERPRETING CORRELATION COEFFICIENTS

Correlation versus Comparison

The interpretation of correlation is based on the concept of *covariance*. If two distributions vary directly, so that a change in X is proportional to a change in Y, then X and Y are said to covary. With great consistency in X and Y scores, covariance is high. This is reflected in a coefficient close to 1.00. This concept must be distinguished, however, from the determination of *differences between* two distributions. To illustrate this point, suppose you were told that exam scores for courses in anatomy and physiology were highly correlated at $r = .98$. Would it be reasonable to infer, then, that a student with a 90 in anatomy would be expected to attain a score close to 90 in physiology?

Let us consider the following table of paired distributions of exam grades. Obviously, the scores are decidedly different. The anatomy scores range from 47 to 60 and the physiology scores from 79 to 90. The mean anatomy grade is 52.9, whereas the mean physiology grade is 82.7; but each student's scores have a proportional relationship, resulting in a high correlation coefficient.

Correlation, therefore, is not going to provide information relative to the difference between sets of data, only to the relative order of scores, whatever their magnitude. A test of statistical significance for differences, like the *t*-test, is required to examine differences. It is inappropriate to make inferences about similarities or differences between distributions based on correlation coefficients.

Student	X Anatomy	Y Physiology
1	50	80
2	56	85
3	52	83
4	57	85
5	47	77
6	48	79
7	60	90

Causation and Correlation

It is also important to distinguish the concepts of causation and correlation in research. The presence of a statistical association between two variables does not necessarily imply the presence of a causal relationship; that is, it does not suggest that X causes Y or Y causes X. In many situations a strong relationship between variables X and Y may actually be a function of some third variable, or a set of variables, that is related to both X and Y. For example, researchers have shown that weak grip strength and slowed hand reaction time are associated with falling in elderly persons.[11] Certainly, we could not infer that decreased hand function causes falls; however, weak hand musculature may be associated with general deconditioning, and slowed reaction time may be related to balance and motor recovery deficits. These associated factors are more likely to be the contributory factors to falls. Therefore, a study that examined the correlation between falls and hand function would not be able to make any valid assumptions about causative factors.

Causal factors are best established under controlled experimental conditions, with randomization of subjects into groups. When this is not possible, researchers may use correlation as a reasonable alternative, but causality must be supported by biological credibility of the association, a logical time sequence (cause precedes outcome), a dose-response relationship (the larger the causal factor, the larger the outcome), and consistency of findings across several studies. Perhaps the most notable example of this approach is the long-term research on the connection between lung cancer and smoking, following numerous studies that confirmed strong correlations, but with a strong physiologic foundation, a clear temporal sequence, and a consistent dose-response relationship.

Willoughby offers a silly example to illustrate the temptation to infer cause and effect from a correlation.[12] In 1940 scholars observed a high positive correlation between vocabulary and college grades, and concluded, therefore, that an improvement in vocabulary would cause an improvement in grades. Willoughby argued that this would be the same as reasoning that a high positive correlation between a boy's height and the length of his trousers would mean that lengthening his trousers would produce taller boys! Clearly, the assumption that one variable causes another cannot be based solely on the magnitude of a correlation coefficient.

Factors Influencing Generalization of Correlation Coefficients

In most situations, a researcher looks at the degree of correlation in sample data as an estimate of the correlation that exists in the larger population. It is important, then, to consider factors that limit the interpretation and consequent generalizability of correlation values.

Range of Test Values

Generalization of correlation values should be limited to the range of values used to obtain the correlation. For example, if age and strength were correlated for subjects between 2 and 15 years old, a strong positive relationship would probably be found. It would not, however, be legitimate to extrapolate this relationship to subjects older than 15, as the sample data are not sufficient to know if the relationship holds beyond that age.

Similarly, the finding of a weak or absent correlation within one age range does not mean that no relationship exists outside that range. Even if we find no relationship between muscle strength and age for subjects aged 30 to 50, we might find a negative relationship for subjects aged 70 to 90. The nature of a relationship may vary dramatically as one varies the range of scores contributing to the correlation. Therefore, it is not safe to assume that correlation values for a total sample validly represent any subgroup of the sample, and vice versa.

Restricting the Range of Scores

The magnitude of the correlation coefficient is a function of how closely a cluster of scores resembles a straight line, based on data from a full range of X and Y values. When the range of X or Y scores is limited in the sample, the correlation coefficient will not adequately reflect the extent of their relationship. By limiting variation in the data, it is difficult to demonstrate covariance. Therefore, r is reduced. It is advisable to include as wide a range of values as possible for correlation analysis.

Assumption of Independence in Correlated Values

Valid correlation also demands that correlated variables be independent of each other. For instance, it would make no statistical sense to correlate a measure of gait velocity with distance walked, as distance is a component of velocity (distance/time). Similarly, it is fruitless to correlate a subscale score on a functional assessment with the total score, as the first variable is included in the second. In each case, correlations will tend to be artificially high because part of the variance in each quantity is being correlated with itself. Researchers should always be familiar with the nature of the variables being studied to avoid spuriously high and misleading correlations.

COMMENTARY

The Stork Was Busy

The application of correlation statistics to clinical decision making must be considered carefully. All statistical analysis is limited by the clinical significance of the data being analyzed. Researchers must be equally aware of the potential danger of using statistical correlation as evidence of a clinical association simply on the basis of numbers. The utility of correlation is limited because it cannot tell us anything about the actual nature of phenomena, and almost any two variables can be correlated numerically.

For example, Snedecor and Cochran cite a correlation of −.98 between the annual birth rate in Great Britain from 1875 to 1920 and the annual production of pig iron in the United States.[13] We can view these variables as related to some general socioeconomic trends, but surely, neither one could seriously be considered a function of the other. Another classic example from many decades ago involves the high positive correlation between the number of storks seen sitting on chimneys in European towns and the number of births in these towns.[14] Could one infer that storks are responsible for an increased birth rate! Obviously, we can offer a more logical explanation based on the increasing number of housing units that are built as the population increases, which provides more chimneys for storks to roost. These types of nonsense correlations help to illustrate the importance of analyzing the clinical credibility of any statistical association and understanding the nature of the variables being studied.

In a more serious vein, Gould describes the lamentable efforts of Sir Ronald Fisher (1890–1962), the father of modern statistics (he invented a little thing called the analysis of variance), who disputed the relationship between smoking and lung cancer.[15] As a smoker, Fisher's statistical argument was first that we could not know if smoking caused cancer or cancer caused smoking. Their undeniable mutual occurrence, he proposed, could reflect a precancerous state that caused a chemical irritation in the lungs that was relieved by smoking, leading to an increased use of cigarettes. More plausibly, however, he later suggested that the association was most likely due to a third factor, a genetic predisposition, which made people more susceptible to lung cancer, and at the same time created personality types that would lead to smoking. Fisher became a consultant for the tobacco companies in 1960, and was apparently instrumental in blocking lawsuits at that time. As this regrettable story illustrates, the often elusive nature of correlation must never allow us to lose sight of logic, and the need to continue to question and examine relationships to truthfully understand clinical phenomena.

KEY TERMS

correlation
correlation coefficient
scatter plot (diagram)
linear relationship
curvilinear relationship
intercorrelations
Pearson product–moment
    coefficient of correlation (r)

covariance
Spearman rank correlation
    coefficient (r_s)
dichotomy
phi coefficient (Φ)
contingency table
point biserial correlation
    coefficient (r_{pb})

rank biserial correlation
    coefficient (r_{rb})
biserial correlation
    coefficient
tetrachoric correlation
    coefficient

REFERENCES

1. Hinkle DE, Wiersma W, Jurs SG. *Applied Statistics for the Behavioral Sciences.* 2d ed. Boston: Houghton Mifflin, 1988.
2. Green SB, Salkind NJ, Akey TM. *Using SPSS for Windows: Analyzing and Understanding Data.* Upper Saddle River, NJ: Prentice-Hall, 1997.
3. Cohen J. *Statistical Power Analysis for the Behavioral Sciences.* 2d ed. Hillsdale, NJ: Lawrence Erlbaum, 1988.
4. Penning MJ. In the middle: Parental caregiving in the context of other roles. *J Gerontol* 1998;53B:S188–S197.
5. Loria C. Relationship of proximal and distal function in motor development. *Phys Ther* 1980;60:167–172.
6. Siegel S, Castellan NJ. *Nonparametric Statistics for the Behavioral Sciences.* 2d ed. New York: McGraw-Hill, 1988.
7. Daniel WW. *Applied Nonparametric Statistics.* Boston: Houghton Mifflin, 1978.
8. Ferguson GA. *Statistical Analysis in Psychology and Education.* 5th ed. New York: McGraw-Hill, 1981.
9. Glass GV. Note on rank-biserial correlation. *Educ Psychol Measur* 1966;26:623–31.
10. Glass GV, Hopkins KD. *Statistical Methods in Education and Psychology.* 3d ed. Boston: Allyn and Bacon, 1996.
11. Nevitt MC, Cummings SR, Hudes ES. Risk factors for injurious falls: A prospective study. *J Gerontol* 1991;46:M164–M170.
12. Willoughby RR. Cum hoc ergo propter hoc. *School and Society* 1940;51:485.
13. Snedecor GW, Cochran WG. *Statistical Methods.* 8th ed. Ames, IA: Iowa State University Press, 1991.
14. Wallis WA, Roberts HV. *Statistics—A New Approach.* Glencoe, IL: Free Press, 1956.
15. Gould SJ. The smoking gun of eugenics: Should we—can we—take a kindly view toward a hero's faults? *Natural History* 1991:8–17.

24

Regression

Correlation statistics are useful for describing the relative strength of a relationship between two variables; however, when a researcher wants to establish this relationship as a basis for prediction, a **regression** procedure is used. The ability to predict outcomes and characteristics is crucial to effective clinical decision making and goal setting. It also has important implications for efficiency and quality of patient care, especially in situations where resources are limited. Regression analysis provides a powerful statistical approach for explaining and predicting quantifiable clinical outcomes. For example, clinicians have looked at the relationship between functional assessments and length of stay to determine which factors are predictive of rehabilitation outcomes and resource use in patients undergoing rehabilitation.[1] Therapists have examined the relationship between the development of postural reactions and age in infants with Down syndrome.[2] Depression in patients with chronic low back pain has been associated with cognitive measures of self-control and perceived interference of back pain in activities of daily living.[3] Such analyses help us explain our empirical clinical observations and provide information that can be used to set realistic goals for our patients. The purpose of this chapter is to describe the process of regression and how it can be used to interpret clinical data.

LINEAR REGRESSION

In its simplest form, linear regression involves the examination of two variables, X and Y, that are linearly related or correlated. The variable designated X is the **independent** or **predictor variable,** and the variable designated Y is the **dependent** or **criterion variable.** For example, we could look at systolic blood pressure (Y) and age (X) in a sample of 10 women. Using regression analysis we can use these data as a basis for predicting a woman's blood pressure by knowing her age. If we plot hypothetical data for this example on a scatter plot, as shown in Figure 24.1, we can see that the data tend to fall in a linear pattern, with larger values of X associated with larger values of Y. The correlation coefficient for these data, $r = .87$, describes a fairly strong association.

If the data were perfectly correlated, all data points would fall along a straight line. This line could then be used to predict values of Y by locating the intersection of points

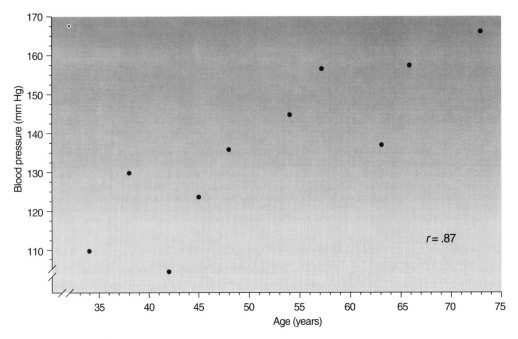

FIGURE 24.1   Scatter plot of age (*X*) and systolic blood pressure (*Y*) for 10 women.

on the line for any given value of *X*. With correlations less than 1.00, however, as in this example, a prediction line can only be *estimated*. If we look at the scatter diagram in Figure 24.1 we might try to plot a line that goes through the middle of the data points—but how do we objectively find the middle? We might try drawing a line through a point that represents the mean of *X* and *Y*, but how do we determine its slope? Clearly, we cannot make this determination without statistical help. The process of regression allows us to find the one line that "best" describes the orientation of all data points in the scatter plot. This line is called the **regression line.**

The Regression Line

The process of linear regression involves first determining an equation for the regression line and then using that equation to predict values of *Y*. The algebraic representation of the regression line is given by

$$\hat{Y} = a + bX \tag{24.1}$$

The quantity $\hat{Y}$ is the *predicted* value of *Y*. The term *a* is the **Y-intercept,** representing the value of *Y* when *X* = 0. Graphically, it is the point at which the line intersects the *Y*-axis (Figure 24.2). This can be a positive or negative value, depending on whether the line crosses the *Y*-axis above or below the *X*-axis. In regression analysis, *a* is also called a **regression constant.** The term *b* is the *slope* of the line, which is the rate of change in *Y* for each one-unit change in *X*. In regression analysis, this term is the **regression coefficient.** When *b* is positive, *Y* increases as *X* increases. When *b* is nega-

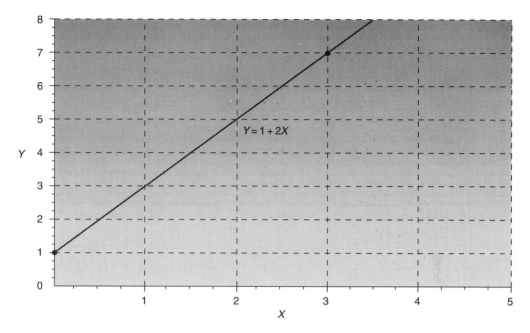

FIGURE 24.2 Graphic presentation of a linear equation.

tive, Y decreases as X increases. If $b = 0$, the slope of the line is horizontal, indicating no relationship between X and Y (Y is constant for all values of X). The positive or negative direction of the slope will correspond to a positive or negative correlation between X and Y.

We can illustrate these concepts by describing the linear equation $Y = 1 + 2X$. This equation represents a straight line that intersects the Y-axis at $Y = 1$. With a slope of 2, Y increases two units for every one-unit change in X. A line can be drawn from this equation by plotting any two points along the line and connecting them with a ruler. We can arbitrarily choose any two values along the X-axis and solve for the corresponding values of Y. The Y-intercept is often used as one of these points. Thus, we can plot one point at $X = 0$, $Y = 1 + 2(0) = 1$. The second point, say at $X = 3$, is determined by $Y = 1 + 2(3) = 7$. This process is illustrated in Figure 24.2.

The Regression Model

Figure 24.3 shows the regression of blood pressure (Y) on age (X), using the data from Figure 24.1. The values that fall on the regression line are the predicted values, $\hat{Y}$, for any given value of X; however, with $r < 1.00$, we can see that this line is only partially useful for predicting Y. Some data points are above the line, some are below, and some fall close to the line. Therefore, if we substitute any X value in the regression equation and solve for $\hat{Y}$, we will obtain a predicted value that will be somewhat different from the actual value of Y. We can visualize this error component in Figure 24.4. The actual Y value for each data point is some positive or negative vertical distance from $\hat{Y}$ on the

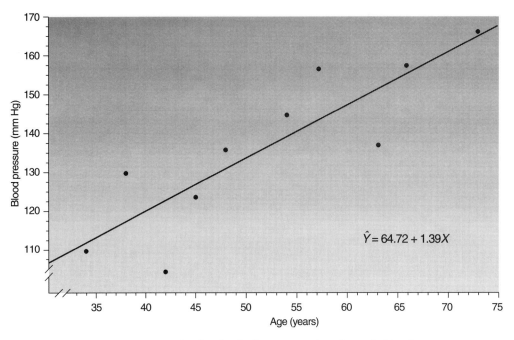

FIGURE 24.3   Least-squares regression line for the linear regression of systolic blood pressure on age.

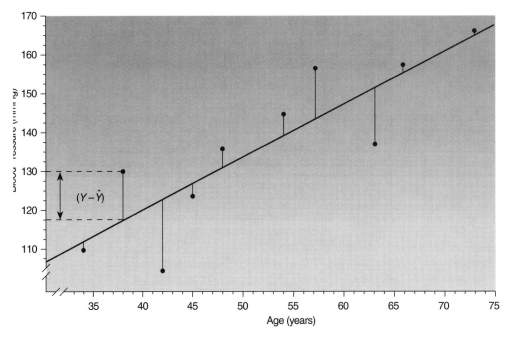

FIGURE 24.4   Deviation of scores from the least-squares regression line for the linear regression of systolic blood pressure on age. Vertical distances represent $Y - \hat{Y}$.

regression line. These distances $(Y-\hat{Y})$ are called **residuals.** Residuals represent the degree of error in the regression line.*

The regression line, or the **line of best fit** for a set of data points, is the unique line that will minimize this error component and yield the smallest residuals. Conceptually, this involves finding the square of all the residuals (to eliminate minus signs) and summing these squares, $\Sigma(Y-\hat{Y})^2$, for every possible line that could be drawn to these data. The one line that gives the smallest sum of squares is the line of best fit. Any other line, with any other values of a and b, would yield a larger sum of the squared residuals. This method of "fitting" the regression line is called the **method of least squares.** Of course, we do not actually go through the process of finding residuals for every possible line. Formulas have been developed that allow us to calculate the line of best fit based on the sample data.

Calculation of the Regression Line and Residuals

We can illustrate the process of regression using the study for predicting systolic blood pressure (SBP) as a function of age. Table 24.1A shows hypothetical data on SBP measurements for a sample of 10 women between 34 and 73 years of age. We calculate the regression coefficient, b, and the regression constant, a, using the computational formulas shown in Table 24.1B.† These values identify a line that intersects the Y-axis at 64.30 with a change of 1.39 units in Y for each unit change in X. Therefore, the line that best fits these data can be drawn from the regression equation $\hat{Y} = 64.30 + 1.39X$ (also see Table 24.3C). This line is superimposed on the scatter plot for these data in Figure 24.3.

We can now calculate the predicted score $(\hat{Y})$ for each subject using the regression equation, as shown in Table 24.2. For example, if we were presented with a woman who was 38 years old, we would predict that her systolic blood pressure would be $\hat{Y} = 64.30 + 1.39(38) = 117.1$. The actual blood pressure value for the 38-year-old subject was, however, 130. Therefore, the residual or error component of prediction is $(Y-\hat{Y}) = 130 - 117.1 = 12.9$. Note that the data point for this subject falls above the regression line; therefore, the regression equation underestimates SBP for this subject, and we have a positive residual.

Residuals are shown under the column labeled $(Y-\hat{Y})$ in Table 24.2. For a woman aged 63, we would predict a SBP of 151.9, where the actual score was 138. Therefore, the regression equation overestimates the SBP score for this subject, and we have a negative residual of –13.9. Most of the errors of prediction in this example are relatively small, because the correlation for these data is high ($r = .87$) and the points cluster close to the regression line. Note that the points for subjects aged 66 and 73 have almost negligible residuals, as these points rest very close to the regression line (Figure 24.4).

The sum of the residuals will always be zero, as the regression line is an average for all data points. Therefore, we take the sum of the squares of these error components, $(Y-\hat{Y})^2$,

---

*We could more accurately represent the regression equation as $Y = a + bX \pm$ error.

†An alternative formula for b can be used: $b = \left(\dfrac{s_y}{s_x}\right)$ where s_y and s_x are the standard deviations for the two variables.

TABLE 24.1. COMPUTATION OF LINEAR REGRESSION: PREDICTION OF SYSTOLIC BLOOD PRESSURE (SBP) AS A FUNCTION OF AGE ($N = 10$)

A. DATA Subject	Age X	SBP Y	X^2	XY
1	34	110	1,156	3,740
2	38	130	1,444	4,940
3	42	105	1,764	4,410
4	45	124	2,025	5,580
5	48	136	2,304	6,528
6	57	145	3,249	8,265
7	57	157	3,249	8,949
8	63	138	3,969	8,694
9	66	158	4,356	10,428
10	73	167	5,329	12,191
	$\Sigma X = 523$	$\Sigma Y = 1,370$	$\Sigma X^2 = 28,845$	$\Sigma XY = 73,725$
	$\overline{X} = 52.3$	$\overline{Y} = 137$		

B. COMPUTATIONS

$$b = \frac{n\Sigma XY - (\Sigma X)(\Sigma Y)}{n\Sigma X^2 - (\Sigma X^2)} = \frac{10(73,725) - (523)(1,370)}{10(28,845) - (523)^2} = \frac{20,740}{14,921} = 1.39$$

$$a = \overline{Y} - b\overline{X} = 137 - 1.39(52.3) = 64.30$$

$$Y = 64.30 + 1.39X$$

TABLE 24.2. PREDICTED SYSTOLIC BLOOD PRESSURE (SBP) SCORES BASED ON THE REGRESSION EQUATION $\hat{Y} = 64.30 + 1.39X$

Subject	Age X	SBP Y	$\hat{Y}$	Residuals $Y - \hat{Y}$	$(Y - \hat{Y})^2$
1	34	110	111.6	−1.6	2.6
2	38	130	117.1	12.9	166.4
3	42	105	122.7	−17.7	313.3
4	45	124	126.9	−2.9	8.4
5	48	136	131.0	5.0	25.0
6	57	145	143.5	1.5	2.3
7	57	157	143.5	13.5	182.3
8	63	138	151.9	−13.9	193.2
9	66	158	156.0	2.0	4.0
10	73	167	165.8	1.2	1.4
				$\Sigma(Y - \hat{Y})^2 =$	898.9

as an estimate of the usefulness of the regression line for prediction. The smaller the sum, the closer the data points are to the regression line and the better the prediction accuracy.

ASSUMPTIONS FOR REGRESSION ANALYSIS

In any regression procedure, we recognize that the straight line we fit to sample data is only an approximation of the true regression line that exists for the underlying population. To make inferences about population parameters from sample data, we must consider the statistical assumptions that affect the validity of the regression equation.

For any given value of X, we can assume that a random distribution of Y scores exists; that is, the observed value of Y in a sample for a given X is actually one random score from the larger distribution of possible Y scores for that X. In the example we have been using, the observed SBP for a given age is a random observation from the larger distribution of all possible blood pressure scores at that age. If we had studied several subjects at each age, we would see a range of blood pressure scores for the same value of X. Some of these Y values would be above the regression line, and some would be below it. For instance, subjects 6 and 7 were both 57 years old in our sample, with different blood pressure scores. As shown in Table 24.2, subject 6 has a predicted score very close to the true score, and subject 7 has a larger residual. If we took many measurements for women at 57 years old, the mean of the distribution of Y scores would fall on the regression line.

Theoretically, we could obtain such a distribution for every value of X, as shown in Figure 24.5. Each of these distributions would have a different mean, $\bar{Y}$. If these means

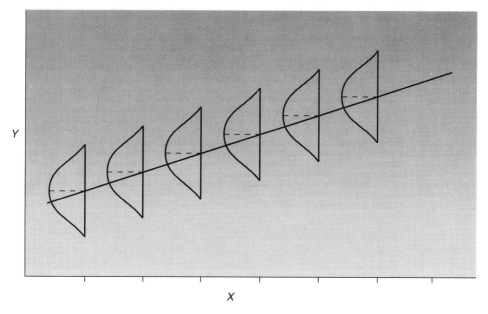

FIGURE 24.5 The linear regression model, showing theoretical normal distributions of Y around the regression line at given values of X. The mean of each distribution lies on the regression line. Therefore, $Y = \hat{Y}$ at each value of X.

were connected, they would fall on a straight line that estimates the population regression line. We assume that each of these distributions is normal and that their standard deviations are equal.

These assumptions help us to understand the relevance of residual error variance to regression analysis. Conceptually, it makes sense that the regression line will contain some degree of error, as it is unlikely that any one score randomly chosen from a distribution will equal the mean. Therefore, we tend to see a scatter of points around the regression line. The least-squares line that is fitted to the sample data is an estimate of the population regression line, and $\hat{Y}$ is an estimate of the population mean for Y at each value of X.

Analysis of Residuals

One way to determine if the assumptions for regression analysis have been met is to examine a plot of residuals, as shown in Figure 24.6. By plotting the residuals (on the Y-axis) against the predicted scores (on the X-axis), we can appreciate the magnitude and distribution of the residual scores. The central horizontal axis represents the mean of the residuals, or zero deviation from the regression line. When the linear regression model is a good fit, the residual scores will be randomly dispersed close to zero. The wider the distribution of residuals around the zero axis, the greater the error.

Several types of patterns can emerge in the residual plot. If the data meet all the basic assumptions, the pattern should resemble a horizontal band of points, as illustrated in Figure 24.6A. The horizontal orientation suggests that the residuals are evenly, but randomly, distributed around the regression line.

Figures 24.6B and C illustrate problematic residual distributions. The pattern in Figure 24.6B indicates that the variance of the residuals is not consistent, but dependent on the value of the predicted variable. Residual error increases as the predicted value gets larger; that is, the degree of accuracy in the regression model varies with the size of the

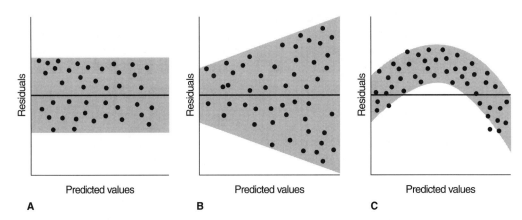

FIGURE 24.6 Patterns of residuals (Y-axis) plotted against predicted scores (X-axis). (A) Horizontal band demonstrates that assumptions for linear regression have been met. (B) Residuals increase as predicted values increase. (C) Curvilinear pattern indicates nonlinear relationship.

predicted value. Therefore, the assumptions of normality and equality of variance are not met. The curvilinear pattern, shown in Figure 24.6C, reflects a nonlinear relationship, negating the validity of the linear model. Other deviant residual patterns may be observed, such as diagonal patterns or a run of positive or negative residuals, indicating some problem in the interpretation of the regression model.

When data do not fall into the horizontal pattern, the researcher may choose to transform one or both sets of data to more closely satisfy the necessary assumptions. Such transformations may stabilize the variance in the data, normalize the distributions, or create a more linear relationship. Methods of data transformation are described in Appendix D. When curvilinear tendencies are observed, polynomial regression models may be used to better represent the data. This approach is discussed later in this chapter.

Most computer programs for linear regression will provide options for calculating, printing, and plotting residuals in a variety of formats. **Standardized residuals,** obtained by dividing each residual score by the standard deviation of the residual distribution, are often used instead of observed residuals to normalize the scale of measurement. Standardized residuals are analogous to z-scores, allowing the residuals to be expressed in standard deviation units. This approach is especially useful when different distributions are compared.

OUTLIERS

If a set of data points represents a distribution of related scores, the points will tend to cluster around their regression line. Sometimes, one or two deviant scores are separated from the cluster, so that they distort the statistical association. For example, the data points in Figure 24.7A show some variability, but most of the points fall within a definite linear pattern ($r = .70$). In Figure 24.7B, this distribution has one additional point, at $X,Y = 1,18$, that does not seem to fit with the rest of the scores. This point is called an **outlier,** because it lies outside the obvious cluster of scores. The correlation for these data with the outlier included is quite low, $r = .06$. One extreme value has significantly altered the statistical description of the data.

What accounts for the occurrence of outliers? Researchers must consider several possibilities. The score may, indeed, be a true score, but an extreme one, because the sample is too small to generate a full range of observations. If more subjects were tested, there might be less of a discrepancy between the outlier and the rest of the scores. There may also be circumstances peculiar to this data point that are responsible for the large deviation. For example, the score may be a function of error in measurement or recording, equipment malfunction, or some miscalculation. It may be possible to review the original data to find and correct this type of error. Other extraneous factors may also contribute to the aberrant score, some of which are correctable, others that are not. For instance, the data may have been collected by a different tester who is not reliable. Or the researcher may find that the subject was inappropriately included in the sample; that is, the subject may have characteristics very different from the rest of the sample, accounting for the deviant response.

Outliers should always be examined in a regression procedure because they can have serious effects on the outcome. Residual plots are often very helpful for identifying outliers. Some researchers consider scores beyond three standard deviations from the mean to be

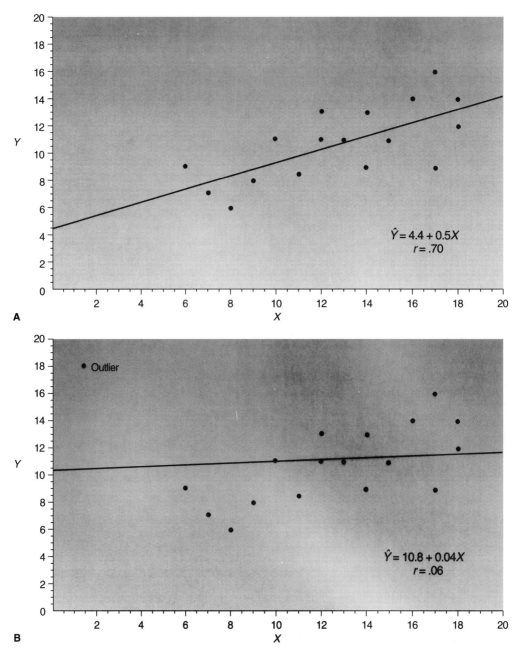

FIGURE 24.7 Regression lines for a distribution of scores (**A**) without and (**B**) with an outlier ($X, Y = 1,18$). In this case, the presence of the outlier causes the regression line to underestimate the degree of association in the data.

outliers. The researcher must determine if the deviant score should be retained or discarded in the analysis. This decision should be made only after a thorough evaluation of the experimental conditions, the data collection procedures, and the data themselves. As a general rule, there is no statistical rationale for discarding an outlier; however, if a causal factor can be identified, the point should probably be omitted, provided that the causal factor is unique to the outlier.[4] It may be helpful to perform the regression with and without the outlier, to demonstrate how inclusion of the outlier changes the conclusions drawn from the data.

ACCURACY OF PREDICTION

Once a regression line is derived, it can be used to predict Y scores based on values of X. It is important to remember that a regression line can be calculated for any set of data, even though it may not represent the data very well. The value of the correlation coefficient, r, is a rough indicator of the "goodness of fit" of the regression line. When r is close to ± 1.00, the regression line provides a strong basis for prediction. As r gets smaller, the errors of prediction will increase; however, the value of r is limited in its interpretation because it represents only the strength of an association. It will not evaluate the accuracy of prediction from the regression line. Several statistical approaches can be used for this purpose.

Coefficient of Determination (r^2)

Statisticians have shown that the square of the correlation coefficient, r^2, is indicative of the percentage of the total variance in the Y scores that can be explained by the X scores. Therefore, r^2 is a measure of proportion, indicating the accuracy of prediction based on X. This term is called the **coefficient of determination.**

For the regression of blood pressure on age, $r = .87$ and $r^2 = .76$ (see Table 24.3A). Therefore, 76% of the variance in systolic blood pressure can be accounted for by knowing the variance in age. We have 76% of the information we would need to make an accurate prediction. Obviously, some other unknown or unidentified factors must account for the remaining variance. The complement of r^2, or $1 - r^2$, reflects the proportion of variance that is not explained by the relationship between X and Y, in this case 24%. Using age as a predictor will result in a reasonable, but not thoroughly accurate, estimate of blood pressure.

Values of r^2 are more meaningful for conceptualizing the extent of an association between variables than values of r alone. For example, with a high correlation like $r = .70$, $r^2 = .49$. This means that less than 50% of the variance in Y is accounted for by knowing X, less than one might think with a correlation coefficient that seems fairly strong. When strength of association is of interest, r will be properly interpreted; however, when Y is predicted from X, r^2 provides a more meaningful description of the relationship. Values of r^2 will range between 0.00 and 1.00. No negative ratios are possible as it is a squared value.

Standard Error of the Estimate (SEE)

Another way to establish the accuracy of prediction is to consider the variance of the errors on either side of the regression line, or the residuals. If the variance in the residuals is high, then the scores are widely dispersed around the regression line, indicating a

TABLE 24.3. OUTPUT FOR REGRESSION ANALYSIS: SYSTOLIC BLOOD PRESSURE AND AGE (N = 10)

A. MODEL SUMMARY

R = .874
R square = .763
Std. Error of the Estimate = 10.611

B. ANALYSIS OF VARIANCE

Source	df	SS	MS	F	Sig.
Regression	1	2882.83	2882.83	25.76	.001
Residual	8	895.17	111.89		
Total	9	3778.00			

C. COEFFICIENTS

Parameter	Unstandardized Coefficients		Standardized Coefficients		
	B	Std. error	Beta	t	Sig.
(Constant)	64.304	14.708		4.372	.002
AGE	1.390	.274	.874	5.076	.001

large error component. The standard deviation of the distribution of errors is called the **standard error of the estimate (SEE)**.[‡]

The better the fit of the regression line, the less variability there will be around it and the smaller the standard error of the estimate. The SEE can be thought of as an indicator of the average error of prediction for the regression equation. Therefore, the SEE is helpful for interpreting the usefulness of a regression equation where reliance on a correlation coefficient can be misleading. To illustrate this with a clinical example, Rothstein and coworkers demonstrated an association between peak torque and isokinetic power of knee extension on a sample of healthy individuals and patients with rheumatic diseases.[5] This relationship is shown in Figure 24.8 for knee movement at a speed of 120 deg/s. Note that correlations are high for both plots (r = .95 and .97), representing patients and normal subjects. Accordingly, the value of r^2 is also high for both distributions. Therefore, r^2 is not helpful in distinguishing between these groups; however, the SEE for the patients' scores is almost twice that of the normals. This is indicative of the greater variability in data points around

---

[‡]The standard error of the estimate is defined by SEE = $\sqrt{\dfrac{\Sigma(Y - \hat{Y})^2}{(n - 2)}}$ where $\Sigma(Y - \hat{Y})^2$ is the sum of the squared residuals, and n represents the number of pairs of scores. For the data in Table 24.2,

SEE = $\sqrt{\dfrac{900.7}{(10 - 2)}}$ = 10.61.

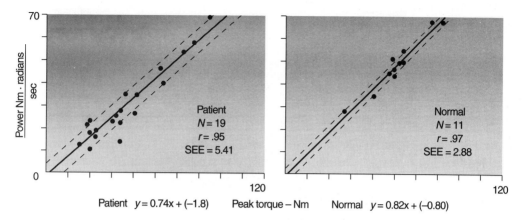

FIGURE 24.8 Relationship of power and peak torque at 120 deg/s of isokinetic movement for a group of patients with rheumatic disease and a normal group. (From Rothstein JM, DeLitto A, Sinacore DR, Rose SJ. Electromyographic, peak torque, and power relationships during isokinetic movement. *Phys Ther* 1983;63:926–33. Reprinted with permission of the American Physical Therapy Association.)

the regression line for the patients. Therefore, predictions obtained with the patients' regression line will be less accurate than those obtained using the line for normals.

Researchers can reduce standard error, and thereby improve accuracy of prediction, by including more than one observation at each value of X within a single study. This improves the estimation of variability at each X, thereby making the regression line a better estimate of the population mean.

ANALYSIS OF VARIANCE OF REGRESSION

Up to this point, we have used regression analysis primarily as a descriptive technique. We can also draw statistical inferences about the regression equation, to document that the observed relationship between X and Y did not occur by chance. We do this by an **analysis of variance of regression.** In essence, this analysis tests the null hypothesis, H_0: $b = 0$, and is analogous to testing the significance of the correlation between X and Y. If H_0 is true, the regression line is essentially horizontal, perhaps with some deviation as a result of sampling error. If H_0 is false, b does not equal zero.[§]

The variance components in a regression analysis are partitioned similarly to those in a regular analysis of variance. The total variance, represented by the total sum of squares (SS_t), reflects the variance explained by the regression of Y on X and the unexplained error variance. These variance components are illustrated in Figure 24.9. For a given X we can locate the observed value of Y and the predicted score $\hat{Y}$, which lies on the regression line. We can also establish the value for $\bar{Y}$, the mean of all Y scores. Without the regression line,

---

[§]The slope of the regression line can also be tested using the *t*-test: $t = \dfrac{b}{(SEE/s_X\sqrt{n-1})}$, where s_X is the standard deviation of the X scores. The results of this test will be the same as for the analysis of variance of regression, based on the relationship $F = t^2$.

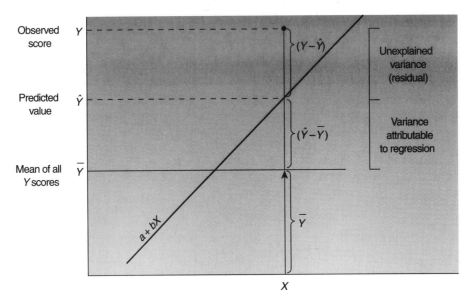

FIGURE 24.9   Illustration of the variance components in an analysis of variance for regression.

the best we can do to predict Y is the mean of the distribution, $\bar{Y}$. For example, if we knew that the mean height for men was 5 ft 8 in., and we wanted to predict the height of any man on the street, our best estimate would be 5 ft 8 in.; but if height is related to weight, then we can improve this estimate if we also know the man's weight. We know more about his height (Y) by knowing his weight (X). Therefore, by using the regression line we have improved our prediction by the amount $\hat{Y}-\bar{Y}$, which is the deviation of the predicted score from the mean. This distance tells us how much better we can predict Y by knowing X.

  If we look at $\Sigma(\hat{Y}-\bar{Y})$ for all the data points in a distribution, we will be able to determine how much of the total variation in the sample is accounted for by knowing the regression of Y on X. The sum of the squares of these differences, $\Sigma(\hat{Y}-\bar{Y})^2$, is called the **regression sum of squares** (SS_{reg}), or that part of Y that is explained by X.

  The rest of the variance is attributed to the deviation of each observed score from the regression line, $(Y-\hat{Y})$, or the residual. It is that part of Y that is not explained by X. This value is an indication of how good or poor a fit the regression line is. When the fit is good, the observed scores will fall close to the line, and the residuals will be small. This means that X is a good predictor of Y. When the fit is poor, X and Y are not strongly related, and these deviations will be large. The term $\Sigma(Y-\hat{Y})^2$ is called the **residual sum of squares** (SS_{res}), or the unexplained variance attributable to the residuals. A linear regression analysis will generate an analysis of variance table that provides these values.

  The ANOVA summary table, shown in Table 24.3B, represents the hypothetical regression of systolic blood pressure (Y) on age (X) for a sample of 10 women (from Figure 24.3). This output follows the format of a standard analysis of variance, with a total of $n-1$ degrees of freedom. In the linear model, 1 degree of freedom is always associated with the regression; therefore, $n-2$ degrees of freedom are attributed to the residuals (the error term). The value of F is equal to $MS_{\text{reg}} / MS_{\text{res}}$.

In this example, the observed *F*-ratio for the regression is 25.76, with 1 and 8 degrees of freedom. As shown in Table 24.3B, this test is significant at .001.[11] This tells us that the relationship between *X* and *Y* is not likely to be the result of chance. It does not indicate how strong this relationship is.

When the analysis of variance of regression results in a nonsignificant *F*-test, the researcher concludes that the observed relationship could have occurred by chance; that is, the regression line does not provide a reasonable basis for predicting values of *Y*. This finding may also occur when the linear model is not an adequate representation of the data. For example, when curvilinear data are subjected to a linear regression analysis, the *F*-test will often be nonsignificant. It is important to examine a scatter plot to determine if this latter explanation is tenable. Methods for interpreting nonlinear regression will be discussed shortly.

RESTRICTIONS ON THE INTERPRETATION OF LINEAR REGRESSION ANALYSIS

Regression equations are derived from a set of known scores, and the accuracy of the regression line for prediction for the individuals in the test sample is reflected in the size of the residuals. The ultimate purpose of regression analysis is not, however, to predict scores we already know. The intent is to predict scores for a new sample of observations from the findings on the known data. Therefore, it is important that the reference population for the analysis be clearly specified, because predictions will not be applicable to those who do not meet population criteria. Most importantly, predictions cannot be validly made for values of *X* that go beyond the range of scores that were used to generate the regression line. If we determine a regression line for predicting blood pressure from age based on a sample of women 34 to 73 years, we cannot apply the equation to males or to younger subjects. We cannot know if the shape of the distribution would be altered with the addition of scores at lower age ranges. Therefore, generalization of a regression procedure is inherently limited by the range of scores used to derive the equation.

A second consideration in the interpretation of regression data is the adequacy of a linear fit. Just as with correlation, linear regression procedures are useful only if the distribution of scores demonstrates a linear association between *X* and *Y*. The lack of a significant slope does not necessarily mean that *X* and *Y* are unrelated, but may indicate that the relationship does not follow a straight line. We discuss the application of regression to curvilinear relationships in the next section.

NONLINEAR REGRESSION

There are obvious limitations inherent in linear regression for describing curvilinear relationships. Because linear regression is the most commonly used regression model, researchers should be wary about interpreting outcomes that demonstrate no relationship between *X* and *Y*. For example, look at the data plotted in Figure 24.10, showing the relationship between psychomotor ability and age for a hypothetical sample of 30 subjects

---

[11]We compare this value with the critical value $_{(.05)}F_{(1,8)} = 5.32$, taken from Appendix Table A.3. Our observed value is greater than the critical value, and, therefore, the variance attributable to the regression is significant.

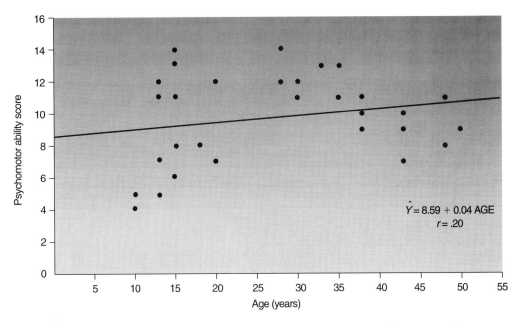

FIGURE 24.10 Linear regression of psychomotor ability (scored 0–15) on age. The regression line appears to be a poor fit.

aged 10 to 50 years. Using linear techniques, the correlation coefficient is low ($r = .20$) and we can demonstrate that the slope of the regression line is not significantly different from zero ($b = 0.04$). Based on this information alone, one would assume that X and Y were not related; however, examination of the scatter plot reveals that the data form a distinctly curved pattern. The measured skill improves until age 25, when a slow decline begins. Therefore, it makes sense to draw a curve that more accurately reflects the relationship between X and Y, as shown in Figure 24.11. We can express this curve statistically in the form of a quadratic equation:

$$\hat{Y} = a + b_1 X + b_2 X^2 \tag{24.2}$$

Equation 24.2 defines a parabolic curve, that is, a curve with one turn. This curve is called a *polynomial of the second order.* (A linear "curve," or straight line, is a polynomial of the first order.) The process of deriving its equation is called **polynomial regression.** Clearly, this fitted curve is more representative of the data points than the linear regression line.

The method of calculating the regression coefficients for this equation goes beyond this text. It is advisable to use a computer to perform these more complex mathematical manipulations; however, the application of this model is similar to that of linear regression. Polynomial regression is also based on the concept of least squares, so that the vertical distance of each point from the curve is minimized. Therefore, the curve can be used for predicting Y scores in the same way as a linear regression line.

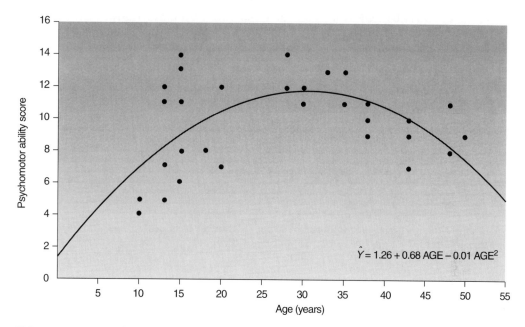

FIGURE 24.11 Curvilinear data for the regression of psychomotor ability on age, and the least-squares curve derived through a second-order polynomial regression.

Polynomials of higher orders can also be derived for curves that take two or more turns. These analyses are very complicated, however, and tend not to be very useful for accurately predicting performance. The polynomial equation can be expanded as necessary. For example, a curve with two turns could be described by

$$\hat{Y} = a + b_1X + b_2X^2 + b_3X^3 \tag{24.3}$$

Researchers often have to decide whether a linear or polynomial regression model best fits their data. This decision is greatly facilitated by examining a scatter plot of the data. The analysis of variance for regression can be applied to determine if the linear or polynomial regression model provides a better fit for a given set of data.[#]

Table 24.4 shows the analysis of variance for both a linear regression (A) and a second-order polynomial regression (B) for the regression of psychomotor ability on age. The F-ratio for the linear regression is not significant ($p = .279$), as we might expect from looking at the data in Figure 24.10. This tells us that the linear model is not adequate for describing this relationship. In the bottom panel we see that the polynomial regression is significant ($p = .007$), indicating that the quadratic curve is a good fit for these data. The equation for the curve is

$$\hat{Y} = 1.261 + .686(\text{AGE}) - .011(\text{AGE}^2)$$

[#]It is also possible to transform nonlinear data to achieve a linear fit by transforming one or both variables, often using log values (see Appendix D).

TABLE 24.4.   OUTPUT FOR ANALYSIS OF VARIANCE FOR LINEAR AND POLYNOMIAL REGRESSION OF PSYCHOMOTOR ABILITY ON AGE ($N = 30$) (See Figures 24.10 and 24.11)

A. LINEAR REGRESSION

ANALYSIS OF VARIANCE

Source	df	SS	MS	F	Sig.
Regression	1	9.33	9.33	1.22	.279
Residual	28	214.04	7.64		
Total	29	223.37			

COEFFICIENTS

Parameter	Unstandardized Coefficients		Standardized Coefficients		
	B	Std. error	Beta	t	Sig.
(Constant)	8.594	1.175		7.315	.000
AGE	.043	.039	.204	1.105	.279

B. POLYNOMIAL REGRESSION (QUADRATIC)

ANALYSIS OF VARIANCE

Source	df	SS	MS	F	Sig
Regression	2	68.11	34.05	5.92	.007
Residual	27	155.26	5.75		
Total	29	223.37			

COEFFICIENTS

Parameter	Unstandardized Coefficients		Standardized Coefficients		
	B	Std. error	Beta	t	Sig.
(Constant)	1.261	2.510		.502	.619
AGE	.686	.204	3.242	3.364	.002
AGE**2	−.011	.003	−3.081	−3.197	.004

Note that the variance attributable to the regression now uses 2 degrees of freedom, because it involves a second-order curve.

A closer look at the analysis of variance helps us see how differently these two approaches explain the data. Note that the total sum of squares for both analyses is the same; that is, the total variability in the sample is the same, regardless of which type of regression is performed. What is different is the amount of that variance that is explained by each of the regression models. The sum of squares attributable to the regression in the linear analysis is 20.3, whereas for the polynomial regression it is 137.2. This clearly demonstrates how a greater proportion of the total variability is explained by the curve.

ANALYSIS OF COVARIANCE

The function of experimental design is to explain the effect of an independent variable on a dependent variable while controlling for the confounding effect of extraneous factors. When extraneous factors are not controlled, the results of measurement cannot be attributed solely to the experimental treatment. Statistically, we speak of controlling the *unexplained variance* in the data, that is, the variance in scores that cannot be explained by the treatment variable. All experiments will have some unexplained variance, sometimes because of the varied individual characteristics of the subjects and sometimes because of unknown or random factors that affect responses. When we cannot control these factors by purposefully eliminating them or manipulating them, we use principles of experimental design to decrease the error variance they cause.

In Chapter 9 we described several design strategies that can reduce chance variability in data, such as using homogeneous groups or matching. Someimes, however, design strategies are not capable of sufficient control. Even when random assignment is used, there is no guarantee that potentially confounding characteristics will be equally distributed, especially when dealing with small samples. The issue of concern is the ability to equate groups at the outset, so that observed differences following treatment can be attributed to the treatment and not to other unexplained factors. When the research design cannot provide adequate control, statistical control can be achieved by measuring one or more confounding variables in addition to the dependent variable, and accounting for the variability in the confounding factors in the analysis. This is the conceptual basis for **analysis of covariance (ANCOVA).**

Adjusting Group Means

The ANCOVA is actually a combination of analysis of variance and linear regression. It is used to compare groups on a dependent variable, where there is reason to suspect that groups differ on some relevant characteristic, called a **covariate,** before treatment. The variability that can be attributed to the covariate is partitioned out, and effectively removed from the analysis of variance, allowing for a more valid explanation of the relationship between the independent and dependent variables.

Example

We can clarify this process with a hypothetical example. Suppose we wanted to compare the effect of two teaching strategies on the clinical performance of students in their first year of clinical training. We hypothesize that training with videotaped cases (Strategy 1) will be more effective than discussion and reading groups (Strategy 2). We randomly assign 12 students to two groups ($n = 6$ per group). We are concerned, however, that the students' academic performance would be a potential confounding factor in making this comparison, based on the assumption that there is a correlation between academic and clinical performance. Therefore, we would want to know if the grade point average

TABLE 24.5.   ANALYSIS OF VARIANCE FOR COMPARISON OF CLINICAL PERFORMANCE FOLLOWING TWO TEACHING STRATEGIES ($N = 12$)

Source	df	SS	MS	F	Sig.
Strategy	1	65.33	65.33	.122	.734
Error	10	5360.33	536.03		
Total	11	5425.66			

(GPA) in the two groups had been evenly distributed. If one group happened to have a higher GPA than the other, our results could be misleading. In this example, teaching strategy is the independent variable, clinical performance is the dependent variable, and GPA is the covariate. By knowing the values of the covariate, we can determine if the groups are different on GPA, and we can use this information to adjust our interpretation of the dependent variable if necessary.

To illustrate how the ANCOVA offers this control, let us first look at a hypothetical comparison between the two teaching groups, without considering GPA. Suppose we obtain the following means for clinical performance on a standardized test (scored 0–100):

Mean clinical score

Strategy 1	43.8 ($\pm$ 24.5)
Strategy 2	48.5 ($\pm$ 21.7)

The analysis of variance comparing these two groups is shown in Table 24.5, demonstrating that these two means are not statistically different ($p = .734$).** Based on this result, is it reasonable to conclude that the teaching strategies are not different? Or might we suspect that GPA may be differentially distributed between the two groups, which has biased the results? To answer these questions, we must take a closer look at the data to see how these variables are related.

Regression

Figure 24.12 shows the distribution of GPA and clinical performance scores for Strategy 1 (•) and Strategy 2 (○) with their respective regression lines. The dependent variable, clinical performance score, is plotted along the Y-axis, and the covariate, GPA, is plotted along the X-axis. We can see from this scatter plot that these variables are highly correlated for both groups ($r = .93$ and $.99$), and that the slopes of the two regression lines are fairly similar ($b = 53.7$ and 46.5).

**An unpaired t-test could also have been performed with the same result ($t = .349, df = 10, p = .734$); however, to adjust scores with a covariate, an analysis of variance must be used. Therefore, we have used the ANOVA here to facilitate comparison of outcomes with the ANCOVA.

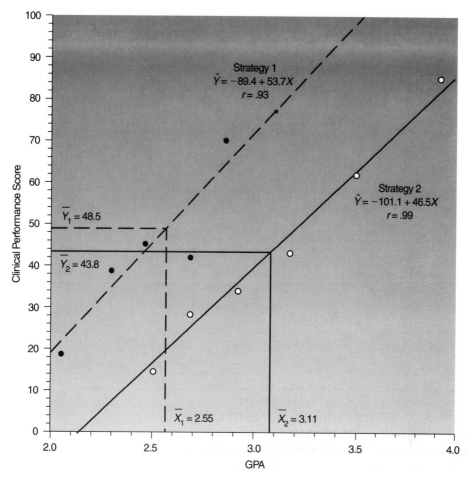

FIGURE 24.12 Regression lines defining the relationship between clinical performance score and grade point average (GPA) for two teaching strategies. GPA is the covariate for an analysis of covariance. The mean GPA for strategy 2 is substantially lower than that for strategy 1.

We can also see that the regression line for Strategy 1 is higher than that for Strategy 2, indicating that Group 1 had higher values of clinical performance for any given GPA than Group 2, even though the sample means for clinical score are not significantly different. There is, however, another important difference. If we look at the mean GPA for each group, we can see that the students using Strategy 1 have substantially lower GPAs than those using Strategy 2 ($\overline{X}_1 = 2.55, \overline{X}_2 = 3.11$). Knowing that GPA is a correlate of clinical performance, it is reasonable to believe that this difference could have confounded the statistical analysis.

Adjusted Means

To eliminate this effect, we want to *artificially equate* the two groups on GPA, using the mean GPA for the total sample as the best estimate for both groups. The mean GPA for both groups combined is 2.84. If we assign this value as the mean GPA for each group, we

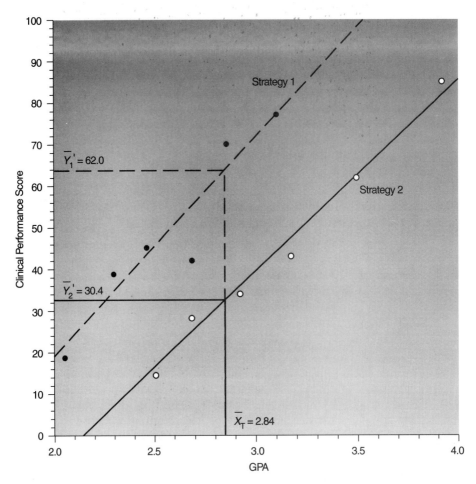

FIGURE 24.13   Adjusted means for clinical score, based on grade point average (GPA) as a covariate. Predicted values of clinical score are based on a common mean GPA for both teaching strategies.

can use the regression lines to predict what the mean score for clinical performance ($\hat{Y}$) would be at that value of X. That is, what average clinical score would we expect for Strategy 1 and Strategy 2 if the groups were equivalent on GPA? As shown in Figure 24.13, we would expect $\overline{Y}'_1 = 62.0$ and $= \overline{Y}'_2 = 30.4$. These are the **adjusted means** for each group.

Note that the adjusted mean for Strategy 1 (62.0) is higher than the observed mean for Strategy 1 (48.5), and the adjusted mean for Strategy 2 (30.4) is lower than the observed mean for Strategy 2 (43.8). These differences reflect variation in the covariate; that is, on average Strategy 2 students had a higher GPA than Strategy 1 students. By setting a common mean GPA, we moved the average GPA up for Strategy 1 (2.55 to 2.84), increasing the corresponding clinical score; and we moved the average GPA down for Strategy 2 (3.11 to 2.84), decreasing the corresponding clinical score. Therefore, we have adjusted scores by removing the effect of GPA differences so we could compare clinical scores as if both groups had the same GPA.

This example illustrates the situation where a covariate obscures the true nature of the difference between group means. This process may also work in the opposite direction, however; that is, the distribution of a covariate can make group means appear significantly different when in fact they are not. In that case, the analysis of covariance may result in no significant difference.

Assumptions for Analysis of Covariance

Before running an ANCOVA, several assumptions should be satisfied to ensure validity of the analysis.

Linearity of the covariate.   The analysis of covariance model is appropriate only if there is a linear relationship between the covariate and the dependent variable. It is most effective when $r > .60$.[6] For example, it would be unreasonable to use height or weight as a covariate for clinical performance. The researcher should check correlations before starting a study, to be sure that data are being collected on a useful covariate. Relationships that are curvilinear will invalidate the analysis of covariance, although the relationship may be made linear by mathematical transformation.

Equality of slopes.   The ANCOVA requires that the slopes of the regression lines for each group be parallel. Therefore, the regression coefficients should not be significantly different. The null hypothesis, H_0: $b_1 = b_2 = ... = b_k$, is tested for **homogeneity of regression,** or **equality of slopes.** This test can be done using a t-test or the analysis of variance.[6] If the slopes are not equal, the analysis of covariance will be misleading, and adjusted scores should not be used. Unequal slopes indicate that the relationship between the covariate and dependent variable is different for each group, and therefore, each group should be analyzed separately. The test for equality of slopes should be done before the ANCOVA is attempted, although some computer programs perform the test as part of the analysis of covariance. The results of the test should be checked before ANCOVA results are used.

Independence of the covariate.   The variable chosen as the covariate must be related to the dependent variable, but must also be independent of the treatment effect; that is, the independent variable cannot influence the value of the covariate. For example, suppose we wanted to study the effect of a general exercise program on balance, using lower extremity strength as a covariate. If we were to measure the subjects' strength after the treatment was completed, we might find that the exercise program increased the strength of the lower extremities. Therefore, the strength value would not be independent of the treatment effect and would not be a valid covariate. To avoid this situation, covariates should always be measured prior to initiation of treatment.

Reliability of the Covariate.   The validity of the ANCOVA is also founded on the assumption that the covariate is not contaminated by measurement error.[7] Any error found in the covariate is compounded when the regression coefficients and adjusted means are calculated. Therefore, justification for using the adjusted scores is based on accuracy of the covariate. Although it may be impossible to obtain totally error-free measurement, every step should be taken to ensure the greatest degree of reliability possible.

Output

After scores are adjusted according to the regression lines, an analysis of variance is run on the adjusted values. Table 24.6A shows the results of this analysis for the teaching strategy data from Figure 24.13. Recall that the analysis of variance showed no significant difference between these strategies (Table 24.5); however, now we find that the difference between groups is significant ($p = .000$), and we can reject the null hypothesis. We conclude that clinical performance does differ between those exposed to videotaped cases and discussion groups when adjusted for their grade point average. We have, therefore, increased the sensitivity of our test by decreasing the unexplained variance. We have accounted for more of the variance in clinical performance by knowing GPA and teaching strategy, than we did by knowing teaching strategy alone.

In the summary table for the ANCOVA, the between-groups effect is based on the adjusted group means (Table 24.6❶). As in a standard analysis of variance, the degrees of freedom will equal $k - 1$. The second line of the table represents the variance attributable to the covariate, or the regression of GPA on clinical score (Table 24.6❷). This component tests the hypothesis that the slope of the regression line is significantly different from zero. If it is not significant, the covariate is not linearly related to the dependent variable, and therefore, the adjusted mean scores will be meaningless. In this example, we can see that the covariate of GPA is significant ($p = .000$). The researcher should always examine the covariate effect first, to determine that the ANCOVA is a reasonable test. The degrees of freedom associated with this factor equal the number of covariates used in the analysis. In this case, with one covariate, we have used 1 degree of freedom.

TABLE 24.6. ANALYSIS OF COVARIANCE FOR ADJUSTED MEANS: COMPARISON OF CLINICAL SCORES FOR STRATEGIES 1 AND 2 (FIGURE 24.13)

A. ANALYSIS OF COVARIANCE

Source	df	SS	MS	F	Sig.
Strategy ❶	1	2083.73	20083.73	48.956	.000
GPA ❷	1	4977.26	4977.26	116.937	.000
Error ❸	9	383.07	42.56		
Total	11	5425.67			

B. ADJUSTED MEANS ❹

Group	Mean	Std. Error
1	30.37	2.94
2	61.96	2.94

❶ The between-groups effect tests the difference between Strategy 1 and Strategy 2, based on adjusted means.
❷ GPA is the covariate. This effect tests if the slope of the regression line for this variable is different from zero.
❸ The error term here is smaller than the error term in Table 24.5, as it does not include the variance accounted for by the covariate.
❹ The adjusted means are based on the regression of GPA on clinical performance (see Figure 24.13).

The third line of the table shows the error variance (Table 24.6❸); that is, all the variance that is left unexplained after the between-groups and covariate sources have been accounted for. When the covariate is a good linear fit, the error variance will be substantially reduced. This is evident if we compare the error sums of squares in Tables 24.5 and 24.6 for the ANOVA and ANCOVA of the same data. In fact, if we look at the error sum of squares for the ANOVA (SS_e = 5360.33), we can see that it is equal to the combined sums of squares for the covariate and the error component in the ANCOVA (4977.26 + 383.07 = 5360.33). By removing the effect of GPA from the unexplained variance, we have left less variance unexplained. Therefore, the ANCOVA allows us to demonstrate a statistical difference between the groups, where the ANOVA did not.

Using Multiple Covariates

The analysis of covariance can be extended to accommodate any number of covariates. There may be several characteristics that are relevant to understanding the dependent variable. For example, if we wanted to compare strength at different age ranges, we might use a combination of height, weight, limb girth, or percentage body fat as covariates. With multiple covariates, the analysis of covariance involves multiple regression procedures, where several X variables are correlated with one Y variable, and a predicted value for Y is determined, based on those covariates that are most highly correlated. Multiple regression techniques are discussed further in Chapter 27.

When several covariates are used, the precision of the analysis can be greatly enhanced, as long as the covariates are all highly correlated with the dependent variable and not correlated with each other. If, however, the covariates are correlated with each other, they provide redundant information and no additional benefit is gained by including them. In fact, using a large number of interrelated covariates can be a disadvantage, because each covariate uses up 1 degree of freedom in the analysis. This decreases the degrees of freedom left for the error term, which increases the F needed for significance between groups. The analysis then loses statistical power. With smaller samples, this could have a detrimental effect.

It is important, therefore, to make educated choices about the use of covariates. Previous research and pilot studies may be able to document which variables are most highly correlated with the dependent variable and which are least likely to be related to each other.

Pretest–Posttest Adjustments

The ANCOVA is often used to control for initial differences between groups based on a pretest measure. When intact groups are tested or when randomization is used with small groups, the initial measurements on the dependent variable are often different enough to be of concern in further comparison. For example, suppose we were studying the effect of two exercise programs on strength. We randomly assign subjects to two groups and would like to assume that their initial strength levels are similar; however, after the pretest we find that one group is much stronger on average than the other, a difference that occurred just by chance. We can use the ANCOVA to equate both groups on their pretest scores and adjust posttest scores accordingly. The analysis between groups is then done using the adjusted posttest scores, as if both groups had started out at the same level of strength.

Researchers are often tempted to control for initial differences by using **difference scores** as the dependent variable in a pretest–posttest design. There are disadvantages to this approach, however, because the potential for measurement error is increased when using difference scores (see Chapter 6). In experimental studies, this situation can reduce the power of a statistical test; that is, the greater the amount of measurement error, the less likely we will find a significant difference between two difference scores, even when the treatment was really effective. Therefore, many researchers prefer the analysis of covariance for statistically controlling initial differences. This approach is not, however, a remedy for a study with poor reliability. Although some research questions may be more readily answered by the use of change scores, the researcher should consider what type of data will best serve the analysis.

Interpreting the ANCOVA

The analysis of covariance is a powerful statistical tool that has often been looked on as a cure-all for design imperfections. Although it has the power to increase the sensitivity of a test by removing many forms of bias, it does not provide an automatic safeguard against problems in the design of a study. The ANCOVA cannot substitute for randomization. Quasi-experimental designs that use intact groups suffer from many interpretive biases, some of which the ANCOVA is able to control better than others. Indeed, unless a covariate is totally reliable, it will introduce some biases of its own. Some researchers have used the ANCOVA to compensate for failures in their design, such as the discovery of uncontrolled variables after data collection has been started, but this is not its intent. The analysis of covariance is correctly used in situations when experimental control of relevant variables is not possible and when these factors are identified and measured at the outset.

The ANCOVA has some limitations that should be considered in this context. One major criticism is that the adjusted means are not real scores, and therefore, the generalization of data from an analysis of covariance is compromised. It is also important to realize that one covariate may be insufficient for removing extraneous effects and that the outcome of an ANCOVA could be significantly altered if different combinations of covariates were used. In addition, researchers must decide which covariates will be most meaningful, and decide early so that data are collected on the proper variables. Covariates that are quantitative variables, such as height, weight, and age, provide the most precision for adjusting scores; however, qualitative variables such as sex and disability can be used as covariates.

COMMENTARY

It's Not That Simple

Two issues related to generalization of regression analysis should be mentioned here. First, as with correlation, it is important to refrain from interpreting predictive relationships as causal. Statistical associations by themselves do not provide sufficient evidence of causality. The researcher must be able to establish the methodological, logical, and theoretical rationales behind such claims; that is, causal inference is a function of how the data were produced, not how they were analyzed.[8] Second, it is important to restrict generalization of predictive relationships to the population on which the data were obtained. The characteristics of subjects chosen for a regression study define this population.

Simple linear regression analysis is limited in that it accounts for the effect of only one independent variable on one dependent variable. Most behavioral phenomena cannot be explained so simply. For instance, when we examined the predictive accuracy of the regression of blood pressure on age, we established that $r^2 = .76$. This indicates that 76% of the variance in blood pressure could be predicted by knowing a woman's age; however, 24% of the variance was unaccounted for. Some other variable or variables must be identified to improve the prediction equation. Multiple regression procedures have been developed that provide an efficient mechanism for studying the combined effect of several independent variables on a dependent variable for purposes of improving predictive accuracy. We present these techniques in Chapter 27.

KEY TERMS

regression
independent (predictor)
   variable (X)
dependent (criterion)
   variable (Y)
linear regression line
   ($\hat{Y} = a + bX$)
Y-intercept (a)
regression constant
regression coefficient (b)
residuals ($Y - \hat{Y}$)
line of best fit

method of least squares
standardized residuals
outlier
coefficient of determination
   (r^2)
standard error of the
   estimate (SEE)
analysis of variance of
   regression
regression sum of squares
   (SS_{reg})

residual sum of squares
   (SS_{res})
polynomial regression
analysis of covariance
   (ANCOVA)
covariate
adjusted means
equality of slopes
   (homogeneity of
   regression)
difference scores

REFERENCES

1. Heinemann AW, Linacre JM, Wright BD, Hamilton BB, Granger C. Prediction of rehabilitation outcomes with disability measures. *Arch Phys Med Rehabil* 1994;75:133–43.
2. Haley SM. Postural reactions in infants with Down syndrome: relationship to motor milestone development and age. *Phys Ther* 1986;66:17–22.
3. Maxwell TD, Gatchel RJ, Mayer TG. Cognitive predictors of depression in chronic low back pain: toward an inclusive model. *J Behav Med* 1998;21:131–43.
4. Snedecor GW, Cochran WG. *Statistical Methods.* 8th ed. Ames, IA: Iowa State University Press, 1991.
5. Rothstein JM, DeLitto A, Sinacore DR, Rose SJ. Electromyographic, peak torque, and power relationships during isokinetic movement. *Phys Ther* 1983;63:926–33.
6. Green SB, Salkind NJ, Akey TM. *Using SPSS for Windows: Analyzing and Understanding Data.* Upper Saddle River, NJ: Prentice-Hall, 1997.
7. Glass GV, Hopkins KD. *Statistical Methods in Education and Psychology.* 3d ed. Boston: Allyn and Bacon, 1996.
8. Cohen J, Cohen P. *Applied Multiple Regression/Correlation Analysis for the Behavioral Sciences.* Hillsdale, NJ: Lawrence Erlbaum Associates, 1975.

25

Analysis of Frequencies: Chi-square

Many research questions in clinical and behavioral science involve categorical variables that are measured on a nominal or ordinal scale. These questions usually deal with the analysis of proportions or frequencies within various categories. For instance, surveys often code responses that represent frequencies, such as the number of yes–no responses to a series of items or the number of respondents who fall into certain age groups. We can then ask questions about the proportion of respondents that fall into each category. In descriptive studies we are often interested in how certain nominal variables are distributed. For example, we might want to determine the proportion of patients with right-sided or left-sided strokes who are functionally dependent or independent at discharge or the proportion of therapists who work in private practice versus institutional settings.

These types of categorical data are analyzed by determining if there is a difference between the proportions *observed* within a set of categories and the proportions that would be *expected* by chance. For example, if therapists are equally likely to work in private or institutional settings, then theoretically we would expect an equal proportion, or 50%, to fall into each category. The null hypothesis states that no difference exists between the actual proportions measured in a sample and this theoretical distribution. If the observed data depart significantly from these expected null values, we reject the null hypothesis.

The purpose of this chapter is to describe the use of several statistics that can be used to analyze frequencies or proportions. These statistics are based on **chi-square, χ^2,** which is a nonparametric statistic used to determine if a distribution of observed frequencies differs from theoretical expected frequencies. Chi-square has many applications in clinical research, in both experimental and descriptive analysis. We concentrate on two general uses of the test. A test of *goodness of fit* is used to determine if a set of observed frequencies differs from a given set of theoretical frequencies that define a specific distribution. A test that compares the proportion of therapists in private and institutional settings fits this model, based on a theoretical distribution of 50:50. *Tests of independence* are used to determine if two classification variables are independent of each other, that is, to examine the degree of association between them. For example, we could study the frequency of left- and right-sided stroke in terms of functional level at discharge to determine if these variables are related or independent of each other. We also discuss the use of a related procedure called the McNemar test, for examining frequencies of correlated samples. In addition, several coefficients of association for categorical data will be described.

THE CHI-SQUARE STATISTIC

As we discuss the different applications of the χ^2 statistic, it is important to keep in mind two general assumptions: (1) *Frequencies represent individual counts*, not ranks or percentages. This means that data in each category represent the actual number of persons, objects, or events in those categories, not a summary statistic. (2) *Categories are exhaustive and mutually exclusive*. Therefore, every subject can be assigned to an appropriate category, but only one. Repeated measurement or assignment is not appropriate; that is, no one individual should be represented in more than one category. The characteristics being measured should be defined with enough specificity to avoid any overlaps in group assignment.

Chi-square is defined by*

$$\chi^2 = \sum \frac{(O - E)^2}{E} \tag{25.1}$$

where O represents the **observed frequency** and E represents the **expected frequency.** As the difference between observed and expected frequencies increases, the value of χ^2 will increase. If observed and expected frequencies are the same, χ^2 will equal zero.

We illustrate the application of this statistic using a simple example. Suppose we tossed a coin 100 times. The null hypothesis states that no bias exists in the coin, and we would expect a theoretical outcome of 50 heads and 50 tails. We observe 47 heads and 53 tails. Does this deviation from the null hypothesis occur because the coin is biased, or is it only a matter of chance? In other words, is the difference between the observed and expected frequencies sufficiently large to justify rejection of the null hypothesis?

We calculate χ^2 by substituting values in the term $(O - E)^2/E$ for each category. For heads,

$$\frac{(O - E)^2}{E} = \frac{(47 - 50)^2}{50} = \frac{(-3)^2}{50} = 0.18$$

For tails,

$$\frac{(O - E)^2}{E} = \frac{(53 - 50)^2}{50} = \frac{(3)^2}{50} = 0.18$$

---

*Although the definitional formula for χ^2 (Equation 25.1) is used most often, there is a computational formula that may be useful: $\chi^2 = \sum \frac{O^2}{E} - N$.

The sum of these terms for all categories is the value of χ^2. Therefore,

$$\chi^2 = \sum \frac{(O - E)^2}{E} = 0.18 + 0.18 = 0.36$$

We analyze the significance of this value using critical values of χ^2 found in Appendix Table A.5. Along the top of the table we identify the desired α level, say .05. Along the side we locate the appropriate degrees of freedom. In this case, $df = 1$. We will discuss rules for determining degrees of freedom for different statistical models shortly. Chi-square tests do not distinguish between one- and two-tailed tests because no negative values are possible.

The calculated value of χ^2 must be *greater than or equal to* the critical value to be significant. In this example, the observed value is less than $_{(.05)}\chi^2_{(1)} = 3.84$. Therefore, H_0 is not rejected, and we would conclude that the coin toss was fair.

GOODNESS OF FIT

In tests for **goodness of fit,** the researcher compares observed frequency counts with a known or theoretical distribution. The classical studies of heredity performed by Mendel illustrate this concept. He observed the color and shape of several generations of peas and compared the frequencies of specific color and shape combinations with a theoretical distribution based on his predictions about the role of dominant and recessive genes. When the observed distributions matched the theoretical model, his genetic theory was supported. Similarly, the coin toss described earlier is essentially a test of goodness of fit to a probability distribution. Chi-square will test the null hypothesis that the proportion of outcomes within each category will not significantly differ from the expected distribution; that is, the observed proportions will fall within random fluctuation of the expected proportions.

There are many models for testing goodness of fit. The three most common applications involve testing observed data against a **uniform distribution** across all categories, a **normal distribution** of scores, and a **known distribution** within the underlying population.

Sample size for goodness of fit tests should be large enough that no expected frequencies are less than 1.0; that is, every category in the theoretical distribution of interest should expect at least one count. When this criterion is not met, sample size should be increased or categories combined to create an appropriate distribution. Note that this criterion applies to the expected frequencies, not the observed counts.

Uniform Distributions

Consider a study designed to determine if the incidence of stroke is greater on the right or the left in people over 70 years of age. If we assume that the causative factors of stroke are not biased to one side, then theoretically we would expect to see a uniform distribution, 50% right-sided and 50% left-sided strokes, in the population. This is the null hypothesis, representing chance occurrence. Suppose we obtain data from a broad sample of 130 patients, and find that 71 were affected on the right and 59 on the left. Is this distribution significantly different from the 50% ratio we expect by chance?

We use chi-square to determine if the observed frequencies fit the uniform distribution model by comparing the observed and expected frequencies using Equation 25.1. First we must establish the expected frequencies. For a uniform distribution we do this simply by dividing the total sample equally among the categories. Therefore, if chance is operating, we would expect 50% of our sample, or 65 people, to have right-sided strokes, and 50%, or 65 people, to have left-sided strokes. We calculate $(O - E)^2/E$ for each category, as shown in Table 25.1.

In the uniform distribution goodness of fit model, degrees of freedom equal $k - 1$, where k is the number of categories. With two categories (right and left), $df = 1$. Therefore, we compare the calculated value, $x^2 = 1.10$, with the critical value $_{(.05)}x^2_{(1)} = 3.84$, obtained from Appendix Table A.5. The calculated value is less than the critical value, and we do not reject the null hypothesis. The difference between the observed and expected frequencies can be attributed to chance, and our sample fits the expected uniform distribution. According to these hypothetical data, the incidence of right- and left-sided strokes can be considered a random event.

By definition, the expected frequencies for a uniform distribution will be evenly divided among the categories. Therefore, if we studied a sample with three or four categories, we would test the observed frequencies in each category against expected frequencies of 33.3% and 25%, respectively. For example, if we assigned 130 cases to three different categories, we would expect 43.33 cases in each category. If we had four categories, we would expect 32.5 cases per category. It may seem strange to be dealing with fractions of a count in expected frequencies, as we obviously cannot have a fraction of an individual in a category; however, these values represent only theoretical values based on an infinite number of possible scores, and cannot be interpreted as representing actual expected counts.

Normal Distributions

The goodness of fit test can also be used to determine if an observed distribution is significantly different from the normal curve. It is often of interest to establish the shape of a distribution as a descriptive procedure. Sometimes it is not obvious if data do indeed

TABLE 25.1.   CALCULATION OF x^2 TO TEST GOODNESS OF FIT TO A UNIFORM DISTRIBUTION: FREQUENCY OF LEFT- AND RIGHT-SIDE STROKE ($N = 130$)

A. DATA AND COMPUTATION					$\dfrac{(O-E)^2}{E}$
Side	O	E	O−E	$(O-E)^2$	
Right	71	65	6	36	.55
Left	59	65	−6	36	.55
	130	130			

$$x^2 = \sum \frac{(O-E)^2}{E} = 1.10$$

B. OUTPUT: HYPOTHESIS TEST

$_{(.05)}x^2_{(1)} = 3.84$ (Table A.5)

Do not reject H_0

```
Chi-square = 1.10
df = 1
p = .293
```

fit the normal model. Chi-square can be used to evaluate if observed data fall within the typical normal distribution.

For example, assume we have a distribution of IQ scores for a sample of 200 individuals. These scores have a sample mean of $\bar{X} = 100$ and standard deviation $s = 15$, as illustrated in Figure 25.1. If these 200 scores fall in a normal distribution, we would expect 34.13% of them to fall within one standard deviation from the mean in either direction; that is, 68.26 scores will fall within the range 85 to 100 and 68.26 scores will fall within the range 100 to 115. Similarly, we would expect 13.59% of the scores to fall within the interval from one standard deviation to two standard deviations; that is, 27.18 scores should fall between 70 and 85 and another 27.18 scores should fall between 115 and 130, and so forth. These values are the expected frequencies. The null hypothesis states that the distribution of scores will match the percentage distribution defined by the normal curve.

We compare these expected frequencies with the observed frequencies by arranging the observed scores in equal and nonoverlapping intervals, covering the full range of observed scores. The cutoff points for these intervals are arbitrary, but we can facilitate the goodness of fit model by using intervals equal to the standard deviations. As shown in Table 25.2, we use the known percentages of the normal curve to calculate the expected frequencies.

If we examine the observed frequencies, we may have some question about the shape of the distribution, as 92 scores fall below the mean and 108 fall above it. In a normal distribution we would expect the median to fall at the mean. Therefore, because more scores fall above the mean, this distribution may be skewed to the left. We cannot make this determination subjectively, however, because we are dealing with a small sample relative to the total population, and differences may be the result of chance. The chi-square test is used to determine if the observed differences from the normal distribution are due to chance or if this distribution is indeed skewed. The calculation of chi-square, using Equation 25.1, is shown in Table 25.2 for these data. For this distribution, $\chi^2 = 6.41$.

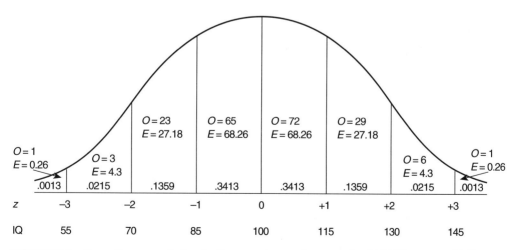

FIGURE 25.1 Proportions expected under the normal curve for a sample of 200 IQ scores, with $\bar{X} = 100$ and $s = 15$. Intervals correspond to standard deviations. Expected frequencies are calculated according to percentages defined by the normal standard distribution.

TABLE 25.2. CALCULATION OF χ^2 FOR GOODNESS OF FIT TO THE NORMAL DISTRIBUTION: SAMPLE OF IQ SCORES ($N = 200, \overline{X} = 100, s = 15$)

A. DATA and COMPUTATION

IQ Score	O	E	Percentage of curve	(O−E)	(O−E)²	$\dfrac{(O-E)^2}{E}$
< 55	1	0.26	1.30	0.74	0.55	2.11
55−69	3	4.30	2.15	−1.30	1.69	0.39
70−84	23	27.18	13.59	−4.18	17.47	0.64
85−99	65	68.26	34.13	−3.26	10.63	0.16
100−114	72	68.26	34.13	3.74	13.99	0.21
115−129	29	27.18	13.59	1.82	3.31	0.12
130−144	6	4.30	2.15	1.70	2.89	0.57
≥145	1	0.26	1.30	0.74	0.55	2.11
	200	200.00				$\chi^2 = 6.41$

B. OUTPUT: HYPOTHESIS TEST

$_{(.05)}\chi^2{}_{(5)} = 11.07$ (Table A.5)

Do not reject H_0

```
Chi-square = 6.41
df = 5
p = .494
```

The degrees of freedom associated with the normal distribution goodness of fit model are equal to $k - 3$.[†] Therefore, with eight intervals, $df = 8 - 3 = 5$. From Table A.5, we locate the critical value $_{(.05)}\chi^2{}_{(5)} = 11.07$. Because the calculated value is smaller than the critical value, we cannot reject the null hypothesis. The observed distribution is not significantly different from the theoretical distribution, and therefore, this sample of IQ scores is normally distributed. The observed differences from expected values are most likely due to chance.

Known Distributions

The third goodness of fit model compares a sample distribution with a known distribution within an underlying population. This is one way to document how well a sample represents its parent population. In many cases, the variable of interest is normally distributed in the population and the goodness of fit test for normal distributions should be used. In other situations, the population shows a unique distribution that can be tested against observed frequencies.

For example, suppose an investigator hypothesizes that thromboembolism is more common in individuals with certain blood types. If this is true, then we can expect to see

---

[†]In addition to the traditional loss of 1 degree of freedom in a set of scores, we must also account for the imposition of a known mean and standard deviation for the normal distribution.[1] Therefore, there are three restrictions on these data and a loss of 3 degrees of freedom.

TABLE 25.3. CALCULATION OF χ^2 FOR GOODNESS OF FIT TO A KNOWN DISTRIBUTION OF BLOOD TYPE ($N = 85$)

A. DATA and COMPUTATION

Blood Type	% in population	O	E	$O-E$	$(O-E)^2$	$\dfrac{(O-E)^2}{E}$	Std. Residual
A	39%	28	33.15	−5.15	26.52	0.80	−0.89
B	9%	19	7.65	11.35	128.82	16.84	4.10
AB	5%	6	4.25	1.75	3.06	0.72	0.85
O	47%	32	39.95	−7.95	63.20	1.58	−1.26
		85	85.00			$\chi^2 = 19.94$	

B. OUTPUT: HYPOTHESIS TEST

$_{(.05)}\chi^2_{(3)} = 7.82$ (Table A.5)

Reject H_0

```
Chi-square = 19.94
df = 3
p = .001
```

those blood types represented among patients with thromboembolism in higher percentages than in the overall population. Suppose we study a sample of 85 patients who have experienced thromboembolism. The null hypothesis states that the disorder is not associated with blood type and that the distribution of blood types in the sample will be similar to that in the overall population. Knowing that 39% of the population has Type A blood, 9% has Type B, 5% has Type AB, and 47% has Type O,[2] we can determine what proportion of the patients should be expected to have each blood type under the null hypothesis. For example, 39% of the sample, or $(0.39)(85) = 33.15$ patients, should have Type A blood. Hypothetical observations and expected values for all four categories are shown in Table 25.3A. By looking at the column labeled $(O - E)$, we can see that there are marked differences between expected and observed frequencies, some showing less than expected and others greater than expected values.

With a known distribution, we test χ^2 with $k - 1$ degrees of freedom. In this case, $df = 4 - 1 = 3$. The calculated value of $\chi^2 = 19.94$, as shown in Table 25.3A. This value exceeds the critical value $_{(.05)} \chi^2_{(3)} = 7.82$, and we can reject the null hypothesis. These hypothetical data do not follow the population distribution, and therefore, there is reason to believe that this disorder has some association with blood type.

INTERPRETING SIGNIFICANT EFFECTS: STANDARDIZED RESIDUALS

When the results of a chi-square test are significant, we can examine the results subjectively, to determine which categories demonstrate the greatest discrepancy between observed and expected values. For this purpose we can look at a residual for each cell, which is the difference between the observed and expected frequencies, given in the column labeled $O - E$. For the blood type study, for instance, the residual for Type A is −5.15. This means that the observed proportion of Type A blood in this sample was less than expected by chance. These raw values may be difficult to interpret, however, as they are effected by the number of observed counts within each cell; that is, cells with larger counts are likely to have larger residuals. Therefore, **standardized residuals** are often used to demonstrate the relative contribution of each cell to the overall value of chi-square:

$$\text{Std. Residual} = \frac{O - E}{\sqrt{E}} \tag{25.2}$$

For example, using the data for Type B blood in Table 25.3A, the standardized residual is

$$\text{Std. Residual} = \frac{11.35}{\sqrt{7.65}} = 4.10$$

Standardized residuals for blood types are listed in the rightmost column in Table 25.3. These residual values can be compared to determine which categories contributed most to the value of χ^2. Residuals that are close to or greater than 2.00 are generally considered important.[3] The values for blood type demonstrate that the difference between observed and expected frequencies for patients with Type B blood shows the greatest discrepancy. The positive sign for the residual indicates that the proportion of individuals with thromboembolism who have Type B blood is greater than expected by chance. The small residuals for the other blood types suggest that they do not contribute appreciably to the value of χ^2. The negative values for Types A and O indicate that those frequencies are actually represented in smaller numbers than would be expected by chance.

TESTS OF INDEPENDENCE

The most common application of chi-square in clinical research is in **tests of independence.** With this approach, researchers examine the association, or lack of association, between two categorical variables. This association is based on the proportion of individuals who fall into each category. These data may be obtained from randomized experiments or from descriptive studies involving classification of subject characteristics.

Many examples of these applications can be found in clinical literature. For example, Vraciu and Vraciu studied patients undergoing open heart surgery, and randomly assigned patients to two groups, one receiving a special program of breathing exercises and the other receiving routine postoperative care.[4] They used χ^2 to determine if the proportion of patients who had pulmonary complications was different for those who did and did not participate in the exercise program. Connolly examined the frequency of lateral dominance problems in a population of children with learning disabilities as compared with the frequency of problems in children with no disability.[5] Tanttula and coworkers used χ^2 to look at the association between location of injury and return to work in patients with burns.[6] Similarly, Deshpande et al. studied the association between specific clinical findings, such as recent surgery, tracheostomy and feeding tube use, and transfer back to an acute care facility in rehabilitation patients with traumatic brain injury.[7] Epidemiologic studies often use chi-square to evaluate the effect of different exposures among diseased and nondiseased individuals.[‡]

In each of the preceding studies, the research question asks if the proportions of subjects observed in each category are independent of each other. Two variables are considered independent if the distribution of one in no way depends on the distribution of the other. For example, if lateral dominance problems are independent of learning disability, then a child with a learning disability is no more likely to have such problems than a nondisabled child. The null hypothesis for a test of independence states that two categorical variables are independent of each other. Therefore, when the null hypothesis is rejected following a significant χ^2 test, it indicates that an association between the variables is present.

Contingency Tables

To test the relationship between two categorical variables, data are arranged in a two-way matrix, called a **contingency table,** with R rows and C columns. To illustrate, consider the data in Table 25.4A, taken from a study by Kleinkort and Wood, who looked at the effect of phonophoresis[§] with 1% versus 10% hydrocortisone for reducing pain associated with subdeltoid bursitis.[9] They studied 70 patients, 39 who received the 1% solution and 31 who received the 10% solution. They assessed each patient's pain level following treatment on an ordinal scale: no pain, minimal, moderate, or severe pain. The 4×2 contingency table shows the observed frequencies as the first entry within each cell (labeled "count"). The marginal totals along the right side of Table 25.4A indicate how many patients experienced each level of pain.

Expected Frequencies

The null hypothesis states that there is no association between the concentration of hydrocortisone and the level of pain following treatment. We begin our analysis by calculating the expected frequencies for each cell in the table. This process is somewhat more complicated when working with a contingency table, because we cannot just evenly divide the total sample among the eight cells. We must account for the observed *proportions* within each variable. First we ask, what proportion of the total sample ($N = 70$) was assigned to the 1% and 10% dosages? According to the observed data, these proportions are

$$1\% \text{ solution:} \qquad 39/70 = 55.71\%$$
$$10\% \text{ solution:} \qquad 31/70 = 44.29\%$$

Therefore, if the null hypothesis is true, and no association exists between concentration of hydrocortisone and pain, we would expect the distribution of treatments at

---

[‡]The *Mantel-Haenszel chi-square* statistic is a variation of the chi-square test for independence, used in case-control and cohort studies, when the association between two variables is considered confounded by a third variable. The data are stratified so that the effect of the confounder is partitioned out. The Mantel-Haenszel statistic essentially adjusts the value of chi-square to account for the differential contribution of each stratum. Formulas for Mantel-Haenszel statistics can be found in most epidemiologic tests.[8] See Chapter 15 for a discussion of confounding in epidemiologic studies.

[§]Phonophoresis is the application of ultrasound to drive a pharmacological agent through the skin.

TABLE 25.4. CALCULATION OF χ^2 FOR A 4 × 2 CONTINGENCY TABLE SHOWING FREQUENCIES OF PAIN LEVEL FOR PATIENTS RECEIVING 1% OR 10% SOLUTIONS OF HYDROCORTISONE ($N = 70$)

A. OUTPUT: DATA

Pain Level		Hydrocortisone 1%	10%	Total
None	Count	14	23	37
	Expected	20.61	16.39	
	Row %	37.8%	62.2%	
	Column %	35.9%	74.2%	
	Total %	20.0%	32.9%	52.9%
	Std. Residual	−1.46	1.63	
Minimal	Count	15	6	21
	Expected	11.70	9.30	
	Row %	71.4%	28.6%	
	Column %	38.5%	19.4%	
	Total %	21.4%	8.6%	30.0%
	Std. Residual	0.97	−1.08	
Moderate	Count	8	2	10
	Expected	5.57	4.43	
	Row %	80.0%	20.0%	
	Column %	20.5%	6.5%	
	Total %	11.4%	2.9%	14.3%
	Std. Residual	1.03	−1.15	
Severe	Count	2	0	2
	Expected	1.11	.89	
	Row %	100.0%	.0%	
	Column %	5.1%	.0%	
	Total %	2.9%	.0%	2.9%
	Std. Residual	.84	−.95	
Total		39	31	70
		55.7%	44.3%	100.0%

B. COMPUTATION

Category		O	E	$O-E$	$(O-E)^2$	$\dfrac{(O-E)^2}{E}$
1%	None	14	20.61	−6.61	43.69	2.12
	Minimal	15	11.70	3.30	10.89	0.93
	Moderate	8	5.57	2.43	5.90	1.06
	Severe	2	1.11	0.89	0.79	0.71
10%	None	23	16.39	6.61	43.69	2.67
	Minimal	6	9.30	−3.30	10.89	1.17
	Moderate	2	4.43	−2.43	5.90	1.33
	Severe	0	0.89	−0.89	0.79	0.89
						$\chi^2 = 10.88$

C. OUTPUT: HYPOTHESIS TEST

$_{(.05)}\chi^2_{(3)} = 7.81$ (Table A.5)   Reject H_0

```
Chi-square = 10.88
df = 3
p = .012
```

Source: Kleinkort JA, Wood F. Phonophoresis with 1 percent versus 10 percent hydrocortisone. *Phys Ther* 1975;55:1320–4.

each level of pain to be the same as the distribution in the total group. This means that within each pain category, 55.71% of the patients should have had the 1% concentration and 44.29% should have had the 10% concentration. For example, of the 37 patients who experienced no pain, 55.71% or (0.5571)(37) = 20.61 cases should have gotten the 1% solution, and 44.29% or (0.4429)(37) = 16.39 cases should have gotten the 10% solution. Similarly, 55.71% of the 21 patients who experienced minimal pain should have gotten 1% (11.70 cases) and 44.29% should have gotten 10% (9.30 cases). These are the frequencies that would be expected if concentration of hydrocortisone and pain are not related. Table 25.4A shows the expected frequencies as the second entry in each cell in the contingency table. Note that the sums of the expected frequencies will always match the marginal totals for observed frequencies.

We can simplify the process of calculating the expected frequency (*E*) for a given cell in the table using the formula

$$E = \frac{f_R f_C}{N} \tag{25.3}$$

where f_R and f_C represent the frequency totals for the row and column associated with that cell, respectively. Therefore, for those with moderate pain, expected frequencies are

1% solution: $E = \dfrac{(10)(39)}{70} = 5.57$

10% solution: $E = \dfrac{(10)(31)}{70} = 4.43$

And for those with severe pain,

1% solution: $E = \dfrac{(2)(39)}{70} = 1.11$

10% solution: $E = \dfrac{(2)(31)}{70} = 0.89$

Interpreting Chi-square

Table 25.4B shows the calculation of χ^2 using these data. These calculations proceed as in previous examples, with all observed and expected frequencies listed in the table (order is unimportant). The test value, $\chi^2 = 10.88$, is compared with the critical value with $(R - 1)$ $(C - 1)$ degrees of freedom. In this case, we have four rows and two columns, with $(4 - 1)$ $(2 - 1) = 3$ degrees of freedom. From Table A.5 we obtain the critical value $_{(.05)}\chi^2_{(3)} = 7.81$. Therefore, χ^2 is significant and the null hyothesis of independence is rejected. These variables are not independent of each other. There is a significant association between the solution of hydrocortisone and the level of pain experienced following treatment.

We can examine the frequencies within each cell to interpret these findings. The output for this analysis allows us to see how each cell contributes to the overall chi-square. As shown in Table 25.4A, the frequency within each cell is also given as a percentage of the column (% solution), the row (pain level), and the total ($N = 70$). For instance, 14 patients in the 1% solution group rated their pain as "none." This represents 37.8% of all those who rated pain as "none" (the row %) and 35.9% of all those who received the 1%

solution (the column %). It also represents 20.0% of the total sample. If we examine the standardized residuals for these data, shown as the last entry in each cell, we can see that the two cells representing patients with no pain contribute most to the significant outcome. Following treatment with the 10% solution, the number of patients experiencing no pain was greater than expected (residual = 1.63). This outcome is just opposite to what was seen with the 1% solution (residual = −1.46). It is reasonable, then, to conclude that the 10% solution was more effective.

Random and Fixed Models for 2 × 2 Tables

When data are arranged in a contingency table, the marginal frequencies can be generated in one of two ways. They may be *fixed effects,* in that the totals are predetermined by the experimenter. If the study were to be repeated, the same frequencies would probably be used. The levels of hydrocortisone treatment can be classified as fixed, in that the subjects were assigned to these groups. The number of subjects in each category of treatment was determined by the researchers. Conversely, the number of subjects appearing in each pain category was not predetermined. This is considered a *random effect,* indicating that the numbers in these categories would probably change with repeated sampling.

   A **fixed model** contingency table is created when both variables of interest are assigned. This approach is rare in clinical studies. The more common **random model** is composed of two random variables. For example, we could analyze a class of 60 students and classify them according to sex and age. The totals in each category would be different for every class that was tested. A **mixed model** is composed of one random and one fixed variable. The hydrocortisone example, in which subjects were assigned to treatment groups and measured on pain, fits this model. Treatment is fixed and pain levels are random. Case-control studies use this approach, choosing a fixed number of cases and control subjects, and then examining how many in each group are exposed to the risk factor. If the study were to be repeated, the same numbers of cases and controls could be chosen, but the exposure data would vary. The significance of analyzing a fixed, random, or mixed model will be discussed shortly when we deal with issues of sample size.

Calculations for 2 × 2 Tables

The 2 × 2 contingency table is a commonly used model in the analysis of frequencies. The cells of the table are traditionally designated by the following notation:

A	*B*	*A* + *B*
C	*D*	*C* + *D*
A + *C*	*B* + *D*	*N*

When using this format, χ^2 can be calculated without expected frequencies, using

$$\chi^2 = \frac{N(AD - BD)^2}{(A + B)(C + D)(A + C)(B + D)} \tag{25.4}$$

   To illustrate this application, consider the data in Table 25.5A showing the number of patients with and without complications following open heart surgery in two groups

TABLE 25.5. CALCULATION OF χ^2 FOR 2× 2 CONTINGENCY TABLE: INCIDENCE OF COMPLICATIONS FOLLOWING OPEN HEART SURGERY FOR GROUPS RECEIVING EITHER BREATHING EXERCISES OR ROUTINE CARE (N= 40)

A. DATA

	Complications		
	Yes	No	Total
Exercise	3	16	19
Routine	8	13	21
Total	11	29	40

B. COMPUTATION

$$\chi^2 = \frac{N\,(AD{-}BC)^2}{(A + B)(C + D)(A + C)(B + D)}$$

$$= \frac{40\,[(3)(13) - (8)(16)]2}{(19)(21)(11)(29)} = \frac{316,840}{127,281} = 2.49$$

C. HYPOTHESIS TEST

$_{(.05)}\chi^2{}_{(1)} = 3.84$ (Table A.5)

Do not reject H_0

```
Chi-square = 2.49
df = 1
p = .115
```

Source: Vraciu JK, Vraciu RA. Effectiveness of breathing exercises in preventing pulmonary complications following open heart surgery. *Phys Ther* 1977;57:1367–71.

receiving breathing exercises or routine postoperative care.[4] Using the preceding computational formula, we determine that $\chi^2 = 2.49$.

There will always be 1 degree of freedom associated with a 2 × 2 table. Therefore, the critical value $_{(.05)}\chi^2{}_{(1)} = 3.84$ is a common standard for significance. In this example, the calculated value, $\chi^2 = 2.49$, does not achieve significance. We do not reject H_0 and we conclude that no association exists between participation in a program of breathing exercises and the number of postsurgical pulmonary complications.

Sample Size Considerations—Yates' Correction for Continuity

Assumptions related to sample size with contingency tables are based on the expected frequencies. In addition to the requirement that each cell contain an expected frequency of at least 1, no more than 20% of the cells should contain expected frequencies less than 5.[10] When this occurs, the researcher may choose to collapse the table (if it is larger than 2 × 2) to combine adjacent categories and increase expected cell frequencies.

A statistical correction, known as **Yates' correction for continuity,** is often recommended to adjust χ^2 to account for small expected frequencies.[10] This procedure reduces the size of χ^2 by subtracting .5 from the absolute value of $O - E$ for each category before squaring:

$$\chi^2 = \sum \frac{(|O - E| - .5)^2}{E} \tag{25.5}$$

The calculation of χ^2 using this method is illustrated in Table 25.6 for the data on hydrocortisone and pain. One cell has an expected frequency less than 1, and two others have expected frequencies less than 5. Therefore, it is appropriate to apply this correction. The calculated value of χ^2 with Yates' correction is now 7.39, which no longer meets the criterion for significance. By correcting for small cell frequencies, we no longer see a statistical association in the data.

With 2×2 tables, Yates' correction for continuity is given as

$$\chi^2 = \frac{N(AD - BC - N/2)^2}{(A + B)(C + D)(A + C)(B + D)} \tag{25.6}$$

A number of statistical sources suggest that Yates' correction for continuity is too conservative and unduly increases the chance of committing a Type II error.[11–13] The potential for this effect is illustrated in the preceding example, where we found no significant difference once the correction was applied. It has been suggested that χ^2 can provide a reasonable estimate of Type I error for 2×2 tables when random or mixed models are used with $N \geq 8$.[14] According to Ferguson, the correction should be applied when a fixed model is used.[15] With expected frequencies less than 5, a related procedure called the **Fisher Exact Test** is often recommended for use with 2×2 tables.[16] This test results in the exact probability of the occurrence of the observed frequencies, given the marginal totals. The calculation of Fisher's Exact Test is quite cumbersome and is best generated by computer analysis.

TABLE 25.6.   CALCULATION OF χ^2 USING YATES' CORRECTION FOR CONTINUITY (DATA FROM TABLE 25.4)

A. DATA and COMPUTATION

O	E	$O-E$	$|O-E|-.5$	$(|O-E|-.5)^2$	$\dfrac{(|O-E|-.5)^2}{E}$
14	20.6	−6.6	6.1	37.21	1.81
15	11.7	3.3	2.8	7.84	0.67
8	5.6	2.4	1.9	3.61	0.65
2	1.1	0.9	0.4	0.16	0.15
23	16.4	6.6	6.1	37.21	2.27
6	9.3	−3.3	2.8	7.84	0.84
2	4.4	−2.4	1.9	3.61	0.82
0	0.9	−0.9	0.4	0.16	0.18
					$\chi^2 = 7.39$

B. HYPOTHESIS TEST $_{(.05)}\chi^2_{(3)} = 7.81$ (Table A. 5)   Do not reject H_0

McNEMAR TEST FOR CORRELATED SAMPLES

One basic assumption required for use of x^2 is that variables are independent; that is, no one subject is represented in more than one cell. There are many research questions, however, for which this assumption will not hold. For instance, we could look at a sample's responses to a question and see how many subjects answered correctly or incorrectly before and after exposure to specific information. Or we could examine the effects of a particular treatment program by looking at the presence or absence of an outcome variable, such as pain, before and after treatment. These studies use nominal variables, but in a repeated measures design. The x^2 test is not valid under these conditions.[17]

The **McNemar test** is a form of the x^2 statistic used with 2 × 2 tables that involve correlated samples, where subjects act as their own controls or where they are matched.[18] This test is especially useful with pretest–posttest designs when the dependent variable is measured as a dichotomy or an ordinal or nominal scale. To illustrate this approach, suppose we asked a group of 35 students whether they are interested in doing research as part of their clinical practice. We ask them this question before and after they complete a research course. The format for such a study is shown in Table 25.7A. In this situation, the cells are not independent, and each subject is represented twice.

The cells in the correlated design follow the standard notation for a 2 × 2 table. The number of students who demonstrate a change in attitude following the research course are reflected in shaded cells *A* and *D*. Students in cell *A* were interested in research before the course, but changed their minds afterward. Those in cell *D* became interested after the course. Students in cells *B* and *C* did not change their attitudes.

TABLE 25.7. McNEMAR TEST: STUDENT ATTITUDES ABOUT RESEARCH BEFORE AND AFTER A RESEARCH COURSE (*N*= 35)

A. DATA

		Before		
		Yes	No	**Total**
After	No	*A*	*B*	
		3	4	7
	Yes	*C*	*D*	
		12	16	28
	Total	15	20	35

B. COMPUTATION

$$x^2 = \frac{(A - D)^2}{(A + D)} = \frac{(3 - 16)^2}{(3 + 16)} = 8.89$$

C. OUTPUT: HYPOTHESIS TEST

$_{(.05}x^2_{(1)} = 3.84$ Reject H_0

```
Chi-square: McNemar Test
  p = .004
  N = 35
```

As A and D represent the total number of students who showed a change in attitude in either direction, these are the only cells of interest for this analysis. Under the null hypothesis, half of those who changed should gain interest in research after the course and half should lose interest. We test this hypothesis using the formula

$$\chi^2 = \frac{(A - D)^2}{A + D} \tag{25.7}$$

which is tested against critical values of χ^2 with 1 degree of freedom (Appendix Table A.5). As shown in Table 25.7B, for this example, $\chi^2 = 8.89$. This value is significant (Table 25.7C). We can see that the proportion of students who became interested in research after the course is substantially higher than for those who lost interest.

COEFFICIENTS OF ASSOCIATION

Sometimes a measure of association, such as a correlation coefficient, is desired as a way of expressing the degree of relationship in a set of categorical data. Chi-square tells us only if the association is significant, not if it is strong or weak.

Phi Coefficient

The **phi coefficient, Φ,** can be used to express the degree of association between two nominal variables in a 2 × 2 table.[16] Its value can range from –1.00 to +1.00, and can be interpreted as a correlation coefficient. It is based on the χ^2 statistic as follows:

$$\Phi = \sqrt{\frac{\chi^2}{N}} \tag{25.8}$$

For the data in Table 25.5,

$$\Phi = \sqrt{\frac{2.49}{40}} = .25$$

This finding indicates a relatively weak association between type of treatment and incidence of pulmonary complications. This test is described in more detail in Chapter 23.

Contingency Coefficient

The **contingency coefficient, C,** is a measure of association that can be used with tables larger than 2 × 2, but with the restriction that the number of rows has to equal the number of columns.[15] This value is given by

$$C = \sqrt{\frac{\chi^2}{N + \chi^2}} \tag{25.9}$$

Once again, using the data in Table 25.5

$$C = \sqrt{\frac{2.49}{40 + 2.49}} = .24$$

As these results show, the phi coefficient and the contingency coefficient will yield similar results with 2 × 2 tables.

The contingency coefficient will range from 0 to a maximum of $\sqrt{(q-1)/q}$ where q represents the number of rows or columns in a symmetrical table. For a 2×2 table the upper limit of C is $\sqrt{(2-1)/2} = .707$. For a 3×3 table, this maximum will be $\sqrt{(3-1)/3} = .816$. Because of these differences, contingency coefficients are not directly comparable unless they are obtained from tables of equal sizes.

Cramer's V

A third measure of association based on χ^2 is **Cramer's V** coefficient, which is an alternative to the contingency coefficient when contingency tables are asymmetrical. This coefficient is designed so that the attainable upper bound is always ± 1.00. The formula is

$$V = \sqrt{\frac{\chi^2}{N(q-1)}} \qquad (25.10)$$

where N is the total number of subjects, and q is the number of rows or columns, *whichever is smaller*. For instance, for the data in Table 25.4, there are two levels of hydrocortisone and four levels of pain. Therefore, $q = 2$. For this example,

$$V = \sqrt{\frac{10.88}{70(2-1)}} = .39$$

which represents a moderate degree of relationship between concentration of cortisone and pain following treatment. The results of the χ^2 test on these data showed that the two variables were not independent. The contingency coefficient indicates the strength of their relationship.

Other Measures of Association

Many computer packages generate a series of coefficients associated with contingency table analyses. These statistics are not based on chi-square.

The **lambda coefficient, λ,** is used to determine how well one can predict membership in one category based on knowledge of another category. Both sets of categories should be at the nominal level. Lambda is reported in asymmetric and symmetric versions. The *asymmetric lambda* is interpreted as the improvement in predicting Y once values of X are known; that is, one nominal variable is designated as the dependent variable (Y) and the other as the independent variable (X). For instance, in the study of hydrocortisone, we could designate the percent solution as the independent variable and predict levels of pain as the dependent variable. In some analyses, however, the researcher is unable to specify which variable is dependent. For example, we might want to look at the relationship between side of stroke and sex, neither of which could necessarily be seen as a dependent variable. In this case, the *symmetric* version of lambda is used. Lambda ranges from 0, when there is no improvement in prediction, to 1.0, when predictions can be made without error.

Kendall's tau-b and **tau-c** are measures of association for ordinal variables that are reported in categories. Tau-b is appropriate with square tables, such 2×2, and tau-c should be used with rectangular tables, where the number of rows and columns differ.

Gamma is based on the tau statistic, but ignores ties; that is, pairs that have the same classification for X and Y are eliminated from the analysis. When tables have three or more dimensions (three or more category variables such as sex, age group, and diagnosis), partial gammas can be calculated.

COMMENTARY

Using Chi-square

Clinical researchers can find many uses for the chi-square statistic—for data analysis and for descriptive purposes. It is often useful as a way of establishing group equivalence following random assignment. For instance, once two groups have been assigned, it may be of interest to compare the numbers of males and females in each group to see if they were assigned in unequal proportions. Or it may be important to determine if certain age groups are equally represented in each experimental group. Chi-square can be used to make these determinations and confirm the validity of the randomization process.

Chi-square should not be used as an alternative to more precise tests, such as the *t*-test or analysis of variance, when data can be measured on a continuous scale. All data can be reduced to categories, but this usually results in a serious loss of information and is not encouraged. For example, if a survey requested information on an individual's age, and the exact age is given, it may not be useful to reduce the data to age intervals.

Issues of sample size are relevant to discussions of chi-square. The statistic is sensitive to increases in sample size when there is a true difference between observed and expected frequencies.[15] With larger samples, the magnitude of these differences will usually increase, thereby increasing the value of χ^2. When samples are very small, these differences can be hidden. It is often useful to consider collapsing categories when this does not compromise the research question, and to reexamine data using larger cell frequencies; however, this should be done only when the combinations of categories are theoretically reasonable and meaningful. It may be helpful to think about potential combinations of categories prior to data analysis. It is never appropriate to make such combinations on the basis of the observed data to achieve significant outcomes. See Appendix C for a discussion of power related to chi-square.

KEY TERMS

chi-square (χ^2)
observed frequency (O)
expected frequency (E)
goodness of fit
uniform distribution
normal distribution
known distribution
standardized residual

tests of independence
contingency table
fixed model
random model
mixed model
Yates' correction for
    continuity
Fisher Exact Test

McNemar test
phi coefficient (Φ)
contingency coefficient (C)
Cramer's V
lambda coefficient (λ)
Kendall's tau
gamma

REFERENCES

1. Snedecor GW, Cochran WG. *Statistical Methods.* 8th ed. Ames, IA: Iowa State University Press, 1991.
2. Volicer BJ. *Multivariate Statistics for Nursing Research.* Orlando, FL: Frune & Stratton, 1984.
3. Haberman SJ. The analysis of residuals in cross-classified tables. *Biometrics* 1984;29:205–220.
4. Vraciu JK, Vraciu RA. Effectiveness of breathing exercises in preventing pulmonary complications following open heart surgery. *Phys Ther* 1977;57:1367–71.
5. Connolly BH. Lateral dominance in children with learning disabilities. *Phys Ther* 1983;63:183–7.
6. Tanttula K, Vuola J, Asko-Seljavaara S. Return to employment after burn. *Burns* 1997;23:341–4.
7. Deshpande AA, Mielis SR, Zafonte RD, Hammond FM, Wood DL. Risk factors for acute care transfer among traumatic brain injury patients. *Arch Phys Med Rehabil* 1997;78:350–2.
8. Hennekens CH, Buring JE. *Epidemiology in Medicine.* Boston: Little, Brown, 1987.
9. Kleinkort JA, Wood F. Phonophoresis with 1 percent versus 10 percent hydrocortisone. *Phys Ther* 1975;55:1320–4.
10. Cochran WG. Some methods for strengthening the common χ^2 tests. *Biometrics* 1954;10:417–51.
11. Conover WJ. Some reasons for not using the Yates continuity correction on 2×2 contingency tables. *J Am Statist Assoc* 1974;69:374–82.
12. Camilli G, Hopkins KD. Applicability of chi-square to 2×2 contingency tables with small expected frequencies. *Psych Bull* 1978;85:163–7.
13. Grizzle JE. Continuity correction on the chi-square test for 2×2 tables. *Am Stat* 1967;21:28–32.
14. Mantel N, Hankey BJ. The odds ratios of a 2×2 contingency table. *Am Stat* 1975;29:143–5.
15. Ferguson GA. *Statistical Analysis in Psychology and Education.* 5th ed. New York: McGraw-Hill, 1981.
16. Siegel S, Castellan NJ. *Nonparametric Statistics for the Behavioral Sciences.* 2d ed. New York: McGraw-Hill, 1988.
17. Ottenbacker KJ. The chi-square test: its use in rehabilitation research. *Arch Phys Med Rehabil* 1995;76:678–81.
18. McNemar Q. *Psychological Statistics.* New York: Wiley, 1969.

CHAPTER

26

Statistical Measures of Reliability

In Chapter 5 we introduced basic concepts of reliability and described how different forms of reliability can be addressed in the planning of research protocols. The purpose of this chapter is to expand on these concepts by presenting the statistical bases for estimates of reliability, including measures of correlation, agreement, internal consistency, response stability, and method comparison for alternate forms. We have waited until this point in the book to present these procedures because they require application of concepts that have been covered in the preceding chapters on statistical analysis.

RELIABILITY THEORY AND MEASUREMENT ERROR

Recall from Chapter 5 that classical reliability theory partitions an observed measurement or score, X, into two components: a *true component, T,* which represents the real value under ideal conditions, and an *error component, E,* which includes all other sources of variance that influence the outcome of measurement. This theoretical relationship is expressed in the equation

$$X = T \pm E \tag{26.1}$$

We can also examine the statistical nature of this relationship by restating it in terms of *variance* (s^2). The total variance within a set of observed scores (s_X^2) is a function of both the **true variance** between scores **(s_T^2)** and the variance in the errors of measurement, or **error variance (s_E^2):**

$$s_X^2 = s_T^2 + s_E^2 \tag{26.2}$$

Although it is an unknown quantity, we assume that s_T^2 is fixed, because true scores will theoretically remain constant. Therefore, in a set of perfectly reliable scores, all observed differences between individual scores should be attributable to true differences between scores; that is, there is no error variance. Conversely, if we look at a set of repeated

TABLE 26.1.   HYPOTHETICAL PAIN MEASURES SHOWING OBSERVED SCORES (X), TRUE SCORES (T), AND ERROR COMPONENTS (E)

Subject		X	T	E	
1		12	10	2	
2		10	10	0	$r_{XX} = \dfrac{s_T^2}{s_X^2} = \dfrac{2.40}{5.60} = .43$
3		8	10	−2	
4		13	11	2	
5		9	11	−2	
6		14	14	0	
	ΣX	66	66	0	
	$\overline{X}$	11	11	0	
	s^2	5.60	2.40	3.20	

measurements from one person, and assume that the true response has not changed, then all observed variance should be the result of error. The essence of reliability, then, is based on the amount of error that is present in a set of scores. A measurement is considered more reliable if a greater proportion of the total observed variance is represented by the true score variance. Thus, reliability is defined by the ratio

$$\frac{\text{true variance}}{\text{true variance} + \text{error variance}} = \frac{\text{true variance}}{\text{total variance}}$$

In statistical terminology, this relationship can be expressed as

$$r_{XX} = \frac{s_T^2}{s_T^2 + s_E^2} = \frac{s_X^2 - s_E^2}{s_X^2} = \frac{s_T^2}{s_X^2} \tag{26.3}$$

where r_{XX} is the symbol for a **reliability coefficient.**

The coefficient of reliability can take values from 0.00 to 1.00. Zero reliability indicates that all measurement variation is attributed to error. Reliability of 1.00 means that the measurement has no error, or $s_E^2 = 0$. As the coefficient nears 1.00, we are more confident that the observed score is representative of the true score.

To illustrate this application, consider the set of hypothetical data presented in Table 26.1. These values represent ratings for six patients on a subjective pain scale, rated from 0 to 20. The first column, labeled X, lists the observed scores and their variance, $s_X^2 = 5.60$; the second column, T, shows the true scores (although in reality these are not known) and their variance, $s_T^2 = 2.40$; the last column, labeled E, shows the error component (the difference between the observed and true scores) and the error variance, $s_E^2 = 3.20$. We can verify that the observed variance is composed of true variance and error variance: $5.60 = 2.40 + 3.20$. These values can be used to calculate the reliability coefficient as follows:

$$r_{XX} = \frac{s_T^2}{s_X^2} = \frac{2.40}{5.60} = 0.43$$

Conceptually, this means that 43% of the variation in the observed scores can be attributed to variation in the true score, and 57% is attributable to measurement error.

TABLE 26.2. A SECOND HYPOTHETICAL SAMPLE OF PAIN MEASURES SHOWING GREATER VARIABILITY IN OBSERVED SCORES

Subject	X	T	E	
1	4	4	0	
2	4	4	0	
3	15	13	2	
4	9	11	−2	$r_{XX} = \dfrac{s_T^2}{s_X^2} = \dfrac{16.00}{19.20} = .83$
5	12	10	2	
6	10	12	−2	
ΣX	54	54	0	
$\overline{X}$	9	9	0	
s^2	19.20	16.00	3.20	

Of course, this approach is completely theoretical, as we can never know the true score or error component within a set of data. Therefore, it is necessary to use observed scores to estimate reliability. Although the procedures for obtaining these estimates will vary, the theory underlying the reliability coefficient is universally applicable; that is, reliability is a function of the amount of error variance in a set of data.

The Effect of Variance on Reliability

As reflected in the definition of reliability, statistical variance is the basis for reliability estimates. We can demonstrate that as the true variance in a set of scores decreases, the reliability coefficient will also decrease. If we look at the differences among the pain scores in Table 26.1, we can see that the patients did not vary greatly from one another. True scores were in a narrow range from 10 to 14. Consequently, the variance within the observed scores is small. We also find that the differences between the observed and true scores (errors) are minimal across the six patients. Based on these observations, we might reason that these measurements should be highly reliable; however, we obtain a reliability coefficient of only .43, much lower than might be expected.

Now let us look at a similar set of hypothetical data for the same variable, shown in Table 26.2. Note that the error components for these scores are identical to those in the first data set. This time, however, the true scores are much more variable ($s_T^2 = 16.00$), with values ranging from 4 to 13. Therefore, the observed scores also exhibit a much higher variance ($s_X^2 = 19.20$). Using these values, we can calculate a second reliability coefficient:

$$r_{XX} = \frac{s_T^2}{s_X^2} = \frac{16.00}{19.20} = 0.83$$

These data demonstrate a much stronger degree of statistical reliability than the first data set, even though the degree of error in the scores is the same! Why does this occur? Recall that reliability is based on the *proportion of the total observed variance that is attributable to error*. Therefore, for a given amount of error variance, it follows that reliability will improve as the total variance increases; that is, as the total variance gets larger, the error component will account for a smaller proportion of it.

This concept is crucial in the interpretation of reliability coefficients and in the design of reliability studies. Suppose we were interested in establishing the reliability of a new device for measuring range of back extension. We gather a large sample of "normal" individuals, all with measurements between 20 and 25 degrees of extension. Even if we are fairly consistent over successive trials, the reliability coefficient will probably be low because the total variance is so small. A low reliability coefficient can be misleading under such conditions. The solution to this problem, of course, is to include subjects that have a wider range of scores in a reliability study. We should be studying normal individuals as well as patients with hypermobility and hypomobility in back extension. Researchers should always consider the range of scores used for estimating reliability in the interpretation of reliability coefficients.

INTRACLASS CORRELATION COEFFICIENT

The historical approach to testing reliability involves the use of correlation coefficients. In Chapter 5 we discussed the problems with this approach, in that it does not provide a measure of agreement, but only covariance (see Figure 5.1 in Chapter 5). Correlations are also limited as reliability coefficients because they are bivariate; that is, only two ratings or raters can be correlated at one time. It is not possible to assess the simultaneous reliability of more than two raters or the relationships among different aspects of reliability, such as raters, test forms, and testing occasions. As these are often important elements in reliability testing, correlation does not provide an efficient mechanism for evaluating the full scope of reliability.

Another objection to the use of correlation as a measure of reliability is based on the statistical definition of reliability; that is, correlation cannot separate out variance components due to error or true differences in a data set. Therefore, the correlation coefficient is not a true reliability coefficient. It is actually more accurate to use the square of the correlation coefficient (the coefficient of determination) for this purpose, because r^2 reflects how much variance in one measurement is accounted for by the variance in a second measurement (see Chapter 24). This is analogous to asking how much of the total variance in a set of data is shared by two measurements (the "true" variance) and how much is not shared (the error variance). If we could correlate true scores with observed scores in a set of data, the square of the correlation coefficient would be the reliability coefficient. We can confirm this interpretation using the data from Table 26.1. For the correlation between observed and true scores, $r = .66$. Therefore, $r^2 = .43$.

To overcome the limitations of correlation as a measure of reliability, many researchers use more than one reliability index within a single study. For instance, in a test–retest situation or a rater reliability study, both correlation and a *t*-test can be performed to assess consistency and average agreement between the data sets. This strategy does address the interpretation of agreement, but it is not useful in that it does not provide a single index to describe reliability. The scores may be correlated but significantly different, or they may be poorly correlated but not significantly different. How should these results be interpreted? It is much more desirable to use one index that can answer this question.

The **intraclass correlation coefficient (ICC)** is such an index. Like other reliability coefficients, the ICC ranges from 0.00 to 1.00. It is calculated using variance estimates obtained through an analysis of variance. Therefore, it reflects both degree of correspondence and agreement among ratings.

Statistically the ICC has several advantages. First, it can be used to assess reliability among two or more ratings, giving it broad clinical applicability. Second, the ICC does not require the same number of raters for each subject, allowing for flexibility in clinical studies.[1] Third, although it is designed primarily for use with interval/ratio data, the ICC can be applied without distortion to data on the ordinal scale when intervals between such measurements are assumed to be equivalent.[2] In addition, with data that are rated as a dichotomy (the presence or absence of a trait), the ICC has been shown to be equivalent to measures of nominal agreement, simplifying computation in cases where more than two raters are involved.[1, 3, 4] Therefore, the ICC provides a useful index in a variety of analysis situations.

Generalizability

Another major advantage of the ICC is that it supports the **generalizability** model proposed by Cronbach as a comprehensive estimate of reliability.[5, 6] The concept of generalizability theory, introduced in Chapter 5, is based on the idea that differences between observed scores are due to a variety of factors, not just true score variance and random error.[7] Differences occur because of variations in the measurement system, such as the characteristics of raters or subjects, testing conditions, alternate forms of a test, administrations of a test on different occasions, and so on. These factors are called **facets** of generalizability.

The essence of generalizability theory is that facets contribute to measurement error as separate components of variance, distinguishable from random error. In classical reliability theory, error variance is undifferentiated, incorporating all sources of measurement error. In generalizability theory, however, the error variance is multivariate; that is, it is further partitioned to account for the influence of specific facets on measurement error. Therefore, the **generalizability coefficient** (the ICC) is an extension of the reliability coefficient:

$$\text{ICC} = \frac{s_T^2}{s_T^2 + s_F^2 + s_E^2} \tag{26.4}$$

where s_T^2 and s_E^2 are the variances in true scores and error components, and s_F^2 is the variance attributable to the facet of interest.[8] The specific facet included in the denominator will vary, depending on whether rater, occasions, or some other facet is the variable of interest in the reliability study. For example, if we include rater as a facet, then the total observed variance would be composed of the true variance between subjects, the variance between raters, and the remaining unexplained error variance.

Equation 26.4 represents a conceptual definition of generalizability. Actual calculations require the use of variance estimates that are obtained from an analysis of variance, which, of course, does not include direct estimates of true variance (as this is unknown). Theoretically, however, we can estimate true score variance by looking at the difference between observed variance among subjects and error variance ($s_T^2 = s_X^2 - s_E^2$). These estimates can be derived from an analysis of variance.

Design Considerations: Models of the ICC

There are actually six different equations for calculating the ICC, differentiated by purpose of the reliability study, the design of the study, and the type of measurements taken. It is necessary to distinguish among these approaches, as under some conditions the results can be decidedly different. To facilitate explanations, we will proceed with this discussion in the context of a reliability study with rater as the facet of interest; however, we emphasize that these applications are equally valid to study other facets.

Shrout and Fleiss describe three *models* of the ICC.[9] They distinguish these models according to how the raters are chosen and assigned to subjects. In Model 1, each subject is assessed by a different set of k raters, and raters are randomly chosen from a larger population of raters. In Model 2, each subject is assessed by the same raters, and raters are randomly chosen. Therefore, the raters are expected to represent the population of raters from which they were drawn, and results can be generalized to other raters with similar characteristics. This randomness may be only theoretical in practice; that is, we choose raters who we believe represent the population of raters, as we do not have access to the entire population. In Model 3, each subject is assessed by the same raters, but the raters represent the only raters of interest. In this latter case, it is not important to generalize findings beyond the raters involved.

Model 1 is rarely useful in clinical reliability studies, as we typically involve multiple raters to measure the same group of subjects. Models 2 and 3 are used most often, and the choice between them represents a major decision about the purpose of the reliability study. In some research situations, the investigator is interested in establishing the intrarater or interrater reliability of a group of clinicians for one specific data collection experience, fitting Model 3. In that case, it is of no interest if anyone else can perform the measurements with equal reliability. If, however, it is important to demonstrate that a particular measuring tool can be used with confidence by all equally trained clinicians, then Model 2 should be used. This approach is appropriate for clinical studies and methodological research, to document that a measuring tool has broad application.

Each of the three ICC models can be expressed in two *forms*, depending on whether the scores are single ratings or mean ratings. Most often, reliability studies are based on comparison of scores from individual raters. In some instances, however, the mean of several raters (or ratings) may be used as the unit of reliability. For instance, when measurements are unstable, it may be necessary to take the mean of several measurements as the individual's score to obtain satisfactory reliability. Using mean scores has the effect of increasing reliability estimates, as means are considered better estimates of true scores, theoretically reducing error variance.

Formulas for the ICC

The six types of ICC are classified using two numbers in parentheses. The first number designates the *model* (1, 2, or 3), and the second number signifies the *form*, using either a single measurement (1) or the mean of several measurements $(k)^*$ as the unit of analysis. We now present the six types of ICC in the context of a reliability study with $k = 4$ raters measuring a random sample of $n = 6$ subjects, as shown in Table 26.3.

Model 1

Model 1 is based on a standard one-way analysis of variance design, in which "subjects" is treated as the independent variable. The one-way ANOVA partitions the total variance into two parts—the variation among subjects (between-subjects) and error, as shown in

---

*The designation of k equals the number of scores used to obtain the mean.

TABLE 26.3. RELIABILITY DATA FOR FOUR RATERS ACROSS SIX SUBJECTS

	RATER			
SUBJECT	**1**	**2**	**3**	**4**
1	7	8	3	5
2	2	4	4	1
3	1	2	6	1
4	5	5	7	2
5	8	9	5	6
6	9	10	6	7

Table 26.4A. The between-subjects component tells us if the subjects are different from each other, which we expect. The error component represents the variation within a subject across raters. Some of this error will be due to true scores changing from trial to trial, some from rater error, and some will be unexplained. This ANOVA does not differentiate these sources of error.

If we assume that each score represents a single rating, we calculate ICC form (1,1) by

$$\text{ICC}(1,1) = \frac{\text{BMS} - \text{WMS}}{\text{BMS} + (k-1)\text{WMS}} \tag{26.5}$$

where BMS is the between-subjects mean square from the analysis of variance, WMS is the within-groups (error) mean square, and k is the number of ratings for each subject.

If these scores represent mean ratings, we use ICC form $(1, k)$:

$$\text{ICC}(1, k) = \frac{\text{BMS} - \text{WMS}}{\text{BMS}} \tag{26.6}$$

Calculations for this model are shown in Table 26.4A.

Model 2

Model 2 is used most often in interrater reliability studies where all n subjects are measured by k raters, and these raters are considered representative of a larger population of similar raters. This model is based on a repeated measures analysis of variance,[9,10] with rater as the independent variable (see Table 26.4B). Therefore, the ANOVA partitions the total variance into effects due to differences between subjects, differences between raters, and error variance.[†] The F-ratio associated with the rater effect reflects the difference among raters, or the extent of agreement or disagreement among them. This effect is significant when the variance due to raters is large, indicating that the raters' scores are different from each other. In this example, the rater effect is not significant ($p = .130$).

[†]Note that the total sum of squares for the within-subjects effect in the repeated measures ANOVA in Panel B of Table 26.5 (between raters + error) is equal to the within subjects sum of squares in Panel A. The error variance in the repeated measures test is smaller because the variance due to raters has been partitioned out.

TABLE 26.4.   COMPUTATION OF ICC BASED ON ANALYSIS OF VARIANCE OF $k = 4$ RATERS ACROSS $n = 6$ SUBJECTS

A. MODEL 1: ONE-WAY ANALYSIS OF VARIANCE

Source of Variance	df	SS	MS	F	Sig.
Between subjects	5	99.38	19.88 (BMS)	5.02	.005
Within subjects	18	71.25	3.96 (WMS)		

$$ICC(1,1) = \frac{BMS - WMS}{BMS + (k-1)WMS} = \frac{19.88 - 3.96}{19.88 + (4-1)3.96} = .50$$

$$ICC(1,k) = \frac{BMS - WMS}{BMS} = \frac{19.88 - 3.96}{19.88} = .80$$

B. MODELS 2 AND 3: REPEATED MEASURES ANALYSIS OF VARIANCE

Source of Variation	df	SS	MS	F	Sig.
Between subjects	5	99.38	19.88 (BMS)	6.03	.002
Within subjects					
Between raters	3	21.79	7.26 (RMS)	2.21	.130
Error	15	49.46	3.30 (EMS)		

$$ICC(2,1) = \frac{BMS - EMS}{BMS + (k-1) + \dfrac{k(RMS - EMS)}{n}}$$

$$= \frac{19.88 - 3.30}{19.88 + (4-1)3.30 + \dfrac{4(7.26 - 3.30)}{6}} = .51$$

$$ICC(2,k) = \frac{BMS - EMS}{BMS + \dfrac{(RMS - EMS)}{n}} = \frac{19.88 - 3.30}{19.88 + \dfrac{(7.26 - 3.30)}{6}} = .81$$

$$ICC(3,1) = \frac{BMS - EMS}{BMS + (k-1)EMS} = \frac{19.88 - 3.30}{19.88 + (4-1)3.30} = .56$$

$$ICC(3,k) = \frac{BMS - EMS}{BMS} = \frac{19.88 - 3.30}{19.88} = .83$$

For single ratings, we use ICC form (2,1):

$$ICC(2,1) = \frac{BMS - EMS}{BMS + (k-1)EMS + \dfrac{k(RMS - EMS)}{n}} \tag{26.7}$$

where BMS is the between-subjects mean square, EMS is the error mean square, RMS is the between-raters mean square, k is the number of raters, and n is the number of subjects tested.

If each rating represents the mean of several scores, we use ICC form (2, k):

$$ICC(2, k) = \frac{BMS - EMS}{BMS + \dfrac{(RMS - EMS)}{n}} \tag{26.8}$$

Calculations using this model are shown in Table 26.4B.

Model 3

Model 3 also uses a repeated measures analysis of variance design.[9, 11] However, in this model, the tested raters are considered the only raters of interest. Shrout and Fleiss suggest that this model is appropriate for testing intrarater reliability with multiple scores from the same rater, as it is not reasonable to generalize one rater's scores to a larger population of raters.[8]

With single ratings, ICC(3,1) is calculated using

$$ICC(3, 1) = \frac{BMS - EMS}{BMS + (k - 1)EMS} \tag{26.9}$$

With mean ratings, we use ICC(3, k)

$$ICC(3, k) = \frac{BMS - EMS}{BMS} \tag{26.10}$$

Calculations are shown in Table 26.4B.

Interpretation of the ICC

Magnitude of the ICC

Like other forms of reliability, there are no standard values for acceptable reliability using the ICC. The ICC ranges between 0.00 and 1.00, with values closer to 1.00 representing stronger reliability. But because reliability is a characteristic of measurement obtained to varying degrees (although rarely to perfection), the researcher must determine "how much" reliability is needed to justify the use of a particular tool. The nature of the measured variable will be a factor, in terms of its stability and the precision required to make sound clinical judgments about it. As a general guideline, we suggest that values above .75 are indicative of good reliability, and those below .75 poor to moderate reliability. For many clinical measurements, reliability should exceed .90 to ensure reasonable validity. These are only guidelines, however, and we urge our readers not to use these as absolute standards. Judgments must be made within the context of each individual study.

Rater Error

When the ICC is high, it is easy to say that reliability is good and to express confidence in the obtained measurements. When reliability is less than satisfactory, however, the researcher is obliged to sort through alternative explanations to determine the contributing sources of error. There are two major reasons for finding low ICC values.

The first explanation is fairly obvious—the raters do not agree. This is not a straightforward interpretation, however, when more than two raters or ratings are analyzed. Because the ICC is an average based on variance across all raters, nonagreement may involve all raters, some raters, or only one rater. The ICC can be considered an *average correlation* across raters and, therefore, does not represent the reliability of any individual rater. For instance, a critical look back at the data in Table 26.3 reveals that Rater 3 seems to be the most out of line with the other raters. In fact, if we obtain the product-moment correlations for all possible pairs of ratings, we find that Raters 1, 2, and 4 demonstrate correlations between .96 and .98, whereas the correlations of Rater 3 with the other three raters are all negative and small, between –.06 and –.19 (Fig. 26.1). The ICC is brought down by the "unreliable" responses of Rater 3.

It is often useful, therefore, to examine the data to determine if there is an interaction between raters and subjects. That is, are the scores dependent on what "level" of rater is doing the measuring? This type of interaction is reflected in the error variance of the repeated measures ANOVA (Models 2 and 3), but cannot be separated out from other sources of error in the one-way ANOVA (Model 1).

When raters are reliable, there should be no interaction between raters and subjects; that is, the error variance should be small. It may be helpful to graph the results, as shown in Figure 26.1. The ratings obtained by Raters 1, 2, and 4 are close and fairly parallel. The scores obtained by Rater 3 are clearly incongruent. By examining both the intercorrelations and graphic evidence, we can determine that there is an interaction between rater and subject. It would be important, then, to review the circumstances of the third rater's tests, to determine why that person's ratings were not consistent with the others.

Variance

A second reason for a low ICC is one that has been discussed before in relation to the reliability coefficient; that is, the variability among subjects' scores must be large to demonstrate reliability. A lack of variability can occur when samples are homogeneous, when raters are all very lenient or strict in their scoring, or when the rating system falls within a restricted range. This effect can be checked by looking for significance of the between-subjects variance in the analysis of variance. If subjects' scores are homogeneous, this source of variance will not be significant. It has been shown that when the between-subjects variance is not significant, the actual limits of the ICC do not match the theoretical limits of 0.00 and 1.00.[12] In fact, it is possible for ratios to range from negative to positive infinity. When a negative ICC is obtained, the value cannot be considered valid. Therefore, it is imperative that researchers be aware of the extent to which scores will naturally vary, and try to obtain heterogeneous samples whenever possible.

Choosing One Model

Although we have calculated all six ICCs for our example, it should be clear that only one type will be appropriate for any one study. The selection of one version should be made before data are collected, based on appropriate design considerations. In most instances, Model 2 or 3 will be the appropriate choice. Some authors have expressed a pref-

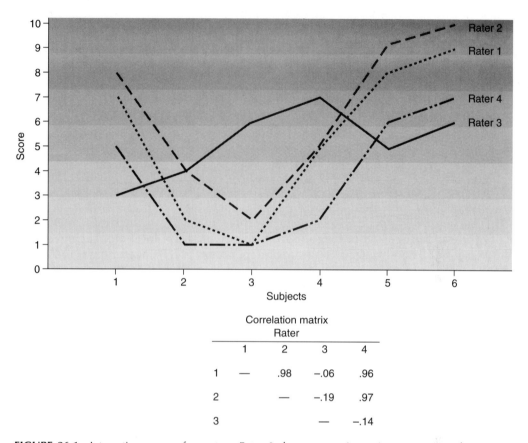

Correlation matrix			
Rater			
	1	2	3	4

	1	2	3	4
1	—	.98	−.06	.96
2		—	−.19	.97
3			—	−.14

FIGURE 26.1 Interaction among four raters. Rater 3 demonstrates inconsistent responses that are responsible for the interaction effect. All other raters show parallel responses, as suggested by the corresponding correlation coefficients.

erence for Model 1, because it provides a more conservative estimate of reliability than the other models;[13] however, the conservative or liberal nature of a statistic is not an adequate rationale for its use if the model is unsuitable for the design.[9] Generally, for the same set of data, Model 1 will give smaller values than Model 2, and Model 2 will yield smaller values than Model 3. Likewise, within each model, the ICC based on mean ratings will always yield a higher correlation than one based on single ratings. Because of these potential differences, the type of ICC used in a particular study should always be reported.

Many statistical programs do not contain procedures for calculating ICCs. Fortunately, they are easy to compute by hand once the analysis of variance is performed.[‡]

[‡]SPSS conveniently runs the appropriate ANOVA for Models 2 and 3 under its SCALE: RELIABILITY ANALYSIS procedure if an *F*-test is requested.[14] All three ICC models can be obtained for single and average ratings.

AGREEMENT

When the unit of measurement is on a categorical scale, reliability is appropriately assessed as a measure of agreement. The simplest index of agreement is **percent agreement,** which is a measure of how often raters agree on scores given to individual subjects (or how often test–retest scores agree). The *coefficient of agreement* represents the total proportion of observations (P_o) on which there is agreement, or

$$P_o = \frac{\text{number of exact agreements}}{\text{number of possible agreements}} = \frac{\Sigma f_o}{N} \qquad (26.11)$$

where Σf_o is the sum of the *frequencies of observed agreements*, and N is the number of pairs of scores that were obtained.

For example, suppose two clinicians wanted to establish their interrater reliability for evaluating level of function for self-care on a 3-point scale. They evaluate 100 patients to determine if they are independent (IND), need some assistance (ASST), or are dependent (DEP). We can summarize these data to show agreements by arranging them in an *agreement matrix,* or frequency table, as shown in Table 26.5A. The quantities along the diagonal represent the number of times both raters agreed on their ratings (f_o). (Ignore values in parentheses for now.) All values off the diagonal represent disagreements. For instance, both raters agreed on ratings of IND for 25 subjects; they agreed on ratings of ASST for 24 subjects; and they agreed on ratings of DEP for 17 subjects. They did not agree on 34 subjects. Of 100 possible agreements, 66 were achieved. Therefore, $P_o = 66/100 = .66$. The two clinicians agreed on their ratings 66% of the time. This value is fair, relative to potential perfect agreement of 100%.

There is a limitation to this interpretation, however. To determine the true reliability of categorical assignment, we must consider the possibility that some portion of the results could have occurred by chance; that is, if two raters were to assign subjects to categories completely at random, some degree of agreement would still be expected. Because of this tendency, percent agreement will often be an overestimate of true reliability. Therefore, a measure is needed that will discount the proportion of agreement that is potentially due to chance alone.

Chance Agreement: The Kappa Statistic

The **kappa** statistic, κ, is a *chance-corrected* measure of agreement.[15] In addition to looking at the proportion of observed agreements (P_o), kappa also considers the proportion of agreements expected by chance (P_c):

$$P_c = \frac{\text{number of expected agreements}}{\text{number of possible agreements}} = \frac{\Sigma f_c}{N} \qquad (26.12)$$

where Σf_c is the sum of the frequencies of agreement expected by chance.

We can illustrate this application using the frequency data for functional assessment shown in Table 26.5. The number of expected chance agreements for each cell along the

TABLE 26.5. COMPUTATION OF PERCENT AGREEMENT AND KAPPA: AGREEMENT MATRIX FOR RATINGS OF FUNCTIONAL ASSESSMENT FOR TWO RATERS (Chance Frequencies in Parentheses)

A. DATA

		Rater 1			
		IND	ASST	DEP	Total
	IND	25 (15.54)	5 (11.10)	7 (10.36)	37
Rater 2	ASST	6 (14.28)	24 (10.20)	4 (9.52)	34
	DEP	11 (12.18)	1 (8.70)	17 (8.12)	29
	Total	42	30	28	100

B. COMPUTATIONS

$$\Sigma f_o = 25 + 24 + 17 = 66 \qquad P_o = \frac{\Sigma f_o}{N} = \frac{66}{100} = .66$$

$$\Sigma f_c = 15.54 + 10.20 + 8.12 = 33.86 \qquad P_c = \frac{\Sigma f_c}{N} = \frac{33.86}{100} = .34$$

$$\kappa = \frac{P_o - P_c}{1 - P_c} = \frac{.66 - .34}{1 - .34} = .49$$

$$\kappa = \frac{\Sigma f_o - f_c}{N - \Sigma f_c} = \frac{66 - 33.86}{100 - 33.86} = .49$$

diagonal is calculated by multiplying the corresponding row and column margin totals, and dividing by the total number of possible agreements, or N.[§] These values are shown in parentheses. For example, for agreements on IND, the row total is 37, and the column total is 42. With $N = 100$, we determine that chance agreements on IND can be expected $(37 \times 42)/100 = 15.54$ times. Similarly, we expect both raters to come up with ratings of ASST $(34 \times 30)/100 = 10.20$ times by chance. The expected frequency for DEP is $(29 \times 28)/100 = 8.12$ times. Therefore, the total number of expected chance frequencies, Σf_c, is 33.86. The proportion of agreement expected by chance for the entire sample is $33.86/100 = 0.34$. This tells us that even if these two raters had no common grading criteria, we could expect agreement between them 34% of the time.

[§]This procedure is identical to calculation of expected frequencies for the χ^2 test. See Chapter 25 for a fuller discussion of this procedure.

Thus, the proportion of observations that can be attributed to reliable measurement is defined by $P_o - P_c$, that is, the proportion of observed agreements less the contribution of chance. The maximum possible nonchance agreements would be $1 - P_c$, or 100% less the contribution of chance. Kappa represents percent agreement based on these correction factors,

$$\kappa = \frac{P_o - P_c}{1 - P_c} \qquad (26.13)$$

which is a ratio of the proportion of observed nonchance agreements to the proportion of possible nonchance agreements.

For the functional assessment data, we know the proportion of observed agreement, $P_o = 66\%$. When we calculate chance observations we note that $P_c = 34\%$. Therefore, to account for the fact that 34% of the agreement could have occurred by chance, we correct our original estimate using the formula for kappa:

$$\kappa = \frac{.66 - .34}{1 - .34} = .49$$

This indicates a lower level of agreement than the 66% obtained using percent agreement. With the effects of chance eliminated, agreement is rated at 49%. This corrected percentage is a more meaningful interpretation of reliability estimates for categorical assignments. Landis and Koch have suggested that values of kappa above 80% represent excellent agreement; above 60%, substantial levels of agreement; from 40% to 60%, moderate agreement; and below 40%, poor to fair agreement.[16] For this example, then, we have achieved only a moderate degree of reliability. The interpretation of this outcome, like any other reliability coefficient, must depend on how the data will be used and the degree of precision required for making rational clinical decisions.

As shown in Table 26.5B, kappa can also be expressed in terms of frequencies to facilitate computation:

$$\kappa = \frac{\Sigma f_o - \Sigma f_c}{N - \Sigma f_c} \qquad (26.14)$$

For all practical purposes, the lower and upper limits of kappa are 0.00 and +1.00.[15] Kappa will be zero if $P_o = P_c$, where agreement equals chance, and positive if $P_o > P_c$, where agreement is better than chance. With perfect agreement, all cells off the diagonal will equal zero; therefore, $P_o = 1.00$ and $\kappa = 1.00$. Kappa can be negative if agreement is worse than chance ($P_o < P_c$), although this is not a likely outcome in clinical reliability studies.

Weighted Kappa

For some applications, kappa is limited in that it does not differentiate among disagreements. Because it is calculated using only the frequencies along the agreement diagonal, kappa assumes that all disagreements (off the diagonal) are of equal seriousness. There may be instances, however, when a researcher wants to assign greater weight to some disagreements than others, to account for differential risks. For example, Jarvik et al. looked at the reliability of classifying disk herniations in patients with lumbar disk disease.[17] They hypothesized that some misclassifications would be more serious than others, if misjudgments were made for those with protruded or extruded disks. In a clinical study, Cooperman et al. examined the reliability of a test for ligamentous stability at the knee, graded 0, +1, +2, or +3, with higher grades indicating less stability.[18] They considered a disagreement between ratings of 0 and +3 to be more serious than a disagreement between 0 and +1 for diagnostic purposes and subsequent treatment decisions. When disagreements can be differentiated in this way, a modified version of the kappa statistic, called **weighted kappa, κ$_w$,** can be used to estimate reliability.[19]

Weighted kappa allows the researcher to specify differential weights for disagreement cells in the agreement matrix. Kappa is actually a special case of weighted kappa, where all cells along the agreement diagonal are given weights of 1 and all disagreements are weighted 0. By assigning different weights to the off-diagonal cells, weighted kappa essentially gives more credit for some disagreements than others.

We can illustrate this procedure once again using the functional assessment data. These data showed 66% observed agreement. In terms of clinical implications, however, we might suggest that disagreements among these grades are not all of the same importance and that weighting them would provide a more practical estimate of reliability.

Assigning Weights

Cohen suggests that the assignment of weights is essentially a judgmental process.[19] Therefore, no one set of weights can be applied universally, and the value of κ$_w$ will be sensitive to the choice of weights.[20] Weights should conform to a hypothesis that defines the relative seriousness of the disagreements.

Incremental Weights.　One approach is to look at a scale as an ordinal continuum with equal intervals, that is, an *incremental scale.*[4] For example, using the functional evaluation scale described in Table 26.5, we might hypothesize that the difference between IND and DEP is twice the difference between ASST and DEP, with IND = 3, ASST = 2, and DEP = 1. If this hypothesis is reasonable, then weights for incremental disagreements can be determined using the formula

$$w = (r_1 - r_2)^2 \tag{26.15}$$

where w is the assigned weight, and r_1 and r_2 are the scores assigned by Rater 1 and Rater 2 to that cell. Therefore, $r_1 - r_2$ represents the *deviation from agreement* for each cell in the agreement matrix. This type of weighting system is shown in Table 26.6A. For instance, a disagreement between IND (3) and ASST (2) would receive a weight of $(3 - 2)^2 = 1$. The same weight would be assigned to disagreements between ASST and DEP; however, a disagreement between IND (3) and DEP (1) would receive a weight of $(3 - 1)^2 = 4$. Weights of zero would automatically be assigned to all the agreement cells on the diagonal, indicating no disagreement.

Asymmetrical Weights.　In many situations, the evaluation of disagreements does not fit a uniform pattern. For instance, we might hypothesize that a disagreement between IND and DEP is more severe than a disagreement between ASST and DEP. We might also suggest that the *direction* of the disagreement is important; that is, assigning a grade of IND to a patient who needs assistance is a more serious error than assigning

TABLE 26.6. TWO SCHEMES FOR WEIGHTING DISAGREEMENTS ON FUNCTIONAL ASSESSMENT DATA

A. Incremental Weights

Cell weights $= (r_1 - r_2)^2$

		Rater 1		
		IND (3)	ASST (2)	DEP (1)
	IND (3)	0	1	4
Rater 2	ASST (2)	1	0	1
	DEP (1)	4	1	0

B. Asymmetrical Weights

		Rater 1		
		IND (3)	ASST (2)	DEP (1)
	IND (3)	0	2	4
Rater 2	ASST (2)	3	0	1
(Criterion)	DEP (1)	6	1	0

DEP to an independent patient. If a patient who is dependent is graded IND, he might be unsafe, left alone without adequate supervision. This is more serious as an evaluation error than unnecessarily supervising a strong patient. Suppose we test the validity of a clinician's assessment of function by comparing her ratings (Rater 1) with those of an "expert" (Rater 2), who acts as the criterion or "gold standard." We would want to assign the highest weight to an error where Rater 1 says IND and Rater 2 says DEP. The next highest weight might go to the converse DEP–IND disagreement. Errors between IND and ASST might be the next most serious, followed by ASST–IND. Errors between ASST and DEP might be perceived as relatively unimportant, as with either rating the patient will receive some supervision. This creates an *asymmetrical pattern* of weights, varying with the direction of disagreement.

For this type of subjective judgment, Cohen suggests first choosing a weight to represent maximum disagreement and then setting the other weights accordingly.[19] For example, as shown in Table 26.6B, we might choose weights of 6 for IND–DEP, 4 for DEP–IND, 3 for IND–ASST, and 2 for ASST–IND disagreements. DEP–ASST errors would be considered least important, with a weight of 1. For convenience, weights of zero are still assigned to all agreements.

Symmetrical Weights. A third pattern of weights can be established when the direction of disagreement is unimportant. For instance, we might argue that any disagreement between IND and DEP is twice as serious as a disagreement between

TABLE 26.7. COMPUTATION OF WEIGHTED KAPPA USING SYMMETRICAL WEIGHTS: TABLE OF AGREEMENTS AND DISAGREEMENTS ON FUNCTIONAL ASSESSMENT DATA*

A. DATA

		Rater 1			
		IND	**ASST**	**DEP**	**Total**
	IND	25 (15.54) $w = 0$	5 (11.10) $w = 3$	7 (10.36) $w = 6$	37
Rater 2	**ASST**	6 (14.28) $w = 3$	24 (10.20) $w = 0$	(9.52) $w = 1$	34
	DEP	11 (12.18) $w = 6$	1 (8.70) $w = 1$	17 (8.12) $w = 0$	29
	Total	42	30	28	100

B. COMPUTATIONS

$\Sigma wf_o = 0(25) + 3(5) + 6(7) + 3(6) + 0(24) + 1(4) + 6(11) + 1(1) + 0(17) = 146$

$\Sigma wf_c = 0(15.54) + 3(11.10) + 6(10.36) + 3(14.28) + 0(10.20) + \ldots + 0(8.12) = 229.60$

$$K_w = 1 - \frac{\Sigma wf_o}{\Sigma wf_c} = 1 - \frac{146}{229.69} = .36$$

*Expected frequencies are in parentheses.

IND and ASST, and that a disagreement between ASST and DEP is only minimally important. To designate a set of weights that reflect this hypothesis, we might choose a weight of 6 to represent any disagreement between IND and DEP, a weight of 3 to represent a disagreement between IND and ASST, and a weight of 1 to represent the less important disagreement between ASST and DEP. These *symmetrical weights (w)* are shown in the center of each cell in Table 26.7A.

Calculation of κ_w

The weights that are assigned to each cell in the agreement matrix are used in the calculation of weighted kappa. An obvious criticism of this procedure is based on the fact that the arbitrary assignment of weights can make the consequent value of κ_w arbitrary as well.[21] This points out the need for the researcher to operate on the basis of a hypothesis that defines the relationship among the rating categories. For instance, each of the preceding weighting systems was based on a different theoretical rationale. The rationale used to define these weights then becomes an integral part of the hypothesis being tested.[2] For this reason, the weights used in calculating κ_w and the rationale for choosing them should be stated in a research report.

We will demonstrate the calculation of κ_w using the functional assessment data with symmetrical weights shown in Table 26.7A. Each cell in the table contains the observed frequency (f_o), the expected chance frequency (f_c, shown in parentheses), and the cell weight (w). The first step is to find the *weighted frequencies* of observed disagreement (wf_o) and chance disagreement (wf_c) for each cell in the matrix by multiplying the observed and chance frequencies by the cell weight. For example, for the first cell in the matrix, wf_o = 0(25) and wf_c = 0(15.54). Note that we are concerned with the *frequencies of disagreements,* not agreements as we were with kappa. Because the cells along the agreement diagonal all have weights of zero, they are effectively eliminated from the calculations.

Next we determine the sum of these terms to find the total weighted observed frequencies, Σwf_o, and the total weighted chance frequencies, Σwf_c. Weighted kappa is given by

$$\kappa_w = 1 - \frac{\Sigma wf_o}{\Sigma wf_c} \tag{26.16}$$

As shown in Table 26.7B, κ_w = .36. This value is somewhat lower than the value obtained for kappa (κ = .41).

Let us consider the implications of weighting this data. According to the frequency data, we find exact agreement in 66 of 100 tests. Kappa reduces this estimate to 49% by correcting for chance, but does not account for any differentiation in the seriousness of the 34 disagreements. Five of these disagreements were between ASST and DEP, which we consider minimally important. Of the 29 more serious disagreements, 18 were between IND and DEP (the most serious) and 11 were between IND and ASST. These serious disagreements account for more than one quarter of the tests and 85% of all the disagreements. By accounting for these serious discrepancies, weighted kappa brings down the level of agreement further to 36%. This gives us a more meaningful estimate of the degree of reliability between these raters than kappa alone, and suggests that these raters demonstrate serious discrepancies too often.

Interpretation of Kappa

Several factors must be considered in the interpretation of kappa or weighted kappa. First, it is important to recognize that kappa represents an *average rate of agreement* for an entire set of scores. It will not indicate if most of the disagreement is accounted for by one specific category or rater. Therefore, in an effort to improve reliability, it is useful to subjectively examine the data when discussing results, to see where the major discrepancies lie.

A second issue, which we continue to stress for all reliability indices, is that of variance among subjects. In measures of agreement, variance is necessary to allow reasonable interpretation of reliability. In a group of subjects with homogeneous characteristics, the percentage of agreements will be necessarily high. Therefore, the reliability analysis is not really showing whether the measurement is capable of differentiating among subjects on that characteristic.

Because kappa is based on proportions, the use of very small samples can provide misleading results. For example, if two raters agree on two observations, the reliability estimate will be 100%. If they disagree on one of those observations, the rating drops to 50%. Such a variation does not accurately reflect reliability when compared with estimates of the same behavior tested many more times.

Kappa is also influenced by the number of categories used. As the number of categories increases, the extent of agreement will generally decrease. This is logical, as with more possibilities of assignment, there is room for greater discrepancy between raters. Therefore, if values of kappa are to be compared, the samples used should contain the same number of categories.

Probably the strongest limitation of kappa is that it is an analysis of exact agreement; that is, it treats agreement as an all-or-none phenomenon with no room for "close" agreement. Therefore, it is appropriate for use with nominal or ordinal data, which require that each subject be placed in an exclusive category. By definition, there can be no doubt as to whether raters achieved the same "score" for each subject. Kappa is less useful for dealing with continuous data on the interval or ratio scales as there is no credit given for scores that remain close over several trials.

Kappa can be used with more than two raters,[1, 22] although an overall kappa is less informative than if separate kappas are computed for pairs of raters.[21] One advantage of using separate analyses is that it is then possible to use different rationales for setting weights for each comparison. A calculation has been derived for using kappa with multiple ratings per subject.[23] It is also possible to use the intraclass correlation coefficient, ICC, as an equivalent of weighted kappa when incremental weights are scaled according to squared disagreements ($w = (r_1 - r_2)^2$).[4]

INTERNAL CONSISTENCY: CRONBACH'S ALPHA

Measuring instruments are often designed as scales, composed of many items that in total should reflect the characteristic being measured. For instance, the quantitative portion of the Graduate Record Examination (QGRE) includes many items to test a student's mathematical ability. Functional scales are designed to include items related to different ADL tasks. In both of these examples, the scales are actually only a sample of the possible items that could be included, although we want to draw a conclusion about an individual's performance based on the total score. If these scales are reliable, we would expect the subject to receive the same score even if we changed the items.

One assumption that is inherent in the use of such scales is the **homogeneity** of the items or their **internal consistency**. A good scale is one that assesses different aspects of the same attribute; that is, the items are homogeneous.[24] Therefore, the QGRE will not include items to assess verbal ability. A scale of physical function will reflect physical performance but not emotional function. Statistically, if the items on the scale are truly measuring the same attribute, they should be moderately correlated with each other and with the total score. These correlations are measures of internal consistency (see Chapter 5 for further discussion of item-total correlations).

The most commonly applied statistical index for internal consistency is **Cronbach's alpha (α)**.[25] It can be used for scales with items that are dichotomous (yes/no) or when there are more than two response choices (such as an ordinal scale or multiple choice items). To illustrate the application of Cronbach's α, we will use hypothetical data from a sample of 14 patients in a rehabilitation hospital who have been assessed for function using six items: walking, climbing stairs, carrying 5 pounds, reaching for a phone, dressing (putting on a shirt), and getting in and out of a car. Each item is scored on an ordinal scale from 1 to 5, with 5 reflecting complete independence. The maximum total score, then, is 30 (see Table 26.8A).

TABLE 26.8.   DETERMINATION OF INTERNAL CONSISTENCY OF A FUNCTIONAL SCALE WITH SIX ITEMS USING CRONBACH'S ALPHA (*N* = 14)

A. DATA

Subject	Car	Carry	Dressing	Reach	Stairs	Walk	Total
1	2	3	4	3	3	4	19
2	1	3	2	3	2	3	14
3	1	1	1	2	1	3	9
4	1	4	3	4	3	3	18
5	1	3	3	4	1	3	15
6	2	4	4	5	3	5	22
7	3	3	2	2	1	2	13
8	2	5	4	5	4	5	25
9	2	4	3	3	5	4	21
10	3	3	3	4	4	5	22
11	3	2	2	2	2	4	15
12	1	1	1	2	1	2	8
13	2	1	1	1	1	2	8
14	2	2	3	2	2	3	14

B. OUTPUT

1. Descriptive Statistics

	Car	Carry	Dress	Reach	Stairs	Walk	Total
Mean	1.857	2.786	2.571	3.000	2.357	3.357	15.929
S.D.	0.770	1.251	1.089	1.240	1.336	1.082	5.567

2. Inter-Item Correlation Matrix

	Car	Carry	Dress	Reach	Stairs	Walk
Car	1.000					
Carry	.125	1.000				
Dress	.196	.830	1.000			
Reach	−.081	.843	.797	1.000		
Stairs	.277	.739	.695	.603	1.000	
Walk	.251	.686	.793	.803	.809	1.000

3. Item-Total Statistics

	Scale mean if item deleted	Scale variance if item deleted	Corrected item-total correlation	Alpha if item deleted
Car	14.071	28.995	.169	.938
Carry	13.143	19.978	.845	.857
Dress	13.357	21.170	.862	.857
Reach	12.929	20.687	.777	.869
Stairs	13.571	19.802	.791	.868
Walk	12.571	21.187	.867	.857

4. Reliability Coefficient   6 items   Alpha = .896

Internal consistency is a reflection of the correlation among these six items and the correlation of each individual item with the total score. Cronbach's α for these data is .896, as shown in panel 4 of Table 26.8B. As with other correlation statistics, this index ranges from 0.00 to 1.00. Therefore, a value that approaches .90 is high, and the scale can be considered reliable. We can interpret this value in two ways. First, it tells us about the correlation among the items on the scale, indicating that overall they are measuring the same attribute. Second, it tells us about the reliability of this scale, or the theoretical correlation of the scale with all other possible scales containing the same number of items drawn from the universe of items on this characteristic.[14] For instance, to measure function we might have used other items such as getting in and out of a chair, putting on pants, or toileting. Of course, we would need a much larger sample to accurately estimate this aspect of the scale's reliability.

Alpha can also be used to examine individual items to determine how well they fit the overall scale. In Panel 1 in Table 26.8B, the means and standard deviations for each item and the total score are displayed. We can see that walking had the highest mean and car transfer the lowest. In Panel 2 we find the inter-item correlations for all six items. All item-pairs have correlations above .60 except for car transfer, which has consistently low correlations with all other items (.277 and lower). Perhaps this one variable should not be part of the scale, representing a different component of function than the other items.

To investigate this possibility, the advantage of α is that it can be computed repeatedly, each time eliminating one item from the analysis. In Panel 3, we see what happens when each item is deleted. In the first column, the mean of the total score is increased when car transfer is deleted, whereas this value remains fairly stable for all other items. The third column in this panel shows the correlation of each item with the sum of the remaining items, or the **item-to-total correlation.** Only car transfer has a low correlation of .17, suggesting that this variable is not related to the other items. Each of the other five items has a correlation of approximately .80 or higher with the total. Finally, in the last column we find that alpha increases to .938 when car transfer is not included, indicating that the scale is more homogeneous when this item is omitted. These statistics suggest that car transfer should be removed from the scale, as it appears to reflect a different dimension of function than the other items.

Interestingly, several sources suggest that a scale with strong internal consistency should only show a moderate correlation among the items, between .70 and .90.[24,26–28] If items have too low a correlation, they are possibly measuring different traits. If the items have too high a correlation, they are probably redundant, and the content validity of the scale might be limited.

RESPONSE STABILITY

In addition to measuring the reliability of instruments and raters, clinical scientists are often interested in assessing the consistency or stability of repeated responses over time. **Response stability** is basic to establishing all other types of reliability, because if the response variable varies from measurement to measurement, it will not be possible to separate out errors due to the rater or instrument. Three statistical methods are commonly used to express response stability: standard error of measurement, coefficient of variation, and method error.

Standard Error of Measurement

Like other forms of reliability, the concept of response stability is related to measurement error. If we were to administer a test to one individual an infinite number of times, we can assume that the responses would vary somewhat from trial to trial. These differences would be a function of random measurement error. Theoretically, if we could plot these responses, the distribution would resemble a normal curve, with the mean equal to the true score and errors falling above and below the mean. This distribution of measurement errors is a theoretical distribution that represents the population of all possible measurement errors that could occur for that variable. With a more reliable measurement, errors will be smaller, and this distribution will be less variable. Therefore, the standard deviation of the measurement errors reflects the reliability of the response. This standard deviation is the **standard error of measurement, SEM.**

We can interpret the SEM according to the properties of the normal curve. For example, suppose we record a series of 25 measurements of grip strength for one subject using a hand dynamometer (assuming sufficient rests so that true values do not change). Let us assume that the mean score is 23 pounds and the SEM is 6. Therefore, there is a 68% chance that this individual's true score falls within ±1 SEM (between 17 and 29 pounds) or a 95% chance that it falls within ±2 SEM (between 11 and 35 pounds). In a subsequent test, if this subject's response is 28 pounds, we can assume that the score does not represent a true change as it falls within the range of measurement error.

When the SEM is based on repeated measurements from a single individual, as in this example, its value will obviously be different for each subject. Therefore, the amount of error, or reliability, associated with a particular measurement will not be a constant estimate. Most often, however, it is not feasible to collect a large enough sample of repeated measurements on each subject. Therefore, we estimate the SEM for a set of scores obtained from a larger sample of subjects as follows:

$$\text{SEM} = s_X\sqrt{1 - r_{XX}} \qquad (26.17)$$

where s_X is the standard deviation of the set of observed test scores, and r_{XX} is the reliability coefficient for that measurement. For example, suppose we administer grip strength tests to a sample of 300 patients, each measured once. Assume the standard deviation of these scores is 12, and the reliability coefficient for this measurement, established by previous test–retest studies, is known to be .85. Therefore,

$$\text{SEM} = 12\sqrt{1 - .85} = 4.65$$

This value can now be used as an estimate of reliability for the entire group. For instance, if the group mean is 30 pounds, then there is a 95% chance that the group's true mean score lies within ±2 SEM, or between 20.7 and 39.3. Therefore, we can estimate that 95% of the time, the errors of measurement using this test will fall within this range. Because the SEM is based on the characteristics of the normal curve, a meaningful estimate can only be made with a large sample of scores.

The interpretation of standard error of measurement is dependent on the type of reliability coefficient that is used in its computation.[29] If the estimate is based on test–retest reliability, then the SEM is indicative of the range of scores that can be expected on retesting. If rater reliability is used, the SEM reflects the extent of expected error in different raters' scores. The choice of reliability coefficient for calculating the SEM must be based on the ultimate purpose of predicting reliability.

Coefficient of Variation

We can also assess response stability across repeated trials by looking at the standard deviation of the responses (for one individual or a group). Variability within the responses should reflect the degree of measurement error. The standard deviation will obviously increase as the repeated scores become more disparate.

The limitation to this approach is that the standard deviation must be interpreted in relation to the size and units of the mean. For example, suppose a distribution of strength scores (in pounds) has a standard deviation of 40 pounds. If the mean of the distribution is 110, reliability will be viewed differently than if the mean is 55. In the first instance the scores are actually less variable relative to the mean. Therefore, on the basis of standard deviation alone, we cannot accurately assess the extent of error in the measurements.

To account for the relationship between the mean and standard deviation, the variability across distributions can be compared using the **coefficient of variation,** *CV*:

$$CV = \frac{s}{\overline{X}} \times 100 \qquad (26.18)$$

This ratio expresses the standard deviation as a *proportion of the mean.* Because both the mean and standard deviation are in the same units, this statistic will be unit free, allowing comparisons across different quantities or different studies.

See Chapter 17 for a more complete discussion and sample calculations of the coefficient of variation.

Method Error

Response stability, or test–retest reliability, can also be expressed in terms of the percentage variation from trial to trial, by analyzing **method error, ME.** Method error is a measure of the discrepancy between two sets of repeated scores, or their difference scores. Larger difference scores reflect greater measurement error.

Method error is calculated using the standard deviation of the difference scores (s_d) between test and retest:

$$ME = \frac{s_d}{\sqrt{2}} \qquad (26.19)$$

This value reflects the amount of variation in the difference scores; however, just like any other standard deviation, it must be interpreted relative to the size of the mean differences. Therefore, it is converted to a percentage using the coefficient of variation:

$$CV_{ME} = \frac{2ME}{\overline{X}_1 + \overline{X}_2} \times 100 \qquad (26.20)$$

Calculation of ME and its associated coefficient of variation is illustrated in Table 26.9B for hypothetical range of motion measurements. The variation in measurement from Test 1 to Test 2 was 6%. The interpretation of this value will depend on the amount of error deemed acceptable by those who must use the information.

TABLE 26.9. COMPUTATION OF METHOD ERROR AND COEFFICIENT OF VARIATION FOR RELIABILITY TESTING

A. DATA

Subject	Test 1	Test 2	Difference (d)
1	18	19	−1
2	17	19	−2
3	17	15	2
4	20	19	1
5	19	18	1
6	19	17	2
7	21	19	2
8	16	16	0
ΣX	147	142	$\Sigma d = 5$
$\overline{X}$	18.38	17.75	$\overline{d} = 0.63$
s	1.58	1.48	$s_d = 1.41$

B. COMPUTATIONS

$$ME = \frac{s_d}{\sqrt{2}} = \frac{1.41}{\sqrt{2}} = 1.00$$

$$CV_{ME} = \frac{2ME}{\overline{X}_1 + \overline{X}_2} = \frac{2(1.00)}{18.38 - 17.75} = .06$$

$$s_{\overline{d}} = \frac{s_d}{\sqrt{n}} = \frac{1.41}{\sqrt{8}} = .50 \qquad\qquad t = \frac{\overline{d}}{s_{\overline{d}}} = \frac{.63}{.50} - 1.26$$

C. HYPOTHESIS TEST　　$H_o: \overline{d} = 0$　　$_{(\alpha_2 = .05)}t_{(7)} = 2.365$　　Do not reject H_o

Method error is often used as an adjunct to test–retest correlation statistics, as it reflects the percentage of variation from trial to trial, which the correlation coefficient does not. In addition, unlike the correlation coefficient, method error is not affected by a lack of variation in raw scores. For instance, for the data in Table 26.9, $r = .58$. This is low, especially considering how close the two pairs of scores are. But we can also see that there is very little variability within these scores, which we know will tend to decrease the correlation coefficient or any reliability coefficient. Method error will not be affected by a restriction in range, because it looks only at the difference scores. Therefore, in situations like this example, where reliability coefficients are misleading, method error provides a useful alternative.

Because method error is based on the variability within difference scores, it will not account for systematic variation between Test 1 and Test 2. Therefore, the researcher may want to check for systematic bias by performing a paired t-test between the test and retest scores.[30] The t-ratio can be obtained directly by dividing the mean of the difference scores, $\overline{d}$, by the standard error of the difference scores, $s_{\overline{d}}$. This computation is illustrated in Table 26.9B. With $n-1$ degrees of freedom, this value demonstrates no significant difference between Test 1 and Test 2.

ALTERNATE FORMS: LIMITS OF AGREEMENT

Reliability is an essential property when measurements are taken with alternate forms of an instrument. For example, clinical researchers have looked at outcomes of measuring joint range of motion with different types of goniometers, inclinometers, electrogoniometers, and radiographs. Even though each instrument is different, they are all intended to result in an accurate recording of joint angles in degrees. We might want to compare different designs of dynamometers for measuring strength, different types of spirometers for assessing pulmonary function, or different types of thermometers for measuring temperature. In each of these examples, we would expect these methods to record similar values. The analysis of reliability in this situation focuses on the agreement between alternative methods. We can consider two methods in agreement when the difference between measurements on one subject is small enough for the methods to be considered interchangeable.[31] This property is an important practical concern as we strive for effective and efficient clinical measurement,[32] as well as a concern for generalization of research findings.

Two analysis procedures have traditionally been applied for method comparisons. The correlation coefficient, *r*, has been used to demonstrate covariance among methods; however, we know this is a poor estimate of reliability, as it does not necessarily reflect the extent of agreement in the data (see Figure 5.1 in Chapter 5 and Table 26.3 in this chapter). The second procedure is the paired *t*-test (or repeated measures ANOVA), which is used to show that mean scores for two (or more) methods are not significantly different. This approach is also problematic, however, as two distributions may show no statistical difference, but still be composed of pairs with no agreement.

An interesting alternative for examining agreement across methods is an index called **limits of agreement.**[31–33] To understand this approach, consider the hypothetical distribution of 10 measurements of range of motion of straight leg raising shown in Table 26.10 for two instruments, a regular goniometer and an inclinometer. The difference between each method for each subject is calculated by subtracting the inclinometer score from the goniometer score (this direction is arbitrary). Therefore, positive difference scores reflect a higher reading for the goniometer. The mean of the difference scores is –0.1 degrees. On average, then, the differences between the methods is quite small, and certainly within acceptable clinical error range. We would be happy to find that the two instruments differed by less than 1 degree. On further examination, however, we can see that the amount of error varied across subjects, from zero to as much as 10 degrees. Therefore, we would be more complete in our estimate of reliability to determine the range of error that would be expected for any individual subject.

A visual analysis can help to clarify this relationship. For example, the scatterplot of these scores is shown in Figure 26.2 (*r* = .86). If we draw a line of identity from the origin, representing agreement of scores, we can see that most of the scores are close, but not in agreement. A further understanding of this relationship can be achieved by looking at a plot of the difference between methods against the mean score for each subject, as shown in Figure 26.3A. The spread of scores around the zero point helps us decide if the observed error is acceptable if we substitute one measurement method for the other. In this example, the error appears unbiased, as differences are spread evenly and randomly above and below the zero point. Other possible patterns are shown in Figures 26.3.B, which shows a pattern with no error, where all differences are zero; 26.3C, which reflects a biased pattern, where the goniometer has consistently resulted in higher

TABLE 26.10.   LIMITS OF AGREEMENT: MEASUREMENT OF STRAIGHT LEG RAISING (IN DEGREES) USING TWO METHODS

A. DATA

Subject	Goniometer	Inclinometer		Difference[a]	Mean[b]
1	55	54		1	54.5
2	58	61		−3	59.5
3	70	80		−10	75.0
4	76	59		7	62.5
5	85	85		0	85.0
6	78	80		−2	79.0
7	72	70		2	71.0
8	80	75		5	77.5
9	63	68		−5	65.5
10	72	68		4	70.0
			Total	−1.0	699.5
			$\overline{X}$	−0.1	69.9
			s	5.09	9.52

B. 95% LIMITS OF AGREEMENT $\overline{X} \pm 2s = -0.1 \pm 10.18 = -10.28$ to 10.08

[a]Goniometer − Inclinometer
[b](Goniometer + Inclinometer)/2

scores, resulting in all positive difference scores; and 26.3D, which shows another biased pattern where error is influenced by the size of the measurement—that is, smaller angles are measured higher by the inclinometer (resulting in a negative difference score) and larger angles are measured higher by the goniometer (resulting in a positive difference score). With a biased pattern, the instruments could not be considered interchangeable.

We can examine the agreement between the two methods by looking at the spread of the difference scores. A larger variability would indicate larger errors. Statistically, this spread is reflected by the standard deviation. Assuming the errors are normally distributed,[ǁ] we would expect that approximately 95% of the difference scores would fall within two standard deviations above and below the mean of the difference scores.[31] This range is considered the *95% limits of agreement.* As shown in Table 26.10A, for the straight leg raise data the mean difference score is −0.1 degrees with a standard deviation of 5.09 degrees. Two standard deviations equal 10.18 degrees. Therefore, the difference between these two methods of measurement of straight leg raise can be expected to vary between −0.1 ± 10.18, or between −10.28 degrees and 10.08 degrees, a range of approximately 20 degrees (see Fig. 26.4).

[ǁ]Because the difference scores represent measurement error, Bland and Altman suggest that they should follow a normal distribution, even if the actual measurements do not.[33] This distribution can be checked by graphing a histogram of the difference scores.[31]

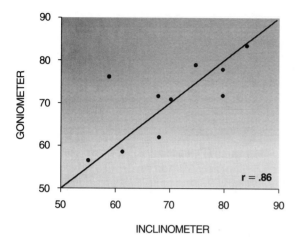

FIGURE 26.2 Example of a method comparison plot, showing the relationship between two different methods for measuring range of motion of straight leg raise. The line of identity emerges from the origin, to show if the two methods agree.

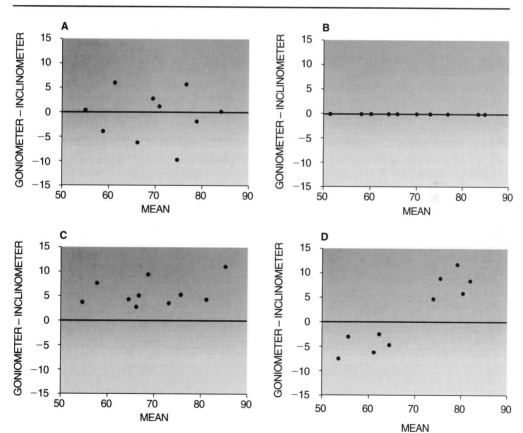

FIGURE 26.3 Plots of difference scores for straight leg raise measurements across mean scores for each subject. The center line represents zero difference. **(A)** Data from Table 26.10. **(B)** Perfect agreement between two methods. **(C)** Pattern with systematic bias in measurement error, in this case with the goniometer consistently producing higher scores than the inclinometer. **(D)** Plot showing bias related to magnitude of the subjects' scores.

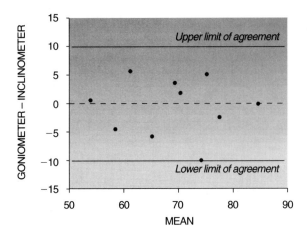

FIGURE 26.4   Difference scores between goniometer and inclinometer, plotted against mean scores for each subject (data from Table 26.10). Dashed line shows the mean difference score (–0.1 degrees). The 95% upper and lower limits of agreement represent 2 standard deviations above and below the mean difference score (–0.1 ± 10.18).

Our question, then, is would we be comfortable using either instrument, if we knew that their difference could be as much as 10 degrees higher or lower? This decision should be based on a clinical criterion and the application of the measurements.[34] We might argue that a potential difference of 20 degrees does not suggest interchangeable methods. We are, of course, assuming that each method is reliable. These considerations have important implications for clinical analyses as well as comparison of research studies.

COMMENTARY

Know Your Reliability Coefficient—Know Your Measurement

Because reliability issues are so important to the validity of clinical science, the statistical bases for interpreting reliability must be understood by those who do the research and those who read research reports. What we learn from looking through professional literature is that preferred methods for analyzing reliability seem to vary with different researchers and within different disciplines. Even though statisticians have been addressing reliability issues for a long time, there is limited consensus on how reliability data are handled.

Choosing a particular approach to reliability testing should be based on an understanding of the nature of the response variable, what types of interpretations are desired, and what measurement issues are of greatest concern. Consideration should be given to the scale of measurement, the amount of variability that can be expected within sample scores, and what units of measurement are used. We should be aware of the intended application of the data and the degree of precision needed to make meaningful clinical decisions. These details are often overlooked, and we allow ourselves to fall into the trap of using specific statistical procedures just because they have been used by others. Researchers should address each of these relevant issues in their reports, so that others can interpret their work properly. Many articles are published with no such discussion, leaving the reader to guess why a particular statistic was used. Because reliability statistics can be applied in so many ways, it is important to maintain an exchange of ideas that promotes such accountability. By having to justify our choices, we are forced to consider what a statistic can really tell us about a variable and what conclusions are warranted.

KEY TERMS

true variance (s_T^2)
error variance (s_E^2)
reliability coefficient (r_{XX})
intraclass correlation
    coefficient (ICC)
generalizability
facets
generalizability coefficient

percent agreement
kappa (κ)
weighted kappa ($κ_w$)
incremental weights
asymmetrical weights
symmetrical weights
homogeneity
internal consistency

Cronbach's alpha (α)
item-to-total correlation
response stability
standard error of
    measurement (SEM)
coefficient of variation (*CV*)
method error (ME)
limits of agreement

REFERENCES

1. Bartko JJ, Carpenter Jr WT. On the methods and theory of reliability. *J Nerv Ment Dis* 1976;163:307–17.
2. Tinsley HEA, Weiss DJ. Interrater reliability and agreement of subjective judgments. *J Counseling Psychol* 1975;22:358.
3. Rae G. On measuring agreement among several judges on the presence or absence of a trait. *Educ Psychol Meas* 1984;44:247.
4. Fleiss JI, Cohen J. The equivalence of weighted kappa on the intraclass correlation coefficient as measures of reliability. *Educ Psychol Meas* 1973;33:613.
5. Mitchell SK. Interobserver agreement: reliability and generalizability of data collected in observational studies. *Psychol Bull* 1979;86:376–90.
6. Cronbach LJ, Gleser GC, Nanda H, Rajaratnam N. *The Dependability of Behavioral Measurements: Theory of Generalizability for Scores and Profiles.* New York: Wiley, 1972.
7. Kazdin AE. Artifact, bias, and complexity of assessment: The ABCs of reliability. *J Appl Behav Anal* 1977;10:141.
8. Berk RA. Generalizability of behavioral observations: a clarification of interobserver agreement and interobserver reliability. *Am J Ment Defic* 1979;83:460–72.
9. Shrout PE, Fleiss JL. Intraclass correlation: uses in assessing rater reliability. *Psychol Bull* 1979;86:420–28.
10. Bartko JJ. On various intraclass correlation reliability coefficients. *Psychol Bull* 1976;83:762–5.
11. Winer BJ. *Statistical Principles in Experimental Design.* 2d ed. New York: McGraw-Hill, 1971.
12. Lahey MA, Downey RG, Saal FE. Intraclass correlations: there's more there than meets the eye. *Psychol Bull* 1983;93:586–95.

13. Riddle DL, Finucane SD, Rothstein JM, Walker ML. Intrasession and intersession reliability of hand-held dynamometer measurements taken on brain-damaged patients. Author's response. *Phys Ther* 1989;69:192–4.
14. Norusis MJ. *SPSS Professional Statistics 6.1.* Chicago: SPSS, 1994.
15. Cohen J. Coefficient of agreement for nominal scales. *Educ Psychol Meas* 1960;20:37–46.
16. Landis JR, Koch GG. The measurement of observer agreement for categorical data. *Biometrics* 1977;33:159–74.
17. Jarvik JG, Haynor DR, Koepsell TD, Bronstein A, Ashley D, Deyo RA. Interreader reliability for a new classification of lumbar disk disease. *Acad Radiol* 1996;3:537–44.
18. Cooperman JM, Riddle DL, Rothstein JM. Reliability and validity of judgments of the integrity of the anterior cruciate ligament of the knee using the Lachman's test. *Phys Ther* 1990;70:225–33.
19. Cohen J. Weighted kappa: nominal scale agreement with provision for scaled disagreement or partial credit. *Psychol Bull* 1968;70:213–20.
20. Graham P, Jackson R. The analysis of ordinal agreement data: beyond weighted kappa. *J Clin Epidemiol* 1993;46:1055–62.
21. Maclure M, Willett WC. Misinterpretation and misuse of the kappa statistic. *Am J Epidemiol* 1987;126:161–9.
22. Fleiss JL. Measuring nominal scale agreement among many raters. *Psychol Bull* 1971;76:378–82.
23. Haley SM, Osberg JS. Kappa coefficient calculation using multiple ratings per subject: a special communication. *Phys Ther* 1989;69:970–4.
24. Streiner DL, Normal GR. *Health Measurement Scales: A Practical Guide to Their Development and Use.* 2d ed. New York: Oxford Press, 1995.
25. Cronbach LJ. Coefficient alpha and the internal structure of tests. *Psychometrika* 1951;16:297–334.
26. Hattie J. Methodology review: assessing unidemensionality of tests and items. *Appl Psychol Meas* 1985;9:139–64.
27. Boyle GJ. Does item homogeneity indicate internal consistency or item redundancy in psychometric scales? *Personality Individ Differences* 1991;12:291–4.
28. Nunally JC. *Psychometric Theory.* 2d ed. New York: McGraw-Hill, 1978.
29. Sechrest L. Reliability and validity. In: Bellack AS, Hersen M, eds. *Research Methods in Clinical Psychology.* New York: Pergamon Press, 1984, 24–54.
30. Francis K. Computer communication: reliability. *Phys Ther* 1986;66:1140–4.
31. Bland M. *An Introduction to Medical Statistics.* 2d ed. New York: Oxford University Press, 1995.
32. Ottenbacher KJ, Stull GA. The analysis and interpretation of method comparison studies in rehabilitation research. *Am J Phys Med Rehabil* 1993;72:266–71.
33. Bland JM, Altman DG. Statistical methods for assessing agreement between two methods of clinical measurement. *Lancet* 1986;Feb 8:307–10.
34. Altman DG. *Practical Statistics for Medical Research.* New York: Chapman and Hall, 1991.

27

Multivariate Analysis

The technological progress of data management systems has provided clinical researchers with a sophisticated statistical framework within which to examine the multifaceted and complex relationships inherent in many clinical phenomena. **Multivariate analysis** refers to a set of statistical procedures that are distinguished by the ability to examine several response variables within a single study and to account for their potential interrelationships in the analysis of the data. These tests are distinguished from **univariate analysis** procedures, such as the *t*-test and analysis of variance, in that univariate methods accommodate only one measured variable.

Given the types of questions being asked today and the types of data being used to examine clinical procedures, multivariate statistics have become quite important for those who do research and those who read research reports. The purpose of this chapter is to introduce the basic concepts behind several of the most commonly used multivariate methods: partial correlation, multiple regression, logistic regression, discriminant analysis, factor analysis, and multivariate analysis of variance.

The application of multivariate procedures necessitates the use of a computer, and may require the assistance of a statistician for more advanced operations. In a short introduction such as this, it is not possible to cover the full scope of these procedures. Therefore, this discussion focuses on a conceptual understanding of multivariate tests and interpretation of the output a computer analysis will generate.

PARTIAL CORRELATION

The product-moment correlation coefficient, r, offers the researcher a simple and easily understood measure of the association between two variables, X and Y. The interpretation of r is limited, however, because it cannot account for the possible influence of other variables on that relationship. For instance, in a study of the relationship between age and length of hospital stay, we might find a correlation of .70, suggesting that older patients tend to have longer hospital stays (as shown by the shaded overlapped portion in Figure 27.1A). If, however, older patients also tend to have greater functional limitations, then the observed relationship between hospital stay and age may actually be the result

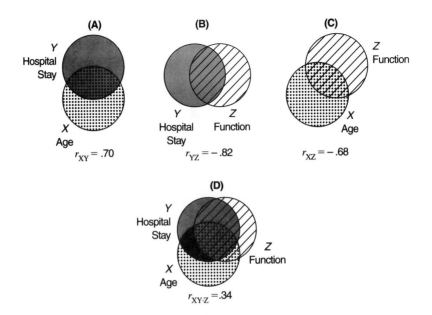

FIGURE 27.1   Representation of partial correlation between hospital stay (*Y*) and age (*X*), with the effect of function (*Z*) removed. In **(A), (B)** and **(C),** the simple correlations between each pair of variables are illustrated. In **(D)** the shaded area represents those parts of hospital stay and age that are explained by function. The black area shows the common variance in hospital stay and age that is not related to function, or their partial correlation.

of their mutual relationship with function; that is, the hospital stay may actually be explained by the patient's functional status. We can resolve this dilemma by looking at the relationship between hospital stay and age with the effect of functional status controlled, using a procedure called **partial correlation.**

The *partial correlation coefficient* is the correlation between two variables, *X* and *Y*, with the effect of a third variable, *Z*, statistically removed. For instance, in the preceding example, assume *X* is age, *Y* is hospital stay, and *Z* is functional status. We would want to know how much of the observed relationship between age and hospital stay (r_{XY}) can be attributed to the confounding influence of function, and how much is purely the relationship between age and hospital stay. The term $r_{XY \cdot Z}$ is used to represent the correlation of *X* and *Y*, with the effect of *Z* eliminated.

For example, suppose we are given the following correlations for a sample of 50 patients:

r_{XY} = .70 (hospital stay with age)

r_{XZ} = –.82 (hospital stay with function)

r_{YZ} = –.68 (function with age)

We "remove" the effect of function from r_{XY} by first determining how much of the variance in both hospital stay and age is explained by function, as shown in Figures 27.1B and C. The overlapped, shaded portions represent the correlation between the two variables. Figure 27.1D shows how these relationships intersect. Once we remove the effect of function, the remaining overlap between hospital stay and age is reduced (the black area in Figure 27.1D). This area represents the relationship between hospital stay and age with the effect of function canceled out. This is the partial correlation.*

For the data in our example, $r_{XY \cdot Z} = .34$. When we compare this partial correlation to the original correlation of X and Y ($r_{XY} = .70$), we can see that age and hospital stay no longer demonstrate as strong a relationship. A large part of the observed association between them could be accounted for by their common relationship with functional status.

The term $r_{XY \cdot Z}$ is called a *first-order partial correlation,* because it represents a correlation with the effect of one variable eliminated. The simple correlation between X and Y is called a *zero-order correlation.* The significance of a first-order partial correlation can be determined by referring to critical values of r in Appendix Table A.4, using $n - 3$ degrees of freedom. Partial correlation can be expanded to control for more than one variable at a time. A *second-order partial correlation* is symbolized by $r_{XY \cdot Z_1 Z_2}$. This value can be checked for significance using Table A.4 with $n - 4$ degrees of freedom. This process can continue with higher-order partial correlations.

Partial correlation is a useful analytic tool for eliminating competing explanations for an association, thereby providing a clearer explanation of the true nature of an observed relationship and ruling out extraneous factors.

MULTIPLE REGRESSION

Multiple regression is an extension of simple linear regression analysis, described in Chapter 24. The multiple regression equation allows the researcher to predict the value $\hat{Y}$ using a set of several independent variables. It can accommodate continuous and categorical independent variables, which may be naturally occurring or experimentally manipulated. The dependent variable, Y, must be a continuous measure. A common purpose of regression analysis is prognostic, predicting a given outcome based on identified factors. For instance, Stineman and Williams developed a model to predict rehabilitation length of stay based on the patient's admitting diagnosis, referral source, and admission functional status.[1] A second purpose of regression is to better understand a clinical phenomenon by identifying those factors associated with it. To illustrate this application, Walker and Sofaer studied sources of psychological distress in patients attending pain clinics.[2] They identified that 60% of the variance associated with psychological distress was explained by a combination of fears about the future, regrets about the past, age, practical help, feeling unoccupied, and personal relationship problems. This type of analysis will often present opportunities for the analysis of theoretical components of constructs.

---

*The partial correlation coefficient is calculated using the formula $r_{XY \cdot Z} = \dfrac{(r_{XY} - r_{XZ} r_{YZ})}{\sqrt{[1 - r_{XZ}^2][1 - r_{YZ}^2]}}$

The Regression Equation

Recall that the regression equation, $\hat{Y} = a + bX$, defines a line that can be used to make predictions, with an inherent degree of random error. This error, or **residual variance,** represents variance in Y that is not explained by the predictor variable, X. For example, suppose we were interested in predicting cholesterol level using body weight as the independent variable, with $r = .48$ and $r^2 = .23$. Based on the limited strength of this relationship, we would expect that a regression equation would provide estimates of cholesterol that would be markedly different from actual values, as body weight by itself does not totally explain cholesterol level. Therefore, the remaining unexplained variance in cholesterol (77%) must be a function of other factors. For instance, cholesterol may also be related to variables such as blood pressure, gender, age, weight, or diet. If we were to add these variables to the regression equation, the unexplained portion of variance would probably be decreased (although not necessarily completely). This expanded analysis results in a *multiple regression equation.*

In multiple regression, the equation accommodates multiple predictor variables:

$$\hat{Y} = a + b_1X_1 + b_2X_2 + b_3X_3 + \ldots + b_kX_k \tag{27.1}$$

where $\hat{Y}$ is the predicted value for the dependent variable, a is a **regression constant** (also called the Y-intercept), and b_1, b_2, b_3, through b_k, are **regression coefficients** for each independent variable. The subscript, k, denotes the number of independent variables in the equation.[†] Like simple linear regression, multiple regression is also based on the concept of least squares, so that the model minimizes deviations of $\hat{Y}$ from Y.

Once regression coefficients and a constant are obtained, we can predict values of $\hat{Y}$ by substituting values for each independent variable in the equation. For instance, suppose we wanted to evaluate the predictive relationship between serum blood cholesterol (CHOL) and potential contributing factors including age (AGE), daily dietary fat intake in grams (DIET), gender (GENDER), systolic blood pressure (SBP), and weight (WT). Table 27.1A lists the intercorrelations among these variables. The coefficients for the regression equation are shown in Table 27.1D❷, including the Y-intercept (constant):

$$\hat{Y} = 19.116 + .012(\text{AGE}) + 3.094(\text{DIET}) + .218(\text{SBP}) + 4.158(\text{GENDER}) + .511(\text{WT})$$

Based on this equation, for a 34-year-old subject, with DIET = 20.0 g, GENDER = 1 (coded for male), SBP = 100 mmHg, and WT = 150 pounds, we can predict cholesterol value as follows:

$$\text{CHOL} = 19.116 + .012(34) + 3.094(20.0) + .218(100) + 4.158(1) + .511(150) = 184.01$$

If this person's true cholesterol level was 175, the residual would be $Y - \hat{Y} = 175 - 184.01 = -9.01$. Scatter plots can also be requested to analyze the residuals, typically plotting the predicted values on the X-axis against the residuals on the Y-axis. Visual analysis of residuals can reveal if the assumption of linearity in the data is violated (see Chapter 24, Figure 24.6).

Regression coefficients are interpreted as *weights* that identify how much each variable contributes to the explanation of Y. As part of the regression analysis, a test of significance is performed on each regression coefficient, to test the null hypothesis,

---

[†]The number of independent variables included in the regression equation is effectively limited by the sample size. Power analysis can be done to estimate the number of subjects that would be needed to identify a significant effect, based on the number of independent variables in the equation. See Appendix C.

TABLE 27.1. OUTPUT FOR MULTIPLE REGRESSION ANALYSIS: PREDICTION OF CHOLESTEROL LEVEL FROM AGE, DIET, BLOOD PRESSURE, GENDER, AND WEIGHT (N = 100)

A. CORRELATIONS

	CHOL	AGE	DIET	SBP	GENDER	WT
CHOL	1.000	.063 ❶ (.266)	.634 (.000)	.109 (.140)	.000 (.500)	.481 (.000)
AGE		1.000	.121 (.116)	−.125 (.108)	.125 (.108)	.010 (.462)
DIET			1.000	.099 (.164)	−.039 (.351)	−.207 (.019)
SBP				1.000	.011 (.455)	−.005 (.482)
GENDER					1.000	−.038 (.353)

B. MODEL

Multiple R = .731   Adjusted R Square = .509

Multiple R Square = .534   Standard Error of the Estimate = 42.613

C. ANALYSIS OF VARIANCE OF REGRESSION

Source	df	SS	MS	F	Sig.
Regression	5	195314.3	39062.86	21.512	.000
Residual	94	170691.0	1815.86		
Total	99	366005.3			

D. COEFFICIENTS

	Unstandardized Coefficients ❷ B	Std Error	Standardized ❸ Coefficients Beta	t ❹	Sig.
Constant	19.116	41.817		.457	.649
AGE	❺ 1.150E-02	.313	.003	.037	.971
DIET	3.094	.410	.553	7.549	.000
SBP	.218	.276	.056	.788	.433
GENDER	4.158	8.612	.034	.483	.630
WT	.511	.100	.368	5.107	.000

❶ Significance level for each correlation coefficient is shown in parentheses.

❷ Regression coefficients for each variable in the equation.

❸ Standardized regression coefficients (beta weights).

❹ Test of significance of regression coefficients for each independent variable. Values for the constant are ignored.

❺ The designation E designates an exponent. A positive exponent moves the decimal place to the right; a negative exponent moves the decimal place to the left. In this case, the decimal place will be moved two places to the left. Therefore, B for AGE is .0115.

H_0: $b = 0$. Depending on the statistical package this will be done using either an F-test or a t-test, as shown in Table 27.1D❹. In this example, the coefficients for AGE, GENDER, and SBP are not significant ($p > .05$). Therefore, these three variables are not making a significant contribution to the prediction of cholesterol level.

Standardized Regression Coefficients

Researchers often want to establish the relative importance of specific variables within a regression equation. The regression coefficients cannot be directly compared for this purpose because they are based on different units of measurement. When it is of interest to determine which variables are more heavily weighted, we must convert the weights to standardized regression coefficients, called **beta weights.** These standardized values are interpreted as relative weights, indicating how much each variable contributes to the value of $\hat{Y}$. For example, the beta weights listed in Table 27.1D❸ show that DIET and WT are the most important variables for predicting cholesterol. The sign of the beta weight indicates the positive or negative relationship between each variable and Y, but only the absolute value is considered in determining the relative weight. Many authors present beta weights in addition to regression coefficients in a research report, to provide the reader with a full and practical interpretation of the observed relationships.

Multicolinearity

A problem occurs in the interpretation of beta weights if the independent variables in the regression equation are correlated with each other. This situation is called **multicolinearity.** The coefficients assigned to variables within the equation are based on the assumption that each variable provides independent information, contributing a unique part of the total explanation of the variance in Y. If independent variables are related to each other, the information they provide to the model is partially redundant. In that case, one variable may be seen as contributing a lot of information, and the second variable may be seen as contributing little; that is, one variable may have a larger beta weight. Each variable may be highly predictive of Y when used alone, but they are redundant when used together. This situation can be avoided by determining the intercorrelations among predictor variables prior to running a regression analysis and selecting independent variables that are not highly correlated with each other.

The interpretation of multicolinearity is based on the concept of partial correlation; that is, each regression coefficient represents the importance of a single variable after having accounted for the effect of all other variables in the equation. Therefore, the value of a regression coefficient is dependent on which other independent variables are in the equation. With different combinations of variables, it is likely that a particular regression coefficient will vary. It is important to remember, therefore, that the relationships defined by a regression equation can be interpreted only within the context of the specific variables included in that equation. When different combinations of variables are examined, the statistical model may change.

Accuracy of Prediction

The overall association between Y and the complete set of independent variables is defined by the **multiple correlation coefficient, R.** This value will range from 0.00 to 1.00; however, because R represents the cumulative association of many variables, its interpretation is obscure. Therefore, its square (R^2) is used more often as an explanation of the functional relationship between Y and a series of X values.

As an analogue of r^2, the value of R^2 represents the proportion of the total variance in Y that is explained by the set of independent variables in the equation; that is, it is the *variance attributable to the regression*. R^2 is the statistic most often reported in journal articles to indicate the accuracy of prediction of a regression analysis. Higher values of R^2 reflect stronger prediction models. The complement, $1 - R^2$, is the proportion of the variance that is left unexplained, or the variance attributable to deviations from the regression. Table 27.1B shows that $R^2 = .534$ for the hypothetical cholesterol analysis, indicating that this group of variables accounts for slightly more than half of the variance in cholesterol.

An *adjusted* R^2 is also generated for the regression (Table 27.1B). This value represents a chance-corrected value for R^2; that is, we can expect some percent of explained variance to be a function of chance. Some researchers prefer to report the adjusted value as a more accurate reflection of the strength of the regression, especially with a large number of variables in the equation.

Many regression programs will also generate a value for the **standard error of the estimate (SEE),** as shown in Table 27.1B. This value represents the degree of variability in the data around the multidimensional "regression line," reflecting the prediction accuracy of the equation (see Chapter 24 for discussion of the SEE).

Analysis of Variance of Regression

A multiple regression analysis generates an analysis of variance to test the linear fit of the equation. The ANOVA partitions the total variance in the data into the variance that is explained by the regression and that part that is left unexplained, or the residual error. The degrees of freedom associated with the regression will equal k, where k represents the number of independent variables in the equation. The probability of F associated with the regression will indicate if the equation provides an explanation of Y that is better than chance. The ANOVA in Table 27.1C demonstrates a significant model for the cholesterol data ($F = 21.512, p < .0001$).

Stepwise Multiple Regression

Multiple regression can be run by "forcing" a set of variables into the equation, as we have done in the cholesterol example. With all five variables included, the equation accounted for 53% of the variance in cholesterol values, although the results demonstrated that the five independent variables did not all make significant contributions to that estimate. We might ask, then, if the level of prediction accuracy achieved in this analysis could have been achieved with fewer variables. To answer this question, we can use a procedure called **stepwise multiple regression,** which uses specific statistical criteria to retain or eliminate variables to maximize prediction accuracy with the smallest number of predictors. It is not unusual to find that only a few independent variables will explain almost as much of the variation in the dependent variable as can be explained by a larger number of variables. This approach is useful for honing in on those variables that make the most valuable contribution to a given relationship, thereby creating an economical model.

Stepwise regression is accomplished in "steps" by evaluating the contribution of each independent variable in sequential fashion.[†] First, all proposed independent variables are correlated with the dependent variable, and the one variable with the highest correlation is entered into the equation at step 1. For our cholesterol example, Table 27.1A shows us that DIET has the highest correlation with CHOL ($r = .634$). Therefore, DIET will be entered first. With this variable alone, $R^2 = .401$ (Table 27.2A). The regression coefficients are shown in Table 27.2C:

$$\hat{Y} = 121.65 + 3.55(\text{DIET})$$

At this point, the remaining variables (those "excluded" from the equation) are examined for their partial correlation with Y, that is, their correlation with CHOL with the effect of DIET removed (Table 27.2D). The variable with the highest significant partial correlation, in this case, is WT (partial $r = .462$, $p = .000$). Therefore, WT is added to the equation in step 2 (Table 27.2E). With the addition of this variable, we have achieved an R^2 of .529 (only slightly lower the value of .543 that was obtained with the full model, see Table 27.1B).[§] There is an increase in R^2 of .128 (sometimes called "R^2 change"). WT improved prediction by almost 13%.

Another criterion for entry of a variable is its **tolerance level.** Tolerance refers to the degree of colinearity in the data. Tolerance ranges from 0.00, indicating that the variable is perfectly correlated with the variables already entered, to 1.00, which means that the other variables are not related (see Table 27.2D and H). The higher the tolerance, the more new information a variable will contribute to the equation. Some computer programs will automatically generate tolerance levels for each variable. Others offer options that must be specifically requested to include tolerance values (colinearity statistics) in the printout.

The stepwise regression continues, adding a new variable at each successive step of the analysis if it meets certain *inclusion criteria;* that is, its partial correlation is highest of all remaining variables, and the test of its regression coefficient is significant. This process continues until, at some point, either all variables have been entered or the addition of more variables will not significantly improve the prediction accuracy of the model. In the current example, Table 27.2H shows us that none of the partial correlations of the remaining three variables is significant. Therefore, no further variables were entered after step 2. As shown in Table 27.2G, the final model for the stepwise regression is

$$\hat{Y} = 48.21 + 3.12 \, (\text{DIET}) + .508 \, (\text{WT})$$

Note that the coefficients in the equation have changed with the addition of WT as a variable. There are times when no variables will be entered if none of them satisfy the min-

---

[‡]Stepwise procedures may be classified as *stepwise, forward,* or *backward* inclusion. Forward inclusion means that the model starts with no variables, and adds variables one by one until the inclusion criterion is satisfied. This procedure is differentiated from stepwise regression in many statistical programs. While both proceed using a forward selection method, adding a new variable at each step, the stepwise procedure can also *remove* a variable at any step, if that variable no longer contributes significantly to the model, given the current variables in the equation. The procedure will specify a significance criterion to enter variables as well as to remove them. In the backward inclusion method, the model starts with all variables in the equation, and partial correlations are calculated as if each one were the last variable to be entered. Using criteria for removal, the variable with the smallest partial correlation is taken out. Steps proceed until no remaining variables are qualified for removal.

[§]Note that the adjusted R^2 is higher with the stepwise analysis (Table 27.2E, adjusted $R^2 = .520$) than with the full model (Table 27.1B, adjusted $R^2 = .509$). This happens because the adjusted R^2 is affected by the number of variables in the equation. With fewer terms in the final stepwise equation, we find that there is actually better prediction than when all four variables were included.

TABLE 27.2. OUTPUT FOR STEPWISE MULTIPLE REGRESSION

Step 1

A. Variable entered: DIET

Multiple R = .634   Adjusted R squared = .395
Multiple R squared = .401   Standard Error of the Estimate = 47.285

B. ANALYSIS OF VARIANCE OF REGRESSION

Source	df	SS	MS	F	Sig.
Regression	1	146890.940	146890.940	65.698	.000
Residual	98	219114.370	2235.861		
Total	99	366005.310			

C. COEFFICIENTS	Unstandardized Coefficients		Standardized Coefficients		
	B	Std Error	Beta	t	Sig.
Constant	121.654	12.378		9.829	.000
DIET	3.547	.438	.634	8.105	.000

D. EXCLUDED VARIABLES	Beta In	t	Sig.	Partial Correlation	Tolerance
AGE	−.014	−.173	.863	−.018	.985
SBP	.047	.599	.550	.061	.990
GENDER	.024	.311	.756	.032	.999
WT	.366	5.134	.000	.462	.957

Step 2

E. Variable entered: WT

Multiple R = .728   Adjusted R squared = .520
Multiple R squared = .529   Standard Error of the Estimate = 42.145

F. ANALYSIS OF VARIANCE OF REGRESSION

Source	df	SS	MS	F	Sig.
Regression	2	193715.449	96857.724	54.531	.000
Residual	97	172289.861	1776.184		
Total	99	366005.310			

G. COEFFICIENTS	Unstandardized Coefficients		Standardized Coefficients		
	B	Std Error	Beta	t	Sig.
Constant	48.210	18.064		2.669	.009
DIET	3.122	.399	.558	7.831	.000
WT	.508	.099	.366	5.134	.000

H. EXCLUDED VARIABLES	Beta In	t	Sig.	Partial Correlation	Tolerance
AGE	−.001	−.011	.991	−.001	.984
SBP	.057	.806	.422	.082	.990
GENDER	.036	.507	.613	.052	.998

imal inclusion criteria. In that case, the researcher must search for a new set of independent variables to explain the dependent variable.

Dummy Variables

One of the general assumptions for regression analysis is that variables are continuous; however, many of the variables that may be useful predictors for a regression analysis, such as gender, occupation, education, and race, or behavioral characteristics such as smoker versus nonsmoker, are measured on a categorical scale. It is possible to include such qualitative variables in a regression equation, although the numbers assigned to categories cannot be treated as quantitative scores. One way to do this is to create a set of coded variables called **dummy variables.**

In statistics, **coding** is the process of assigning numerals to represent categorical or group membership. For regression analysis we use 0 and 1 to code for the absence and presence of a dichotomous variable, respectively. All dummy variables are dichotomous. For example, with a variable such as smoker – nonsmoker, we code 0 = nonsmoker and 1 = smoker. For sex, we can code male = 0 and female = 1. In essence we are coding 1 for female and 0 for anyone who is not female. We can use these codes as scores in a regression equation and treat them as interval data.

For instance, we can include gender as a predictor of cholesterol level, to determine if men or women can be expected to have higher cholesterol levels. Assume the following regression equation was obtained:

$$\hat{Y} = 220 - 27.5X$$

Using the dummy code for females, $\hat{Y} = 220 - 27.5\,(1) = 194.5$, and for males $\hat{Y} = 220 - 27.5$ $(0) = 220$. With only this one dummy variable, these predicted values are actually the means for cholesterol for females and males. The regression coefficient for X is the difference between the means for the groups coded 0 and 1.

When a qualitative variable has more than two categories, more than one dummy variable is required to represent it. For example, consider the variable of college class, with four levels: freshman, sophomore, junior, and senior. We could code these categories with the numbers 1 through 4 on an apparent ordinal scale; however, these numerical values would not make sense in a regression equation, because the numbers have no quantitative meaning. A senior is not four times more of something than a freshman. Therefore, we must create a dichotomous dummy variable for each category, as follows:

$$X_1 = 1 \text{ if a freshman}$$
$$0 \text{ if not a freshman}$$

$$X_2 = 1 \text{ if a sophomore}$$
$$0 \text{ if not a sophomore}$$

$$X_3 = 1 \text{ if a junior}$$
$$0 \text{ if not a junior}$$

Each variable codes for the presence or absence of a specific class membership. We do not need to create a fourth variable for seniors, because anyone who has zero for all three variables will be a senior. We can show how this works by defining each class with a unique combination of values for X_1, X_2, and X_3:

	X_1	X_2	X_3
Freshman	1	0	0
Sophomore	0	1	0
Junior	0	0	1
Senior	0	0	0

The number of dummy variables needed to define a categorical variable will always be one less than the number of categories.

Suppose we wanted to predict a student's attitude toward the disabled, on a scale of 0 to 100, based on class membership. An analysis might develop an equation such as

$$\hat{Y} = 85 - 55X_1 - 25X_2 - 15X_3$$

Therefore, the predicted values for each class would be

Freshman: $\hat{Y} = 85 - 55(1) - 25(0) - 15(0) = 30$
Sophomore: $\hat{Y} = 85 - 55(0) - 25(1) - 15(0) = 60$
Junior: $Y = 85 - 55(0) - 25(0) - 15(1) = 70$
Senior: $Y = 85 - 55(0) - 25(0) - 15(0) = 85$

Several dummy variables can be combined with quantitative variables in a regression equation. Because so many variables of interest are measured at the nominal level, the use of dummy variables provides an important mechanism for creating a fuller explanation of clinical phenomena. Some computer programs will automatically generate dummy codes for nominal variables. For others, the researcher must develop the coding scheme.

LOGISTIC REGRESSION

Many questions of prediction or explanation involve outcomes that are categorical. For example, we might ask why some individuals experience recurrent falls. VanSwearingen et al. identified mobility and functional characteristics that could predict whether a person did or did not have a history of falls.[3] We might look for factors related to whether or not a patient returns to work following rehabilitation. Cifu et al. examined several measures of physical and psychological function as predictors of successful return to work 1 year after traumatic brain injury.[4] These examples illustrate the application of **logistic regression,** where the dependent variable has only two values—the occurrence or nonoccurrence of a particular event, or the presence or absence of a condition, typically coded 0 and 1.[ǁ] We cannot use multiple regression for this purpose, as a categorical dependent variable cannot meet the assumption of a normal distribution (see Chapter 24, Figure 24.5). The independent variables in logistic regression may be

---

[ǁ]Logistic regression can be used when the outcome variable has more than two categories, an approach that is beyond the scope of this text.

continuous, ordinal, or categorical. Logistic regression can be run using a full set of independent variables, or it may be run using a stepwise procedure.

The Logistic Regression Model

In logistic regression, rather than predicting a value for an outcome variable, we are actually predicting the probability of an event occurring. Using the regression equation, we determine if the independent variables can predict whether an individual is likely to belong to the group coded 0 (the reference group) or the group coded 1 (the target group). Consider the following hypothetical example. Suppose we wanted to predict the discharge disposition for patients following rehabilitation, as either "return to home" (coded 0) or "long-term care" (coded 1). We would like to set appropriate goals and begin suitable discharge planning as soon as possible, and we would like to determine if characteristics upon admission will be useful predictors of discharge status. We will use the following variables, coded as present (1) or absent (0), except for age which is continuous:

Functional status	ADL	0 = independent; 1 = limited
Age	AGE	Continuous
Marital status	MAR	0 = married; 1 = not married
Gender	GENDER	0 = male; 1 = female

We will examine hypothetical data from 100 patients, 46 of whom went to long-term care (LTC). The statistical question is, what is the likelihood that an individual will be discharged to LTC given this combination of factors? The results of a logistic regression for these variables are shown in Table 27.3.

The Logistic Function

We can think of the **logistic function** as a linear combination of these variables, similar to linear regression analysis. The likelihood of the predicted outcome is based on the odds of being discharged to LTC, or more accurately, the logarithm of the odds:

$$Z = a + b_1X_1 + b_2X_2 + b_3X_3 + b_4X_4 + b_5X_5 \tag{27.2}$$

where Z is the natural logarithm of the odds, called a **logit**, a is a regression constant, and b is the regression coefficient. Even though we are using a different mathematical base (logarithms), this equation is conceptually the same as the multiple regression equation—but with two major differences. First, the dependent variable (the logit) is a dichotomous outcome, resulting in prediction of group membership. Second, where multiple regression uses the least squares criterion for finding the equation with the smallest residuals, logistic regression uses the concept of **maximum likelihood,** which means that the equation will present the "most likely" solution that demonstrates the best odds of achieving accurate prediction of group membership.

Coefficients for the logistic regression for our discharge status question are shown in Table 27.3B❷. This logistic regression equation would, therefore, be written:

$$Z = -11.167 + 2.384(ADL) + .104(AGE) + 2.935(MAR) - .018(GENDER)$$

TABLE 27.3. SELECTED OUTPUT FOR LOGISTIC REGRESSION ANALYSIS: RISK FACTORS ASSOCIATED WITH DISCHARGE DISPOSITION IN ELDERLY PATIENTS ($N = 100$)

A. CLASSIFICATION TABLE FOR DISCHARGE

Cut Value is .50

		Predicted 0	Predicted 1	Percent Correct ❶
Observed	0	46	8	85.19%
	1	9	37	80.43%
			Overall	83.00%

B. COEFFICIENTS

Variable	B ❷	S.E.	df	Sig ❸	Exp(B) ❹	95% CI for Exp(B) ❺ Lower	Upper
ADL	2.384	.656	1	.0003	10.848	3.000	39.192
AGE	.104	.046	1	.0236	1.110	1.014	1.215
MAR	2.935	.662	1	.0000	18.822	5.147	68.808
GENDER	−.018	.642	1	.9778	.982	.279	3.459
Constant	−11.167	3.984	1	.0051			

❶ Classification results compare predictions using the logistic regression to actual observed results. (See Figure 27.2).

❷ Regression coefficients for the logistic regression.

❸ Significance levels (*p*) for each regression coefficient.

❹ Odds ratios associated with each independent variable, adjusted for the presence of all other variables in the equation. The odds ratio is equal to e^B.

❺ The 95% confidence interval (CI) for the odds ratio. If a CI contains the null value (1.0), the odds ratio is not significant. For these data, only the odds ratios for ADL, AGE, and MAR are significant.

Predicted Probabilities

We can use the coefficients in the logistic regression equation to predict the probability that an individual belongs to the target group, as follows:

$$\text{Probability} = \frac{e^z}{1+e^z} \ or \ \frac{1}{1+e^{-z}} \tag{27.3}$$

where e is the base of the natural logarithm.[#] The probability associated with the outcome will be 0 if the subject is discharged home, and 1 if long-term care. We can expect, however, that the logistic regression will yield probabilities between 0 and 1. A value closer to 1.0 (above .5) will suggest a probability in favor of discharge to long-term care, and a value closer to zero (below .5) would predict that this event is not likely to occur;

[#]Find the key marked e^x on your scientific calculator.

that is, the subject is likely to be discharged home. A probability of .5 would mean that the individual has an equal likelihood of either outcome.

When this model is applied to an individual's data, we obtain the probability of that individual being discharged to long-term care. Consider, for example, a subject who ultimately was discharged to LTC, whose scores were ADL = 1, AGE = 78, MAR = 1, and GENDER = 0;

$$Z = -11.167 + 2.384(1) + .104(78) + 2.935(1) - .018(0) = 2.264$$

Therefore,**

$$\text{Probability (discharge to LTC)} = \frac{e^{2.264}}{1 + e^{2.264}} \text{ or } \frac{1}{1 + e^{-2.264}} = .91$$

Using this model, we would have correctly predicted that this individual would be discharged to LTC, as the probability is greater than .5.

Let's look at another example for a subject who was also discharged to LTC, with scores of ADL = 1, AGE = 80, MAR = 0, and GENDER = 0:

$$Z = -11.167 + 2.384(1) + 2.935(0) - .018(0) + .104(80) = -0.463$$

Therefore,

$$\text{Probability (discharge to LTC)} = \frac{e^{-0.463}}{1 + e^{-0.463}} \text{ or } \frac{1}{1 + e^{-(-0.463)}} = .39$$

We would incorrectly predict that this individual would be discharged home because the probability is less than .5.

A histogram helps us visually understand how these predictions are interpreted. In Figure 27.2 we see such a graph of the predictions for subjects in this example, where the symbol "0" represents those who were actually discharged home, and the symbol "1" represents those who went to long-term care. The X-axis shows the predicted probabilities associated with each individual's scores. In this instance, probabilities above .5 are assigned to group 1, whereas probabilities of .5 or below are assigned to the group coded 0. Therefore, on the left half of the graph we can see that nine of those who actually went to long-term care (coded 1) were predicted to go home, whereas on the right half we find that eight of those who went home (coded 0) were predicted to go to long-term care. These incorrect classifications are shaded on the graph. Classification results are also given in Table 27.3A. A total of 83% of the sample was correctly classified using this logistic model. Over 80% of those who actually went to long-term care (1) were correctly classified; approximately 85% of those who went home (0) were correctly assigned using the logistic regression model.

The histogram also allows us to see the effect of using this model and the consequences of misclassification. For instance, in this example we can see that most of the misclassifications occur in the region around .5. In setting discharge plans, we might want to reserve judgment for this group. We would be more confident, however, in setting up home discharge plans for those with probabilities below .25, and similarly confident in securing a bed in a skilled nursing facility for those with probabilities above .75.

---

*The value $e^{2.264} = 9.62$ and $e^{-2.264} = .104$.

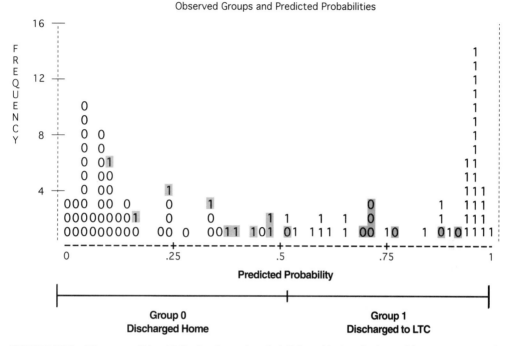

FIGURE 27.2 Histogram (*N* = 100) of estimated probabilities of being discharged home (0) versus discharged to long-term care (1), derived from logistic regression. Each symbol represents one subject. Shaded symbols represent misclassifications using a cutoff score of .50. (*Histogram obtained using SPSS 8.0 logistic regression procedure.*)

The Odds Ratio

It is generally more useful to interpret logistic regression coefficients in terms of *odds* rather than probability. Odds tell us how much more likely it is that an individual belongs to the target group than the reference group. If the odds are 1.00, then either outcome is equally likely. With odds greater than 1.00, the individual is more likely to belong to the target group; conversely, with odds less than 1.00, the individual is more likely to belong to the reference group.

The *odds ratio* is used to estimate the odds of membership in the target group, given the presence of specific independent variables (see Chapter 15 for discussion of the odds ratio). The regression coefficient in the logistic equation is the logarithm of the odds for each independent variable. Therefore, an odds ratio can be computed for each variable by using the regression coefficient as the exponent of *e* (see Table 27.3 ❹). For a subject who is limited in ADL (ADL = 1), the odds of going to LTC are $e^{2.384}$ = 10.848. This number represents the odds of going to LTC with a one-unit change in the value of *X*. With a dichotomous variable, this means that an individual who is limited in ADL is almost 11 times more likely to go LTC as compared with one who is independent (a change from 0 to 1 for ADL). Confidence intervals can also be determined for each odds ratio (Table 27.3 ❺). A significant odds ratio will not contain the null value, 1.0, within the confidence interval. We can see that this is true for the odds ratios associated with ADL, AGE, and MARital status.

TABLE 27.4. ODDS RATIOS (OR) ASSOCIATED WITH DISCHARGE STATUS AND FUNCTIONAL INDEPENDENCE (ADL)

ADL		Discharge		TOTAL
		Long-Term Care (1)	Home (0)	
Limited	1	35	9	44
Independent	0	11	45	56
TOTAL		54	46	100

$$OR = \frac{ad}{bc} = \frac{(35)(45)}{(9)(11)} = 15.909$$

Adjusted Odds Ratio

When the logistic regression equation includes several independent variables, as in our example, each odds ratio is actually corrected for the influence of the other variables. Just as independent variables in multiple regression exhibit colinearity, independent variables in logistic regression will affect each other. This is an important consideration for prediction models. For instance, if we were to look at the simple association between discharge status and ADL, we would find an odds ratio of 15.909 (see Table 27.4). This means that individuals who are limited in ADL are almost 16 times more likely to be discharged to long-term care than those who are independent. However, if we look at the results of the logistic regression in Table 27.3B, we find that the odds ratio associated with ADL is 10.848. This discrepancy is a function of the other variables in the equation; that is, the odds ratio for ADL is *adjusted* for the influence of the other factors. Therefore, the odds ratios shown in Table 27.3❹ are considered **adjusted odds ratios.**

Continuous Variables

When an independent variable is continuous, this interpretation is more complex. Consider the effect of AGE on discharge status, with an odds ratio of 1.11. Remember that an odds ratio of 1.0 indicates that either outcome is equally likely. Because the odds ratio relates to the relative increase in odds with a one-unit increase in X, we can interpret this value as the odds associated with a 1-year difference in age, such as from 87 to 88, or any other 1-year difference. Therefore, with a 1-year difference in age, the odds of going home or to long-term care are essentially even. As the unit difference increases, however, we must multiply the regression coefficient for age ($B = .104$, Table 27.3B❷) to obtain the odds ratio. With a 2-year difference in age, then, we determine the odds ratio by $e^{(2 \times .104)} = 1.23$. Not much of a change. To determine the odds related to a 10-year difference in age, we find $e^{(10 \times .104)} = 2.83$. Now the odds of going to long-term care are almost 3 times greater for someone who is 80 as compared with someone who is 70, or for someone who is 75 compared with someone who is 65. Many researchers choose to categorize continuous variables to simplify this interpretation.

Presentation of Results

The presentation of results from a logistic regression will depend on the research question. In many research situations, the investigator is actually interested in one particular variable, but wants to control for potential confounders. Using our discharge study, we might be specifically interested in the effect of function on discharge status, but we would want to account for the influence of demographic factors. In that case we might report that the odds ratio for ADL was 10.848, adjusted for age, marital status, and gender.

Alternatively, we could approach this analysis using a broader question, asking which of these four factors is related to discharge status. For this approach, we would summarize results, suggesting that ADL, AGE, and MARital status are most influential in predicting discharge status, adjusted for age and gender (Table 27.3B). In addition to the increased likelihood of going to LTC if the patient is functionally limited, those who are not married are almost 19 times more likely to be sent to LTC than those who are married.

Another consideration in presenting results is the significance associated with each independent variable. In the current example, only ADL, AGE, and MARital status have significant regression coefficients (Table 27.3B❸). Some authors will present coefficients and odds ratios for all independent variables, regardless of their significance. Others will provide odds ratios only for significant variables.

DISCRIMINANT ANALYSIS

Discriminant analysis is another form of regression, also used when the dependent variable is categorical. It is a technique for distinguishing between two or more groups based on a set of characteristics that are predictors of group membership. Based on the equation generated by the discriminant analysis, subjects are classified according to their scores, and the model is then examined to see if the classifications were correct, similar to logistic regression. Discriminant analysis has an important distinction from logistic regression, however, in that the independent variables are assumed to be normally distributed, and variances are assumed to be equal across groups. Dichotomous independent variables can be used, but with a mixture of continuous and dichotomous variables, discriminant analysis may be less than optimal.[5]

The ability to classify individuals into distinct groups can be useful in many areas of clinical and behavioral science, for purposes of prevention, evaluation, screening, and diagnosis. For example, Ermer and Dunn studied three groups of children: with autism, attention deficit disorder, and without disabilities.[6] The researchers conducted a discriminant analysis to determine if these groups could be differentiated on the basis of their scores on nine factors of a Sensory Profile. Nearly 90% of the cases were correctly classified using the resulting model.

The discriminant analysis develops a statistical model, called a **discriminant function,** that will allow us to describe the existing groups and to assign new individuals to a group when it is not known to which group they belong. Discriminant analysis can be performed using a fixed set of variables or in a stepwise manner to reduce the discriminant function to a minimum of relevant variables.

To demonstrate this process, consider a hypothetical example in which we are interested in distinguishing between athletes who are likely to sustain an injury over the

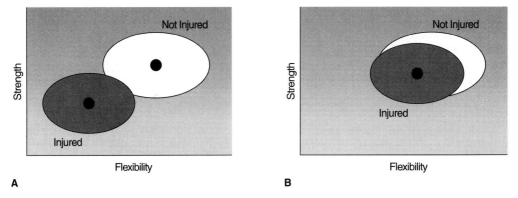

FIGURE 27.3 Basis for discriminant analysis. In **(A)** groups are different in levels of strength and flexibility. In **(B)** the variables do not discriminate between the groups.

course of a season (designated group 1) versus those who will remain uninjured (designated group 0). Using a group of athletes from one school, we will consider overall strength, flexibility, balance, and time in play as risk factors. To illustrate these relationships, consider only the first two variables for a moment. In Figure 27.3 we have plotted scores representing strength (Y) and flexibility (X) for injured and noninjured groups. In Figure 27.3A, the variables clearly discriminate between the groups, with those who were not injured demonstrating greater strength and flexibility; however, even with this degree of separation, we can see that discrimination will not be totally accurate because there is some overlap between the groups. Figure 27.3B represents a different situation, where there is much less differentiation between the groups, and it is likely that the independent variables would not be successful in distinguishing between them. When we incorporate many more variables into the analysis, we cannot visualize discrimination in a two-dimensional plot, but we can extend this illustration conceptually to visualize the discrimination between groups in multiple planes.

The Discriminant Function

Any number of predictor variables can be used to develop the **discriminant function,** which is analogous to the multiple regression prediction equation. The equation takes the form:

$$D = a + d_1X_1 + d_2X_2 + d_3X_3 + \ldots + d_kX_k \tag{27.4}$$

where D is the *discriminant score, a* is a constant, d is the *discriminant function coefficient,* and k is the number of predictor variables in the equation. The discriminant score for each subject is calculated by substituting scores for each predictor variable into the equation (see Table 27.5C❺). The purpose of the discriminant function is to determine the linear combination of variables that makes the groups as statistically distinct as possible; that is, it provides maximum discrimination between the groups. Discriminant function coefficients are often expressed as *standardized coefficients,* without a constant in the equation, similar to a beta weight in linear regression (see Table 27.5C❺).

TABLE 27.5. SELECTED OUTPUT FOR DISCRIMINANT ANALYSIS: RISK FACTORS ASSOCIATED WITH ATHLETIC INJURY (N = 109)

A. GROUP MEANS ❶

		BALANCE	FLEXIBILITY	STRENGTH	TIME in PLAY
No injury	Mean	33.37	65.44	14.23	19.03
	Std. Dev.	10.25	13.70	5.48	8.26
Injury	Mean	21.64	40.38	22.94	26.78
	Std. Dev.	4.78	16.32	8.56	6.74

B. EIGENVALUES

Function	Eigenvalue ❷	% Variance	Canonical ❸ Correlation	Wilks' Lambda	Chi- ❹ Square	df	Sig.
1	1.898	100.00	.809	.345	111.711	4	.000

C. CANONICAL DISCRIMINANT FUNCTION COEFFICIENTS

Factor	Function 1 Unstandardized Coefficients	Function 1 Standardized Coefficients
BALANCE	.055 ❺	.448
FLEXIBILITY	.040	.592
STRENGTH	−.081	−.572
TIME in PLAY	−.052	−.395
Constant	−1.016	

D. CLASSIFICATION RESULTS

	Predicted Group Membership		
Actual Group	No Injury	Injury	Total
No injury	56 (94.9%)	3 (5.1%)	59
Injury	7 (14.0%)	43 (86.0%)	50

90.8% of original grouped cases correctly classified

❶ Group means for each variable in the analysis.

❷ The eigenvalue is a reflection of the proportion of variance that is accounted for by the discriminant function.

❸ The canonical correlation is the correlation between the two sides of the equation, that is, between group membership and the discriminant function (the weighted sum of the independent variables).

❹ Chi-square tests the significance of the canonical correlation. In this case, $p = .000$, which is significant. If p is greater than .05, it would suggest that the discriminant function does not significantly account for differences between groups.

❺ The unstandardized coefficients are used to create the discriminant function, including a constant:
$D = -1.016 + .055(BALANCE) + .04(FLEXIBILITY) - .081 (STRENGTH) - .052(TIME)$
The standardized coefficients are similar to beta weights in a multiple regression analysis, with no constant:
$D = .448(BALANCE) + .592(FLEXIBILITY) - .572(STRENGTH) - .395(TIME)$
where each variable is expressed as a standardized z-score.

When more than two criterion groups are used, discriminant analysis becomes more complex, necessitating the development of more than one discriminant function. With k groups, we will require $k - 1$ discriminant functions. For example, in the previously described study by Ermer and Dunn, where three groups were used, two discriminant functions were generated, one distinguishing normal children from the two disabled groups, and the second distinguishing the two disabled groups from each other.[6]

The ability of the discriminant function to distinguish between groups can be assessed in several ways. The statistics associated with the equation are shown in Table 27.5B. An **eigenvalue** (Table 27.5B❷) is a measure of variance, indicating how well the discriminant function discriminates between the groups; the higher the eigenvalue, the greater the discrimination.[††] This value is difficult to interpret, however, as it has no upper limit. Therefore, it is usually preferable to use a measure of correlation that ranges from 0 to 1, similar to the interpretation of R^2. The **canonical correlation** expresses this relationship, conceptually serving as a correlation of group membership with the discriminant function (Table 27.5B❸). The square of the canonical correlation reflects the extent to which the variance in scores in the discriminant function accounts for differences among the groups. In this example, with a canonical correlation of .809, approximately 66% of the variability in scores is accounted for by the differences between injured and noninjured athletes. A chi-square test is used to determine the significance of this relationship (Table 27.5B❹).

Classification

Probably the most useful test of the discriminant function is the degree to which it accurately predicts group membership. Obviously, when we calculate D it will not be exactly equal to 1 or 0. Therefore, a cutoff score must be defined, below which subjects are assigned to group 0 and above which they are assigned to group 1. The discriminant analysis will establish the coefficients and cutoff score that will maximize accuracy of classification. Unless the predictor variables are completely different from each other, with no overlapping variance (correlation), we can anticipate that this classification will not be 100% correct. A summary of classification results is included as the final step in the discriminant analysis. Because we know the true group assignment for each subject, we can determine if the discriminant function has correctly classified each individual. For example, Table 27.5D shows the results of the discriminant analysis for classifying athletes who were and were not injured. This summary shows that of those who actually had no injury, 94.9% were correctly classified, and of those who were injured, 86.0% were correctly classified. In the entire sample of 109 subjects, 90.8% were placed in the correct group by the discriminant function. This would be considered excellent discrimination. Therefore, based on these hypothetical data, measures of strength, flexibility, balance, and time in play will be useful predictors of an athlete's risk of injury.

[††]An eigenvalue is analogous to an F-ratio, the ratio of the between-groups sum of squares to the within-groups sum of squares that would be generated in an analysis of variance, with group as the independent variable and the discriminant function as the dependent variable (the discriminant function is interpreted as a weighted sum of the values on the predictor variables).

In essence, analysis of variance and the *t*-test for independent samples are special forms of discriminant analysis. Questions that are analyzed using these tests would often be equally well suited to discriminant analysis, and results would be identical; that is, where groups are significantly different using an analysis of variance, the discriminant analysis would show that the predictor variables are capable of discriminating among the groups. For instance, using the current example, we could have done five separate *t*-tests to determine if the injured and noninjured athletes were different from each other for each of the five identified risk factors. The discriminant analysis approach is more useful, however, when several measured variables are studied, accounting for their interdependence in the analysis, and controlling for potential Type I errors with multiple univariate analyses.

FACTOR ANALYSIS

The technique of **factor analysis** is quite different from any of the statistical procedures we have examined thus far. Rather than using data for comparison or prediction, factor analysis takes an exploratory approach to data analysis. Its purpose is to examine the structure within a large number of variables, in an attempt to explain the nature of their interrelationships. This procedure is more controversial than other analytic methods because it leaves room for subjectivity and judgment; however, factor analysis makes an important contribution to multivariate methods because it can provide insights into the nature of abstract constructs, and allows us to superimpose order on complex phenomena.

The concept of factor analysis is illustrated in Figure 27.4. The larger set of variables at the top is composed of several overlapping circles with various degrees of "stripedness" or "dottedness." We can assume that there is some relationship among circles that have similar patterns. Through factor analysis, these variables are reorganized into two relatively independent circles, each one representing a set of related variables. Each set of striped and dotted variables represents a unique **factor**. A factor consists of a cluster of variables that are highly correlated among themselves, but poorly correlated with items on other factors. Therefore, we assume that circles with stripes are related to other circles with stripes, but not to circles with dots, and vice versa.

In real terms, we use factor analysis to examine a large set of variables that represents elements of an abstract construct, and to reduce it to a smaller, more manageable set of underlying concepts. For example, we could examine a large set of behaviors within an individual and categorize them as representing different conceptual elements of the person's psychological state. Loss of appetite, lack of motivation, and withdrawal might reflect underlying "depression." Sleeplessness, inability to concentrate, and nail biting might be indicative of "anxiety." Depression and anxiety would each be composed of a set of related elements, with each set of elements unrelated to the other set. The intercorrelation of variables within a factor suggests that those variables, taken together, represent a singular concept that can be distinguished from other factors. Therefore, depression can be distinguished from anxiety.

We might also be interested in the relative strength of the association between each of the variables within a factor and the concept that the factor represents. For instance,

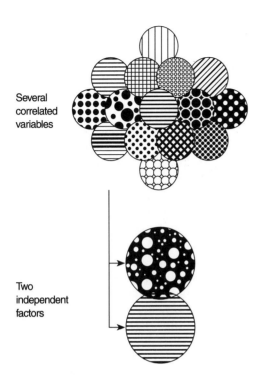

FIGURE 27.4   Conceptual representation of factor analysis.

Several correlated variables

Two independent factors

what is the relationship between sleeplessness and the concept of anxiety? In addition to grouping variables into factors, factor analysis also weights each variable within a factor. These coefficients, called **factor loadings,** are measures of the correlation between the individual variable and the overall factor.

The determination of what variables make up a factor is not determined a priori. The factor analysis approaches a set of data by calculating the intercorrelations among all the variables and arranging them into sets of statistically related variables. Through a complex series of manipulations that can only be envisioned by a computer, the analysis derives the factors and shows which variables fit best into each factor. To demonstrate this application using a practical example, suppose we are interested in studying behaviors that are related to chronic pain in a sample of 150 patients with low back pain. For this hypothetical example, we will examine seven variables (although many more would probably be of interest in such a study). These variables have all been measured on a 5-point Likert scale, based on the frequency with which each behavior is observed, from 1 = "never observed" to 5 = "almost always observed." The seven variables are (1) COMPLAINs about pain; (2) CHANGES position frequently while sitting; (3) GROANS, moans, or sighs; (4) RUBS painful body parts; (5) ISOLATEs herself or himself; (6) MOVES rigidly and stiffly; and (7) drags feet when WALKING. We will interpret a computer printout for a factor analysis on these seven variables.

Extraction of Factors

The first step in a factor analysis is the creation of a correlation matrix for all the test items. On the basis of these correlations, the factor analysis attempts to identify the **principal components**[‡‡] of the data; that is, the analysis proceeds to identify sets of variables that are linearly correlated with each other. Conceptually, this method looks at the data in a multidimensional space and configures the variables in all possible combinations to determine groupings that "go together" statistically; that is, they demonstrate strong correlations. These clustered variables represent "components" of the total data set and are derived through a process called *extraction.* The process is as mathematically complex as it sounds.

Principal components analysis "extracts" a factor from the overall data matrix by determining what combination of variables shows the strongest linear relationship and accounts for a large portion of the total variance in the data. The first factor that is "extracted" will account for as much of the variance in the data as possible. The second factor represents the extraction of the next highest possible amount of variance from the remaining variance. Each successive factor that is identified "uses up" another component of the total variance, until all the variance within the test items has been accounted for. These factors are abstract statistical entities only. This process does not indicate which variables are related to which factors.

As shown in the printout in Table 27.6A❶, this analysis has extracted seven factors. The number of factors derived from a set of variables will always equal the number of variables, as it does here. These factors are statistical representations of variance and cannot be interpreted as any real concept yet. The computer is simply looking at patterns within the data and manipulating numbers. It will not be until the end of the analysis that these "factors" will make sense.

Even though seven factors have been identified, several of these factors account for small amounts of variance, and do not really contribute in any way to an understanding of the structure of the data. We can usually characterize the data most efficiently using only the first few components. Therefore, we need to establish a cutoff point to limit the number of factors for further analysis. The statistic used to set this cutoff is called an **eigenvalue** (Table 27.6A❷), which tells us how much of the total variance is explained by a factor. Factor 1 will always account for more variance than the other factors (in this example 27.1%). The most common approach restricts retaining factors to those with an eigenvalue of at least 1.00. Using this criterion, then, we limit further analysis to the first four factors, which taken together account for 72.5% of the variance in the data (Table 27.6A❸).

The result of a principal components analysis is a factor matrix (Table 27.6B), which contains the factor loadings for each variable on each factor. Loadings are interpreted like correlation coefficients, and range from 0.00 to ±1.00. Ideally we want each variable to have a loading close to 1.00 on one factor and loadings close to 0.00

[‡‡]There are actually several different approaches to factor analysis, of which *principal components analysis (PCA)* is one. As this is the more common approach reported in the literature, we have chosen to present it here. Those interested in other approaches should consult manuals for different statistical packages, as well as references listed at the end of this chapter.

TABLE 27.6.   SELECTED OUTPUT FOR FACTOR ANALYSIS: SEVEN MEASURES RELATED TO CHRONIC PAIN BEHAVIOR (*N* = 100)

A. EIGENVALUES

❶ Factor	❷ Eigenvalue	Percent of Variance	Cumulative Percent
1	1.89	27.1	27.1
2	1.12	15.9	43.0
3	1.06	15.1	58.1
4	1.01	14.4	72.5 ❸
5	0.84	11.9	84.4
6	0.78	11.1	95.5
7	0.30	4.5	100.0

B. FACTOR MATRIX USING PRINCIPAL COMPONENTS SOLUTION

	Factor 1	Factor 2	Factor 3	Factor 4
COMPLAIN	0.55	−0.28	0.27	−0.42
CHANGES	0.19	−0.74	0.05	−0.32
GROANS	0.31	−0.60	0.29	−0.17
RUBS	0.27	0.36	0.73	−0.01
ISOLATE	0.28	0.01	0.34	0.80
MOVES	0.87	0.04	−0.25	−0.06
WALKING	0.75	0.08	−0.43	0.24

C. VARIMAX ROTATED FACTOR MATRIX

		Factor 1	Factor 2	Factor 3	Factor 4
1	COMPLAIN	0.24	**0.72**	0.19	−0.11
2	CHANGES	0.19	−0.24	**0.74**	−0.24
3	GROANS	0.01	**0.73**	−0.17	0.08
4	RUBS	−0.12	0.25	**0.71**	0.38
5	ISOLATE	0.14	−0.04	0.00	**0.90**
6	MOVES	**0.86**	0.27	0.14	−0.00
7	WALKING	**0.89**	−0.02	−0.05	0.14

❶ Seven factors are identified in the data, corresponding to the number of variables entered.
❷ The eigenvalues reflect the amount of variance accounted for by each factor, commonly with a cutoff at 1.0.
❸ Using the 1.0 cutoff for the eigenvalue, we will stop at four factors, accounting for a cumulative 72.5% of the variance in the data.

on all other factors.[§§] Factor loadings greater than .30 or .40 are generally considered indicative of some degree of relationship. We consider only the absolute value of the

---

[§§]The ideal outcome of a factor analysis would be the generation of factors that are composed of variables with high loadings on only that one factor. These would be considered "pure" factors. This does not always happen, however. When one variable loads heavily on two factors, those factors do not represent unique concepts, and there is some correlation between them. The researcher must then reconsider the nature of the variables included in the analysis and how they relate to the construct that is being studied.

loading in this interpretation. The sign indicates if the variable is positively or negatively correlated with the factor.

Unfortunately, this factor matrix is usually difficult to interpret because it does not provide the most unique structure possible; that is, several variables may be "loaded" on more than one factor. For instance, if we look across the row for COMPLAIN, we can see that factor loadings are moderately strong for both Factors 1 and 4. Therefore, the next step is to develop a unique statistical solution so that each variable relates highly to only one factor. This process is called *factor rotation.*

Factor Rotation

Factor rotation is also a complex, multidimensional concept. Envision multiple axes in space, all intersecting at a central point, each one representing one factor. In this example, we would imagine four planes, or axes, one for each of the four factors we have identified. Each of the seven variables sits somewhere in this four-dimensional space, with factor loadings that identify its location relative to each of the four axes. The factor loadings can be considered multidimensional coordinates. In the ideal solution to this analysis, each of the variables would be located directly on one of the axes, which would indicate that the variable was "loaded" on that factor. We would then be able to identify which variables "belonged" to each factor.

We can illustrate this concept more simply using a two-dimensional example. Assume we have identified only two factors, Factor 1 and Factor 2. We could plot each of the seven variables against these two axes, as shown in Figure 27.5A.[‡‡] The vertical axis represents Factor 1 and the horizontal axis represents Factor 2. As we can see, none of the variables sits directly on either of the axes. Some variables are located close to the origin, indicating that they are not related to either factor (their factor loading is small). The other variables sit in space somewhere between the two factors. This plot does not present a clear "structure" in the data in terms of specific factor assignments. If, however, we could rearrange the orientation of axes and variables, we might be able to create a structure that will help us interpret these relationships. We do this by *rotating* the two axes in such a way as to maximize the orientation of variables near one of the axes. There are actually several ways that factor axes can be statistically rotated to arrive at this solution. In this example, we have used the most common approach, called **varimax rotation,** which tries to minimize the complexity of the loadings within each factor.[##]

[‡‡]For this illustration, the factor loadings are hypothetical. We cannot use the factor loadings given in Table 27.6, as these represent coordinates in a four-dimensional space.

[##]Other forms of rotation that are used less often are *quartimax rotation,* which is based on simplifying row loadings, and *equimax rotation,* which simplifies loadings on rows and columns. Each of these methods will result in a slightly different positioning of the axes. Varimax rotation is used most often because it generally presents the clearest factor structure. For some analyses it may be necessary to try different solutions to develop the one that best differentiates factors. Fortunately, these processes are easily requested in a computer analysis. It is important to recognize that different mathematical solutions can be generated, depending on the rotation approach used.

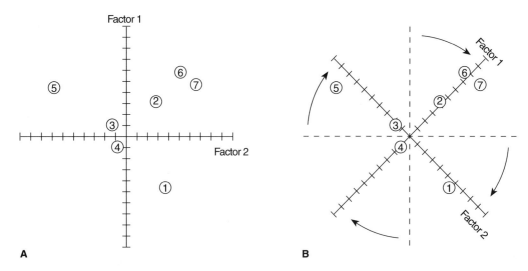

FIGURE 27.5 Orthogonal rotation of factor axes.

This rotation is shown in Figure 27.5B. The rotation improves the spatial structure of the variables so that distinct factors are now visible; that is, several of the variables lie directly on or close to one of the axes. We find that variables 2, 6, and 7 now have the closest orientation to Factor 1, and variables 1 and 5 have the closest orientation to Factor 2. Variables 3 and 4, still clustered around the origin, show little or no relationship to either factor. This type of two-dimensional plot can be requested as part of a computer analysis for combinations of factors.

This form of rotation is called **orthogonal rotation** because the axes stay perpendicular to each other as they are rotated. This means that the two factors are independent of each other (*orthogonal* means "independent"); that is, they maintain maximal separation. **Oblique rotation,** used less often, allows the axes to change their orientation to each other. Therefore, some variables could be close to both factors, and the factors would be correlated. This might lead to a more realistic solution in some cases; however, the orthogonal solution will typically be easier to interpret, and in many cases will provide a comparable solution to oblique rotation.

In the actual factor analysis, this rotation process is carried out for all four planes simultaneously. Clearly, it would be impossible to conceive of this type of analysis without a computer. We must visualize a spatial solution that provides the one best linear combination for all variables.

This process results in the creation of a *rotated factor matrix* shown in Table 27.6C. This matrix provides new factor loadings that represent the spatial coordinates of each variable in the reoriented multiaxial rotated solution. This new configuration should provide a cleaner statistical picture. We interpret this information by looking across each row of the matrix to determine which factor has the highest loading for that variable. We have highlighted the one loading for each variable that shows the strongest relationship to one of the factors. MOVES and WALKING load highest on Factor 1; COMPLAIN and

GROAN load highest on Factor 2; CHANGES and RUBS load highest on Factor 3; and ISOLATE is loaded highest on Factor 4.

Naming Factors

The final solution to a factor analysis is the naming of factors according to a common theme or theoretical construct that characterizes the important variables in the factor. This is a subjective and sometimes difficult task, especially in situations where the variables within a factor do not have obvious ties. The computer runs the analysis without any preconceived judgments on its part as to what "should" go together or what combinations "make sense." The researcher must look for commonalties and theoretical relationships that will explain the statistical outcome. When the factor labels are not so obvious, it may be necessary to reexamine the very nature of the construct being studied.

Table 27.7 shows how we have assigned the seven variables to four factors, using the strongest factor loadings for each variable as the criterion. Factor 1 could be called "mobility." Factor 2 could be labeled "verbal complaints." Factor 3 is concerned with "nonverbal complaints," and Factor 4 may be associated with "nonsocial behavior." We are able to specify the percentage of the total variance in the data that each factor explains, using the information given in Table 27.6A. Together, these four factors account for 72.5% of the total variance. Table 27.7 illustrates the type of information that is often included in a published report of factor analysis.

What we have, then, is a set of variables that contribute to a construct we are calling "chronic pain behavior." The variables demonstrate different components of this construct. We can begin to understand the structure of pain behavior by focusing on four elements that we have called mobility, verbal complaints, nonverbal complaints, and nonsocial behavior. As we move forward in this research, we can explore how each of these elements contributes to a patient's reactions to treatment, interactions with family, participation in social activities, and so on. The factor analysis has provided a framework from which we can better understand these types of theoretical relationships.

TABLE 27.7. FACTOR LOADINGS ON FOUR FACTORS RELATED TO CHRONIC PAIN BEHAVIOR

Factor 1: Mobility		Factor 2: Verbal Complaints	
Variable	**Loading**	**Variable**	**Loading**
MOVES	.86	COMPLAIN	.72
WALKING	.89	GROANS	.73
% Variance: 27.1%		% Variance 15.9%	

Factor 3: Nonverbal Complaints		Factor 4: Nonsocial Behavior	
Variable	**Loading**	**Variable**	**Loading**
CHANGES	.74	ISOLATE	.90
RUBS	.71		
% Variance: 15.1%		% Variance: 14.4%	

Applications of Factor Analysis

Exploratory Analysis

Factor analysis can be used to answer many types of research questions. As an exploratory approach, it can be used to sort through a large number of variables in an effort to reveal patterns of relationships that were not obvious before. This type of analysis may represent early stages of inquiry, when concepts and relationships are not yet sufficiently understood to propose relevant hypotheses. A classic example of this approach was presented by Thurstone and Thurstone in their studies of intelligence.[7] They factor analyzed 60 tests and identified six primary abilities: verbal, number, spatial, word fluency, memory, and reasoning. Through repeated testing, these have come to be accepted as some of the elements that underlie the construct of intelligence, and are used as the basis for many intelligence tests.

Reduction of Data

Factor analysis can also be used to simplify a test battery, by determining which elements of the test are evaluating the same concepts. This approach can result in reducing the number of items that are used, or it may provide the basis for creating composite summary scores for each concept. For example, Jette used factor analysis to look at a set of 45 items on a functional capacity evaluation, with the intent of reducing the number of items without sacrificing the comprehensiveness of the assessment.[8] The test items were structured into factors that identified distinct functional constructs, such as physical mobility, personal care, home chores, transfers, and kitchen chores. Jette suggested that two or more items from each functional category should be assessed as part of the evaluation, substantially reducing the time needed to complete the test, while maintaining the validity of the information it produces. This method of sorting through a large number of items is preferable to the intuitive or empirical classification of functional tasks into categories.

Factor Scores

One of the most interesting uses of factor analysis is the creation of a smaller set of composite scores, to be used as evaluative data or to be used as data in a statistical analysis. Subscores are created for each factor by multiplying each variable value by a weighting, and then summing the weighted scores for all variables within the factor. This result is called a **factor score.** The advantage of using composite scores is that the total number of variables needed for further analysis is decreased. This, in turn, will improve variance estimates for analyses such as regression or discriminant analysis. For example, Warren and Davis used a discriminant analysis to differentiate patients with and without running-related injuries.[9] They started with 72 anatomical variables and performed a factor analysis to reduce these data to nine factors. Factor scores were then used as independent variables in a discriminant analysis to predict membership in six pain groups. This simplified the analysis, which would have been quite cumbersome with 72 variables. Unfortunately, their classification was successful for only 29.1% of their cases, and they concluded that the identified factors were not good predictors of type of pain.

Construct Validity

Many experimental and clinical constructs, such as intelligence or motor development, cannot be measured directly. Therefore, they must be defined by relevant measurable variables that together form a conceptual package, indicative of the construct. Most tests of this sort contain many items that supposedly evaluate different components of the construct. These components can be considered factors, each one addressing a separate concept within the total construct. The construct validity of these tests must be established to document that they are indeed measuring the abstract behavior they supposedly define. This approach is basically one of theory testing; that is, the results of testing should conform to the specific hypotheses for the construct. For example, suppose we developed a new intelligence test to evaluate children with delayed cognitive development. If we accept the theoretical premise of intelligence defined by Thurstone and Thurstone,[7] then we could hypothesize, a priori, which items on the new test should go together to reflect each of the six primary elements of intelligence, as previously described. After the test is administered to a large sample, the scores can be factor analyzed, and we should see factors emerge that fit with this theory. If the factors do not match the hypothesized variable groupings, the test items are probably not measuring what they were intended to measure. This approach to construct validity testing is an important one that should be replicated on several samples before any conclusions are drawn about the appropriate or inappropriate inclusion of test items.

Limitations of Factor Analysis

Although factor analysis has a unique statistical role in multivariate analysis, its subjectivity is often the basis for serious criticism. Researchers must be cautious about how "factors" are interpreted, as they are not real measurement entities, but only hypothetical statistical concepts. Naming a factor does not make it real. Similar analyses on different samples may organize data differently, as will other approaches to a single analysis, such as different methods of extraction or rotation. These differences can alter a factor's essential meaning. Indeed, factor analysis may generate factors that are totally uninterpretable within the framework of the research question. Because of the subjective and judgmental nature of some decisions, we recommend consulting an experienced statistician to document the rationale for using particular methods under specific research conditions.

MULTIVARIATE ANALYSIS OF VARIANCE

Many experimental research designs incorporate tests for more than one dependent variable. For example, if we were interested in the physiological effects of exercise, we might measure heart rate, blood pressure, respiration, oxygen consumption, and other related variables on each subject at the same time. Or if we wanted to document muscle activity during a particular exercise, we might record electromyographic data from several muscles in the upper and lower extremities simultaneously. It makes sense to do this because it is efficient to collect data on as many relevant variables as possible at one time, and because it is useful to see how one person's responses vary on all these parameters concurrently. These types of data are usually analyzed using *t*-tests or analyses of variance, with each dependent variable being tested in a separate analysis.

This approach to data analysis presents two major problems. First, the use of multiple tests of significance within a single study can increase the probability of a Type I error. This means that the more tests we perform, the more likely we are to find significant differences, just by chance. The second problem is related to the univariate basis of the *t*-test and analysis of variance. The validity of these tests is based on the assumption that each test represents an independent event; however, if we measure heart rate, blood pressure, and respiration on one person, we cannot assume that the responses are unrelated. Most likely, changes in one variable will influence the others. Therefore, these responses are not independent events and should not be analyzed as if they were.

The purpose of a **multivariate analysis of variance (MANOVA)** is to account for the relationship among several dependent variables when comparing groups. This test can be applied to all types of experimental designs, including repeated measures, factorial designs, and analyses of covariance. In many situations, a MANOVA can be more powerful than multiple analyses of variance if the dependent variables are correlated.

Statistical Hypotheses for Multivariate Analyses

To illustrate the concept of multivariate analysis, suppose we wanted to measure systolic blood pressure (SBP) and diastolic blood pressure (DBP) to study the effects of three different medications for reducing hypertension. Hypothetical means for such a study are shown in Table 27.8. If we were to use a standard analysis of variance for this study, we would perform two separate analyses, one for systolic and one for diastolic pressure. In each analysis, we would compare means across the three treatment groups. In a multivariate model, we no longer look at a single value for each treatment group, but rather we are concerned with the overall effect on both dependent variables. We conceptualize this effect as a multidimensional value, called a **vector**. The mean vector, $\bar{V}$, for each group represents the means of all dependent variables for that group. In statistical terms, a vector can be thought of as a list of group means. In this example, there would be two values in each of the three vectors, representing systolic and diastolic blood pressure measures for each medication group. Therefore, $\bar{V}_1 = (50,120)$, $\bar{V}_2 = (60,110)$, and $\bar{V}_3 = (90,135)$. Figure 27.6 illustrates how these values would be oriented in a two-dimensional framework. The center point in each group, called the **group centroid,** represents the intersection of the means for both dependent variables, or the spatial location

TABLE 27.8.   MEANS FOR SYSTOLIC AND DIASTOLIC BLOOD PRESSURE FOR THREE TREATMENT GROUPS

	Treatment Group		
	1	**2**	**3**
Systolic	120	110	135
Diastolic	50	60	90

of the mean vector. The purpose of the MANOVA is to determine if there is a significant difference among the group centroids.

The multivariate null hypothesis states

$$H_0: \bar{V}_1 = \bar{V}_2 = \ldots = \bar{V}_k$$

where $\bar{V}$ represents the mean vector for each group. The alternative multivariate hypothesis states that at least one group has a population centroid that is different from the others. Just as with an ANOVA, follow-up tests are necessary to explain significant differences.

Multivariate Test Statistics

The concept behind the multivariate analysis of variance is really the same as that for the analysis of variance. The total variance in the sample is partitioned into parts that represent between-groups and error effects, although in the multivariate case, variability is measured against centroids rather than individual group means.

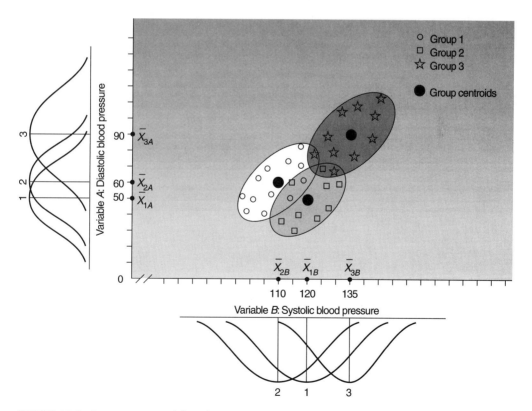

FIGURE 27.6 Representation of diastolic and systolic blood pressure for three groups in a multivariate model.

The statistics associated with multivariate analysis of variance are not as clear-cut as using F or t in univariate models. When two groups are compared, *Hotelling's T^2* can be used, which is a multivariate extension of Student's t-test. With more than two groups, four statistical procedures are usually reported in a computer analysis: Wilks' lambda, the Hotelling-Lawley trace, the Pillai-Bartlett trace, and Roy's maximum characteristic root (MCR). Each of these tests is a variance ratio, although each has a slightly different interpretation. For the sake of consistency in generating critical values for these statistics, most programs convert these values to F-values.

Unfortunately, statisticians are not in agreement as to which one of these procedures should be used. In most cases, the tests yield similar results. The rationale for choosing one test over the others is based on a complex consideration of statistical power and how well the assumptions underlying each test are met.[10] Rather than attempt to define these rationales, a task that goes beyond the scope of this text, we encourage researchers to consult with a statistician to make these decisions based on the specific research situation. We advise that Wilks' lambda is used most often, and will probably be the most easily interpreted.[10, 11]

When the MANOVA demonstrates a significant effect, follow-up analyses are usually based on univariate analyses of variance or a discriminant analysis. The latter procedure is considered preferable, because it maintains the integrity of the multivariate research question. Discriminant analysis will show if the values for the response variables, in this example SBP and DBP, can discriminate among the treatment groups. Some MANOVA programs will offer discriminant analysis or univariate analyses of variance as an optional part of the output.

COMMENTARY

Can We Keep It Simple?

Multivariate analyses have become popular in behavioral research because of the increased availability of computer programs to implement them. Their applications are, however, not well understood by many clinical researchers, and many studies using multivariate designs are still analyzed using univariate methods.

Multivariate techniques can accommodate a wide variety of data and are able to account for the complex interactions and associations that exist in most clinical phenomena. Many research questions could be investigated more thoroughly if investigators considered multivariate models when planning their studies. We have limited this chapter to a discussion of the conceptual elements of multivariate analysis, but with enough of an introduction to terminology and application that the beginning researcher should be able to communicate effectively with a statistician and follow the computer output. This information will also facilitate understanding research reports that present the results of these analyses.

Although we have emphasized the potential for improving explanations of clinical data using multivariate methods, we must also include the caveat that clinical research need not be complicated to be meaningful. A problem is not necessarily better solved by a complex analysis, nor should such an approach be taken just because computer programs are available. The indiscriminate use of multiple measurements will not substitute for a well-defined study with a select number of variables. To be sure, the results of multivariate analyses are harder to interpret and involve some risk of judgmental error, such as in factor analysis. In addition, multivariate tests require the use of larger samples. Many important and concise research questions can be answered using simpler methods and designs. Many clinical variables can be studied effectively using a single criterion measure. On the other hand, simple analysis is not necessarily better just because the interpretation of results will be easier and clearer. The choice of analytic method should be based on the research problem and the theoretical foundation behind it. When dealing with constructs that reflect several abstract phenomena, multivariate methods offer the most powerful means for developing and explaining theory. The purpose of this chapter was to present alternatives that provide the researcher with useful choices for planning the most effective study possible.

KEY TERMS

multivariate analysis
univariate analysis
partial correlation
multiple regression
residual variance
regression constant (*a*)
regression coefficient (*b*)
beta weights
multicolinearity
multiple correlation
  coefficient (*R*)
standard error of the
  estimate (*SEE*)

stepwise multiple
  regression
dummy variables
coding
logistic regression
logistic function
logit
maximum likelihood
adjusted odds ratio
discriminant analysis
discriminant function
eigenvalue
canonical correlation

factor analysis
factor
factor loading
principle components
varimax rotation
orthogonal rotation
oblique rotation
factor score
multivariate analysis of
  variance (MANOVA)
vector
group centroid

REFERENCES

1. Stineman MG, Williams SV. Predicting inpatient rehabilitation length of stay. *Arch Phys Med Rehabil* 1990;71:881–7.
2. Walker J, Sofaer S. Predictors of psychological distress in chronic pain patients. *J Adv Nurs* 1998;27:320–6.
3. VanSwearingen JM, Paschal KA, Bonino P, Chen T. Assessing recurrent fall risk of community-dwelling frail older veterans using specific tests of mobility and the Physical Performance Test of Function. *J Gerontol* 1998;53A:M457–M464.
4. Cifu DX, Keyser-Marcus L, Lopez E et al. Acute predictors of successful return to work 1 year after traumatic brain injury: a multicenter analysis. *Arch Phys Med Rehabil* 1997;78:125–31.

5. Norusis MJ. *SPSS Professional Statistics 6.1.* Chicago: SPSS Inc., 1994.
6. Ermer J, Dunn W. The sensory profile: a discriminant analysis of children with and without disabilities. *Am J Occup Ther* 1998;52:283–90.
7. Thurstone L, Thurstone T. *Factorial Studies of Intelligence.* Chicago: University of Chicago Press, 1941.
8. Jette AM. Functional capacity evaluation: an empirical approach. *Arch Phys Med Rehabil* 1980;61:85–9.
9. Warren BL, Davis V. Determining predictor variables for running-related pain. *Phys Ther* 1988;68:647–51.
10. Bray JH, Maxwell SE. *Multivariate Analysis of Variance.* Beverly Hills, CA: Sage Publications, 1986.
11. Kerlinger FN, Pedhazur EJ. *Multiple Regression in Behavioral Research.* New York: Holt, Rinehart & Winston, 1973.

28

Data Management

An important part of the research process is the development of a data management plan that specifies how data will be recorded, organized, reduced, and analyzed. This planning requires a knowledge of data coding and format requirements, statistics, and computers. The number of statistical packages for use on a microcomputer has grown dramatically, many at reasonable prices. The two most commonly used programs are SPSS (Statistical Package for the Social Sciences) and SAS (Statistical Analysis System). SPSS has traditionally been used more for the social and behavioral sciences, although its use has increased in health care research. SAS is used most often in medicine and epidemiology as a biostatistics program. These packages, once available only on main frames, have been adapted for use on personal computers. Many other programs are also on the market, and it would be useless to name them here as we are sure more will be published by the time this chapter is done! Even though these packages are all slightly different, they adhere to certain standards that are important for data management. The purpose of this chapter is to describe procedures for setting up data to be entered into a computer and analyzed with statistical programs.

RECORDING DATA

An essential part of the data collection plan is the development of a scheme for recording data. As part of the formulation of the research proposal, the researcher must determine what variables will be studied and how they will be measured. Some measurements produce quantitative data, such as range of motion and blood pressure. Variables such as sex, group, and race produce qualitative categorical data.

A data recording system must be carefully developed. Typically, data are collected from each subject and recorded on a separate sheet. The subject's identification code is listed (not the name—a list of subjects' names and codes can be kept separately). The subject code should be generated by the researcher, as opposed to using potentially identifying information such as a unit number or social security number. Other relevant information might include the date, the individual collecting the data (if there is more than one investigator), and demographic information such as age and gender. If possible, data should be listed in the order they will be included in the data file, to facilitate data entry.

The importance of a well-organized data collection scheme becomes most evident when the researcher begins to type data into a computer. If data are not clearly recorded and in a consistent format, data entry will be a difficult and potentially error-ridden process.

DATA CODING

Types of Variables

Data can be entered into the computer as numerals or characters. Quantitative data are **numeric,** having values of single or multiple digits, sometimes including decimal points, and composed of only numbers. Numeric values can be preceded by a plus or minus sign, although plus signs are usually assumed and not entered. Character variables, called **alphanumeric** or **string variables,** are composed of letters or characters (but may include digits). String variables may be letters or words that represent variable values, such as male/female or the names of states or cities. Variables can also be entered as dates, using one of many acceptable forms, such as MM-DD-YY, where month, day, and year are entered as two digits separated by dashes. Money values can be coded for different monetary units, with or without decimal places.

Codes for Categorical Variables

Data for categorical variables are entered as labels. For instance, if gender is a variable, we enter either male or female as the data value. Although we can enter the full label as the data, it is much easier to code these labels. Using character codes, for instance, sex could be coded F for female and M for male. It is generally recommended, however, that codes be entered as numeric data to facilitate statistical analysis, such as coding 1 for female and 0 for male. For dichotomous variables it is conventional to use 1 and 0 as codes, usually signifying the absence of a trait as zero. As a pure label it does not matter whether we code gender as 1 and 0, as 1 and 2, or any other number; however, many statistical procedures will only manipulate categorical data with 1 and 0 as the category codes (see discussion of dummy variables in Chapter 24). As much as possible, decisions about coding categorical variables should be made before data are collected. Codes should be used on data collection forms to expedite transfer of data to the computer.

Missing Data

It is not unusual for some pieces of data to be missing from a subject's record because of errors in recording, unavailability of information, nonresponses on surveys, or problems in data collection. To identify missing values, blanks are used as the default in many computer programs. Others have specific rules for identifying missing values, such as the use of a period in place of a missing datum. It is not advisable to use zeros to code missing values, as zeroes will be read as a number and there may be true zeroes in the data. Most often, missing data are coded using numeric values that are out of range of any actual data values. For example, the code of –9 or 99 is commonly used. Sometimes several codes are identified for missing values, depending on the reason for the missing information. For instance, a separate code might be used for a survey respondent refusing to answer a question versus one who is undecided about an answer.

DATA ENTRY

Statistical packages have grown up with the computer, and today most programs provide a format for data entry similar to a spreadsheet. Each variable is entered in a separate column, and each row represents an individual subject. Most programs will allow you to enter data in a spreadsheet program, such as Excel® or Lotus®, and then import it into the statistical format. When data originate as a spreadsheet, the first row in each column should contain the variable name, which will then be read by the statistical program. To facilitate this transfer, the variable names should conform to the restrictions of the statistical program.

Variable Names

Many programs require that a variable name be no more than 8 characters (numbers or letters), and that it begin with a letter and have no spaces. Some allow hyphens, underscores, or periods within a variable name, but some do not. Each variable must have a unique name. For example, a pretest and posttest value for pain could be coded PAIN1 for the pretest and PAIN2 for the posttest. Researchers should be familiar with the requirements for the statistical package they use.

Variable Fields

Each row of data, representing a single subject's scores, is called a **record** or **case.** Each individual score, or variable value, is identified as a **field.** A case is composed of several fields of data. Fields are described according to their *width,* that is, the number of digits or spaces needed for the maximum possible value. The field width is described according to the format *w.d,* where *w* is the total number of spaces (or field width) and *d* is the number of digits within the field that follow a decimal point. For example, the value 7.8 takes up three spaces (including the decimal point), for a field width of 3.1. The value 360 also takes up three spaces with no decimal places, for a field width of 3.0. The value 136.45 takes up six spaces, described as a field width of 6.2. Data can also be entered without the decimal point. For instance, with a specified field width of 5.2, the value 13645 will be read 136.45.

Code Books

Code books are used to organize data and to catalog the order of entry of all variables. Variable names are listed with their abbreviations. Codes are listed to identify their values. Figure 28.1 shows a sample page from a code book for a study comparing two types of exercise programs for improving range of motion in patients with frozen shoulder. Data were collected on subjects' age, sex, weight, and their pretest and posttest range of motion. Two trials were performed for each test. Codes were developed for sex and for group assignment. The code book is a necessary reference for all those who are involved with the study, most especially those who will analyze the data.

Data Formats

Data are entered in a file so that each subject's record looks the same; that is, all variables are entered in the same order along a row of data. The format can be described as free or fixed. **Free format** requires only that a space be inserted between each variable entry.

VARIABLE	Variable Name	Codes	Field Width	Locations
		CODE BOOK		
1. Subject number	SUBJ		2.0	1–2
2. Age	AGE		2.0	3–4
3. Sex	SEX	1 = male 2 = female	1.0	5
4. Weight	WT		4.1	6–9
5. Group	GROUP	1 = exercise 0 = control	1.0	10
6. Pretest ROM- Trial 1	PRE1		4.1	11–14
7. Pretest ROM- Trial 2	PRE2		4.1	15–18
8. Posttest ROM- Trial 1	POST1		4.1	19–22
9. Posttest Rom- Trial 2	POST2		4.1	23–26

FIGURE 28.1 Sample page from a code book.

Variable fields do not need to line up. Data entered in spreadsheets are read as free format, with each variable located in a new column.

Fixed format is used when the number of spaces within each variable field is consistent for every subject. This format is often used with large databases to save space. Fixed format data can be imported into spreadsheet format by identifying variable locations. Fixed format requires that values for each variable be recorded in the same columns. In this context, a column equals a space. Code books for fixed data will specify the variable locations by column number, as shown in the rightmost column in Figure 28.1. For example, consider the following data entry for these nine variables:

> 00114109751075508001200 1250
> 00235012051055006300850 0900
> 00351015050080508501155 1180

Each variable is lined up so that numerals are right justified within each field. For example, subject number (columns 1–3) contains three digits with leading zeroes, in expectation of more than 99 subjects. The code book shows that values for weight and range of motion are based on four digits with one decimal place (field width 4.1). Therefore, several of these values also contain leading zeroes. These same data are shown in free format in Figure 28.2A.

Data must be organized so that they match the requirements of the specific statistical procedures being used. Consider the hypothetical data shown in Figure 28.2A. The

A. ORIGINAL DATA

	SUBJ	AGE	SEX	WT	GRP	PRE1	PRE2	POST1	POST2
1	001	14	1	97.5	1	75.5	80.0	10.0	125.0
2	002	35	0	120.5	1	55.0	63.0	85.0	90.0
3	003	51	0	150.5	2	80.5	85.0	115.5	118.0

B. MODIFIED DATA

PREMEAN	POSTMEAN	AGEGRP
77.75	122.50	1
59.00	87.50	2
82.75	116.75	3

FIGURE 28.2 Data file for a pretest–posttest control group design. **(A)** The original nine variables are entered (see Figure 28.1); **(B)** three new variables are created through data modification: PREMEAN, POSTMEAN, and AGEGRP.

independent variable in this study is exercise group, an independent factor with two levels, coded 1 and 2. This variable is considered a **grouping variable,** one that divides the subjects into separate groups. The computer program will require specification of these group codes. If there are more than two grouping variables, as in a factorial design, each one is assigned a column for its own group code. The same code values (i.e., 1 and 2) can be used for each variable. The dependent variable is range of motion, measured in a pretest and posttest. Each of these scores is entered in a separate column.

Labels

Because variable names must be kept short and categories are coded, it is sometimes cumbersome to read a printout of an analysis. We have to remember so many codes and abbreviations. To facilitate reading the output, most programs will allow the researcher to specify **labels** for variables and for category codes. These labels can usually extend from 40 to 60 characters or longer, and allow the researcher to customize the printout in a way that will be convenient for interpretation. To make this happen, however, the researcher must first type in all the labels, which is time consuming, but worthwhile when reams of paper are sitting in front of you and you cannot remember whether males are coded 1 or 0! Labels are not required, but with large data sets they are extremely useful.

Data Cleaning

Once data are typed into the computer, and before analyses are run, the entered data should be checked against the raw data to be sure there are no discrepancies or coding errors. This process is called **data cleaning,** and although it may be time consuming and tedious, it is essential to ensure validity of the data analysis. The data file can be printed out or displayed on a computer screen and visually checked for accuracy against the original data. Frequency counts should be checked for all categorical variables. The output will list all the codes for each variable and the number of times that code appears in the data. It will also indicate how many subjects are counted, and if there are missing data for that variable. This allows the researcher to determine if there are mistakes in codes, or if the variable has too few entries to be useful. For continuous variables, descriptive statistics should be run to analyze means, minimums, and maximums, to be sure that the range of scores is appropriate. In this way, the researcher can ascertain if values out of the possible range have been entered. For instance, if the maximum blood pressure score is printed as 560, the researcher knows there is an error and can go back and correct that entry. Because computers are not able to interpret data, the researcher must be confident in the accuracy of the numbers the computer will process.

DATA MODIFICATION

All statistical programs include processes for **data modification** and **transformation** to create new variables or to assign new codes to existing variables. For example, we might want to compute the mean of several trials to use for data analysis; or we might have scores for several items on a scale and want to get the sum. Perhaps a continuous variable will be converted to categories. When these types of transformations are performed, a new variable is created, and must be given a new and unique variable name.

Computing New Variables

Computing a new variable requires that some arithmetic operation be performed on the existing data. All programs use the same symbols to represent logical operations. These symbols, known as **operators**, are used to create expressions that are instructions to the computer. The following symbols are used for arithmetic operations:

$+$	add	$A + B$
$-$	subtract	$A - B$
$/$	divide	A/B
$*$	multiply	$A * B$
$**$	exponent	$A**2$

These expressions are considered **simple expressions** because they contain one operator. When more than one operator is used, a **compound expression** is created, for instance,

$$A**2*B/(C + 1.0)$$

is a compound expression. This expression is equal to

$$\frac{(A^2)\,(B)}{C + 1.0}$$

When compound expressions are used, specific rules apply to the order in which operations take place. First, all expressions within parentheses are carried out. Second, adjacent operations are carried out in the following order: (1) exponentiation, (2) division and multiplication, and (3) addition and subtraction. Within each of these levels, operations proceed from left to right. For example, in the preceding expression, the first operation will be to complete the addition $(C + 1.0)$ within the parentheses. Next, the value of A will be squared. This value will then be multiplied by B. Lastly, this product will be divided by the sum $(C + 1.0)$. If the parentheses had been left out, the expression would be read differently. Using

$$A**2*B/C + 1.0$$

the expression would read

$$\frac{(A^2)\,(B)}{C} + 1.0$$

To illustrate the application of these arithmetic operators, we might want to compute a mean pretest and posttest score to use for analysis for the data in Figure 28.2. To do this, we tell the computer we want to create two new variables called PREMEAN and POST-MEAN using the following expressions:

$$PREMEAN = (PRE1 + PRE2)/2$$

$$POSTMEAN = (POST1 + POST2)/2$$

Note the importance of the parentheses, so that the sum of all three items is divided by 2, and not just the value for PRE2 or POST2. When these computations are done, the values for the new variables will appear as new columns in the data file, as shown in Figure 28.2B. These new variables can now be used in statistical procedures. We could, for instance, get a difference score between PREMEAN and POSTMEAN, and subject these values to a *t*-test. This type of data modification can also be done within spreadsheet programs.

Recoding Variables

We can also use **comparison operators** to recode variables by specifying relationships between them. Comparison operators may be specified as symbols or letter combinations:

$=$	EQ	equal to
$^=$	NE	not equal to
$>$	GT	greater than
$<$	LT	less than
$>=$	GE	greater than or equal to
$<=$	LE	less than or equal to

Comparison operators are usually used with an IF statement, which specifies a specific operation to be carried out if a given relationship exists. For instance, we have a variable called AGE entered in a data set, and we want to create three age groups for a comparison analysis. We would indicate that *if* age is less than 30 (AGE < 30), *then* we want to assign that subject to Age Group 1. If age is between 30 and 50 (AGE $>= 30$ and AGE $<= 50$), the subject should be assigned to Age Group 2. Over 50 (AGE > 50), subjects are in Age Group 3. These statements specify values for a new variable called AGEGRP (shown in the last column in Figure 28.2B). When assigning values to a new variable, the researcher must be careful not to overlap any categories, or the computer will not be able to perform the desired functions. In addition, groupings should reflect the full range of values that is present in the data.

Statistical Procedures

Many statistical procedures also provide a mechanism for creating and saving new variables. For example, when running a factor analysis, factor scores are created for each subject on each factor. These values can be saved and used as variables in future analyses. When regression procedures are run, residual scores can be calculated and saved. Most programs require specific instructions for these options.

DATA MANAGEMENT

Data collection is complete, all the data are entered, and we are ready to begin data analysis. If the research proposal was done well, we are ready to approach this phase of the research process in an organized way. It is a good idea to start by becoming familiar with the data by looking at descriptive statistics—frequencies for categorical variables and means for continuous variables. Sometimes histograms or line plots are helpful to visually assess the shape of a distribution. For correlational data scatterplots should be created to get a sense of the linearity and degree of relationship in the data. These initial steps are necessary to understand the scope of the data, and may suggest alternative statistical approaches. For example, transformations may be needed for nonlinear variables (see Appendix D), or outliers may be identified.

The next step is the culmination of all the research efforts—to apply statistical procedures to answer the research question. This is the fun part! Some helpful hints:

To make this process efficient, prepare a list of specific hypotheses, variables, and appropriate statistical procedures to guide your time at the computer. Be specific. For instance, if you intend to compare two groups, specify the *t*-test, paired or unpaired, and which variables will be used. If you run several regressions, list which are the independent and dependent variables for each one. Then you won't have to sit at the computer, faced with columns and columns of data, and wonder where to start.

Look at the output as you generate it. Examine your findings. Often, additional questions emerge and you may choose to run further tests. For instance, you may find relationships among some variables that you did not anticipate. Groups may end up having different characteristics than planned or a characteristic may be too rare to warrant further study. It may be of interest to perform certain analyses on subgroups within the data. Statistical programs provide different filtering options to select subjects according to a specified criterion. You might specify that an analysis be done only on those coded 1 for gender, or only those coded for group 1.

Sometimes it is useful to sort data, reordering the subjects according to the value of a particular variable. For instance, subjects may be entered into the database in order of their testing, but not necessarily in order of their subject number. The data may be sorted in ascending or descending order, and may have primary and secondary keys. Suppose we collect data on gender and age. We could instruct the program to first sort on gender, putting all females and males together. Then within gender we can sort on age, so we could see the spread of ages for females and males. We could look at age from youngest to oldest or vice versa.

Finally, most statistical programs include choices for creating tables or charts directly from the data. Many of these programs provide fairly sophisticated options, with a variety of fonts and colors to customize your presentation. These charts and tables can be imported into wordprocessing or presentation programs. Many different types of charts are usually available, and it is often helpful to try out different formats to see which presents the data best. Be sure you save your data and output so you can play with options and prepare your project for the final phase of the process—presentation as a platform or poster, or a published paper.

COMMENTARY

"Anyone can analyze data, but to really mess things up takes a computer!"

Because of the seemingly overwhelming power of computers for statistical analysis, it may seem unnecessary to become proficient in statistics. The computer seems to be able to handle the job of running statistical procedures with infinite ease, and can provide answers to statistical questions without the researcher ever having to crack a formula. The days of writing out a program and searching for the misplaced semicolon are gone. Today you need a mouse and a keyboard, and once you have entered your data and variable names you have very little else to do. Most programs will guide you through analyses by clicking on the appropriate buttons.

This is an oversimplification of the situation, however, for two reasons. First, the researcher must know the conceptual foundations for the statistical tests that will be used to make the appropriate choices. The computer can only carry out the instructions it is given. Programs require that the researcher sort through different options that will dictate how the procedures will be carried out. Most run at **default settings,** that is, parameters that are set at a certain level unless they are specifically changed. For instance, to run a stepwise regression procedure, variables will be included in the equation if partial correlations reach a specific level of significance. The default setting may be .05 or .15. The analysis will run at that level unless the researcher specifies a different level in the program. In addition, there are several approaches to stepwise analysis, and these may have to be specified. Some programs will print out certain summary statistics by default, such as mean, standard deviation, and range. These programs may require additional options to request different information. The researcher must know how the data should be analyzed, and what summary values are of interest, and then must be able to instruct the computer to perform the desired operations.

Second, there is an enormous amount of information generated by a computer analysis, and the interpretation of that output must be based on an understanding of the statistical procedures that were run. In many instances, only portions of the printout will be useful. If data are entered incorrectly, the output will be useless. If the data are inappropriate for a particular procedure, the computer may still be able to run an analysis, but the output will be uninterpretable. The wise researcher will have sufficient knowledge of both computers and statistics to be able to make the appropriate choices and ensure statistical conclusion validity for the study. When this knowledge is not sufficient, advice should be obtained from a statistical consultant.

KEY TERMS

numeric variables
alphanumeric (string)
    variables
record (case)
field
code book
free format

fixed format
grouping variable
labels
data cleaning
data modification
    (transformation)
operators

simple expression
compound expression
comparison operators
default settings

PART **V**

Communication

C H A P T E R

29

Writing a Research Proposal

The initial stages of the research process include development of the research question and delineation of methods of data collection. The success of the project depends on how well these elements have been developed and defined in advance, so that the proper resources are gathered and methods proceed with reliability and validity. The plan that describes all these preparatory elements is the **research proposal.** The proposal describes the purpose of the study, the importance of the research question, and the research protocol and justifies the feasibility of the project.

The proposal serves several purposes. First, it represents the synthesis of the researcher's critical thinking and the scientific literature to ensure that the research question is refined enough to be studied, that the assumptions and theoretical rationale on which the study is based are logical, and that the method is appropriate for answering the question. Second, the well-prepared proposal constitutes the body of a grant application when external funding is required. Third, it serves as an application for review by peer or administrative committees. This document will be carefully scrutinized by the **Institutional Review Board (IRB)** (see Chapter 3). Fourth, the proposal enhances communication among colleagues who may be coinvestigators and with consultants whose advice may be needed. Finally, the careful, detailed account of the study procedures serves as a guide throughout the data collection phase to ensure that the researchers follow the outlined rules of conduct. The research proposal, therefore, is an indispensable instrument in initiating and implementing a project.

When proposals are written as part of a grant application for funding from foundations or governmental agencies, the researcher must obtain the guidelines of the agency to which the proposal will be submitted. Generally, requirements and components of a proposal will be the same for grant applications as they are for academic and clinical institutions; however, to write a successful grant application, the researcher must understand the interests of the funding agency, the extent of available funds, the deadlines for submitting proposals, and the proper format of the application.*

---

*A reference, such as the *Foundation Reporter,*[1] can be used to aid in selecting an appropriate agency. This reference provides information about an agency's contact individual, foundation philosophy, typical recipients, application, review procedures, and restrictions. Other resources may be found on the Internet, such as *A Bibliography of State and Local Foundations Directories.*[2]

The purpose of this chapter is to discuss the process of developing and writing a research proposal. The exact format of a research proposal depends on the requirements or instructions of the individuals, clinics, faculty, or agencies that will review the project. The order of presentation of material may vary, as may the extent of the information required. The following guidelines are meant to reflect the most common elements of a proposal. A research proposal has two basic parts, as shown in Table 29.1. The first part provides details of the research plan, and the other describes the administrative and personnel support required to carry out the project.

TABLE 29.1.   WORKING PLAN FOR DEVELOPING A RESEARCH PROPOSAL

I. THE RESEARCH PLAN

    A. Title

    B. Abstract

    C. Statement of the research problem

        1. Rationale and justification for the study

        2. Significance of the study

    D. Statement of the purpose of the study

        1. Specific aims or objectives

        2. Research hypotheses or guiding questions

    E. Background of the study

        1. Topics for the review of literature related to:

           a. Theory and supportive rationale

           b. Related studies

           c. Methods

        2. Previous work by the investigator that supports the project

    F. Method

        1. Subjects: characteristics, sampling method, plans for recruitment

        2. Materials: instrumentation, plans to establish reliability and validity

        3. Procedures

           a. Study design

           b. Details of test and treatment administration

           c. Data collection methods

           d. Timetable and organizational chart

        4. Data management and analysis

    G. Literature cited

    H. Documentation of informed consent

II. PLAN FOR ADMINISTRATIVE SUPPORT

    A. Budget: personnel, equipment, facilities, and supplies

    B. Resources and environment

    C. Personnel: qualifications, time commitment, job descriptions, consultants

COMPONENTS OF THE RESEARCH PLAN

Before writing one word, the researcher spends considerable time thinking, gathering facts, and consulting with individuals who are knowledgeable in the content and methodology of interest. Students should also review guidelines for preparing their proposal with faculty advisors. Researchers who are seeking funding may find it helpful to read other proposals that were submitted to and funded by the agencies that are being considered. As one proceeds with the development of the project and considers its feasibility, it is helpful to follow an organized working plan that focuses on the important elements of the project. Although this outline will vary for some agencies, the following sections reflect the basic components required for most research studies.

Title

The title of a research proposal will be the first thing readers see, although it is often easier for the researcher to develop an appropriate title after the study design has been formulated. The title will become the project's "public identity."[3] It is the first impression of what the reviewers should expect to read in the subsequent pages. It must be concise and informative. A title such as "Bronchopulmonary Dysplasia" is certainly concise, but the reader is likely to say, "What about it?" Expanded, this title could be "Cardiovascular Problems in Bronchopulmonary Dysplasia." This is better, but does not yet suggest a research focus. With a few more words, this title will say much more: "Cardiovascular Effects of Physical Therapy Intervention in Infants with Bronchopulmonary Dysplasia." We now know that this proposed research has an *independent variable* and a *dependent variable* and that the sample will be infants.

Abstract

A summary or **abstract** of the project or program, often limited to one page, is required by most funding agencies and institutional review boards, and may be required for student projects. When a proposed project is to be reviewed by faculty, administrative, or foundation committees, all members of these committees will receive the summary, whereas only selected members of such committees may review the full proposal. The abstract should highlight the purpose and importance of the proposed project. A brief description of the method should identify the study subjects, procedures, and methods for data analysis. The proposed duration of the study and overall projected costs may be stated. Because the summary is likely to be read before the detailed proposal, it must make a positive impression, conveying specifically what is to be done and why the study is important.

Body of the Proposal

The body of the research proposal is the narrative portion that will explain the purpose and importance of the study and describe the design and procedures in detail.

Statement of the Problem

The opening statement of the proposal identifies the subject area to be studied. As an introduction, this statement should convey a clear sense of the importance of the problem in terms of applicability of potential findings to clinical practice and patient care. It may begin as a broad definition but should lead the reader logically toward a definition of the specific delimited topic, which will become the focus of the present project.

As an example, Rudd and coworkers compared a specialist community rehabilitation program with a standard hospital and home care program for patients with stroke.[4] The statement of the problem, as it might have been written in a proposal, would first establish why the study was needed by defining the problems related to costs of hospitalization and psychosocial aspects of managing these patients. By acknowledging these problems and alternative approaches to rehabilitation, the researchers justify the need to further examine the effectiveness of different treatment settings.

The problem statement, therefore, presents a rationale for the specific question being addressed by the project. In the preceding example, the authors have created a rationale for examining the difference between the structured specialist community program and standard care. No single project can be expected to solve a problem in its entirety. On the other hand, each project should clearly contribute to the solution. Each study expands the evidence that can be used to support the body of knowledge related to the research problem. The content of the opening section of the proposal should clearly demonstrate this contribution.

Purpose, Hypotheses, and Specific Aims

In a brief statement, the researcher must state precisely what the project is expected to accomplish. The **purpose** of the study should follow clearly from the justification presented earlier. If the research is to be experimental or correlational, the purpose is translated here into research hypotheses. Research **hypotheses** are stated in positive terms; they reflect the expectations of outcome. Null hypotheses that serve a statistical function do not belong in the text, unless the purpose of the research is specifically to show that no relationship exists between variables. If the research is descriptive in nature, the author will state the characteristics or behaviors that will be documented in the work and what questions the data will answer about the target population.

Many granting agencies require a statement of **specific aims** or **objectives** for a project. For instance, a study's objectives might be to add to the body of knowledge in a certain content area, to test a theoretical proposition, to demonstrate differences between certain treatments to develop more effective and efficient intervention strategies, to document the reliability of an instrument, or to establish the relationship between specific variables as a basis for making treatment planning decisions. These objectives are derived from the research hypotheses or descriptive questions. Objectives help reviewers focus on the description of methods and will often help the researcher guide the discussion of results when the study is completed.

Background

The presentation of background information includes the theoretical rationale for the study and pertinent facts, observations, or claims that have led the investigator to the proposed research question. This information is derived from the literature review and from previous or related work done by the investigator. Funding agencies look favorably on projects that are built on previous work by the investigator.

The literature review is difficult to present concisely, and much effort is usually required to integrate published material to make relevant points. While preparing for a project, the researcher will have read and catalogued many references, typically many more than will or should be included in the written proposal. Authors must continually ask, "Is this reference or point of information directly related to this study?" "Does it contribute to the rationale or clarify the basic assumptions that underlie the research question?" If the answer is "No," then the reference should be set aside or discarded. When the references have been selected, they should be organized by topic areas to facilitate organization of the paper (see Chapter 7).

The presentation of the review of literature includes the main points that serve as the background of the proposed study. A meaningful review of literature provides a clear representation of the author's thought processes in developing the proposed study. It is not simply a series of abstracts of papers on the topic. The author must convey an integration of content that supports the need, importance, and rationale for the proposed study. The need and importance of the proposed study are defined in relationship to existing clinical or scientific reports. The first elements of the review may include relevant epidemiological factors, demographics, the impact of the research issue on health care policy or practice, and the potential impact on patients. For instance, for the example cited earlier, the investigators might focus on the rising costs of care resulting from the increased incidence of stroke, and the potential psychosocial advantages of the patients' early return to community living. The major portion of the background focuses on prior research that has been done to address the same or related questions, reflecting current knowledge or lack of knowledge. This includes a synthesis of consistencies and conflicts found in prior reports. The possible reasons for inconsistencies and identifiable limitations of previous studies should be elucidated to provide further evidence that more study is required. The content of this section should show the logic for selecting the subjects, the variables to be studied, and the methods of measurement. This section should end with a summary of the facts, problems, or controversies found in the literature and the relevant perspectives of the researcher that lead directly back to the specific need and stated purpose of the proposed study.

Method

The method section is probably the most important part of the proposal, and should be both concise and clear. The author should include enough detailed information so that reviewers can judge the soundness of the work, so that members of the institutional review board can determine exactly what the subjects will be asked to do, and so that the researcher can determine the feasibility of the study. The opening section identifies the overall study design that will be employed to test the research hypothesis or answer the research question. For example,

> *This study will be a randomized controlled trial to compare the effects of a specialized community rehabilitation program and a standard hospital-based program on motor abilities, cognition, aphasia, activities of daily living, anxiety, and depression in patients who have had a stroke.*

The details of the research methods are usually presented in four subsections: Subjects, Materials, Procedures, and Data Analysis.

Subjects.   The description of *subjects* used in human studies is extremely important because of the inherent variability among them and the vast number of extraneous factors that may affect human behavior or performance. The author must describe who the subjects will be in terms of *inclusion* and *exclusion* criteria, how many and from where subjects will be recruited, how they are to be selected, and the method by which they will be assigned to groups for the study. Characteristics such as age, sex, height, weight, disability, diagnosis, and duration of hospitalization should be defined if they are relevant to the study. The author must include all, and only, those factors that could influence the results and the ability to generalize the findings to the target population or to compare findings with other similar studies. Funding agencies and institutional review boards may require a power analysis to demonstrate the appropriateness of the proposed sample size.

Materials.   *Materials* refers to the equipment, instruments, or measuring tools that will be used in the study. Materials should be described according to important characteristics such as brand name and model and should be documented for reliability and validity. If measurement tools are new, relatively unknown, or developed by the researcher, they should be described in sufficient detail and a figure should be included. If the measurement tool is a survey, the entire document may be presented as an appendix to the proposal or a set of sample questions may be included in the narrative.

Procedures.   The *procedures* section describes precisely what is to be done from beginning to end of the investigation, in chronological sequence. Procedures also include how, and by whom, data are to be collected. Operational definitions should be provided for independent and dependent variables. If these procedures are extensive and lengthy, they may be briefly described in the text with references to appendices which will present the details in full. The researcher should include strategies for controlling extraneous variables.

A chart or flow sheet, presented in tabular form, will serve to summarize the procedural sequence. Figure 29.1 illustrates the timetable for a hypothetical 2-year study. The study is a pretest–posttest design with subjects randomly assigned to two treatment groups. The treatment intervention period lasts 6 months. Measurement data for evaluation of outcomes will be collected initially, each month for 6 months, and 9 months after the initial evaluation of each patient. This written description is consistent with the graph, as it should be. The last patients will be admitted to the study in month 15; their treatment period, lasting 6 months, will end in month 21, and their follow-up assessment will be made 3 months later, in month 24. Such a display of the "work schedule" will assist reviewers in evaluating the feasibility of the investigation in terms of time and available funding.

Data Analysis.   The plan for *data analysis* should outline specific procedures for recording, storing, and reducing data and for statistically analyzing the data. Reviewers will examine both descriptive and analytical methods to determine their

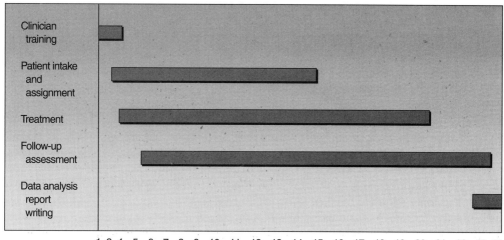

FIGURE 29.1 Graphic display of a hypothetical study timetable.

appropriateness for the design of the study and the type of measurement. It is often helpful to obtain the services of a statistician to be sure that this section is accurate and complete. The funding agency will probably have a statistician review it.

The final part of the narrative portion of the proposal should be a listing of literature cited in the paper. Some agencies require the use of a specific bibliographic style, but often this is left to the discretion of the researcher.

Documentation of Informed Consent

A copy of the informed consent form must accompany the proposal when subjects will be directly involved in the study. The informed consent form may not be required for secondary analysis studies. Most funding agencies and sponsoring institutions require IRB approval before a proposal is submitted and reviewed. The time delays inherent in obtaining this approval must be built into the timetable for submitting the proposal. Documentation of IRB approval must accompany the proposal. The process and elements of obtaining informed consent are discussed in Chapter 3.

PLAN FOR ADMINISTRATIVE SUPPORT

Budget

Every proposal, even those written for student research, should include an estimate of projected expenses to demonstrate the feasibility of the project. For a grant application, the budget is an extremely important part of the proposal, and must be complete and detailed according to the instructions of the funding agency. Students may need to show how resources will be made available to them if there are no costs associated with the project. Many schools provide small grants that will assist students with their thesis projects. The format and content of the budget will vary depending on the type of research proposal. Generally, the budget is presented by category as a summary of totals and as an itemized budget. For grants that are expected to run more than 1 year, only the first year's budget is itemized, and summaries of projected expenses for additional years are provided. A narrative section, called the **budget justification,** should be included to explain the projected costs in each category. The typical budget categories are personnel, equipment, facilities, supplies, and travel.

The itemized *personnel budget* identifies the name of each individual who will participate in the study, their proposed title (such as principal investigator, consultant, statistician, research assistant, secretary), the salary for each individual, and the percentage of full time or number of hours that will be devoted to the project. Dollar amounts may be based on percentage of the individual's full-time salary or an hourly wage for a specified number of hours. Some personnel may be asked to participate in the project with no remuneration. These individuals should also be listed, showing no salary request. Associated fringe benefit amounts are listed separately based on the total amount of projected salaries and wages. Reviewers will scrutinize the personnel budget particularly to evaluate the appropriateness of the time commitment of each participant. The budget justification should explain the responsibilities of each participant and should show that the personnel will realistically be able to achieve the desired outcomes.

Equipment costs are given for all equipment that will be purchased with grant funds. Costs should reflect current prices and any charges related to installation, calibration, and maintenance. Most granting agencies define "equipment" as items costing at least $300 and having an extended life expectancy of at least 3 to 5 years. The narrative should provide details of equipment, such as manufacturer, model number, and special accessories that are needed for the study. The researcher should indicate if some of the necessary equipment is already available, to show the funding agency that the project can be completed with some contribution by the researcher's institution.

The budget may include a request for funds for *alteration* or *renovations* to facilities. If space must be altered to accommodate equipment or to provide a work area, the contractors' estimates should be confirmed before specifying those costs in the budget. Explanations of all construction costs should be provided in detail, justifying why they are necessary for the study.

The category called *supplies* usually refers to consumable materials as opposed to capital equipment. Questionnaires and survey instruments, materials used for presentations (e.g., slides or posters), data books, floppy diskettes, and equipment items costing less than $300 are examples of "supply" items. Specific quantities of these supplies should be given with justification. A category of "other expenses" may also be included to account for miscellaneous items such as telephone costs and photocopying.

Depending on the nature of the project and the regulations of the funding agency, *travel expenses* may be budgeted. Travel to and from the institutional "home base" to collect data is certainly part of conducting a project and is likely to be an acceptable expense. Travel to meetings where data may be presented is more indirectly related to the project, but can often be justified. Travel costs may also be applied to patients who must be transported for purposes of the research.

All of the preceding budget categories are defined as **direct costs. Indirect costs** relate principally to the overhead charged by the sponsoring institution for administrative activities, facility maintenance, and any other support services. Funding agencies usually limit the amount of support that may be used for indirect costs based on some defined percentage of the total budget. In cases when the customary institutional charge exceeds the set limit, the budget narrative should specify the manner in which such a discrepancy will be handled. In some cases, granting agencies will negotiate this percentage. The total budget for the project is the sum of all direct and indirect costs.

In every institution where research is conducted, there is an administrative officer responsible for grants and contracts. This individual will be able to assist researchers with the general "anatomy" of a proposal budget and will provide information about fringe benefits, indirect costs, and institutional support. Consultation with this individual is essential and should begin early in the process of developing a research proposal budget. The administrative officer must sign off on the proposal before it is submitted, reflecting institutional approval of the proposed project.

Resources and Environment

Many funding agencies and academic or clinical institutions will also ask for information regarding existing resources for carrying out the proposed project. The investigator will be asked to describe available laboratory facilities, equipment, clinical sites, computer capability, office space, and so on, to demonstrate that the project is feasible within the institution's environment. The areas in which data collection will take place should be described, as should the areas where equipment will be housed. In addition, administrative support services may need to be described. Documentation of secretarial or technical assistance or the need to acquire such support will be evaluated by reviewers in regard to the feasibility and justification of the applicant's budget request.

Personnel

Identification of the investigators and their qualifications is an important element of a proposal, especially when external funding is being sought. Personnel will probably not be a factor in student research, except when expert assistance is required for carrying out parts of the project. Funding agencies will examine investigators' education, experience, track record of research, and prior publications to determine that they have appropriate qualifications. This information is most often provided in the form of biographical summaries for each person working on the project. Some institutions offer a variety of funding programs and the eligibility requirements differ for each program. For example, the Arthritis Foundation offers several programs ranging from postdoctoral fellowships for individuals with 3 to 7 years of research experience to health professions traineeships to support the research of individuals with master's degrees. Grants through the National Institutes of Health usually require that someone with an MD or PhD and research experience act as primary investigator. Foundations that support new investigators often require that the proposed work be supervised by an experienced, competent researcher. Because of these kinds of criteria, the inclusion of information about the participants in a proposed study is essential to the process of evaluation by an agency or foundation.

PRESENTATION OF THE PROPOSAL

Style

The research proposal is a forward-looking document. The researcher's thinking begins with the present, acknowledges and draws from the past, but primarily leads to the future. Therefore, the statement of the problem is written in the present tense, the background is written in the past tense, and the method (which is the proposed research) is written in the future tense.

The actual format required for the proposal varies among agencies and schools. The researcher must follow the specific instructions provided by the sponsoring agency. The method of citing references should be consistent throughout, and tables and appendices should be clearly labeled and cited in the text.

The tone or mood of the document should be positive, persuasive, and scholarly. The researcher must convince reviewers that the proposed research is important, that there is a need to conduct the proposed research, and that the research team has the knowledge and ability to accomplish the study objectives. Phrases such as "perhaps the results will contribute" and "we hope to demonstrate" convey hesitation and insecurity. Conversely, the use of superlatives, implying that this work will be the greatest of all, will detract from the substance. A proposal that is sensible, factual, and realistic will receive the attention it deserves.

Printing

The final draft of the completed proposal must be neat and readable, and printed on a laser-quality printer. Review committees require several copies; each copy should be clear with high contrast.

COMMENTARY

Review, Revise, Edit, Revise, Review

The author of a research proposal should expect to edit and revise sections of the entire document through the full process. Indeed, the original draft may not be recognizable when the process is finished. To the author, the "final" version may be perfectly clear and complete; however, one final step should be taken: enlisting others to read the whole proposal. Graduate students have "built-in" readers; this is one of the responsibilities of thesis and dissertation advisory committees. Those who are not students should seek three kinds of individuals to review the proposal. One who is knowledgeable about the topic and the relevance of the project should be asked to evaluate the appropriateness, accuracy, and thoroughness of the presentation. Another who understands research design and methodology will concentrate on the validity of the research methods relative to the research question and specific aims. The third should be someone who is unfamiliar with the subject matter and who will react to the readability of the paper. All three may notice inconsistencies, instances of unnecessary professional jargon, or redundancy. This kind of preliminary review by colleagues is valuable for inspiring the researcher's confidence that the proposal is ready for formal review and subsequent successful implementation.

KEY TERMS

research proposal
Institutional Review Board
  (IRB)

abstract
hypothesis
specific aims (objectives)

budget justification
direct costs
indirect costs

REFERENCES

1. *Foundation Reporter.* 29th ed. Detroit, MI: The Taft Group Comprehensive Profiles and Guiding Analyses of America's Major Private Foundations, 1998.
2. *A Bibliography of State and Local Foundations Directories.* The Foundation Center, 23 June 1998. <http://fdncenter.org/onlib/director.html>
3. Meador R. *Guidelines for Preparing Proposals. A Manual on How to Organize Winning Proposals.* Chelsea, MI: Lewis Publishers, 1985, p. 19.
4. Rudd AG, Wolfe CDA, Tilling K, and Beech R. Randomised controlled trial to evaluate discharge scheme for patients with stroke. *BMJ* 1997;315:1039–44.

30

Reporting the Results of Clinical Research

The culmination of the research process is the communication of results. This final stage may be the most important part of the process in that only shared information can clarify, amplify, and expand the professional body of knowledge. Research reports can be developed in a variety of ways. The written article published in a refereed journal provides a permanent record of research that will be available to a large audience. Oral reports and poster presentations at professional meetings serve to disseminate research information in a timely fashion, although the audience is limited and the record of research findings will be found only in abstract form. Students are usually required to document their work in the form of a thesis or dissertation, but may be given the option of writing the paper in the form of a journal article. The purpose of this chapter is to describe the process of preparing manuscripts for publication in scientific journals, poster presentations, and oral reports.

THE JOURNAL ARTICLE

Selecting a Journal

The researcher should decide where the manuscript will be submitted before writing the final paper. The expansion of the scope of practice in the health professions has been accompanied by a proliferation of publications serving specialized areas of practice. The choices are numerous and selection of the appropriate one deserves careful thought.

Some journals have a clearly defined focus with priorities explicitly stated. This focus is often stated in a journal's masthead or instructions to authors. For example, the journal *Physical Therapy* "contributes to and documents the evolution and expansion of the scientific and professional body of knowledge related to physical therapy." When a journal's focus is not so obvious, the contents of several issues of that journal should be read to determine if a particular study is consistent with the subject matter and type of research that the journal tends to publish. It is an unfortunate waste of time, effort, and perhaps money to make the wrong choice and to have a manuscript returned because it "is not suitable for publication" in a particular journal. This is almost verbatim what the rejection letter will say.

Another consideration in selecting a journal is the readership. The product of a research project should reach the people who will best be able to use the information. If, for example, a study documents the functional outcome of an orthopedic surgical procedure, the report should be in a journal that orthopedists read. If, on the other hand, the study focuses on the postoperative physical or occupational therapy intervention, journals devoted to these professions will be more appropriate.

Submitting the Article

Every journal publishes **Instructions to Authors** which must be followed in the preparation of a manuscript. Although the general format of a research report is fairly consistent in medical and scientific writing,[1] each journal has its own particular rules about organization of a manuscript; preparation of tables, illustrations, or graphs; and method of reference citation. Look carefully at articles published in the journal to follow the format. Failure to follow the instructions is a reason for rejection; or, at least, the manuscript will be returned for corrections.

Authors must expect delays in responses when their article is being reviewed. Some journal editors are more rigorous about turnaround time than others. Standard policy for scientific journals states that authors should submit an article to only one journal at a time, to protect journals from conflicts in copyright. If an article is rejected, the author can then submit it to a different journal.

Structure and Content of the Written Research Report

The sections of a research report are the abstract, introduction, methods, results, discussion, conclusion, and references, as shown in Table 30.1. The introduction and methods sections serve the same purpose as in the project proposal; that is, they describe the rationale for the study and the specific procedures used to collect the data (see Chapter 29). Although the content of these sections will be similar to the proposal, the author will have to do some serious editing to fit the journal article format. The "forward-looking" statements must be changed to past tense because the project is now completed. The last three sections of the article will be completely new.

Although no universal rules apply, generally manuscripts for journal articles should not exceed 15 pages, and should be typed and double spaced. Journals have limited space, and will not publish papers that are too long, unless they are especially important contributions to the literature. Many authors publish the results of large studies in two parts.

Abstract

Most journals require an **abstract** of the report which the author usually prepares *after* the manuscript is complete. The abstract summarizes the content of the article including the purpose of the study, the number and type of subjects, the basic procedures used, a summary of the results, and the major conclusion. The abstract must be concise. The prescribed limit may be 150 words, occasionally less. Readers will refer to the abstract first to decide

TABLE 30.1. STRUCTURE OF A JOURNAL ARTICLE FOR REPORTING RESEARCH

Section	Should contain
Abstract	• Overview and purpose of the study • General description of methods • Highlights of results • Statement of significance of results • General conclusions
Introduction	• Statement of the problem • Clinical relevance • Review of literature • Rationale and theoretical framework • Specific purpose and hypotheses (or guiding questions)
Methods	• Study design • Criteria for and methods of subject selection • Description and number of subjects • Measurement methods and data collection techniques • Data analysis procedures
Results	• Narrative description of statistical outcomes • Tables and figures that summarize findings • Statements to support or reject hypotheses
Discussion (and Conclusions)	• Interpretation of statistical outcomes • Discussion of clinical significance of outcomes • Importance of the work • Comparison of results with work of others • How results support or conflict with theory • Critique of the study limitations and strengths • Suggestions for further study
References	• List of all references cited in the article

whether to read the complete report. Computerized retrieval systems store author-written abstracts. Therefore, they must be able to stand alone, despite their brevity.

Introduction

The *introduction* can be drawn from the statement of purpose, the background, and specific aims included in the research proposal. As in the proposal, the introduction of an article should provide a description of the research question and the context within which the author intended to answer it. After reading the first one or two paragraphs of the introduction, the reader should have a clear understanding of the problem being studied and why it is important. The literature review should reflect the relevant background that is necessary to support the theoretical rationale for the study, and should provide sufficient information for the reader to understand how the research question will be answered. The introduction should end with a statement of the specific purpose of the study, delineating the variables that were studied and the research hypotheses or guiding questions that have been investigated in this study.

Methods

The *methods* section should begin by describing the subjects, including how many were studied, what criteria were used to recruit them, how they were selected, and how they were assigned to groups. Relevant characteristics of subjects, especially age and sex, should be summarized using means, ranges, and frequencies. Many journals now require a statement documenting that subjects read and signed an informed consent form and that the project was approved by the appropriate committees.

The methods section continues with a description of equipment and data collection procedures, presented in chronological order so that the reader can follow the procedural flow of the project. If the measurement or treatment procedures are standardized and well known, they can be described briefly and the author can refer the reader to the original sources for a more detailed description. When manufactured instruments are used, the company name and address should be cited. Operational definitions should be provided for all variables, with the intent that someone could replicate the data collection procedures. Many researchers develop a written protocol that they use as a guide during data collection to be sure that all procedures are followed properly. This protocol can easily serve as an outline for this section of the paper.

Diagrams, photographs, and tables can clarify and simplify the presentation of methods. For example, demographic information and special characteristics of subjects can be summarized in a table, and photographs of a unique procedural setup may make a lengthy verbal description unnecessary.

The methods section ends with a full description of the procedures used to reduce and analyze the data, including specific statistical procedures. If unique or new statistical methods are used, they should be referenced.

Results

The *results* section contains *only* a report of results, that is, a narrative description of exactly what happened in order of importance relative to the specific aims or hypotheses of the study. In the course of the study, the researchers may have gained considerable amounts of information, but unless it relates specifically to the stated purpose of the project, such information should not be included in this section. If one simple hypothesis has been proposed, the results section may be stated in a few succinct sentences.

The outcomes of statistical tests must be included to demonstrate or support the statement of results. Although the inclusion of calculated values, degrees of freedom, and the significance level is important, the narrative portion of the results section should emphasize the variables of interest rather than just statistics. For example, in a study of gait comparing elderly and young women, the statement, "The differences in step length were significant, $t = -3.13$ ($p < .01$)," is not as meaningful to the reader as, "The elderly women demonstrated a significantly shorter step length than the younger group ($t = -3.13, p < .01$)." When detailed statistical or descriptive information related to the study variables is needed in the paper, it is usually easier and often clearer for the reader to refer to tables or graphs that summarize such information.

Two major principles should guide the structure of the results section. One is that tables and figures should not duplicate the narrative; that is, if the author includes values for group means and standard deviations in the body of the text, there is no need to repeat them in a table. The author can refer the reader to the tables and figures for details and should only summarize these details in the text. The reader should be able to understand the results without referring to the tables and should be able to understand the tables without referring to the text. Therefore, the tables and figures should complement but be independent of the text. Second, the author should not discuss results in this section. Statements related to how this information could be applied to practice or interpretation of outcomes should be left to the discussion section.

Discussion

The *discussion* section is the heart of a research report. It reflects the researcher's interpretation of the results in terms of the purpose of the study and the outside world. In this part of the paper the author can express opinions. The author should comment on the importance of the results, limitations of the study, suggestions for future research, and clinical implications.

The commentary about the importance of results should not be a reiteration of the results section, but should focus on alternative explanations of the observed outcomes, emphasizing how they either support or refute previous work or clinical theories. All results should be addressed, including those that were not statistically significant. The author should provide perspectives on the applicability of results to practice or further study.

The limitations of the study, including possible extraneous variables that could have affected the outcomes, should be identified and explained. Some of these factors may have been identified before the study began and others will have become evident during the course of data collection or analysis. These may include a small sample size, attrition of subjects, or lack of subject adherence to the protocol. The author must consider the relative importance of these limitations to the interpretations of results. It is essential that the author delineates all major extraneous factors so that the reader can examine the results realistically.

Every research endeavor leads to further questions. Sometimes these questions arise out of the expressed limitations of a study and the need to clarify extraneous factors. In clinical research, alternative methods exist for studying the same or similar research questions and these may need to be examined. Given the results of a study, the author may want to reconsider a particular theory and how it may be applied. Suggestions for future research will develop from these ideas and should be expressed.

The immediate or potential applicability of results to clinical practice should be acknowledged by authors. Their perspectives on the clinical relevance of studies are important whether the research focus is primarily on theory, applied science, or clinical effectiveness.

Conclusion

The *conclusion* is a brief restatement of the purpose of the study and its principal findings. It is often written in such a way that the author states the deductions made from the results. Phrases such as "the results of this study indicate" and "this study demonstrates" serve to link the summary of results and the meaning of those results.

References

The style of citing *references* throughout the text and in the listing of references at the end of a manuscript must follow the Instructions to Authors. Many journals use the style suggested by the published "Uniform Requirements."[1] Others may follow the American Psychological Association or the American Medical Association guidelines.[2, 3]

The Internet is an important new source of references. Journals may eventually include instructions for such citations. The Modern Language Association of America (MLA) has published a full array of methods for citing documents that have been obtained from websites.[4]

Tables and Graphs

Tables and graphs are frequently used in the results section of an article to facilitate explanation of statistical findings and to provide visual explanations. To be effective, the tables and graphs must follow guidelines for the specific journal and general considerations for developing visual materials. The narrative portion of the paper will often present general descriptions of findings, and the tables and figures will present the details.

Tables

The customary table has five components: the title, column headings (horizontally displayed), row headings (vertically displayed), the "field" within which the data are arranged by columns and rows, and footnotes. Most journals use a format whereby horizontal lines can be drawn to frame the column headings and the bottom of the table, but no other lines (horizontal or vertical) are permitted. The well-constructed table of research results will present numeric or descriptive data demonstrating the relationships between independent and dependent variables. The title should identify those relationships. For example, for a table presenting the effect of ultrasound on shoulder range of motion, the title could read: "Pretest and Posttest Range of Motion Values. . . ."

Whether data are oriented vertically or horizontally may depend on the size and format requirement of the journal; however, logically, related numeric data should be presented in the columns, particularly when they will be summarized with totals or means and standard deviations in the last row. The sequence of column headings should progress logically from left to right based on the order of events. In the display of pretest and posttest data, the pretest should come first. The column headings should specify what was measured and the units of measurement, such as "(degrees)." The source of column data must be identified by the row headings, such as subjects by number or code when individual data points are displayed, or with labels, such as "control" and "experimental" when the table represents grouped summaries.

Footnotes may be used to present *p*-values, to explain abbreviations, or to cite references. A journal's Instructions to Authors may specify the style for sequentially labeling footnotes. Some may use small italic arabic letters (*a,b,c*). Others may use symbolic keys. For example, the American Medical Association style requires a common symbolic sequence: * (asterisk), † (dagger), ‡ (double dagger), § (section mark), ‖ (parallels), ¶ (paragraph symbol), and # (number sign).[3]

Specialized tables are constructed to present statistical test summaries. Many examples are presented in this text. A tabular presentation of a frequency distribution is shown in Table 17.3. A typical analysis of variance table, called a "source table," is shown in Table 20.1.

Graphs

Graphs provide a visual demonstration of research results. Trends, relationships, and comparisons may be presented more effectively and more concisely by constructing a graph than by writing a detailed text. Graphs can be drawn in a number of ways. Frequency data are commonly represented using a histogram or a frequency polygon. Figures 17.1 and 17.2 in this text are examples. In a *histogram* the bars are contiguous, and in a *frequency polygon,* the data points are connected by lines because these graphs display the distribution of a group of scores. A *pie chart* graphically can display the proportional distribution of selected characteristics of a whole sample where the percentage of each characteristic is drawn to scale as a piece of the whole pie. A *bar graph,* which is a series of separate bars, may be used to show frequency or magnitude data derived from separate samples, such as control versus experimental group values, or experimental events, such as pretest and posttest values.

In constructing graphs, the author must pay careful attention to the scaling of the units of measurement. Graphs are intended to represent meaningful trends, relationships, or comparisons; therefore scales should be realistic and drawn to illustrate important, true differences in the data. They can, however, be drawn to present a false impression—either exaggerating or diminishing real differences. For example, Figure 30.1 displays shoulder abduction range of motion before and after treatment intervention. The data in both graphs are the same: a mean of 100 degrees for both groups before treatment, 110 degrees for the control group, and 120 degrees for the experimental group following treatment. The magnitude of change appears to be greater in Figure 30.1A as compared with Figure 30.1B. Especially considering that normal shoulder abduction range is somewhere between 160 and 180 degrees, Figure 30.1A seems to be an exaggeration of the comparative effectiveness of the treatment intervention.

In deciding what content to present in narrative form or in tables or graphs, the author should consider a general rule that each element of the results section must stand alone and each must contribute to the complete and accurate presentation of the research findings.

Converting Theses and Dissertations for Publication

Most theses and dissertations are written on the basis of a six-chapter format: statement of the problem, review of the literature, methods, results, discussion, and conclusion. Journal articles contain the same elements, but are honed carefully by authors to avoid all but the essential content presented succinctly. The full document that is prepared to meet degree requirements is usually too long and over referenced to be acceptable as a journal article. The challenge for the student is to condense content considerably while retaining substance and meaning.

This task is not a simple undertaking; therefore, the student must consider seriously the decision and commitment to proceed. The selection of the thesis or dissertation topic

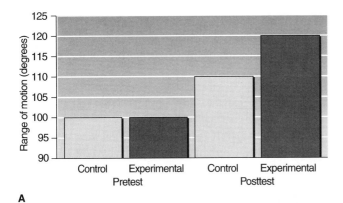

A

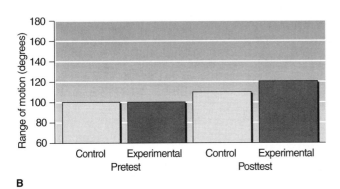

B

FIGURE 30.1 Two bar graphs showing shoulder abduction range of motion before and after treatment for two groups, illustrating the effect of vertical axis scaling: (**A**) Scale from 90 to 125 degrees; (**B**) Scale from 60 to 180 degrees.

often depends on the specific educational objectives of the student. The research project offers the student an opportunity to study in depth a particular, and perhaps very limited, topic that will contribute to the overall purpose of the selected course of study. The student should consider whether the outcome of the project will also offer the journal readers new and useful information or new insight and perspectives on the subject. Only if the answer is affirmative should the process of editing begin. The review of literature, presentation of methods and results, and discussion will require the most work.

The review of the literature in the full document is usually extremely lengthy. The student does not want to miss any citation even remotely related to the topic, and must demonstrate to the faculty that indeed a complete search of the literature was made. The author who writes solely for publication is obliged to make the same thorough search, but must be more selective, including in the manuscript only those references that provide necessary, contemporary information and explicitly relevant background for the work. Here is a sample statement that might be found in a thesis:

> *Electromyography is the procedure of detecting and recording action potentials propagated along muscle membranes.*[8–10, 12–16, 18, 20]

For publication, the number of references cited could be reduced to one comprehensive review article on electromyography. Even more importantly, the entire statement can be omitted as it reflects common knowledge and contributes nothing new to the background of a study.

The author of every research paper is obliged to clearly and explicitly describe the method of study; however, a "blow-by-blow" description is usually unnecessary in a journal article, and can be very tedious for the reader. Often, minute details of the protocol are delineated in appendices of a thesis. For the journal article, the content of appendices must be explained in a few sentences.

Other appendices may contain all the raw data gathered during the investigation. Whereas the faculty advisor may need this information to guide the student or assess the work, journal readers do not need or want to see the raw data. Therefore, all the important information contained in those appendices must be synthesized and incorporated into the results section of the journal article.

The student turned journal author must carefully consider the emphasis of the discussion section. Two problems arise in preparing the discussion. First, perhaps because of a lack of confidence, the student hesitates to firmly interpret results and accomplishes nothing more than to reiterate the results. Second, implications of the findings and suggestions for further study are often confined to a description of what went wrong. Although presentation of the limitations of the study is important, it cannot be the only source of discussion. Indeed, if the limitations are overwhelming, the reader will begin to question the validity of the study.

Regarding style and organization of the adapted thesis or dissertation, one unique problem requires careful attention. In attempting to summarize or condense the lengthy document, the temptation is to "lift" sentences and paragraphs and to string these together to construct a shorter paper. The shorter paper may appear complete and clear to the authors because of their long-standing familiarity with the full document. Unfortunately, for the reader, snatches of information taken out of context may not be understandable. The text loses coherence and meaning. The solution to this problem is for the author to write a completely new document; and, when this new manuscript is prepared, it should be reviewed by colleagues who have not been involved with the study or the writing of the original thesis or dissertation.

Writing Style

The process of scientific writing "is not primarily a 'literary,' effort, but is an exercise in organization and clarity of expression."[5] The final written report should be strong, reflecting the objectivity and logic of the research project. We have reviewed the customary format and content of the research report to guide the author through the structural elements; however, the readability of the report depends on the author's skill in communicating with precision.[6] Readers complain that research reports are boring and difficult to follow. These complaints may have nothing to do with the subject but with sentence structure or the flow of ideas—the personal writing style of the author. Writing does not come easily to many of us; for some, it is most painful, but necessary to serve the goal of communicating the results of research.

We will not present a "style manual" in this text, but will highlight a few common problems and current issues that interfere with clear writing. A selection of useful references for developing and improving writing skills are cited at the end of this chapter. Even the most accomplished author may benefit from consulting such references, especially when the early drafts of a paper seem cumbersome.

People-First Consideration

Our patients or clients are indeed people first! It is incumbent on all of us to be sensitive to this basic human issue. We can easily reflect this in the description of subjects who have been studied. As examples, "Stroke patients" are patients who have had a stroke. "Learning-disabled children" are children who have learning disabilities. Attention to people-first language demonstrates an underlying respect that should be reflected in our scientific publications.

Active versus Passive Voice

A sentence written in **active voice** is powerful and concrete. **Passive voice** tends to make sentences ponderous and dull. The writer must create sentences that make the intended point most clearly. At times, the choice between active and passive voice is not so obvious. The following sentences illustrate the choices.

> *Passive*   One hour was spent by the raters to observe the patient's movement patterns so that the number of changes in static posture could be documented.

> *Active*   The raters spent one hour observing the patient's movement patterns to document the number of changes in static posture.

The emphasis is different in these two sentences. The amount of time is emphasized in the passive example, whereas the raters and their activity are highlighted in the active example. In addition, the active example is shorter by six words! Consider the following examples as well:

> *Passive*   Increased tension throughout the upper extremity and neck is produced by constant pain in the wrist.

> *Active*   Constant pain in the wrist increases tension throughout the upper extremity and neck.

The focus is very different in these two sentences. If the author is addressing the potential for dysfunction at sites remote from the pathology, then the first (passive) example may be best. If the author is developing a rationale for eliminating wrist pain, the active example may be more appropriate.

Passive voice may be appropriate when the subject of the sentence is unimportant or the object or action should be emphasized. For example, "Patients were randomly assigned . . ." conveys an important action, and the subject (who assigned) may not be important.

Superfluous passive expressions, such as "it has been suggested . . ." or "it is thought that . . ." usually distract the reader because they dilute the strength of the message. Who suggested? Who thought? In citing the work of others, authors should acknowledge the *who*, for example, "Jones and Brown suggested. . . ." In discussing present work, the authors might write "Our preliminary results indicate. . . ." Using active voice in such cases is direct and clear.

One special case should be discussed—the use of first-person active voice. For many years, authors went out of their way to avoid using first-person active voice with the notion that to use it detracts from the "scientific," "objective" nature of research reports. Now, the use of first person is acceptable in selected instances. When authors (researchers) are emphasizing their own actions, experiences, assumptions, or opinions, their writing may be more readable and indeed more accurate if they say "We think the logical interpretation of this finding is . . ." or "We found that this technique is. . . ." On the other hand, overuse of "I" and "we" can be intrusive, calling unnecessary attention to the authors, especially when purely scientific information is being conveyed. Presentation of techniques, procedures, and results requires attention to what was done and how, not who. Therefore, it is stronger to say "The subjects were asked to complete the questionnaire," rather than "I asked the subjects to complete the questionnaire."

Simplicity of Language

In conversation, we tend to use expressions and phrases that are spontaneous, but often superfluous to the point we are making. Many such expressions will be found in the early drafts of written work because of the natural effort to "speak" the text. Authors must, however, remain cognizant of the need to be concise in scientific writing. Many of the elements of creative writing that we learned in school, designed to create metaphors and add color to our words, should be discarded for scientific writing. Many authors try to use different words for the same concept to avoid being repetitious; however, where one word will make the point best, it is better to be repetitious than to be unclear or ambiguous. Adjectives and adverbs are especially useless for describing scientific findings. There is no need to say that an outcome is "very practical" or "extremely useful." It would be sufficient to be practical or useful for clinical care.

The use of expressions should also be tempered for scientific reports. Although it is certainly more interesting to read a paper that is written with variations in sentence structure, the purpose of an article is to communicate findings, not to create poetry. Here are a few examples of complex phrases that can usually be avoided:

in light of the fact that = because
with the exception of = except
in spite of the fact that = although
is designed to improve = improves
due to the fact that = because
was found to have = had
immediately prior to = before

In early drafts, there may be redundant phrases, such as "exactly identical" and "grouped together," and unnecessary qualifiers, such as "blue in color" and "end result." Correcting these kinds of errors is easy, if the author is looking for them.

Bates has presented a summary of "formulas" that can be employed to evaluate the "readability" of a manuscript.[6] One of these formulas is Gunning's "Fog Index," which was originally described in 1952. The Fog Index uses the average length of sentences and the percentage of "difficult" words to calculate a number that Gunning equated to a reader's school grade level. His formula is calculated as follows:

1. Choose a sample of 100 words or more.
2. Divide the number of words in the sample by the number of sentences to determine the average number of words in a sentence.
3. Divide the number of words of three or more syllables by the number of words in the sample to find the percentage of difficult words.
4. Add the average number of words in a sentence to the percentage of difficult words.
5. Multiply this total by 0.4 to obtain the Fog Index.

If we take a sample of 110 words, with 6 sentences and 18 words of three or more syllables, the average number of words per sentence is 18, and 16% are difficult words. The total would be 34 for a Fog Index of 13.6, rounded to 14. This sample with the score of 14 would be considered appropriate to the reading level of a college sophomore, according to Gunning. No one would mathematically evaluate an entire research report! When a manuscript seems tedious, however, the author might sample a few paragraphs. This process may be useful in editing to ensure that the "message" is not buried in verbiage.

THE POSTER PRESENTATION

A poster presentation is a report of research that is displayed on a large board so that it can be read and viewed by large groups in a casual atmosphere. Posters afford a special opportunity for researchers and their professional colleagues to exchange ideas in conference settings. Poster sessions are organized so that each poster is available for several hours. Sessions may be somewhat formalized by asking researchers to present a brief oral summary to an assembled group, with a moderator who guides a discussion around each poster in a symposium format. In another format, the open session, posters are displayed in an exhibit hall where interested participants view the posters in a less formal manner. In this case, the researcher is available to answer questions or engage in discussion. A major advantage of the poster presentation is that interested members of the audience can study the content and contemplate the implications of a study at a comfortable pace. The researcher has an opportunity to clarify or amplify details of the study. Observers' reactions or questions may be helpful in guiding future work and stimulating new ideas.

Content and Layout

The poster should contain the major elements of the study in a clear, brief series of statements including title, purpose, hypothesis or specific aims, method, results and discussion, and conclusions. The poster should be self-explanatory, but "telegraphic" in style; that is, content should include key words and phrases and not necessarily complete sentences. Tables, graphs, or photographs should summarize and illustrate important findings or unique aspects of the method. The most effective posters do not contain so much written material that the observer gets lost, but should be complete enough to allow the observer to understand the full intent of the study.

The conference sponsor will provide guidelines about the size and composition of the board that will be available. The customary size is 4 ft high and 6 or 8 ft wide. The composition is usually cork or particle board, so that thumb tacks can be used to hang sections of the poster.

In preparing a poster, a scaled template should be drawn, showing the arrangement of text and figures. The content elements can be moved about the template to find the best arrangement for the logical flow of information. Ordinarily, the eye follows from left to right as in reading. The introductory materials should be placed at the top left and the conclusion at the bottom right. Methods and results should be displayed prominently in the center. Figure 30.2 is a sample template for the arrangement of a poster.

Materials

Many facilities employ or have contracts with medical illustrators who have the appropriate materials and expertise to construct posters. Enlisting their help or consultation may be the most efficient way to create a poster; however, medical illustrations are usually quite

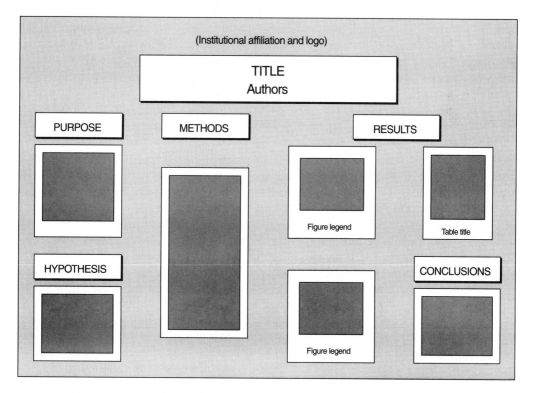

FIGURE 30.2 A sample template for the arrangement of a poster presentation.

expensive. Fortunately, computer software and laser printers can readily create text and graphics, so that mounting a poster can be greatly facilitated.

The effective poster should be legible and uncluttered with content presented in sharp contrast to its background. Text and figures can be mounted on colored poster board so that there is a contrasting border around each section. Letters for the title should be 2 in. high, headings should be at least 1 in. high, and text letters should be at least 0.5 in. high. The size and type of the text should be readable from 4 feet away.[7] The print should be bold with clear sharp edges. Sharp-contrast laser printers produce excellent images that can be photographically enlarged, or may be produced in large enough font to display directly.

THE ORAL PRESENTATION

Oral presentation of research findings in an open forum of colleagues is a time-honored tradition in medicine and science. This avenue of communication offers immediate, timely dissemination of new information. Like the poster presentation, it encourages direct interchange of ideas and stimulates consideration of new directions in research.

The notion of oral reporting is particularly attractive to those who consider writing a difficult task and speaking a much "freer," more comfortable, process; however, the oral report of research is not at all the same as conversational speaking. In conversation, ideas are conveyed spontaneously, with facial expressions or gestures for emphasis and opportunities to repeat or reconstruct a thought to clarify a point. In a formal presentation, which usually has a time limit of 10 or 15 minutes, each word and phrase must be carefully chosen to convey the speaker's message correctly. The message is emphasized and illustrated visually with slides or overhead transparencies. Unlike conversational speaking, the oral presentation of research is highly structured. Thorough planning and preparation, including practice, are required to ensure success.

Planning and Preparation

Most organizations select individuals to present oral papers on the basis of written abstracts submitted by the researchers. That written abstract can be the skeleton of the presentation because it contains the major elements of the research project. Indeed, the presenter is obliged to adhere to the topic as written in the abstract.

Because content must be well organized and because of the customary time limits, we suggest that the talk be written. From an initial draft, the speaker can adapt and refine the talk. Key words and phrases can be manipulated to improve precision and emphasis. Logical sequencing and transitions from thought to thought can be refined.

Most organizations require that speakers strictly adhere to the prescribed time limit. Therefore, even at this early stage, the text should be read aloud so the speaker begins to develop a sense of timing. Practice should include using visual materials. The experienced presenter may know that eight pages of double-spaced text including references to slides will be about a 10-minute talk. Each individual must acquire this sense of timing, for which there is no common formula. If the talk is too lengthy, the presenter must abbreviate the content. What can be eliminated? Is the background or introductory material too extensive? Have any extraneous, albeit interesting, sidelights been included? Is the talk complicated by falsely fancy words or jargon?

Editing may continue until the final product is ready, but the major elements must be in place early, so that the slides or overheads can be planned and prepared.

Visual Presentation

Visual aids are essential to the success of an oral presentation. Effective slides or overhead transparencies emphasize and illustrate the content of the presentation and focus the audience's attention to important details. On the other hand, a presentation can be destroyed by poorly constructed, overwhelming, or confusing slides. In this section, we discuss a few important guidelines for planning and preparing slides. These guidelines also apply to making overhead transparencies. As with poster presentations, slide preparation can be facilitated by consulting a medical illustrator or photographer.

The type and number of slides to use should be determined by identifying the key points of the written text. The most effective presentations use slides to accompany all parts of the paper, so that the listener is guided through each section of the presentation. Factors of production cost and the time allotted for the presentation may dictate how slides are used. Four types of slides may be presented: words or phrases (text), photographs, graphs, and tables. Word slides are customarily used to present the title of the presentation, the statement of the purpose or objectives, important background material, hypotheses, description of subjects and study protocol, summary of results, and conclusions. Photographs can illustrate aspects of the method such as the equipment setup or subject activity. Graphs and tables are used to demonstrate the results.

Word slides must be legible and should contain no more than six lines of text or 45 characters per line.[7] The distance between lines should be at least the height of the tallest letter. The choice of uppercase or lowercase lettering and typeface depends on the number of words and the spacing of phrases. Ornate, italic, and open typefaces are usually difficult to read. One guideline for the size of print for projection suggests that if the words and numbers on a slide can be read directly from a slide without a magnifier, people in the back of the room should be able to read them when projected. Figure 30.3A illustrates a slide that contains too many words to be an effective source of information to a large audience. Figure 30.3B shows how this information can be reduced to present major points, which would then be discussed by the presenter in greater detail. By highlighting each point, the listener can focus on each one as the presenter addresses it. In addition, the text is larger and less cluttered so that the listener can read it quickly and easily without being drawn away from the spoken material. The border of each of these "slides" is an example of a template drawn in proportion to a 34-mm slide.

The content of each slide and the verbal commentary must be synchronized. The audience cannot take in two separate subjects at one time. Because many of us are "visual learners," the presenter's remarks will be lost if the slide does not fit the talk. An uncoordinated presentation is distracting and will be received negatively.

Graphs and tables must be simple and easily understood. The amount of information included, of course, depends on how much is needed to present the results adequately. When a study has generated much data, the presenter may have to be selective in what to include in the presentation because listeners cannot absorb mounds of data in such a short time span. Generally, three comparison lines, or six bars on a graph, or four rows and columns in a table is a sensible limit. Legends, headings, and numbers should be large enough to be read easily.

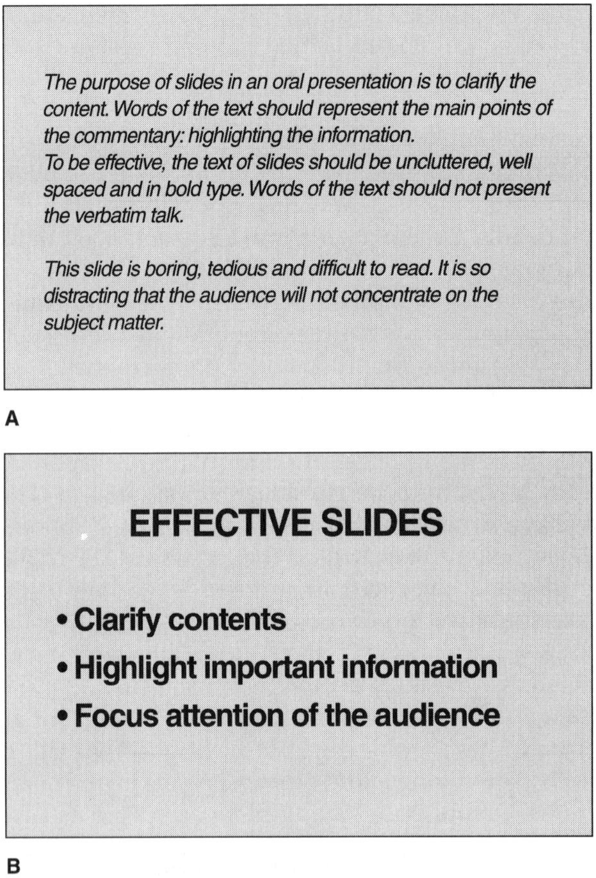

A

B

FIGURE 30.3 Illustration of slide content: (**A**) overcrowded; (**B**) summarized.

Many computer programs are now available for making slides and transparencies. These programs provide an array of background colors and print styles, as well as designs and patterns that can make slides more attractive. Researchers should be wary of making slides too busy or "glitzy." The background of the slide should not detract from the information it is trying to convey.

Rehearsal

After the presentation is written and slides are keyed to the text, rehearsal can begin. First, the presenter should go through the talk incorporating the slide presentation to be sure that the slides are synchronized properly with the verbal commentary and to confirm the length of the talk. Then, presentation to the "hometown" audience is warranted. Not only will staff members, fellow students, and faculty comment on or make suggestions for the presentation, but also they should be encouraged to ask questions, which may indicate the kind of questions that will come up in discussion following the formal conference presentation. Being well prepared for both the talk and the discussion will inspire confidence and ensure a professional performance.

COMMENTARY

Taking the Final Step

According to DeBakey, a written report of research findings should provide information that is new, true, important, and comprehensible.[9] These criteria can be applied to poster and oral presentations, as well. New treatment or measurement techniques may have been developed and tested. Effectiveness of intervention may have been demonstrated, reaffirmed, or refuted. The process of a study may have been valid and objective. The findings may have important implications for clinical practice. But who will know if the report is poorly prepared? Sheen presented the point this way: "As a scientific author, you must write so that you are understood or, perhaps more important, so that you are not misunderstood."[8]

The final step in the research process—to communicate the results—requires time: time to plan, time to write, time to revise. Early drafts of reports and presentations should be put away for awhile and then later reread with the intention of editing. The editorial board of a journal and sponsors of a conference establish rules and restrictions for the format and organization, but only the author can make a presentation clear, precise, and alive.

KEY TERMS

Instructions to Authors   active voice   passive voice
abstract

REFERENCES

1. International Committee of Medical Journal Editors. Uniform requirements for manuscripts submitted to biomedical journals. *JAMA* 1997;277:927.
2. American Psychological Association. *Publication Manual of the APA.* 3d ed. Washington, DC: APA, 1983.
3. American Medical Association. *Manual of Style.* 8th ed. Baltimore: Williams & Wilkins, 1989.
4. Gibaldi J. *MLA Style Manual and Guide to Scholarly Publishing.* 2d ed. New York: The Modern Language Association of America, 1998.
5. Staheli LT. *Speaking and Writing for the Physician.* New York: Raven Press, 1986.
6. Bates JD. *Writing with Precision.* Reston, VA: Acropolis Books Ltd., 1990.
7. *Creative Solutions Poster Presentation.* <http://www.best4health.org/html/poster4.htm> 14 May 1998.
8. Sheen AP. *Breathing Life into Medical Writing. A Handbook.* St. Louis: CV Mosby, 1982.
9. DeBakey L. *The Scientific Journal. Editorial Policies and Practices.* St. Louis: CV Mosby, 1976.

SUGGESTED ADDITIONAL READINGS

Alley M. *The Craft of Scientific Writing.* Englewood Cliffs, NJ: Prentice-Hall, 1987.
American Medical Association. *Manual of Style.* 8th ed. Baltimore: Williams & Wilkins, 1989.
Day RA. *How to Write and Publish a Scientific Paper.* 5th ed. Phoenix: Oryx Press, 1998.

Gibaldi J. *MLA Style Manual and Guide to Scholarly Publishing.* 2d ed. New York: The Modern Language Association of America, 1998.

Huth EJ. *How to Write and Publish Papers in the Medical Sciences.* 2d ed. Baltimore: Williams & Wilkins, 1990.

Portney L, Craik R. Sharing your research: platform and poster presentations. *PT Magazine* 1998;6:72–81.

Strunk W, White EB. *The Elements of Style,* 3d ed. New York: MacMillan, 1979.

Zinsser W. *On Writing Well,* 3d ed. New York: Harper & Row, 1988.

31

Evaluating Research Reports

The link between research and clinical practice in health professions must be made by those who read reports of completed research. As consumers of research, we have a responsibility to evaluate research reports to determine whether the findings provide sufficient evidence to support the effectiveness of current practices or offer alternatives that will improve patient care. Our professional advancement depends on incorporating research findings into our scheme of making clinical judgments and treatment decisions.

For most of us, it is neither practical nor possible to read the plethora of material presented each month in professional journals. Therefore, the first step in effective reading is to select publications and articles that offer the most useful information. When a particular topic is important to practice, readers may consider going to the library to find textbooks or review articles that cite many references from the research literature. Books and review articles are useful for acquiring a basic, often in-depth, understanding of a topic; however, we have to realize that the information is secondhand, presented from the perspective of another: the textbook or review article author. The problem is one of interpretation; the original research may be misrepresented or inadequately described. The solution is that consumers of research must study the firsthand reports of researchers to judge the merits of the work.

The purpose of this chapter is to present a practical approach for critically reading and evaluating published literature. Authors may use this approach to review their own manuscripts before submitting them for publication. Although this chapter focuses on the written research report, the approach also applies to the evaluation of oral and poster presentations.

ANALYZING CONTENT OF AN ARTICLE

The purpose of critical analysis of a research report is to determine its worth, which depends on the validity of the project as it is reported. The structure and content elements of research reports have been described in Chapter 30. In this chapter we outline the kinds of questions readers should ask during their critical reviews.

One of the first considerations in evaluating the scientific merit of an article is the reputation of the journal. Scientific journals are generally *refereed,* which means that the articles have been subjected to review by content experts and accepted for publication on the basis of reviewer evaluation. The editors and reviewers of refereed journals follow policies and procedures designed to ensure that published articles meet defined criteria. De-Bakey[1] has outlined the elements of a manuscript that reviewers are customarily asked to evaluate. These include importance of the research, originality, appropriateness of the research design, adequacy of the method, soundness of conclusions and interpretation, relevance of the discussion, and clarity of writing. The manuscript review process is similar, in fact, to the way in which responsible readers will evaluate published articles. Important information is presented in nonrefereed journals; however, readers must realize that the contents of those publications have not been scrutinized in the same way as those in refereed journals.

Title and Abstract

Readers begin their evaluation of an article at the top, by reading the title and abstract. Titles should be informative, but are often so abbreviated that the reader is unable to learn much about content other than the general topic. If the reader is interested in the topic, then the next step is to read the abstract. Abstracts of research papers will include fairly specific information about the purpose, method, results, and major conclusions of the presented work. When readers decide that the results and conclusions stated in the abstract could be useful and could be applied to their practice, their decision should be to continue into the body of the paper. The abstract should never be taken at face value. Without studying the details of the report, there is no way to be sure that the study was valid. There is simply not enough substance to make that judgment.

Introduction

By the time the introductory paragraphs of an article have been read, readers should understand the overall problem that provided the impetus for the study. The following questions focus the evaluation of the introduction:

- What is the problem? Has it been clearly stated? Why is it important?
- How has the author used the literature to form a sound and logical rationale?
- What is the theoretical context for the study?
- Are references appropriate and comprehensive?
- Is the study descriptive, exploratory, or experimental?
- What is the specific purpose?
- What are hypotheses or guiding questions?

In the opening sentences of an article, the author should establish the problem being investigated. The reader should not have to search to figure out what the study is all about. The background material should demonstrate that the researchers have thoughtfully and thoroughly reviewed the relevant literature. They should have synthesized the literature, the related theoretical models, their experiences, and their perspectives of the problem. This synthesis should provide a rationale for pursuing this line of research. Readers should be convinced that the study was needed. Most important, the specific purpose or aims of the study should have been clearly stated and the research question should be evident early in the article. The authors of an experimental study may have explicitly stated the hypotheses that were to be tested. If not, readers should be able to determine what the researchers expected to find, based on the content of the introduction. From these statements, readers should know whether the study is designed to be descriptive, exploratory, or experimental research.

If the answers to the preceding questions are satisfactory, readers should be content that the direction of this work is correct and meaningful. They should be able to anticipate the methods that would be appropriate to answer the research question. If any of these questions cannot be answered, readers must wonder about the critical thinking of the researchers and the validity of everything that follows.

Methods

Each part of the methods section must be evaluated. Readers may be tempted to slide through this section because of its detail, but this is not fair and may lead readers to accept the findings and conclusions with inappropriate certainty. This section contains the essential information that allows the reader to judge the validity of the study. Flaws or omissions detected in the methods section affect the usefulness of interpretations derived from the study.

Subjects

Readers must know who the subjects were, to interpret the validity of conclusions and to understand the extent to which the findings can be applied to clinical situations. The following questions should be considered:

- Who were the subjects?
- What were inclusion and exclusion criteria?
- How were subjects selected, and from what population were they chosen?
- How many subjects were studied? Is the sample size adequate?

The answers to these questions will help to determine whether sampling bias might have existed and to identify other potential confounding factors. Age, gender, diagnosis, and level of function of the subjects are among the many factors that may affect both the internal and external validity of findings. Inclusion and exclusion criteria should be specified so that the target population for the study is clearly identified. If readers want to apply the findings to their clinical practice, the attributes of the study's subjects must fit with their clinical population or, at least, should not be so different as to be irrelevant. For example, many research studies, especially those done by students, use normal, healthy individuals who are convenient subjects, but results from such studies are probably not applicable to patients. Readers will be able to make the decision about applicability if the authors have defined the sample well enough. It is also essential to know if the subjects form a sample of convenience, or if they represent a random sample of a larger population. In studies using surveys, the respondents who return their questionnaires may have characteristics different from those who did not choose to respond.

The number of subjects in a study is an important consideration when interpreting the results of the statistical analysis. Specifically, failure to demonstrate statistically significant differences should not be assumed to mean that no difference truly exists. The possibility of a Type II error resulting from an inadequate sample size should be considered.

Design

The researchers will have chosen from the number of true experimental, quasi-experimental, or nonexperimental designs and should have clearly described their choice. Part III of this book describes these research designs with examples of their application. Based on the specific stated purpose of the project, readers should be able to judge the appropriateness of the choice that the researchers made.

> - What is the research design? Is it appropriate for answering the research question?
> - How many groups were tested?
> - How were subjects assigned to groups?
> - Was a randomization procedure used?
> - Was a control group used?
> - What are the independent variables? How many levels do they have?
> - How often were treatments and measurements applied?

There are at least three important reasons for readers to pay attention to the design of a study. First, the balance between issues of internal validity and generalizability has to be scrutinized. When true experimental designs are employed with the strict control inherent in these designs, readers should consider how to relate the findings to their "real world." In the "experimental" setting, where confounding factors and internal validity are rigorously controlled, the effects of manipulating or imposing the independent variable can be accepted with a high degree of confidence. But, have these controls created such an "artificial" situation that it would be unrealistic to expect the same outcome when methods or procedures are implemented in clinical practice? On the other hand, if quasi-experimental designs or descriptive methods are employed, readers must be alert to the possibility that extraneous variables have interfered with the interpretation of the results. The validity of an experimental or quasi-experimental study will depend in large part on how subjects are assigned to groups and whether a control group was included in the design. As an example, when intact groups are used, the author should specify the basis on which the subjects were grouped. Patients may be recruited from a particular hospital, or children may be assigned to groups based on reading readiness. The author should then consider what differences might exist between hospitals or reading groups that might influence how the subjects will respond. Second, the number of groups, the number or levels of independent variables, the number of dependent variables, and the frequency of measurements will influence the selection of statistical analysis procedures. Part IV of this book illustrates the integral relationship between research design and statistical analysis. Third, if the researchers have chosen a single-case design (Chapter 12) or the sequential clinical trials model (Chapter 11), readers should be aware of the special rules that apply and can then determine whether the study procedures follow those rules.

Instrumentation

The instrumentation section should describe the measurement tools or equipment used in the study.

- Is instrumentation described in sufficient detail?
- How have the authors documented the reliability and validity of the instruments?

Readers should know what specific devices were used. If these are standard and commercially available, the model numbers and names and addresses of manufacturers must be included. If they are standardized questionnaires or survey instruments, references must be cited.

The question of reliability relates to the reproducibility and consistency of measurements. Three aspects of reliability need to be evaluated.

1. The reliability of the instrument itself, as a piece of "hardware" or as a "paper" instrument, should be documented. Hardware, such as strain gauges and electrogoniometers, must be calibrated regularly and tested against standards such as calibrated weights and angles. Paper instruments, such as attitudinal surveys and health status questionnaires, must also be tested for internal consistency. Readers should find evidence that instrumental reliability has been determined.
2. Evidence of intra- or interrater reliability should be discussed when the measurement method involves direct participation of testers. This should be

determined through replicate testing performed by the researchers and the data subjected to analysis using appropriate reliability statistics.

3. Reliability should be established for the specific population being studied, for the dependent variable being measured, and for the conditions of the research project. For example, a procedure for testing grip strength using a dynamometer may be highly reliable when used to test normal subjects, but will it be reliable when used to test patients with wrist pain? Does reliability differ if measurements are taken at home or in the clinic? If functional status is being reported, was it determined by self-report, interview, or observation?

Validity of measurement instruments or procedures refers to their ability to measure what they are supposed to measure. The concept of validity is complex, but, at least, readers should be satisfied that the instruments used to collect data are designed to do so in an accurate, relevant manner. Where validity is questionable, the author should provide examples of the instrument's use in other studies that may support its use for this project.

Procedures

The description of procedures should report the sequence of events from beginning to end. The following questions should be asked about the data collection methods:

- Are data collection procedures described clearly and in sufficient detail to allow replication?
- What are operational definitions for all variables?
- How have threats to internal validity been controlled?

The data collection methods should include who performed the measurements, what the subjects were asked to do, what the data collectors did, and when and how often measurements were taken. In observational studies, the circumstances surrounding measurement will be important. In experimental studies, the control group subjects may have been undergoing a comparison treatment or may have been asked to follow particular rules, such as to rest or to refrain from eating for 2 hours before testing. Experimental group subjects will have been subjected to the independent variable(s) as operationally defined. All of these activities must be described in sufficient detail so that readers could, in a similar setting with similar subjects, replicate the study procedures.

Most authors do not address issues of internal validity directly in their description of procedures. It is the reader's responsibility to consider if the effects of history, maturation, attrition, instrumentation, testing, and selection are affecting the observed changes (see Chapter 9).

Data Analysis

Both descriptive and inferential statistical analyses should be identified. The researcher should satisfy the following questions:

- What statistical procedures were used? Are they appropriate to analyze the data?
- Has the author justified the use of any unique or unusual statistical tests?
- Has the author addressed each research question in the analysis?
- What alpha level was used for the level of significance?

If inferential statistics were used, the acceptable significance level, such as $\alpha = .05$, should have been established by the researchers and reported. The statistical tests should be described not merely by name, but by specifying to which data the analyses were applied. This information is necessary for readers to evaluate the appropriateness of the analyses. The use or misuse of statistics should be judged on the basis of two major factors: the nature of measurements (scale, reliability, linearity, and so on) and the study design (the number of groups or variables and frequency of measurement). For example, the reader should determine if parametric statistics were used when nonparametric procedures would have been more appropriate, or if multiple t-tests were used to compare several groups when an analysis of variance should have been used. Discrepancies in the proper application of statistical tests interfere with the statistical conclusion validity of the study and detract from the interpretation of the data.

Results

The results section must report the findings of the study without interpretation or commentary.

- Do the results address the research question?
- Are figures and tables presented accurately? Do they complement the text?
- Has each hypothesis or specific aim been addressed?
- Are the results statistically significant?

Readers should find a narrative description presented in the order of the stated purposes, aims, or hypotheses. The results should be used to clearly answer each research question. Either in the text or in graphs and tables, the outcome of statistical analyses must be reported. Typically, the author includes the test statistic value, such as the t or F, the degrees of freedom, and the associated p-value (if not significant, the abbreviation

"NS" may be used). Readers should be able to associate the findings and the statistical significance of the results by reading that information.

The narrative description of findings may be illustrated or complemented with figures and tables to clarify and summarize the descriptive characteristics of the data. Readers should study graphs and tables carefully. They should be complete, but not too complex. It is a useful exercise to compare data from tables with information found in the text, to be sure that the discussion of results follows what was actually reported.

Readers should also note whether all subjects are accounted for in the statistical results. When the displayed data show a different (usually fewer) number of subjects than stated in the subjects section, the authors should explain. Were some lost to follow-up, did they drop out of the study, or did something go wrong with the data collection process? Missing information that is unexplained should lead readers to suspect a biased presentation. Authors should include information on subject adherence to the research protocol and data analysis strategies to deal with noncompliant subjects.

Discussion and Conclusions

Before studying the authors' discussion and conclusions, readers should carefully review the methods and results, to judge the validity of the study and the outcome and to have the necessary information to answer these questions.

- How does the author interpret results?
- Did the author clarify if hypotheses were rejected or accepted?
- What alternative explanations does the author consider for the obtained findings?
- How are the findings related to prior reports?
- What limitations are described? Are there limitations that are not addressed?
- If results are not significant, does the author consider the possibility of Type II error?
- Regardless of the statistical outcome, are the results clinically important?
- Does the author discuss how the results apply to practice?
- Does the author present suggestions for further study?
- Do the stated conclusions flow logically from the obtained results?

Readers should find a clear statement of the authors' major conclusions based on their interpretation of the results and research hypotheses. Throughout the discussion section, readers should find answers. The authors should compare and contrast results with other related work, to offer support for existing clinical theory or propose an alternative theory or explanation. The authors should acknowledge factors about the subjects, materials, or methods that could have complicated the interpretation of the results. As the authors discuss the limitations, they should share their ideas for approaching the research question differently. On the other hand, if the authors expressed confidence in the design and execution of the study and, therefore, have confidence in the results, they should suggest a direction that future studies might take. Finally, and perhaps most important, the authors should discuss the impact of the results on clinical practice. Is their evidence strong enough to suggest a need to change some aspect of treatment intervention or practice models? As critical consumers of the products of clinical research, readers should study the discussion and conclusion sections of the research report to decide whether the authors' answers to these kinds of questions are true, appropriate, and justified.

COMMENTARY

The Reader's View

The final published report of research does not end the story of the project. Readers have an opportunity to comment in the journal that published the report by submitting a letter to the editor or by being invited by the editor to present a formal commentary that will accompany the report at the time of publication. The purpose of responding or reacting to reports through the journal is to offer points of view that may differ from those of the researchers or to raise questions about some aspect of the research design, methods, or interpretation of results. Comments should never be confrontational or degrading, but should provide constructive criticisms or may offer evidence to support the published findings. Written dialogue between researchers and respondents may stimulate new ideas for keeping their line of research alive. Readers should look for and evaluate letters or commentaries with the same kind of scrutiny that they applied to the evaluation of the original report.

Critical analysis of research reports is a skill that must be developed and practiced. We offer one caveat. As one develops this ability, there is a tendency to be overly critical, finding many flaws, major and minor, real and potential. Because of the nature of clinical research, there will always be some aspects of the design that could have been tighter or cleaner. The important element is whether the limitations in the design are so great that the findings are useless. In refereed journals these flaws are not likely to be "fatal"; that is, the articles that make it to the publication stage have been screened. Regardless of the imperfections that exist in the clinical research process, we must remember to find the merits of each project and accept them in the context of the entire endeavor. With careful attention to the details of all research reports we choose to read, we should expect to learn something valuable from each one.

REFERENCES

1. DeBakey L. *The Scientific Journal. Editorial Policies and Procedures.* St. Louis: CV Mosby, 1976.

A

Statistical Tables

TABLE A.1   AREAS UNDER THE NORMAL CURVE (z)

z	Area between 0 and z	Area above z	z	Area between 0 and z	Area above z	z	Area between 0 and z	Area above z
0.00	.0000	.5000	0.40	.1554	.3446	0.80	.2881	.2119
0.01	.0040	.4960	0.41	.1591	.3409	0.81	.2910	.2090
0.02	.0080	.4920	0.42	.1628	.3372	0.82	.2939	.2061
0.03	.0120	.4880	0.43	.1664	.3336	0.83	.2967	.2033
0.04	.0160	.4840	0.44	.1700	.3300	0.84	.2995	.2005
0.05	.0199	.4801	0.45	.1736	.3264	0.85	.3023	.1977
0.06	.0239	.4761	0.46	.1772	.3228	0.86	.3051	.1949
0.07	.0279	.4721	0.47	.1808	.3192	0.87	.3078	.1922
0.08	.0319	.4681	0.48	.1844	.3156	0.88	.3106	.1894
0.09	.0359	.4641	0.49	.1879	.3121	0.89	.3133	.1867
0.10	.0398	.4602	0.50	.1915	.3085	0.90	.3159	.1841
0.11	.0438	.4562	0.51	.1950	.3050	0.91	.3186	.1814
0.12	.0478	.4522	0.52	.1985	.3015	0.92	.3212	.1788
0.13	.0517	.4483	0.53	.2019	.2981	0.93	.3238	.1762
0.14	.0557	.4443	0.54	.2054	.2946	0.94	.3264	.1736
0.15	.0596	.4404	0.55	.2088	.2912	0.95	.3289	.1711
0.16	.0636	.4364	0.56	.2123	.2877	0.96	.3315	.1685
0.17	.0675	.4325	0.57	.2157	.2843	0.97	.3340	.1660
0.18	.0714	.4286	0.58	.2190	.2810	0.98	.3365	.1635
0.19	.0753	.4247	0.59	.2224	.2776	0.99	.3389	.1611
0.20	.0793	.4207	0.60	.2257	.2743	1.00	.3413	.1587
0.21	.0832	.4168	0.61	.2291	.2709	1.01	.3438	.1562
0.22	.0871	.4129	0.62	.2324	.2676	1.02	.3461	.1539
0.23	.0910	.4090	0.63	.2357	.2643	1.03	.3485	.1515
0.24	.0948	.4052	0.64	.2389	.2611	1.04	.3508	.1492
0.25	.0987	.4013	0.65	.2422	.2578	1.05	.3531	.1469
0.26	.1026	.3974	0.66	.2454	.2546	1.06	.3554	.1446
0.27	.1064	.3936	0.67	.2486	.2514	1.07	.3577	.1423
0.28	.1103	.3897	0.68	.2517	.2483	1.08	.3599	.1401
0.29	.1141	.3859	0.69	.2549	.2451	1.09	.3621	.1379
0.30	.1179	.3821	0.70	.2580	.2420	1.10	.3643	.1357
0.31	.1217	.3783	0.71	.2611	.2389	1.11	.3665	.1335
0.32	.1255	.3745	0.72	.2642	.2358	1.12	.3686	.1314
0.33	.1293	.3707	0.73	.2673	.2327	1.13	.3708	.1292
0.34	.1331	.3669	0.74	.2704	.2296	1.14	.3729	.1271
0.35	.1368	.3632	0.75	.2734	.2266	1.15	.3749	.1251
0.36	.1406	.3594	0.76	.2764	.2236	1.16	.3770	.1230
0.37	.1443	.3557	0.77	.2794	.2206	1.17	.3790	.1210
0.38	.1480	.3520	0.78	.2823	.2177	1.18	.3810	.1190
0.39	.1517	.3483	0.79	.2852	.2148	1.19	.3830	.1170

TABLE A.1 *Continued*

z	Area between 0 and z	Area above z	z	Area between 0 and z	Area above z	z	Area between 0 and z	Area above z
1.20	.3849	.1151	1.60	.4452	.0548	2.00	.4772	.0228
1.21	.3869	.1131	1.61	.4463	.0537	2.01	.4778	.0222
1.22	.3888	.1112	1.62	.4474	.0526	2.02	.4783	.0217
1.23	.3907	.1093	1.63	.4484	.0516	2.03	.4788	.0212
1.24	.3925	.1075	1.64	.4495	.0505	2.04	.4793	.0207
			1.645	**.4500**	**.0500**			
1.25	.3944	.1056	1.65	.4505	.0495	2.05	.4798	.0202
1.26	.3962	.1038	1.66	.4515	.0485	**2.054**	**.4800**	**.0200**
1.27	.3980	.1020	1.67	.4525	.0475	2.06	.4803	.0197
1.28	.3997	.1003	1.68	.4535	.0465	2.07	.4808	.0192
1.29	.4015	.0985	1.69	.4545	.0455	2.08	.4812	.0188
						2.09	.4817	.0183
1.30	.4032	.0968	1.70	.4554	.0446	2.10	.4821	.0179
1.31	.4049	.0951	1.71	.4564	.0436	2.11	.4826	.0174
1.32	.4066	.0934	1.72	.4573	.0427	2.12	.4830	.0170
1.33	.4082	.0918	1.73	.4582	.0418	2.13	.4834	.0166
1.34	.4099	.0901	1.74	.4591	.0409	2.14	.4838	.0162
1.35	.4115	.0885	1.75	.4599	.0401	2.15	.4842	.0158
1.36	.4131	.0869	**1.751**	**.4600**	**.0400**	2.16	.4846	.0154
1.37	.4147	.0853	1.76	.4608	.0392	2.17	.4850	.0150
1.38	.4162	.0838	1.77	.4616	.0384	2.18	.4854	.0146
1.39	.4177	.0823	1.78	.4625	.0375	2.19	.4857	.0143
			1.79	.4633	.0367			
1.40	.4192	.0808	1.80	.4641	.0359	2.20	.4861	.0139
1.41	.4207	.0793	1.81	.4649	.0351	2.21	.4864	.0136
1.42	.4222	.0778	1.82	.4656	.0344	2.22	.4868	.0132
1.43	.4236	.0764	1.83	.4664	.0336	2.23	.4871	.0129
1.44	.4251	.0749	1.84	.4671	.0329	2.24	.4875	.0125
1.45	.4265	.0735	1.85	.4678	.0322	2.25	.4878	.0122
1.46	.4279	.0721	1.86	.4686	.0314	2.26	.4881	.0119
1.47	.4292	.0708	1.87	.4693	.0307	2.27	.4884	.0116
1.48	.4306	.0694	1.88	.4699	.0301	2.28	.4887	.0113
1.49	.4319	.0681	**1.881**	**.4700**	**.0300**	2.29	.4890	.0110
			1.89	.4706	.0294			
1.50	.4332	.0668	1.90	.4713	.0287	2.30	.4893	.0107
1.51	.4345	.0655	1.91	.4719	.0281	2.31	.4896	.0104
1.52	.4357	.0643	1.92	.4726	.0274	2.32	.4898	.0102
1.53	.4370	.0630	1.93	.4732	.0268	**2.326**	**.4900**	**.0100**
1.54	.4382	.0618	1.94	.4738	.0262	2.33	.4901	.0099
						2.34	.4904	.0096
1.55	.4394	.0606	1.95	.4744	.0256	2.35	.4906	.0094
1.56	.4406	.0594	**1.96**	**.4750**	**.0250**	2.36	.4909	.0091
1.57	.4418	.0582	1.97	.4756	.0244	2.37	.4911	.0089
1.58	.4429	.0571	1.98	.4761	.0239	2.38	.4913	.0087
1.59	.4441	.0559	1.99	.4767	.0233	2.39	.4916	.0084

Continued

z	Area between 0 and z	Area above z	z	Area between 0 and z	Area above z	z	Area between 0 and z	Area above z
2.40	.4918	.0082	**2.75**	**.4970**	**.0030**	3.10	.49903	.00097
2.41	.4920	.0080	2.76	.4971	.0029	3.11	.49906	.00094
2.42	.4922	.0078	2.77	.4972	.0028	3.12	.49910	.00090
2.43	.4925	.0075	2.78	.4973	.0027	3.13	.49913	.00087
2.44	.4927	.0073	2.79	.4974	.0026	3.14	.49916	.00084
2.45	.4929	.0071	2.80	.4974	.0026	3.15	.49918	.00082
2.46	.4931	.0069	2.81	.4975	.0025	3.16	.49921	.00079
2.47	.4932	.0068	2.82	.4976	.0024	3.17	.49924	.00076
2.48	.4934	.0066	2.83	.4977	.0023	3.18	.49926	.00074
2.49	.4936	.0064	2.84	.4977	.0023	3.19	.49929	.00071
2.50	.4938	.0062	2.85	.4978	.0022	3.20	.49931	.00069
2.51	.4940	.0060	2.86	.4979	.0021	3.21	.49934	.00066
2.52	.4941	.0059	2.87	.4979	.0021	3.22	.49936	.00064
2.53	.4943	.0057	**2.88**	**.4980**	**.0020**	3.23	.49938	.00062
2.54	.4945	.0055	2.89	.4981	.0019	3.24	.49940	.00060
2.55	.4946	.0054	2.90	.4981	.0019	3.25	.49942	.00058
2.56	.4948	.0052	2.91	.4982	.0018	3.26	.49944	.00056
2.57	.4949	.0051	2.92	.4982	.0018	3.27	.49946	.00054
2.576	**.4950**	**.0050**	2.93	.4983	.0017	3.28	.49948	.00052
2.58	.4951	.0049	2.94	.4984	.0016	**3.29**	**.49950**	**.00050**
2.59	.4952	.0048						
2.60	.4953	.0047	2.95	.4984	.0016	3.30	.49951	.00048
2.61	.4955	.0045	2.96	.4985	.0015	3.31	.49953	.00047
2.62	.4956	.0044	2.97	.4985	.0015	3.32	.49955	.00045
2.63	.4957	.0043	2.98	.4986	.0014	3.33	.49957	.00043
2.64	.4959	.0041	2.99	.4986	.0014	3.34	.49958	.00042
2.65	**.4960**	**.0040**	3.00	.4987	.0013	3.35	.49960	.00040
2.66	.4961	.0039	3.01	.4987	.0013	3.36	.49961	.00039
2.67	.4962	.0038	3.02	.4987	.0013	3.37	.49962	.00038
2.68	.4963	.0037	3.03	.4988	.0012	3.38	.49964	.00036
2.69	.4964	.0036	3.04	.4998	.0012	3.39	.49965	.00035
2.70	.4965	.0035	3.05	.49886	.00114	3.40	.49966	.00034
2.71	.4966	.0034	3.06	.49889	.00111	3.45	.49972	.00028
2.72	.4967	.0033	3.07	.49893	.00107	3.50	.49977	.00023
2.73	.4968	.0032	3.08	.49896	.00104	3.60	.49984	.00016
2.74	.4969	.0031	**3.09**	**.49900**	**.00100**	3.70	.49989	.00011
						3.80	.49993	.00007
						3.90	.49995	.00005
						4.00	.49997	.00003

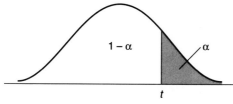

One-tailed test (α_1)

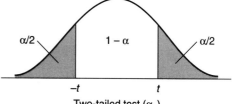

Two-tailed test (α_2)

TABLE A.2 CRITICAL VALUES OF *t*

df	α_1	.10	.05	.025	.01	.005	.0005
	α_2	.20	.10	.05	.02	.01	.001
1		3.078	6.314	12.706	31.821	63.657	636.619
2		1.886	2.920	4.303	6.965	9.925	31.598
3		1.638	2.353	3.182	4.541	5.841	12.924
4		1.533	2.132	2.776	3.747	4.604	8.610
5		1.476	2.015	2.571	3.365	4.032	6.859
6		1.440	1.943	2.447	3.143	3.707	5.959
7		1.415	1.895	2.365	2.998	3.499	5.405
8		1.397	1.860	2.306	2.896	3.355	5.041
9		1.383	1.833	2.262	2.821	3.250	4.781
10		1.372	1.812	2.228	2.764	3.169	4.587
11		1.363	1.796	2.201	2.718	3.106	4.437
12		1.356	1.782	2.179	2.681	3.055	4.318
13		1.350	1.771	2.160	2.650	3.012	4.221
14		1.345	1.761	2.145	2.624	2.977	4.140
15		1.341	1.753	2.131	2.602	2.947	4.073
16		1.337	1.746	2.120	2.583	2.921	4.015
17		1.333	1.740	2.110	2.457	2.898	3.965
18		1.330	1.734	2.101	2.552	2.878	3.922
19		1.328	1.729	2.093	2.539	2.861	3.883
20		1.325	1.725	2.086	2.528	2.845	3.850
21		1.323	1.721	2.080	2.518	2.831	3.819
22		1.321	1.717	2.074	2.508	2.819	3.792
23		1.319	1.714	2.069	2.500	2.807	3.767
24		1.318	1.711	2.064	2.492	2.797	3.745
25		1.316	1.708	2.060	2.485	2.787	3.725
26		1.315	1.706	2.056	2.479	2.779	3.707
27		1.314	1.703	2.052	2.473	2.771	3.690
28		1.313	1.701	2.048	2.467	2.763	3.674
29		1.311	1.699	2.045	2.462	2.756	3.659
30		1.310	1.694	2.042	2.457	2.750	3.646
40		1.303	1.684	2.021	2.423	2.704	3.551
60		1.296	1.671	2.000	2.390	2.660	3.460
120		1.289	1.658	1.980	2.358	2.617	3.373
∞		1.282	1.645	1.960	2.326	2.576	3.291

For unpaired *t*-test $df = (n_1-1) + (n_2-1)$. For paired *t*-test, $df = n - 1$. Test statistic must be greater than or equal to critical value to reject H_b.

Abridged from Table III in Fisher FA, Yates F. *Statistical Tables for Biological, Agricultural, and Medical Research.* Published by Longman Group UK, Ltd, 1974. Used with permission.

TABLE A.3(I) CRITICAL VALUES OF F, $\alpha = .05$

df_e for denominator	df_b for numerator															
	1	2	3	4	5	6	7	8	9	10	12	15	20	30	60	∞
1	161.4	199.5	215.7	224.6	230.2	234.0	236.8	238.9	240.5	241.9	243.9	245.9	248.0	250.1	252.2	254.3
2	18.51	19.00	19.16	19.25	19.30	19.33	19.35	19.37	19.38	19.40	19.41	19.43	19.45	19.46	19.48	19.50
3	10.13	9.55	9.28	9.12	9.01	8.64	8.89	8.85	8.81	8.79	8.74	8.70	8.66	8.62	8.57	8.53
4	7.71	6.94	6.59	6.39	6.26	6.16	6.09	6.04	6.00	5.96	5.91	5.86	5.80	5.75	5.69	5.63
5	6.61	5.79	5.41	5.19	5.05	4.95	4.88	4.82	4.77	4.74	4.68	4.62	4.56	4.50	4.43	4.36
6	5.99	5.14	4.76	4.53	4.39	4.28	4.21	4.15	4.10	4.06	4.00	3.94	3.87	3.81	3.74	3.67
7	5.59	4.74	4.35	4.12	3.97	3.87	3.79	3.73	3.68	3.64	3.57	3.51	3.44	3.38	3.30	3.23
8	5.32	4.46	4.07	3.84	3.69	3.58	3.50	3.44	3.39	3.35	3.28	3.22	3.15	3.08	3.01	2.93
9	5.12	4.26	3.86	3.63	3.48	3.37	3.29	3.23	3.18	3.14	3.07	3.01	2.94	2.86	2.79	2.71
10	4.96	4.10	3.71	3.48	3.33	3.22	3.14	3.07	3.02	2.98	2.91	2.85	2.77	2.70	2.62	2.54
11	4.84	3.98	3.59	3.36	3.20	3.09	3.01	2.95	2.90	2.85	2.79	2.72	2.65	2.57	2.49	2.40
12	4.75	3.89	3.49	3.26	3.11	3.00	2.91	2.85	2.80	2.75	2.69	2.62	2.54	2.47	2.38	2.30
13	4.67	3.81	3.41	3.18	3.03	2.92	2.83	2.77	2.71	2.67	2.60	2.53	2.46	2.38	2.30	2.21
14	4.60	3.74	3.34	3.11	2.96	2.85	2.76	2.70	2.65	2.60	2.53	2.46	2.39	2.31	2.22	2.13
15	4.54	3.68	3.29	3.06	2.90	2.79	2.71	2.64	2.59	2.54	2.48	2.40	2.33	2.25	2.16	2.07

TABLE A.3(l)—Continued

| df_e for denominator | \multicolumn{16}{c}{df_b for numerator} |
	1	2	3	4	5	6	7	8	9	10	12	15	20	30	60	∞
16	4.49	3.63	3.24	3.01	2.85	2.74	2.66	2.59	2.54	2.49	2.42	2.35	2.28	2.19	2.11	2.01
17	4.45	3.59	3.20	2.96	2.81	2.70	2.61	2.55	2.49	2.45	2.38	2.31	2.23	2.15	2.06	1.96
18	4.41	3.55	3.16	2.93	2.77	2.66	2.58	2.51	2.46	2.41	2.34	2.27	2.19	2.11	2.02	1.92
19	4.38	3.52	3.13	2.90	2.74	2.63	2.54	2.48	2.42	2.38	2.31	2.23	2.16	2.07	1.98	1.88
20	4.35	3.49	3.10	2.87	2.71	2.60	2.51	2.45	2.39	2.35	2.28	2.20	2.12	2.04	1.95	1.84
21	4.32	3.47	3.07	2.84	2.68	2.57	2.49	2.42	2.37	2.32	2.25	2.18	2.10	2.01	1.92	1.81
22	4.30	3.44	3.05	2.82	2.66	2.55	2.46	2.40	2.34	2.30	2.23	2.15	2.07	1.98	1.89	1.78
23	4.28	3.42	3.03	2.80	2.64	2.53	2.44	2.37	2.32	2.27	2.20	2.13	2.05	1.96	1.86	1.76
24	4.26	3.40	3.01	2.78	2.62	2.51	2.42	2.36	2.30	2.25	2.18	2.11	2.03	1.94	1.84	1.73
25	4.24	3.39	2.99	2.76	2.60	2.49	2.40	2.34	2.28	2.24	2.16	2.09	2.01	1.92	1.82	1.71
26	4.23	3.37	2.98	2.74	2.59	2.47	2.39	2.32	2.27	2.22	2.15	2.07	1.99	1.90	1.80	1.69
27	4.21	3.35	2.96	2.73	2.57	2.46	2.37	2.31	2.25	2.20	2.13	2.06	1.97	1.88	1.79	1.67
28	4.20	3.34	2.95	2.71	2.56	2.45	3.26	2.29	2.24	2.19	2.12	2.04	1.96	1.87	1.77	1.65
29	4.18	3.33	2.93	2.79	2.55	2.43	2.35	2.28	2.122	2.18	2.10	2.03	1.94	1.85	1.75	1.64
30	4.17	3.32	2.92	2.69	2.53	2.42	2.33	2.27	2.21	2.16	2.09	2.01	1.93	1.84	1.74	1.62
40	4.08	3.23	2.84	2.61	2.45	2.34	2.25	2.18	2.12	2.08	2.00	1.92	1.84	1.74	1.64	1.51
60	4.00	3.15	2.76	2.53	2.37	2.25	2.17	2.10	2.04	1.99	1.92	1.84	1.75	1.65	1.53	1.39
120	3.92	3.07	2.68	2.45	2.29	2.17	2.09	2.02	1.96	1.91	1.83	1.75	1.66	1.55	1.43	1.25
∞	3.84	3.00	2.60	2.37	2.21	2.10	2.01	1.94	1.88	1.83	1.75	1.67	1.57	1.46	1.32	1.00

df_b = between-groups degrees of freedom.
df_e = error (within-groups) degrees of freedom.
Test statistic must be greater than or equal to critical value to reject H_0.

TABLE A.3(II) CRITICAL VALUES OF F, $\alpha = .01$

df_e for denominator	df_b for numerator															
	1	2	3	4	5	6	7	8	9	10	12	15	20	30	60	∞
1	4052	5000	5403	5625	5764	5859	5928	5982	6022	6056	6106	6157	6209	6261	6313	6366
2	98.50	99.00	99.17	99.25	99.30	99.33	99.36	99.37	99.39	99.40	99.42	99.43	99.45	99.47	99.48	99.50
3	34.12	30.82	29.46	28.71	28.24	27.91	27.67	27.49	27.35	27.33	27.05	26.87	26.69	26.50	26.32	26.13
4	21.20	18.00	16.69	15.98	15.52	15.21	14.98	14.80	14.66	14.55	14.37	14.20	14.02	13.84	13.65	13.46
5	16.26	13.27	12.06	11.39	10.97	10.67	10.46	10.29	10.16	10.05	9.89	9.72	9.55	9.38	9.20	9.02
6	13.75	10.92	9.78	9.15	8.75	8.47	8.26	8.10	7.98	7.87	7.72	7.56	7.40	7.23	7.06	6.88
7	12.25	9.55	8.45	7.85	7.46	7.19	6.99	6.84	6.72	6.62	6.47	6.31	6.16	5.99	5.82	5.65
8	11.26	8.65	7.59	7.01	6.63	6.37	6.18	6.03	5.91	5.81	5.67	5.52	5.36	5.20	5.03	4.86
9	10.56	8.02	6.99	6.42	6.06	5.80	5.61	5.47	5.35	5.26	5.11	4.96	4.81	4.65	4.48	4.31
10	10.04	7.56	6.55	5.99	5.64	5.39	5.20	5.06	4.94	4.85	4.71	4.56	4.41	4.25	4.08	3.91
11	9.65	7.21	6.22	5.67	5.32	5.07	4.89	4.74	4.63	4.54	4.40	4.25	4.10	3.94	3.78	3.60
12	9.33	6.93	5.95	5.41	5.06	4.82	4.64	4.50	4.39	4.30	4.16	4.01	3.86	3.70	3.54	3.36
13	9.07	6.70	5.74	5.21	4.86	4.62	4.44	4.30	4.19	4.10	3.96	3.82	3.66	3.51	3.34	3.17
14	8.86	6.51	5.56	5.04	4.69	4.46	4.28	4.14	4.03	3.94	3.80	3.66	3.51	3.35	3.18	3.00
15	8.68	6.36	5.42	4.89	4.56	4.32	4.14	4.00	3.89	3.80	3.67	3.52	3.37	3.21	3.05	2.87

TABLE A.3(II)—Continued

df_e for denominator	\multicolumn{16}{c}{df_b for numerator}
	1	2	3	4	5	6	7	8	9	10	12	15	20	30	60	∞
16	8.53	6.23	5.29	4.77	4.44	4.20	4.03	3.89	3.78	3.69	3.55	3.41	3.26	3.10	2.93	2.75
17	8.40	6.11	5.18	4.67	4.34	4.10	3.93	3.79	3.68	3.59	3.46	3.31	3.16	3.00	2.83	2.65
18	8.29	6.01	5.09	4.58	4.25	4.01	3.84	3.71	3.60	3.51	3.37	3.23	3.08	2.92	2.75	2.57
19	8.18	5.93	5.01	4.50	4.17	3.94	3.77	3.63	3.52	3.43	3.30	3.15	3.00	2.84	2.67	2.49
20	8.10	5.85	4.94	4.43	4.10	3.87	3.70	3.56	3.46	3.37	3.23	3.09	2.94	2.78	2.61	2.42
21	8.02	5.78	4.87	4.37	4.04	3.81	3.64	3.51	3.40	3.31	3.17	3.03	2.88	2.72	2.55	2.36
22	7.95	5.72	4.82	4.31	3.99	3.76	3.59	3.45	3.35	3.26	3.12	2.98	2.83	2.67	2.50	2.31
23	7.88	5.66	4.76	4.26	3.94	3.71	3.54	3.41	3.30	3.21	3.07	2.93	2.78	2.62	2.45	2.26
24	7.82	5.61	4.72	4.22	3.90	3.67	3.50	3.36	3.26	3.17	3.03	2.89	2.74	2.58	2.40	2.21
25	7.77	5.57	4.68	4.18	3.85	3.63	3.46	3.32	3.22	3.13	2.99	2.85	2.70	2.54	2.36	2.17
26	7.72	5.53	4.64	4.14	3.82	3.59	3.42	3.29	3.18	3.09	2.96	2.81	2.66	2.50	2.33	2.13
27	7.68	5.49	4.60	4.11	3.78	3.56	3.39	3.26	3.15	3.06	2.93	2.78	2.63	2.47	2.29	2.10
28	7.64	5.45	4.57	4.07	3.75	3.53	3.36	3.23	3.12	3.03	2.90	2.75	2.60	2.44	2.26	2.06
29	7.60	5.42	4.54	4.04	3.73	3.50	3.33	3.20	3.09	3.00	2.87	2.73	2.57	2.41	2.23	2.03
30	7.56	5.39	4.51	4.02	3.70	3.47	3.30	3.17	3.07	2.98	2.84	2.70	2.55	2.39	2.21	2.01
40	7.31	5.18	4.31	3.83	3.51	3.29	3.12	2.99	2.89	2.80	2.66	2.52	2.37	2.20	2.02	1.80
60	7.08	4.98	4.13	3.65	3.34	3.12	2.95	2.82	2.72	2.63	2.50	2.35	2.20	2.03	1.84	1.60
120	6.85	4.79	3.95	3.48	3.17	2.96	2.79	2.66	2.56	2.47	2.34	2.19	2.03	1.86	1.66	1.38
∞	6.63	4.61	3.78	3.32	3.02	2.80	2.64	2.51	2.41	2.32	2.18	2.04	1.88	1.70	1.47	1.00

TABLE A.4   CRITICAL VALUES OF *r*

df	α_1 α_2	.05 .10	.025 .05	.01 .02	.005 .01	.0005 .001
1		.988	.997	.9995	.9999	.9999
2		.900	.950	.980	.990	.999
3		.805	.878	.934	.959	.991
4		.729	.811	.882	.917	.974
5		.669	.755	.833	.875	.951
6		.622	.707	.789	.834	.925
7		.582	.666	.750	.798	.898
8		.549	.632	.716	.765	.872
9		.521	.602	.685	.735	.847
10		.497	.576	.658	.708	.823
11		.476	.553	.634	.684	.801
12		.458	.532	.612	.661	.780
13		.441	.514	.592	.641	.760
14		.426	.497	.574	.623	.742
15		.412	.482	.558	.606	.725
16		.400	.468	.543	.590	.708
17		.389	.456	.529	.575	.693
18		.378	.444	.516	.561	.679
19		.369	.433	.503	.549	.665
20		.323	.381	.445	.487	.597
25		.360	.423	.492	.537	.652
30		.296	.349	.409	.449	.554
35		.275	.325	.381	.418	.519
40		.257	.304	.358	.393	.490
45		.243	.288	.338	.372	.465
50		.231	.273	.322	.354	.443
60		.211	.250	.295	.325	.408
70		.195	.232	.274	.302	.380
80		.183	.217	.257	.283	.357
90		.173	.205	.242	.267	.338
100		.164	.195	.230	.254	.321

$df = n - 2$.

Test statistic must be greater than or equal to critical value to reject H_0.

Adapted from Table VII in Fisher RA, Yates F. *Statistical Tables for Biological, Agricultural, and Medical Research.* Published by Longman Group UK, Ltd. 1974. Used with permission.

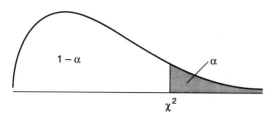

TABLE A.5   CRITICAL VALUES OF CHI-SQUARE, χ^2

df	α	.05	.02	.01	.005	.001
1		3.84	5.02	6.64	7.88	10.83
2		5.99	7.38	9.21	10.60	13.82
3		7.82	9.35	11.35	12.84	16.27
4		9.49	11.14	13.28	14.86	18.47
5		11.07	12.83	15.09	16.75	20.52
6		12.59	14.45	16.81	18.55	22.46
7		14.07	16.01	18.48	20.28	24.32
8		15.51	17.53	20.09	21.96	26.13
9		16.92	19.03	21.67	23.59	27.88
10		18.31	20.48	23.21	25.19	29.59
11		19.68	21.92	24.73	26.76	31.26
12		21.03	23.34	26.22	28.30	32.91
13		22.36	24.74	27.69	29.82	34.53
14		23.69	26.12	29.14	31.32	36.12
15		25.00	27.49	30.58	32.80	37.70
16		26.30	28.85	32.00	34.27	39.25
17		27.59	30.19	33.41	35.72	40.79
18		28.87	31.53	34.81	37.16	42.31
19		30.14	32.85	36.19	38.58	43.82
20		31.41	34.17	37.57	40.00	45.32
21		32.67	35.48	38.93	41.40	46.80
22		33.92	36.78	40.29	42.80	48.27
23		35.17	38.06	41.64	44.18	49.73
24		36.42	39.36	42.98	45.56	51.18
25		37.65	40.65	44.31	46.93	52.62
26		38.89	41.92	45.64	48.29	54.05
27		40.11	43.19	46.96	49.65	55.47
28		41.34	44.46	48.28	50.99	56.89
29		42.56	45.72	49.59	52.34	58.30
30		43.77	46.98	50.89	53.67	59.70
40		55.76	59.34	63.69	66.77	73.40
50		67.51	71.42	76.15	79.49	86.66
60		79.08	83.30	88.38	91.95	99.61
70		90.53	95.02	100.43	104.22	112.32
80		101.88	106.63	112.33	116.32	124.84
90		113.15	118.14	124.12	128.30	137.21
100		124.34	129.56	135.81	140.47	149.45

For one-sample test, $df = k-1$. For two-sample test, $df = (R-1)(C-1)$. Test statistic must be greater than or equal to critical value to reject H_0.

Adapted from Table 8 in Pearson and Hartley (eds): *Biometrika Tables for Statisticians,* ed. 3. New York: Cambridge, 1966, by permission of the Biometrika Trustees.

TABLE A.6   CRITICAL VALUES OF THE STUDENTIZED RANGE STATISTIC, *q*, FOR TUKEY'S HONESTLY SIGNIFICANT DIFFERENCE (HSD) AND NEWMAN-KEULS (NK) COMPARISONS

df_e	α	\multicolumn{11}{c}{*r* = number of means (HSD) or size of comparison interval (NK)}
		2	3	4	5	6	7	8	9	10	11	12
5	.05	3.64	4.60	5.22	5.67	6.03	6.33	6.58	6.80	6.99	7.17	7.32
	.01	5.70	6.98	7.80	8.42	8.91	9.32	9.67	9.97	10.24	10.48	10.70
6	.05	3.46	4.34	4.90	5.30	5.63	5.90	6.12	6.32	6.49	6.65	6.79
	.01	5.24	6.33	7.03	7.56	7.97	8.32	8.61	8.87	9.10	9.30	9.48
7	.05	3.34	4.16	4.68	5.06	5.36	5.61	5.82	6.00	6.16	6.30	6.43
	.01	4.95	5.92	6.54	7.01	7.37	7.68	7.94	8.17	8.37	8.55	8.71
8	.05	3.26	4.04	4.53	4.89	5.17	5.40	5.60	5.77	5.92	6.05	6.18
	.01	4.75	5.64	6.20	6.62	6.96	7.24	7.47	7.68	7.86	8.03	8.18
9	.05	3.20	3.95	4.41	4.76	5.02	5.24	5.43	5.59	5.74	5.87	5.98
	.01	4.60	5.43	5.96	6.35	6.66	6.91	7.13	7.33	7.49	7.65	7.78
10	.05	3.15	3.88	4.33	4.65	4.91	5.12	5.30	5.46	5.60	5.72	5.83
	.01	4.48	5.27	5.77	6.14	6.43	6.67	6.87	7.05	7.21	7.36	7.49
11	.05	3.11	3.82	4.26	4.57	4.82	5.03	5.20	5.35	5.49	5.61	5.71
	.01	4.39	5.15	5.62	5.97	6.25	6.48	6.67	6.84	6.99	7.13	7.25
12	.05	3.08	3.77	4.20	4.51	4.75	4.95	5.12	5.27	5.39	5.51	5.61
	.01	4.32	5.05	5.50	5.84	6.10	6.32	6.51	6.67	6.81	6.94	7.06
13	.05	3.06	3.73	4.15	4.45	4.69	4.88	5.05	5.19	5.32	5.43	5.53
	.01	4.26	4.96	5.40	5.73	5.98	6.19	6.37	6.53	6.67	6.79	6.90
14	.05	3.03	3.70	4.11	4.41	4.64	4.83	4.99	5.13	5.25	5.36	5.46
	.01	4.21	4.89	5.32	5.63	5.88	6.08	6.26	6.41	6.54	6.66	6.77
15	.05	3.01	3.67	4.08	4.37	4.59	4.78	4.94	5.08	5.20	5.31	5.40
	.01	4.17	4.84	5.25	5.56	5.80	5.99	6.16	6.31	6.44	6.55	6.66
16	.05	3.00	3.65	4.05	4.33	4.56	4.74	4.90	5.03	5.15	5.26	5.35
	.01	4.13	4.79	5.19	5.49	5.72	5.92	6.08	6.22	6.35	6.46	6.56
17	.05	2.98	3.63	4.02	4.30	4.52	4.70	4.86	4.99	5.11	5.21	5.31
	.01	4.10	4.74	5.14	5.43	5.66	5.85	6.01	6.15	6.27	6.38	6.48
18	.05	2.97	3.61	4.00	4.28	4.49	4.67	4.82	4.96	5.07	5.17	5.27
	.01	4.07	4.70	5.09	5.38	5.60	5.79	5.94	6.08	6.20	6.31	6.41
19	.05	2.96	3.59	3.98	4.25	4.47	4.65	4.79	4.92	5.04	5.14	5.23
	.01	4.05	4.67	5.05	5.33	5.55	5.73	5.89	6.02	6.14	6.25	6.34

TABLE A.6—*Continued*

df_e	α	\multicolumn{11}{c}{r = number of means (HSD) or size of comparison interval (NK)}
		2	3	4	5	6	7	8	9	10	11	12
20	.05	2.95	3.58	3.96	4.23	4.45	4.62	4.77	4.90	5.01	5.11	5.20
	.01	4.02	4.64	5.02	5.29	5.51	5.69	5.84	5.97	6.09	6.19	6.28
24	.05	2.92	3.53	3.90	4.17	4.37	4.54	4.68	4.81	4.92	5.01	5.10
	.01	3.96	4.55	4.91	5.17	5.37	5.54	5.69	5.81	5.92	6.02	6.11
30	.05	2.89	3.49	3.85	4.10	4.30	4.46	4.60	4.72	4.82	4.92	5.00
	.01	3.89	4.45	4.80	5.05	5.24	5.40	5.54	5.65	5.76	5.85	5.93
40	.05	2.86	3.44	3.79	4.04	4.23	4.39	4.52	4.63	4.73	4.82	4.90
	.01	3.82	4.37	4.70	4.93	5.11	5.26	5.39	5.50	5.60	5.69	5.76
60	.05	2.83	3.40	3.74	3.98	4.16	4.31	4.44	4.55	4.65	4.73	4.81
	.01	3.76	4.28	4.59	4.82	4.99	5.13	5.25	5.36	5.45	5.53	5.60
120	.05	2.80	3.36	3.68	3.92	4.10	4.24	4.36	4.47	4.56	4.64	4.71
	.01	3.70	4.20	4.50	4.71	4.87	5.01	5.12	5.21	5.30	5.37	5.44
∞	.05	2.77	3.31	3.63	3.86	4.03	4.17	4.29	4.39	4.47	4.55	4.62
	.01	3.64	4.12	4.40	4.60	4.76	4.88	4.99	5.08	5.16	5.23	5.29

From Table 29 in Pearson ES, Hartley HO (eds). *Biometrika Tables for Statisticians,* ed 3. New York: Cambridge, 1966, by permission of the Biometrika Trustees.

TABLE A.7   CRITICAL VALUES OF $t(B)$ FOR BONFERRONI'S MULTIPLE COMPARISON

df_e	α_2	Number of comparisons (c)								
		2	3	4	5	6	7	8	9	10
2	.10	4.243	5.243	6.081	6.816	7.480	8.090	8.656	9.188	9.691
	.05	6.164	7.582	8.774	9.823	10.769	11.639	12.449	13.208	13.927
	.01	14.071	17.248	19.925	22.282	24.413	26.372	28.196	29.908	31.528
3	.10	3.149	3.690	4.115	4.471	4.780	5.055	5.304	5.532	5.744
	.05	4.156	4.826	5.355	5.799	6.185	6.529	6.842	7.128	7.394
	.01	7.447	8.565	9.453	10.201	10.853	11.436	11.966	12.453	12.904
4	.10	2.751	3.150	3.452	3.669	3.909	4.093	4.257	4.406	4.542
	.05	3.481	3.941	4.290	4.577	4.822	5.036	5.228	5.402	5.562
	.01	5.594	6.248	6.751	7.166	7.520	7.832	8.112	8.367	8.600
5	.10	2.549	2.882	3.129	3.327	3.493	3.638	3.765	3.880	3.985
	.05	3.152	3.518	3.791	4.012	4.197	4.358	4.501	4.630	4.747
	.01	4.771	5.243	5.599	5.888	6.133	6.346	6.535	6.706	6.862
6	.10	2.428	2.723	2.939	3.110	3.253	3.376	3.484	3.580	3.668
	.05	2.959	3.274	3.505	3.690	3.845	3.978	4.095	4.200	4.296
	.01	4.315	4.695	4.977	5.203	5.394	5.559	5.704	5.835	5.954
7	.10	2.347	2.618	2.814	2.969	3.097	3.206	3.302	3.388	3.465
	.05	2.832	3.115	3.321	3.484	3.620	3.736	3.838	3.929	4.011
	.01	4.027	4.353	4.591	4.782	4.941	5.078	5.198	5.306	5.404
8	.10	2.289	2.544	2.726	2.869	2.987	3.088	3.176	3.254	3.324
	.05	2.743	3.005	3.193	3.342	3.464	3.569	3.661	3.743	3.816
	.01	3.831	4.120	4.331	4.498	4.637	4.756	4.860	4.953	5.038
9	.10	2.246	2.488	2.661	2.796	2.907	3.001	3.083	3.155	3.221
	.05	2.677	2.923	3.099	3.237	3.351	3.448	3.532	3.607	3.675
	.01	3.688	3.952	4.143	4.294	4.419	4.526	4.619	4.703	4.778
10	.10	2.213	2.446	2.611	2.739	2.845	2.934	3.012	3.080	3.142
	.05	2.626	2.860	3.027	3.157	3.264	3.355	3.434	3.505	3.568
	.01	3.580	3.825	4.002	4.141	2.256	4.354	4.439	4.515	4.584
11	.10	2.186	2.412	2.571	2.695	2.796	2.881	2.955	3.021	3.079
	.05	2.586	2.811	2.970	3.094	3.196	3.283	3.358	3.424	3.484
	.01	3.495	3.726	3.892	4.022	4.129	4.221	4.300	4.371	4.434

TABLE A.7—*Continued*

df_e	α_2	\multicolumn{9}{c}{Number of comparisons (c)}
		2	3	4	5	6	7	8	9	10
12	.10	2.164	2.384	2.539	2.658	2.756	2.838	2.910	2.973	3.029
	.05	2.553	2.770	2.924	3.044	3.141	3.224	3.296	3.359	3.416
	.01	3.427	3.647	3.804	3.927	4.029	4.114	4.189	4.356	4.315
13	.10	2.146	2.361	2.512	2.628	2.723	2.803	2.872	2.933	2.988
	.05	2.526	2.737	2.886	3.002	3.096	3.176	3.245	3.306	3.361
	.01	3.371	3.582	3.733	3.850	3.946	4.028	4.099	4.162	4.218
14	.10	2.131	2.342	2.489	2.603	2.696	2.774	2.841	2.900	2.953
	.05	2.503	2.709	2.854	2.967	3.058	3.135	3.202	3.261	3.314
	.01	3.324	3.528	3.673	3.785	3.878	3.956	4.024	4.084	4.138
15	.10	2.118	2.325	2.470	2.582	2.672	2.748	2.814	2.872	2.924
	.05	2.483	2.685	2.827	2.937	3.026	3.101	3.166	3.224	3.275
	.01	3.285	3.482	3.622	3.731	3.820	3.895	3.961	4.019	4.071
16	.10	2.106	2.311	2.453	2.563	2.652	2.726	2.791	2.848	2.898
	.05	2.467	2.665	2.804	2.911	2.998	3.072	3.135	3.191	3.241
	.01	3.251	3.443	3.579	3.684	3.771	3.844	3.907	3.963	4.013
18	.10	2.088	2.287	2.426	2.532	2.619	2.691	2.753	2.808	2.857
	.05	2.439	2.631	2.766	2.869	2.953	3.024	3.085	3.138	3.186
	.01	3.195	3.379	3.508	3.609	3.691	3.760	3.820	3.872	3.920
20	.10	2.073	2.269	2.405	2.508	2.593	2.663	2.724	2.777	2.824
	.05	2.417	2.605	2.736	2.836	2.918	2.986	3.045	3.097	3.143
	.01	3.152	3.329	3.454	3.550	3.629	3.695	3.752	3.802	3.848
25	.10	2.047	2.236	2.367	2.466	2.547	2.614	2.672	2.722	2.767
	.05	2.379	2.558	2.683	2.779	2.856	2.921	2.976	3.025	3.069
	.01	3.077	3.243	3.359	3.449	3.521	3.583	3.635	3.682	3.723
30	.10	2.030	2.215	2.342	2.439	2.517	2.582	2.638	2.687	2.731
	.05	2.354	2.528	2.649	2.742	2.816	2.878	2.932	2.979	3.021
	.01	3.029	3.188	3.298	3.384	3.453	3.511	2.561	3.605	3.644

Continued

TABLE A.7   CRITICAL VALUES OF $t(B)$ FOR BONFERRONI'S MULTIPLE COMPARISON TEST—*Continued*

df_e	α_2	**2**	**3**	**4**	**5**	**6**	**7**	**8**	**9**	**10**	**15**	**20**	**25**	**30**
								Number of comparisons (c)						
40	.10	2.009	2.189	2.312	2.406	2.481	2.544	2.597	2.644	2.686	2.843	2.952	3.036	3.103
	.05	2.323	2.492	2.608	2.696	2.768	2.827	2.878	2.923	2.963	3.113	3.218	3.298	3.363
	.01	2.970	3.121	3.225	3.305	3.370	3.425	3.472	3.513	3.549	3.689	3.787	3.862	3.923
60	.10	1.989	2.163	2.283	2.373	2.446	2.506	2.558	2.603	2.643	2.793	2.897	2.976	3.040
	.05	2.294	2.456	2.568	2.653	2.721	2.777	2.826	2.869	2.906	3.049	3.148	3.223	3.284
	.01	2.914	3.056	3.155	3.230	3.291	3.342	3.386	3.425	3.459	3.589	3.679	3.749	3.805
120	.10	1.968	2.138	2.254	2.342	2.411	2.469	2.519	2.562	2.600	2.744	2.843	2.918	2.978
	.05	2.265	2.422	2.529	2.610	2.675	2.729	2.776	2.816	2.852	2.987	3.081	3.152	3.209
	.01	2.859	2.994	3.087	3.158	3.215	3.263	3.304	3.340	3.372	3.493	3.577	3.641	3.693
∞	.10	1.949	2.114	2.226	2.311	2.378	2.434	2.482	2.523	2.560	2.697	2.791	2.862	2.920
	.05	2.237	2.388	2.491	2.569	2.631	2.683	2.727	2.766	2.300	2.928	3.016	3.083	3.137
	.01	2.806	2.934	3.022	3.089	3.143	3.186	3.226	3.260	3.289	3.402	3.480	3.539	3.587

TABLE A.8 CRITICAL VALUES FOR THE MANN-WHITNEY U-TEST

n_1	α_1	α_2	3	4	5	6	7	8	9	10	11	12	13	14	15	16	17	18	19	20	21	22	23	24	25
													n_2 (larger sample size)											
3	.005	.01	—	—	—	—	—	—	0	0	0	1	1	1	2	2	2	2	3	3	3	4	4	4	5
	.01	.02	—	—	—	—	0	0	1	1	1	2	2	2	3	3	4	4	4	5	5	6	6	6	7
	.025	.05	—	—	0	1	1	2	2	3	3	4	4	5	5	6	6	7	7	8	8	9	9	10	10
	.05	.10	0	0	1	2	2	3	4	4	5	5	6	7	7	8	9	9	10	11	11	12	13	13	14
4	.005	.01	—	—	—	0	0	1	1	2	2	3	3	4	5	5	6	6	7	8	8	9	9	10	10
	.01	.02	—	—	0	1	1	2	3	3	4	5	5	6	7	7	8	9	9	10	11	11	12	13	13
	.025	.05	—	0	1	2	3	4	4	5	6	7	8	9	10	11	11	12	13	14	15	16	17	17	18
	.05	.10	—	1	2	3	4	5	6	7	8	9	10	11	12	14	15	16	17	18	19	20	21	22	23
5	.005	.01	—	—	0	1	1	2	3	4	5	6	7	7	8	9	10	11	12	13	14	14	15	16	17
	.01	.02	—	—	1	2	3	4	5	6	7	8	9	10	11	12	13	14	15	16	17	18	19	20	21
	.025	.05	—	1	2	3	5	6	7	8	9	11	12	13	14	15	17	18	19	20	22	23	24	25	27
	.05	.10	1	2	4	5	6	8	9	11	12	13	15	16	18	19	20	22	23	25	26	28	29	30	32
6	.005	.01	—	—	—	2	3	4	5	6	7	9	10	11	12	13	15	16	17	18	19	21	22	23	24
	.01	.02	—	—	—	3	4	6	7	8	9	11	12	13	15	16	18	19	20	22	23	24	26	27	29
	.025	.05	—	—	—	5	6	8	10	11	13	14	16	17	19	21	22	24	25	27	29	30	32	33	35
	.05	.10	—	—	—	7	8	10	12	14	16	17	19	21	23	25	26	28	30	32	34	36	37	39	41
7	.005	.01	—	—	—	—	4	6	7	9	10	12	13	15	16	18	19	21	22	24	25	27	29	30	32
	.01	.02	—	—	—	—	6	7	9	11	12	14	16	17	19	21	23	24	26	28	30	31	33	35	36
	.025	.05	—	—	—	—	8	10	12	14	16	18	20	22	24	26	28	30	32	34	36	38	40	42	44
	.05	.10	—	—	—	—	11	13	15	17	19	21	24	26	28	30	33	35	37	39	41	44	46	48	50
8	.005	.01	—	—	—	—	—	7	9	11	13	15	17	18	20	22	24	26	28	30	32	34	35	37	39
	.01	.02	—	—	—	—	—	9	11	13	15	17	20	22	24	26	28	30	32	34	36	38	40	42	45
	.025	.05	—	—	—	—	—	13	15	17	19	22	24	26	29	31	34	36	38	41	43	45	48	50	53
	.05	.10	—	—	—	—	—	15	18	20	23	26	28	31	33	36	39	41	44	47	49	52	54	57	60

Continued

TABLE A.8 CRITICAL VALUES FOR THE MANN-WHITNEY U-TEST—Continued

n_1	α_1	α_2	9	10	11	12	13	14	15	16	17	18	19	20	21	22	23	24	25
									n_2 (larger sample size)									
9	.005	.01	11	13	16	18	20	22	24	27	29	31	33	36	38	40	43	45	47
	.01	.02	14	16	18	21	23	26	28	31	33	36	38	40	43	45	48	50	53
	.025	.05	17	20	23	26	28	31	34	37	39	42	45	48	50	53	56	59	62
	.05	.10	21	24	27	30	33	36	39	42	45	48	51	54	57	60	63	66	69
10	.005	.01	—	16	18	21	24	26	29	31	34	37	39	42	44	47	50	52	55
	.01	.02	—	19	22	24	27	30	33	36	38	41	44	47	50	53	55	58	61
	.025	.05	—	23	26	29	33	36	39	42	45	48	52	55	58	61	64	67	71
	.05	.10	—	27	31	34	37	41	44	48	51	55	58	62	65	68	72	75	79
11	.005	.01	—	—	21	24	27	30	33	36	39	42	45	48	51	54	57	60	63
	.01	.02	—	—	25	28	31	34	37	41	44	47	50	53	57	60	63	66	70
	.025	.05	—	—	30	33	37	40	44	47	51	55	58	62	65	69	73	76	80
	.05	.10	—	—	34	38	42	46	50	54	57	61	65	69	73	77	81	85	89
12	.005	.01	—	—	—	27	31	34	37	41	44	47	51	54	58	61	64	68	71
	.01	.02	—	—	—	31	35	38	42	46	49	53	56	60	64	67	71	75	78
	.025	.05	—	—	—	37	41	45	49	53	57	61	65	69	73	77	81	85	89
	.05	.10	—	—	—	42	47	51	55	60	64	68	72	77	81	85	90	95	99
13	.005	.01	—	—	—	—	34	38	42	45	49	53	57	60	64	68	72	75	79
	.01	.02	—	—	—	—	39	43	47	51	55	59	63	67	71	75	79	83	87
	.025	.05	—	—	—	—	45	50	54	59	63	67	72	76	80	85	89	94	98
	.05	.10	—	—	—	—	51	56	61	65	70	75	80	84	89	94	98	103	108
14	.005	.01	—	—	—	—	—	42	46	50	54	58	63	67	71	75	79	83	87
	.01	.02	—	—	—	—	—	47	51	56	60	65	69	73	78	82	87	91	95
	.025	.05	—	—	—	—	—	55	59	64	69	74	78	83	88	93	98	102	107
	.05	.10	—	—	—	—	—	61	66	71	77	82	87	92	97	102	107	113	118
15	.005	.01	—	—	—	—	—	—	51	55	60	64	69	73	78	82	87	91	96
	.01	.02	—	—	—	—	—	—	56	61	66	70	75	80	85	90	94	99	104
	.025	.05	—	—	—	—	—	—	64	70	75	80	85	90	96	101	106	111	117
	.05	.10	—	—	—	—	—	—	72	77	83	88	94	100	105	111	116	122	128
16	.005	.01	—	—	—	—	—	—	—	60	65	70	74	79	84	89	94	99	104
	.01	.02	—	—	—	—	—	—	—	66	71	76	82	87	92	97	102	108	113
	.025	.05	—	—	—	—	—	—	—	75	81	86	92	98	103	109	115	120	126
	.05	.10	—	—	—	—	—	—	—	83	89	95	101	107	113	119	125	131	137

TABLE A.8—Continued

n_1	α_1	α_2	17	18	19	20	21	22	23	24	25
						n_2 (larger sample size)					
17	.005	.01	70	75	81	86	91	96	102	107	112
	.01	.02	77	82	88	93	99	105	120	126	132
	.025	.05	87	93	99	105	111	117	123	129	135
	.05	.10	96	102	109	115	121	128	134	141	147
18	.005	.01	—	81	87	92	98	104	109	115	121
	.01	.02	—	88	94	100	106	112	118	124	130
	.025	.05	—	99	106	112	119	125	132	138	145
	.05	.10	—	109	116	123	130	136	143	150	157
19	.005	.01	—	—	93	99	105	111	117	123	129
	.01	.02	—	—	101	107	113	120	126	133	139
	.025	.05	—	—	113	119	126	133	140	147	154
	.05	.10	—	—	123	130	138	145	152	160	167
20	.005	.01	—	—	—	105	112	118	125	131	138
	.01	.02	—	—	—	114	121	127	134	141	148
	.025	.05	—	—	—	127	134	141	149	156	163
	.05	.10	—	—	—	138	146	154	161	169	177
21	.005	.01	—	—	—	—	118	125	132	139	146
	.01	.02	—	—	—	—	128	135	142	150	157
	.025	.05	—	—	—	—	142	150	157	165	173
	.05	.10	—	—	—	—	154	162	170	179	187
22	.005	.01	—	—	—	—	—	133	140	147	155
	.01	.02	—	—	—	—	—	143	150	158	166
	.025	.05	—	—	—	—	—	158	166	174	182
	.05	.10	—	—	—	—	—	171	179	188	197
23	.005	.01	—	—	—	—	—	—	148	155	163
	.01	.02	—	—	—	—	—	—	158	167	175
	.025	.05	—	—	—	—	—	—	175	183	192
	.05	.10	—	—	—	—	—	—	189	198	207
24	.005	.01	—	—	—	—	—	—	—	167	172
	.01	.02	—	—	—	—	—	—	—	175	184
	.025	.05	—	—	—	—	—	—	—	192	201
	.05	.10	—	—	—	—	—	—	—	207	217
25	.005	.01	—	—	—	—	—	—	—	—	180
	.01	.02	—	—	—	—	—	—	—	—	192
	.025	.05	—	—	—	—	—	—	—	—	211
	.05	.10	—	—	—	—	—	—	—	—	227

The test statistic must be equal to or less than the critical value to reject H_0.

When groups are of unequal size, n_1 is the smaller group.

Adapted from Table 1 in Verdooren LR. Extended tables of critical values for Wilcoxon's test statistic. *Biometrika* 1963; 50 (1 and 2): 177, with the permission of the Biometrika Trustees.

TABLE A.9   PROBABILITIES* ASSOCIATED WITH VALUES OF x IN THE BINOMIAL TEST

n	0	1	2	3	4	5	6	7	8	9	10	11	12	13	14	15	16
4	.062	.312	.688	.938	—												
5	.031	.188	.500	.812	.969	—											
6	.016	.109	.344	.656	.891	.984	—										
7	.008	.062	.227	.500	.773	.938	.992	—									
8	.004	.035	.145	.363	.637	.855	.965	.996	—								
9	.002	.020	.090	.254	.500	.746	.910	.980	.998	—							
10	.001	.011	.055	.172	.377	.623	.828	.945	.989	.999	—						
11	—	.006	.033	.113	.274	.500	.726	.887	.967	.994	—	—					
12	—	.003	.019	.073	.194	.387	.613	.806	.927	.981	.997	—					
13	—	.002	.011	.046	.133	.291	.500	.709	.867	.954	.989	.998	—				
14	—	.001	.006	.029	.090	.212	.395	.605	.788	.910	.971	.994	.999	—			
15	—	—	.004	.018	.059	.151	.304	.500	.696	.849	.941	.982	.996	—			
16	—	—	.002	.011	.038	.105	.227	.402	.598	.773	.895	.962	.989	.998	—		
17	—	—	.001	.006	.025	.072	.166	.315	.500	.685	.834	.928	.975	.994	—		
18	—	—	.001	.004	.015	.048	.119	.240	.407	.593	.760	.881	.952	.985	.996	—	
19	—	—	—	.002	.010	.032	.084	.180	.324	.500	.676	.820	.916	.968	.990	.998	—
20	—	—	—	.001	.006	.021	.058	.132	.252	.412	.588	.748	.868	.942	.979	.994	.999
21	—	—	—	.001	.004	.013	.039	.095	.192	.332	.500	.668	.808	.902	.961	.987	.996
22	—	—	—	—	.002	.008	.026	.067	.143	.262	.416	.584	.738	.857	.933	.974	.992
23	—	—	—	—	.001	.005	.017	.047	.105	.202	.339	.500	.661	.798	.895	.953	.983
24	—	—	—	—	.001	.003	.011	.032	.076	.154	.271	.419	.581	.729	.846	.924	.968
25	—	—	—	—	—	.002	.007	.022	.054	.115	.212	.345	.500	.655	.788	.885	.946
26	—	—	—	—	—	.001	.005	.014	.038	.084	.163	.279	.423	.577	.721	.837	.916
27	—	—	—	—	—	.001	.003	.010	.026	.061	.124	.221	.351	.500	.649	.779	.876
28	—	—	—	—	—	—	.002	.006	.018	.044	.092	.172	.286	.425	.575	.714	.828
29	—	—	—	—	—	—	.001	.004	.012	.031	.068	.132	.229	.356	.500	.644	.771
30	—	—	—	—	—	—	.001	.003	.008	.021	.049	.100	.181	.292	.428	.572	.708

*Tabled probabilities are for one-tailed tests. Double values in table for a two-tailed test.

Adapted from Table D in Siegel S, Castellan, N.J.: Nonparametric Statistics for the Behavioral Sciences, ed 2. New York: McGraw-Hill, 1988, with permission.

TABLE A.10   CRITICAL VALUES OF *T* FOR THE WILCOXON SIGNED-RANKS TEST

N	α_1 .025 α_2 .05	.01 .02	.005 .01
6	0	—	—
7	2	0	—
8	4	2	0
9	6	3	2
10	8	5	3
11	11	7	5
12	14	10	7
13	17	13	10
14	21	16	13
15	25	20	16
16	30	24	20
17	35	28	23
18	40	33	28
19	46	38	32
20	52	43	38
21	59	49	43
22	66	56	49
23	73	62	55
24	81	69	61
25	89	77	68

The test statistic must be equal to or less than the critical value to reject H_0.

TABLE A.11   CRITICAL VALUES OF SPEARMAN'S RANK CORRELATION COEFFICIENT, r_s

n	α_2 0.10 α_1 0.05	0.05 0.025	0.02 0.01	0.01 0.005	0.005 0.0025	0.002 0.001	0.001 0.0005
4	1.000						
5	0.900	1.000	1.000				
6	0.829	0.886	0.943	1.000	1.000		
7	0.714	0.786	0.893	0.929	0.964	1.000	1.000
8	0.643	0.738	0.833	0.881	0.905	0.952	0.976
9	0.600	0.700	0.783	0.833	0.867	0.917	0.933
10	0.564	0.648	0.745	0.794	0.830	0.879	0.903
11	0.536	0.618	0.709	0.755	0.800	0.845	0.873
12	0.503	0.587	0.671	0.727	0.776	0.825	0.860
13	0.484	0.560	0.648	0.703	0.747	0.802	0.835
14	0.464	0.538	0.622	0.675	0.723	0.776	0.811
15	0.443	0.521	0.604	0.654	0.700	0.754	0.786
16	0.429	0.503	0.582	0.635	0.679	0.732	0.765
17	0.414	0.485	0.566	0.615	0.662	0.713	0.748
18	0.401	0.472	0.550	0.600	0.643	0.695	0.728
19	0.391	0.460	0.535	0.584	0.628	0.677	0.712
20	0.380	0.447	0.520	0.570	0.612	0.662	0.696
21	0.370	0.435	0.508	0.556	0.599	0.648	0.681
22	0.361	0.425	0.496	0.544	0.586	0.634	0.667
23	0.353	0.415	0.486	0.532	0.573	0.622	0.654
24	0.344	0.406	0.476	0.521	0.562	0.610	0.642
25	0.337	0.398	0.466	0.511	0.551	0.598	0.630
26	0.331	0.390	0.457	0.501	0.541	0.587	0.619
27	0.324	0.382	0.448	0.491	0.531	0.577	0.608
28	0.317	0.375	0.440	0.483	0.522	0.567	0.598
29	0.312	0.368	0.433	0.475	0.513	0.558	0.589
30	0.306	0.362	0.425	0.467	0.504	0.549	0.580
31	0.301	0.356	0.418	0.459	0.496	0.541	0.571
32	0.296	0.350	0.412	0.452	0.489	0.533	0.563
33	0.291	0.345	0.405	0.446	0.482	0.525	0.554
34	0.287	0.340	0.399	0.439	0.475	0.517	0.547
35	0.283	0.335	0.394	0.433	0.468	0.510	0.539
36	0.279	0.330	0.388	0.427	0.462	0.504	0.533
37	0.275	0.325	0.383	0.421	0.456	0.497	0.526
38	0.271	0.321	0.378	0.415	0.450	0.491	0.519
39	0.267	0.317	0.373	0.410	0.444	0.485	0.513
40	0.264	0.313	0.368	0.405	0.439	0.479	0.507
41	0.261	0.309	0.364	0.400	0.433	0.473	0.501
42	0.257	0.305	0.359	0.395	0.428	0.468	0.495
43	0.254	0.301	0.355	0.391	0.423	0.463	0.490
44	0.251	0.298	0.351	0.386	0.419	0.458	0.484
45	0.248	0.294	0.347	0.382	0.414	0.453	0.479

TABLE A.11—*Continued*

n	α_2 α_1	0.10 0.05	0.05 0.025	0.02 0.01	0.01 0.005	0.005 0.0025	0.002 0.001	0.001 0.0005
46		0.246	0.291	0.343	0.378	0.410	0.448	0.474
47		0.243	0.288	0.340	0.374	0.405	0.443	0.469
48		0.240	0.285	0.336	0.370	0.401	0.439	0.465
49		0.238	0.282	0.333	0.366	0.397	0.434	0.460
50		0.235	0.279	0.329	0.363	0.393	0.430	0.456
60		0.214	0.255	0.300	0.331	0.360	0.394	0.418
70		0.198	0.235	0.278	0.307	0.333	0.365	0.388
80		0.185	0.220	0.260	0.287	0.312	0.342	0.363
90		0.174	0.207	0.245	0.271	0.294	0.323	0.343
100		0.165	0.197	0.233	0.257	0.279	0.307	0.326

TABLE A.12   LATIN SQUARES

3 × 3

```
A B C        A B C
B C A        C A B
C A B        B C A
```

4 × 4

```
A B C D      A B C D      A B C D
B A D C      C D A B      D C B A
C D A B      D C B A      B A D C
D C B A      B A D C      C D A B
```

5 × 5

```
A B C D E        A B C D E
B C D E A        C D E A B
C D E A B        E A B C D
D E A B C        B C D E A
E A B C D        D E A B C
```

6 × 6

```
A B C D E F      A B C D E F
B C D E F A      C D E F A B
C D E F A B      E F A B C D
D E F A B C      B C D E F A
E F A B C D      F A B C D E
F A B C D E      D E F A B C
```

7 × 7

```
A B C D E F G    A B C D E F G    A B C D E F G
B C D E F G A    C D E F G A B    E F G A B C D
C D E F G A B    E F G A B C D    B C D E F G A
D E F G A B C    G A B C D E F    F G A B C D E
E F G A B C D    B C D E F G A    C D E F G A B
F G A B C D E    D E F G A B C    G A B C D E F
G A B C D E F    F G A B C D E    D E F G A B C
```

8 × 8

```
A B C D E F G H    A B C D E F G H    A B C D E F G H
B A D C F E H G    E F G H A B C D    D C B A H G F E
C D A B G H E F    B A D C F E H G    H G F E D C B A
D C B A H G F E    F E H G B A D C    E F G H A B C D
E F G H A B C D    G H E F C D A B    F E H G B A D C
F E H G B A D C    C D A B G H E F    G H E F C D A B
G H E F C D A B    H G F E D C B A    C D A B G H E F
H G F E D C B A    D C B A H G F E    B A D C F E H G
```

TABLE A.12—*Continued*

9×9

A	B	C	D	E	F	G	H	I
B	C	A	E	F	D	H	I	G
C	A	B	F	D	E	I	G	H
D	E	F	G	H	I	A	B	C
E	F	D	H	I	G	B	C	A
F	D	E	I	G	H	C	A	B
G	H	I	A	B	C	D	E	F
H	I	G	B	C	A	E	F	D
I	G	H	C	A	B	F	D	E

A	B	C	D	E	F	G	H	I
G	H	I	A	B	C	D	E	F
D	E	F	G	H	I	A	B	C
B	C	A	E	F	D	H	I	G
H	I	G	B	C	A	E	F	D
E	F	D	H	I	G	B	C	A
C	A	B	F	D	E	I	G	H
I	G	H	C	A	B	F	D	E
F	D	E	I	G	H	C	A	B

10×10

A	B	C	D	E	F	G	H	I	J
B	G	A	E	H	C	F	I	J	D
C	H	J	G	F	B	E	A	D	I
D	A	G	I	J	E	C	B	F	H
E	F	H	J	I	G	A	D	B	C
F	E	B	C	D	I	J	G	H	A
G	I	F	B	A	D	H	J	C	E
H	C	I	F	G	H	D	E	A	B
I	J	D	A	C	H	B	F	E	G
J	D	E	H	B	A	I	C	G	F

12×12

A	B	C	D	E	F	G	H	I	J	K	L
B	L	G	C	D	J	K	E	H	A	F	I
C	K	A	B	F	L	I	D	G	H	J	E
D	F	I	A	L	E	C	G	J	B	H	K
E	D	F	G	J	K	A	L	C	I	B	H
F	H	K	E	G	C	D	B	A	L	I	J
G	I	D	F	K	H	J	A	L	C	E	B
H	E	L	J	C	A	B	I	K	D	G	F
I	J	B	L	H	G	F	K	D	E	A	C
J	C	E	K	A	I	H	F	B	G	L	D
K	G	J	H	I	B	L	C	E	F	D	A
L	A	H	I	B	D	E	J	F	K	C	G

Adapted from Tables XV and XVI in Fisher RA, Yates F. *Statistical Tables for Biological, Agricultural, and Medical Research.* Published by Longman Group UK, Ltd, 1974. Used with permission.

B

Summary of Statistical Procedures

Equation numbers in text are given in parentheses.

DESCRIPTIVE STATISTICS (Sample Data)

Mean $\qquad\qquad \overline{X} = \dfrac{\Sigma X}{n}$ (17.1)

Variance $\qquad\qquad s^2 = \dfrac{\Sigma(X - \overline{X})^2}{n - 1} = \dfrac{\Sigma X^2 - \dfrac{(\Sigma X)^2}{n}}{n - 1}$ (17.3,17.4)

Standard deviation $\qquad s = \sqrt{\dfrac{\Sigma(X - \overline{X})^2}{n - 1}} = \sqrt{\dfrac{\Sigma X^2 - \dfrac{(\Sigma X)^2}{n}}{n - 1}}$ (17.5,17.6)

Coefficient of variation $\qquad CV = \dfrac{s}{\overline{X}} \times 100$ (17.7)

z-score $\qquad\qquad z = \dfrac{X - \overline{X}}{s}$ (17.8)

Standard error of the mean $\qquad s_{\overline{X}} = \dfrac{s}{\sqrt{n}}$ (18.1)

CONFIDENCE INTERVALS

For the mean
　Large samples $\qquad CI = \overline{X} \pm (z)s_{\overline{X}}$ (18.2,18.3)

　Small samples $\qquad CI = \overline{X} \pm (t)s_{\overline{X}}$ (18.4)

For the difference between
　sample means $\qquad CI = (\overline{X}_1 - \overline{X}_2) \pm (t)s_{\overline{X}_1 - \overline{X}_2}$ (19.6)

MEASURES OF ASSOCIATION AND CORRELATION

Design conditions	Level of measurement	Test	Statistic
Two continuous variables	Ratio/interval	Pearson product—moment correlation	r
	Ordinal	Spearman rho	r_s
One categorical variable (goodness of fit)	Nominal	Chi square	χ^2
Two (or more) independent samples	Nominal	Chi square	χ^2
Two correlated samples	Nominal	McNemar test	χ^2
Two dichotomies	Nominal	Phi coefficient	ϕ
One dichotomy and one continuous variable	Nominal and ratio/interval	Point biserial correlation	r_{pb}
	Nominal and ordinal	Rank biserial correlation	r_{rb}
One independent variable and one dependent variable	Ratio/interval (ordinal)	Linear regression	r^2
Two or more independent variables and one dependent variable	Ratio/interval (ordinal)	Multiple correlation	R^2

Pearson correlation coefficient

$$r = \frac{n\Sigma XY - (\Sigma X)(\Sigma Y)}{\sqrt{[n\Sigma X^2 - (\Sigma X)^2][n\Sigma Y^2 - (\Sigma Y)^2]}} \tag{23.1}$$

Spearman rank correlation

$$r_s = 1 - \frac{6\Sigma d^2}{n(n^2 - 1)} \tag{23.2}$$

Chi square

$$\chi^2 = \Sigma \frac{(O - E)^2}{E} \tag{25.1}$$

McNemar test

$$\chi^2 = \frac{(A - D)^2}{A + D} \tag{25.7}$$

Phi coefficient

$$\phi = \frac{BC - AD}{\sqrt{(A + B)(C + D)(A + C)(B + D)}} \tag{23.3}$$

Point biserial correlation

$$r_{pb} = \frac{\overline{Y}_1 - \overline{Y}_0}{S_Y} \sqrt{\frac{n_1 n_0}{N(N - 1)}} \tag{23.5}$$

Rank biserial correlation

$$r_{rb} = \frac{2}{n}(\overline{R}_1 - \overline{R}_0) \tag{23.6}$$

COMPARISON OF MEANS: ONE INDEPENDENT VARIABLE TWO LEVELS ($k = 2$)

Design conditions	Level of measurement	Test	Statistic
Independent groups	Ratio/interval	Unpaired t-test	t
	Ordinal	Mann–Whitney U test	U
		Rank sum test	T
Repeated measure	Ratio/interval	Paired t-test	t
(correlated samples)	Ordinal	Sign test	x
		Wilcoxon signed-ranks test	T

INFERENTIAL STATISTICS

Unpaired t-test (equal variances)

$$t = \frac{\overline{X}_1 - \overline{X}_2}{s_{\overline{X}_1 - \overline{X}_2}} \tag{19.1}$$

Pooled variance estimate

$$s_p^2 = \frac{s_1^2 (n_1 - 1) + s_2^2 (n_2 - 1)}{n_1 + n_2 - 2} \tag{19.2}$$

Standard error of the difference

$$s_{\overline{X}_1 - \overline{X}_2} = \sqrt{\frac{s_p^2}{n_1} + \frac{s_p^2}{n_2}} \tag{19.3}$$

Unpaired t-test (unequal variances)

$$t = \frac{\overline{X}_1 - \overline{X}_2}{\sqrt{\frac{s_1^2}{n_1} + \frac{s_2^2}{n_2}}} \tag{19.4}$$

Paired t-test

$$t = \frac{\overline{d}}{s_{\overline{d}}} \tag{19.5}$$

Mann–Whitney U test

$$U_1 = R_1 - \frac{n_1(n_1 + 1)}{2} \tag{22.1}$$

or

$$U_2 = R_2 - \frac{n_2(n_2 + 1)}{2}$$

COMPARISON OF MEANS: ONE INDEPENDENT VARIABLE THREE OR MORE LEVELS (k ≥ 3)

Design conditions	Level of measurement	Test	Statistic
Independent groups	Ratio/interval	Analysis of variance	F
	Ordinal	Kruskal–Wallis ANOVA by ranks	H (χ^2)
Repeated measure	Ratio/interval	Repeated measures ANOVA	F
	Ordinal	Friedman two-way ANOVA by ranks	χ_r^2 (χ^2)

Analysis of variance

$$F = \frac{MS_b}{MS_e} \tag{20.5}$$

$$MS = \frac{SS}{df} \tag{20.4}$$

Total sum of squares

$$SS_t = \Sigma(X - \overline{X})^2 = \Sigma X^2 - \frac{(\Sigma X)^2}{n} \tag{20.1, Table 20.1}$$

Between-groups sum of squares

$$SS_b = \Sigma \frac{(\Sigma X_i)^2}{n} - \frac{(\Sigma X)^2}{N} \tag{20.2, Table 20.1}$$

Error sum of squares

$$SS_e = \Sigma X^2 - \Sigma \frac{(\Sigma X_i)^2}{n} \tag{20.3, Table 20.1}$$

Kruskal–Wallis ANOVA

$$H = \frac{12}{N(N + 1)} \Sigma \frac{R^2}{n} - 3(N + 1) \tag{22.4}$$

Friedman two-way ANOVA

$$\chi_r^2 = \frac{12}{nk(k + 1)} \Sigma R^2 - 3n(k + 1) \tag{22.19}$$

COMPARISON OF MEANS: TWO OR THREE INDEPENDENT VARIABLES (ANY NUMBER OF LEVELS IN EACH VARIABLE)

Design conditions	Level of Measurement	Test	Statistic
Independent groups	Ratio/interval	Two-way (or three-way) ANOVA	F
One repeated measure (mixed design)	Ratio/interval	Two-way (or three-way) ANOVA with one repeated factor	F
All repeated measures	Ratio/interval	Two-way (or three-way) repeated measures ANOVA	F

RELIABILITY STATISTICS

Intraclass correlation coefficients

$$ICC(1, 1) = \frac{BMS - WMS}{BMS + (k + 1)WMS} \tag{26.5}$$

$$ICC(1, k) = \frac{BMS - WMS}{BMS} \tag{26.6}$$

$$ICC(2,1) = \frac{BMS - EMS}{BMS + (k - 1)EMS + \dfrac{k(RMS - EMS)}{n}} \tag{26.7}$$

$$ICC(2, k) = \frac{BMS - EMS}{BMS + \dfrac{(RMS - EMS)}{n}} \tag{26.8}$$

$$ICC(3, 1) = \frac{BMS - EMS}{BMS + (k - 1)EMS} \tag{26.9}$$

$$ICC(3, k) = \frac{BMS - EMS}{BMS} \tag{26.10}$$

Kappa

$$\kappa = \frac{P_o - P_c}{1 - P_c} = \frac{\Sigma f_o - \Sigma f_c}{N - \Sigma f_c} \tag{26.13} \tag{26.14}$$

Weighted kappa

$$\kappa_w = 1 - \frac{\Sigma w f_o}{\Sigma w f_c} \tag{26.16}$$

Standard error of measurement

$$SEM = s_X \sqrt{1 - r_{XX}} \tag{26.17}$$

Method error

$$ME = \frac{s_d}{\sqrt{2}} \tag{26.19}$$

C

Power and Sample Size

In Chapter 18 we introduced the concept of power as an important consideration in testing the null hypothesis. The purpose of this appendix is to describe statistical procedures for power analysis and estimation of sample size for studies using the *t*-test, analysis of variance, correlation, multiple regression, and chi-square for contingency tables. These procedures are based on the work of Cohen.[1] For each procedure, formulas are provided, followed by specific examples of their use.

THE EFFECT SIZE INDEX

In power analysis we are concerned with five statistical elements: the significance criterion (α), the sample size (n), sample variance (s^2), effect size (ES), and power ($1 - \beta$). These elements are related in such a way that given any four, the fifth is readily determined.

Effect size is a measure of the magnitude of difference or correlation. The larger the observed effect, the more likely it will result in a significant statistical test (given a specific alpha level). An *effect size index* is a statistic that represents effect size using a standardized value that is universally applicable for all units of data, just as *t*, *F* and *r* are unit free. A different form of effect size index is used for each statistical procedure.

It is a simple process to calculate a sample effect size index following completion of a study. We know the sample size, and we can calculate the actual variance, means, correlations, or proportions in the data. This information can then be used to determine the degree of power achieved.

During planning stages of a study we use effect size to determine how many subjects will be needed. But because data are not yet available, the researcher must make an educated guess as to the expected effect size. This hypothesis is often based on previous research or pilot data, where studies can provide reasonable estimates for mean differences, correlations and variances. When such data are not available, the effect size estimate may be based on the researcher's opinion of a clinically meaningful difference; that is, the researcher can determine how large an effect would be important. For example, suppose we were interested in studying two treatments for improving shoulder range of motion in patients with adhesive capsulitis. We might say that the results of the treatments should differ by at least 20 degrees, or we would not consider the difference to be meaningful. Therefore, if we observed a difference this large, we would want it to be significant. This would be the effect size we would propose. Similarly, for a correlational study we could propose that a correlation of at least .60 would be important. These types of clinical judgments can then be used to guide the estimation of sample size.

Conventional Effect Sizes

When the researcher wants to establish the required sample size prior to data collection, and no clinical judgment or previous data provide a reasonable guide, Cohen proposes the use of conventional values, which are based on operational definitions for "small," "medium," and "large" effect sizes.[1] Although these definitions are purely relative and somewhat intuitive, Cohen suggests that they represent reasonable estimates for planning purposes. Specific values for small, medium, and large effects are proposed for each statistical procedure. Cohen emphasizes, however, that these descriptions are necessarily relative, and must be operationalized for a given research situation. A small effect size for tests of movement may be quite different from a small effect for psychological phenomena.

As a starting point then, a *small effect size* is considered small enough so that changes are not perceptible to the human eye, but not so small as to be minute. In new areas of inquiry, effect sizes are likely to be small because the phenomenon under study is typically not well understood and perhaps not under good experimental control. Many behavioral effects are likely to fall into this category, because of the influence of extraneous variables and the subtleties of human performance.

A *medium effect size* is conceived as large enough to be visible to the naked eye, so that one would be aware of the change in the course of normal observation.

A *large effect size* represents a great degree of separation, so that there is very little overlap between population distributions. Differences should be grossly observable. Large effect sizes are often seen in sociology, economics, and physiology, fields characterized by studies with large samples and good experimental control.

One way to conceptualize these definitions is to think of effect size in terms of variance. Using a simple framework involving two group means, the difference between means would be considered small if it is 20% of one standard deviation (assuming both groups have the same standard deviation). A medium effect would be equivalent to half a standard deviation, and a large effect would be 80% of a standard deviation. It is useful to think of effect size, then, as a ratio of the variance between groups relative to the variance within groups.

Estimating Sample Size

So what happens if the estimate of effect size is incorrect? What happens if we predict a large effect size and choose the appropriate sample, but the actual scores reveal a small effect, which turns out to be nonsignificant? Well, then we go back and determine the probability of a Type II error, and what level of power was actually achieved. This information can then be used for interpreting the study's results and in planning future studies. It is usually more prudent to be conservative in effect size estimates, so that a large enough sample will be recruited. If several analyses are planned for a given set of data (such as several regression equations or multiple analyses of variance), the sample size must be large enough to support the smallest hypothesized effect for the most complex analysis.[2]

Tables

Tables are provided for power and sample size estimates at the end of this appendix. Power can be determined by knowing effect size and sample size, and sample size can be determined by knowing the expected effect size and the desired level of power. Tables are included for $\alpha = .05$, for one- and two-tailed test where appropriate. Each statistical procedure requires its own set of tables. We have limited these tables to basic configurations for the t-test, analysis of variance, correlation, regression, and chi-square. The reader is referred to Cohen for additional tables.[1]

POWER ANALYSIS FOR THE t-TEST

Power analysis for the t-test is based on the effect size index, d, which expresses the difference between the two sample means in standard deviation units.

Unpaired t-Test: Equal Variances

For the unpaired t-test with equal variances, the effect size index is calculated according to:

$$d = \frac{\overline{X}_1 - \overline{X}_2}{s} \tag{C.1}$$

where $\overline{X}_1$ and $\overline{X}_2$ are the group means, and s is their common standard deviation. Assuming equality of variance, s can be the standard deviation from either group, or it can be their arithmetic average, the square root of the pooled variance, $\sqrt{s_p^2}$ (see Equation 19.2).

If used after data analysis, the d index can also be computed using the calculated value of t:

$$d = t\sqrt{\frac{n_1 + n_2}{n_1 n_2}} \tag{C.2}$$

With a nondirectional alternative hypothesis, only the absolute value of d is considered. With a directional hypothesis, the sign of d must correspond to the predicted direction.

Unpaired t-Test: Unequal Variances

When the assumption of homogeneity of variance is not met, the calculation of d is based on the *root mean square (s')* of s_1 and s_2 as follows:

$$s' = \sqrt{\frac{s_1^2 + s_2^2}{2}} \tag{C.3}$$

The value of s' is used in the denominator of Equation C.1.

Paired *t*-Test

When data are collected in a repeated measures design, calculation of d is based on paired scores. In this case, we first calculate d' using the means for the two test conditions and a common standard deviation:

$$d' = \frac{\overline{X}_1 - \overline{X}_2}{s} \tag{C.4}$$

We account for the fact that these values are correlated by adjusting d as follows:

$$d = \frac{d'}{\sqrt{1 - r}} \tag{C.5}$$

where r is the correlation coefficient for the paired data.

When no estimate of r can be made, we can substitute the formula

$$d' = \frac{\overline{d}}{s_d} \tag{C.6}$$

where $\overline{d}$ is the mean of the difference scores, and s_d is the standard deviation of the difference scores. The value of d to be used in the power tables is then determined by

$$d = d'\sqrt{2} \tag{C.7}$$

Conventional Effect Sizes

When d cannot be computed directly, the following conventions can be used to assign value to the effect size index: small $d = .20$, medium $d = .50$, and large $d = .80$.

Power and Sample Size Tables

To determine the power achieved for a given sample size and effect size, we use Tables C.1.1 and C.1.2, found at the end of this appendix, for estimates at α_1 and $\alpha_2 = .05$. Along the top of the table we locate the appropriate value of d, and down the side, the known sample size, n. For the unpaired test, sample size refers to the number of subjects in *each group* (assuming equal groups), not both groups combined. For the paired *t*-test, this is the number of subjects in the study. Power levels, in percentages, are given in the body of the table.

Unequal Samples. When sample sizes are different for the two groups being compared, the *harmonic mean* of the two sample sizes, n', is computed:

$$n' = \frac{2n_1 n_2}{n_1 + n_2} \tag{C.8}$$

The value of n' is then used to locate n in the power table.

Table C.2 is used to determine the sample size needed for the *t*-test to achieve a desired level of power for one- and two-tailed tests at $\alpha = .05$ and $.01$. For each subtable, the value of d is located across the top, and the desired power is given at the left. Power levels are listed for .70, .80, and .90. The sample sizes found in the body of the table represent the number of subjects required *in each group,* or the total number of subjects for paired observations.

When the exact value of d is not provided in the table, an adequate approximation of n can be given by

$$n = \frac{n_{.10}}{100d^2} + 1 \tag{C.9}$$

where $n_{.10}$ is the sample size given for $d = .10$ in Table C.2, and d is the exact calculated value of the effect size index.*

Examples

Unpaired *t*-Test: Equal Variances.   Consider the data from Table 19.1 in Chapter 19. In that hypothetical study, we measured change in pinch strength in two groups, with $\bar{X}_1 = 10.11$, $\bar{X}_2 = 5.45$, and $s_p^2 = 14.695$. A directional hypothesis was proposed. Therefore, using Equation C.1,

$$s = \sqrt{s_p^2} = \sqrt{14.695} = 3.83 \qquad\qquad d = \frac{10.11 - 5.45}{3.83} = 1.22$$

Alternatively, $t = 2.718$, with $n = 10$ per group. Therefore, using Equation C.2,

$$d = 2.718\sqrt{\frac{10 + 10}{(10)(10)}} = 2.718\sqrt{.20} = 1.22$$

To determine the power achieved with this test, we refer to Table C.1.1 for $\alpha_1 = .05$ and $n = 10$. With $d = 1.2$, we achieve 83% power. If we use these values to determine sample size for 80% power, we refer to Table C.2 for $\alpha_1 = .05$, where we find that we would need 9 subjects per group.

Now suppose we are planning this study. We state a nondirectional hypothesis and propose that a difference of 5 pounds would be important. We guess that a standard deviation of 8.0 would be expected. Therefore, we estimate that $d = 5/8 = .625$. Referring to Table C.2 for $\alpha_1 = .05$ and $d = .60$, we would estimate that we will need 35 subjects *per group* (a total of 70) to achieve 80% power. If once the study is completed, we obtain an effect size index of 1.2 with $n = 35$, we would then have achieved more than 99% power (Table C.1.1).

Unpaired *t*-Test: Unequal Variances.   Consider the data in Table 19.2 in Chapter 19 for change in pinch strength, where $\bar{X}_1 = 10.80$, $\bar{X}_2 = 5.65$ and $s_1^2 = 25.17$, $s_2^2 = 4.89$. Therefore, using Equations C.3 and C.1,

$$s' = \sqrt{\frac{25.17 + 4.89}{2}} = 3.88 \qquad\qquad d = \frac{10.80 - 5.65}{3.88} = 1.33$$

---

*When using an average value for n the power estimates will be underestimates; that is, the power value in the table will be slightly lower than the true power. This underestimate will be trivial when $n' > 25$. Note that when sample sizes and variances are both unequal, the estimates of power using these tables may be inaccurate.[1]

Because the samples are of unequal size, we compute the harmonic mean to determine n' using Equation C.8. With $n_1 = 10$ and $n_2 = 15$:

$$n' = \frac{2n_1 n_2}{n_1 + n_2} = \frac{2(10)(15)}{10 + 15} = \frac{300}{25} = 12$$

Using $n = 12$ in Table C.1.1, we find for $d = 1.2$ power is 89%, and for $d = 1.4$ power is 96%. We can, therefore, estimate that power is approximately 93% for $d = 1.3$.

To determine sample size requirements with $d = 1.3$ we can use Table C.2. For 80% power with $\alpha_1 = .05$, we would need between 9 and 7 subjects (between $d = 1.2$ and 1.4). To calculate the exact sample size for $d = 1.3$, we use Equation C.9:

$$n = \frac{n_{.10}}{100d^2} + 1 = \frac{1237}{100(1.3)^2} + 1 = 7.32 + 1 = 8.32$$

These results should always be rounded up to the nearest whole number. We would need 9 subjects per group to achieve 80% power with this effect size.

Paired t-Test.   Consider the data in Table 19.3 in Chapter 19 for paired data. We examined the angle of the pelvis with and without a lumbar pillow in a sample of 8 subjects. For the paired t-test, we found that $\overline{X}_1 = 112.25$, $\overline{X}_2 = 98.00$ and $s_1 = 9.18$, $s_2 = 8.16$. A nondirectional hypothesis was proposed. The analysis also showed that $r = .86$ for the paired scores. Therefore, we use Equations C.4 and C.5:

$$s = \frac{9.18 + 8.16}{2} = 8.67 \qquad d' = \frac{112.25 - 98.00}{8.67} = 1.64 \qquad d = \frac{1.64}{\sqrt{1 - .86}} = 4.38$$

Alternatively, using $\overline{d} = 14.250$ and $s_d = 4.621$, with Equations C.6 and C.7:

$$d' = \frac{14.250}{4.621} = 3.084 \qquad d = 3.084\sqrt{2} = 4.36$$

To determine power at $\alpha_2 = .05$, we use Table C.1.2. For $n = 8$ we can see that we essentially achieve 100% power, as the effect size index of 4.36 is off the chart. Even though this sample is small, the effect size is extremely large, providing substantial statistical power.

POWER ANALYSIS FOR THE ANALYSIS OF VARIANCE

For the analysis of variance (ANOVA) the effect size index, f, is defined by

$$f = \sqrt{\frac{SS_b}{SS_e}} \tag{C.10}$$

where SS_e is the error sum of squares from the ANOVA summary table.[†] For a one-way ANOVA, SS_b is the between-groups sum of squares. For a two-way ANOVA, SS_b can

---

[†]Some statistical programs report this effect size index as eta squared (η^2):[3] $\eta^2 = \dfrac{SS_b}{SS_b + SS_e}$

These indices are related:[1] $f = \sqrt{\dfrac{\eta^2}{1 - \eta^2}}$ and $\eta^2 = \dfrac{f^2}{1 + f^2}$

represent either an individual main effect or the interaction effect; that is, a separate effect size index can be computed for each effect.[‡] This index can be applied to independent samples and repeated measures designs.

If we do not have access to the ANOVA summary, we can also calculate f using the following formula:

$$f = \frac{s_m}{s} \tag{C.11}$$

where s_m is the standard deviation of the group means around the grand mean, and s is the common standard deviation for each group. For planning purposes, to estimate f, researchers may be able to hypothesize values for group means and their common standard deviation, based on theory and previous research. With equal sample sizes, s_m is obtained by

$$s_m = \sqrt{\frac{\Sigma (\overline{X}_i - \overline{X}_G)^2}{k}} \tag{C.12}$$

where $(\overline{X}_i - \overline{X}_G)$ represents the deviation of each individual group mean ($\overline{X}_i$) from the grand mean ($\overline{X}_G$) and k is the number of groups.[§] Equation C.12 will work for the between-groups effect in a one-way ANOVA and for the main effects in a factorial design.

For two-way interactions, the f index must account for the variability among the interaction means with reference to the main effects (A and B) and the grand mean as follows:

$$s_{m(AB)} = \sqrt{\frac{\Sigma (\overline{X}_{AB} - \overline{X}_A - \overline{X}_B + \overline{X}_G)^2}{df_{AB} + 1}} \tag{C.13}$$

where $\overline{X}_{AB}$ is the individual cell mean, $\overline{X}_A$ is the marginal mean for variable A and $\overline{X}_B$ is the marginal mean for variable B for that cell, and $\overline{X}_G$ is the grand mean for the sample. The term df_{AB} represents the degrees of freedom associated with the interaction term $(A–1)(B–1)$.

Conventional Effect Sizes

When effect sizes cannot be estimated from existing data, conventional values are as follows: Small $f = .10$, medium $f = .25$, large $f = .40$.[‖]

Power and Sample Size Tables

Power tables for the analysis of variance are arranged according to the degrees of freedom associated with each F-test (df_b). In a one-way ANOVA, this is the between-groups effect. In a two-way ANOVA (or larger) these effects will include each main effect and an

---

[‡]Alternatively, an effect size index can also be computed for the overall two-way ANOVA model, combining all between-groups effects. The term SS_b would then be the sum of all between-groups sums of squares (i.e., SS_A, SS_B, and $SS_{A \times B}$).

[§]If groups are not of equal size, the difference between each group mean and the grand mean must be weighted

by the sample size, using $S_m = \sqrt{\dfrac{\Sigma n_i (\overline{X}_i - \overline{X}_G)^2}{N}}$ where n_i is the number of subjects in each group and N is the

total sample size for all groups combined.

[‖]Using η^2 these conventional effect sizes are equivalent to small $\eta^2 = .01$, medium $\eta^2 = .06$, Large $\eta^2 = .14$.

interaction effect. Tables C.3.1 through C.3.4 give power estimates for different values of the effect size index, f, at $df_b = 1, 2, 3$, and 4 at $\alpha = .05$. See Cohen for additional tables.[1]

Sample sizes can be found using Table C.4 for various levels of α and df_b. These tables are used in the same way as the tables for the t-test.

To find n for a value of f that is not tabled, we use

$$n = \frac{n_{.05}}{400f^2} + 1 \tag{C.14}$$

where $n_{.05}$ is the sample size for $f = .05$ at the desired level of power and f is the exact value of the effect size index.

Examples

One-Way Analysis of Variance.   Consider the data for a one-way analysis of variance presented in Table 20.1 in Chapter 20. In this study we examined the effect of different assistive devices on step length in 15 patients with above-knee amputations. Three groups were compared ($k = 3$). Using data from the ANOVA output summary table, we found that $SS_b = 130$ and $SS_e = 90$. Therefore, using Equation C.10,

$$f = \sqrt{\frac{SS_b}{SS_e}} = \sqrt{\frac{130}{90}} = \sqrt{1.44} = 1.20$$

Given conventional effect sizes for f, this is an extremely large effect.

To determine the power achieved with this test, we refer to Table C.3.2 for $df_b = 2$. The sample size used in the table refers to the number of subjects *in each group,* in this case $n = 5$. In this example, the f index is larger than .80, which is the highest value listed in the table. If we look across the row for $n = 5$, for $f = .80$ the power is 69%. Therefore, we can expect that power is substantially higher for $f = 1.2$, and should approach at least 80%, if not close to 100%. Note that we actually would not do a power analysis for this study, as it resulted in a significant F-test. We use it here for illustration only.

Suppose we did not know these results, but we wanted to plan this study to determine the needed sample size. We hypothesize that step length will be greatest for those using a cane, slightly less for those using crutches, and much less for those using no device. As an estimate, based on our knowledge of gait, we guess that the means will be 15, 10, and 5, respectively. Using the literature as a guide, we also estimate that the standard deviation will be 5.0. With these values, we estimate a grand mean of $(15 + 10 + 5)/3 = 10$. Therefore, we can estimate f using Equations C.12 and C.11 as follows:

$$s_m = \sqrt{\frac{\Sigma(\overline{X}_i - \overline{X}_G)}{k}} = \sqrt{\frac{(15 - 10)^2 + (10 - 10)^2 + (5 - 10)^2}{3}} = 4.08$$

$$f = \frac{s_m}{s} = \frac{4.08}{5.0} = .82$$

We turn to Table C.4 ($df_b = 2$) to determine the sample size needed to achieve 80% power with this estimated effect size. Using $f = .80$, we find that we would need

6 subjects per group, or a total sample of 18 subjects. Based on conventional effect sizes, this is considered a large effect, achieving high power even with a relatively small sample.

Two-Way Analysis of Variance.   In a two-way ANOVA, power can be determined for each of the main effects and interaction effects. Consider the data presented in Table 20.2 in Chapter 20, for a study comparing the effect of three types of stretch (*A*) in two knee positions (*B*) for increasing ankle range of motion. A total of 60 subjects were assigned to six unique treatment groups. This analysis resulted in a significant interaction as well as a significant main effect for Stretch, but no significant effect for Position.

Main Effect.   To look at the main effect of Position (variable *B*), we estimate effect size using Equation C.10 as follows:

$$f_B = \sqrt{\frac{SS_B}{SS_e}} = \sqrt{\frac{2.12}{697.36}} = \sqrt{.003} = .055$$

where SS_B is the sum of squares associated with Position (variable *B*).[#] Based on conventional values, this would be considered an extremely small effect. To determine the power of this test with two levels, we use Table C.3.1 for $df_B = 1$. Each level of Position includes 30 subjects. This test achieves 6% power. Therefore, we have a 94% chance that we committed a Type II error. However, we must also consider the fact that the difference between main effect means for the two positions was 0.36 degrees (see Figure 20.4); that is, the observed effect size was extremely small. Given that we are measuring range of motion, such an effect would not be considered important. Therefore, it is unlikely that we have truly committed a Type II error. It is more likely that these positions are not different.

How many subjects would we have needed to achieve 80% power with this effect? We use Table C.4 for $df_b = 1$. For $f = .05$ at 80% power, we would need 1,571 subjects *per group*. As this is surely unreasonable, we might reconsider the inclusion of this variable in our research hypothesis.

Interaction Effect.   To determine power for the interaction effect (an illustration, as this effect was significant), we use Equation C.10 as follows:

$$f_{AB} = \sqrt{\frac{SS_{AB}}{SS_e}} = \sqrt{\frac{707.72}{697.36}} = \sqrt{1.02} = 1.01$$

We refer to Table C.3.2 for $df_b = 2$ (the degrees of freedom associated with the interaction effect). The effect size values do not go as high as 1.00, but for $n = 10$ at $f = .80$, power is 97%. Therefore, we know that we have achieved maximal power for this effect.

In planning this study, suppose we hypothesized that prolonged stretch would be most effective, and that the control group would not change. We also believe that greater

---

[#] For these examples, please do not confuse subscripts *A* and *B*, which represent values associated with factors *A* and *B*, and subscript *b* which indicates the between-groups effect.

ankle range of motion will be achieved when stretch is given with the knee extended. We project the following means:

Stretch		Knee Position		Marginal Means
		Flexion B_1	Extension B_2	
Prolonged	A_1	15	20	$\bar{X}_{A_1} = 17.5$
Quick	A_2	10	10	$\bar{X}_{A_2} = 10$
Control	A_3	0	0	$\bar{X}_{A_3} = 0$
Marginal Means		$\bar{X}_{B_1} = 8.3$	$\bar{X}_{B_2} = 10$	$\bar{X}_G = 9.15$

From the literature we estimate that the standard deviation in our data will be 5.0. Using these values, we compute $s_{m(AB)}$ using Equation C.13 as follows:

$$s_{m(AB)} = \sqrt{\frac{(15 - 17.5 - 8.3 + 9.15)^2 + (20 - 17.5 - 10 + 9.15)^2 + \ldots + (0 - 0 - 10 - 9.15)^2}{2 + 1}} = \sqrt{2.78} = 1.67$$

Therefore, according to Equation C.10,

$$f_{AB} = \frac{1.67}{5.0} = .33$$

To determine sample size, we look at Table C.4 for $df_b = 2$, power = 80%, and $f = .30$. We would need 36 subjects *per group*, or a total of 72 subjects. If we were doing this type of planning for a two-way design, we would project sample sizes for each main effect and interaction, and use the largest sample size as our guideline.

POWER ANALYSIS FOR CORRELATION

Power analysis for correlations is based on the magnitude of association, or the correlation coefficient. Because the correlation coefficient is a unit-free index, the effect size index does not need to be adjusted, and is simply the value of r.

Conventional Effect Sizes

Cohen addresses the dilemma that often surfaces when interpreting values of r; that is, even small correlations are often considered meaningful.[1] This is especially common in the behavioral and clinical sciences, where significant correlations will often be less than .60. Therefore, how does one conceptualize a "large" or "small" effect? This must be a relative frame of reference, based on knowledge of the literature and clinical hypotheses; that is, how much of the variance in clinical phenomena can we truly expect to predict?

Based on this understanding, Cohen hesitates to offer conventional effect sizes for r, but does suggest the following may be used when no other statistical rationale is obvious: Small $r = 1.0$, medium $r = .30$, large $r = .50$.

Power and Sample Size Tables

Tables C.5.1 and C.5.2 can be used to estimate power for the Pearson and Spearman correlations for one- and two-tailed tests at $\alpha = .05$. Table C.6 provides estimated sample sizes required to achieve various levels of power for the same significance levels. The values of n in the tables represent the number of paired observations.

Example

Refer to Table 23.2 in Chapter 23, showing the correlation of proximal and distal behaviors in a sample of 12 normal infants, with a resulting correlation of $r = .37$, which was not significant at $\alpha_1 = .05$. To determine the level of power achieved, we refer to Table C.5.1. With $r = .40$ and 12 subjects, we attained 38% power; that is, there is a 62% chance we committed a Type II error. To find how many subjects we needed for 80% power, we use Table C.6 ($\alpha_1 = .05$). We should have recruited a sample of 37 subjects. In planning a study, we simply hypothesize a meaningful value for r and use this value in Table C.6.

POWER ANALYSIS FOR REGRESSION

In regression analysis, a quantitative dependent variable (Y) is correlated with a set of independent variables (X_1, X_2, through X_k). As with correlation, the degree of association within the regression equation represents the effect size, in this case R^2. The independent variables may represent quantitative or categorical variables (see Chapters 24 and 27).

In determining power, however, we must convert R^2 to another index that will account for both the number of subjects and the number of independent variables in the regression. This index, called lambda (λ)** is calculated as follows:

$$\lambda = \frac{R^2}{1 - R^2} (N) \tag{C.15}$$

Power and Sample Size Tables

Table C.7 is used to determine the power of the regression for $\alpha = .05$. To use this table we must know three elements: (1) the number of independent variables, k, in the leftmost column, (2) the number of residual degrees of freedom, df_{res}, in the analysis of variance of regression (equal to $N - k - 1$), in the second column, and (3) the value for λ, along the top. For values of λ that fall between the values in the table, power can be determined by linear interpolation. Four values for df_{res} are given: 20, 60, 120, and ∞. Although not strictly

---

**Lambda is the *noncentrality parameter* of the F-test. Some statistical programs, such as SPSS, will generate a value for the noncentrality parameter as part of a power analysis for an analysis of variance. This value by itself is not used to represent power, but is needed to obtain power estimates.

linear, for degrees of freedom that fall between these values, power can be estimated with reasonable accuracy.

To determine sample size, we specify a level of power, the number of independent variables, and a projected R^2. We then use Table C.8 to determine a value for lambda and substitute that value in the formula:

$$N = \frac{\lambda(1 - R^2)}{R^2} \qquad (C.16)$$

The obvious dilemma in this process is that finding a value for lambda requires estimating df_{res}, which is a function of sample size, which we are trying to determine! Therefore, the process becomes one of limited trial and error. We start with one value for lambda, determine the associated sample size, and then calculate df_{res} for that sample ($df_{res} = N - k - 1$). If the numbers do not correspond, we go back and choose a different value for df_{res} and try again. One choice in the table will provide a reasonable estimate.

Example

To illustrate power analysis for multiple regression, consider a hypothetical study involving five independent variables ($k = 5$) as predictors of hospital length of stay (LOS). Suppose our sample consists of 30 patients, and results show that $R^2 = .20$ ($p = .176$). Because this is not significant, we want to determine the power of the test. First we calculate lambda for $k = 5$, $R^2 = .20$, $df_{res} = 24$, and $N = 30$, using Equation C.15:

$$\lambda = \frac{R^2}{1 - R^2} (N) = \frac{.20}{1 - .20} (30) = 7.5$$

We refer to Table C.7. Using the closest values for $df_{res} = 20$, $k = 5$, and $\lambda = 8$, we find that our test achieved approximately 44% power, indicating a 56% probability of committing a Type II error.

Table C.7 also shows us how the number of independent variables included in the regression will influence the number of subjects needed. As k increases, we can see that power decreases for a given value of λ. Just to illustrate, look at $k = 3$ for $\lambda = 14$ at $df_{res} = 20$. Power is 82%. If we double the number of independent variables, $k = 6$, power decreases to 66%. With 10 independent variables, we are down to 51%. Researchers will often use stepwise regression or factor analysis to decrease the number of independent variables in a regression analysis, which clearly will have the effect of improving power.

Now let us suppose we are planning this study and we want to determine how many subjects would be needed to achieve 80% power in the analysis with five independent variables. A literature search suggests that the hypothesized effect will be $R^2 = .40$. We start by referring to Table C.8 to determine the value for lambda. Since we do not know how many subjects we need, we must first choose a trial value for df_{res}. Cohen suggests that, as the values of lambda do not vary greatly among the four choices for residual degrees of freedom, using a trial value for $df_{res} = 120$ will generally yield an

N of sufficient accuracy.[1] Starting there, for $k = 5$ at 80% power, we find $\lambda = 13.3$. Using Equation C.16, we determine N as follows:

$$N = \frac{\lambda(1 - R^2)}{R^2} = \frac{13.3(1 - .40)}{.40} = 19.95$$

This projection tells us we would need 20 subjects to achieve 80% power.[††] If we use this estimate, the residual degrees of freedom would then be $N - k - 1 = 20 - 5 - 1 = 14$. Obviously, a great disparity exists between this value and $df_{res} = 120$, which we used to calculate N. This is the trial and error part. Now we return to Table C.8 and find $\lambda = 16.7$ for $k = 5$ and 80% power at $df_{res} = 20$, which we guess will be closer to our required N. This time we find

$$N = \frac{\lambda(1 - R^2)}{R^2} = \frac{16.7(1 - .40)}{.40} = 25.05$$

If we use a sample of 25 subjects, df_{res} will be $25 - 5 - 1 = 19$, which corresponds with the tabled values, so we can be comfortable with the outcome. Note that in planning this study, we hypothesized a value for R^2 that is much higher than the value we actually obtained, and therefore, the sample size estimate would not have been adequate for finding a significant effect. Projections of sample size are only as good as the projected effect size.

POWER ANALYSIS FOR CHI-SQUARE

We can establish power for the chi-square test for goodness of fit tests as well as contingency tables. The effect size index is given the symbol w.

For a 2 × 2 contingency table,[‡‡]

$$w = \sqrt{\frac{\chi^2}{N}} \tag{C.17}$$

For a contingency table with more than two rows or columns,[§§]

$$w = \sqrt{\frac{\chi^2}{N(q - 1)}} (\sqrt{q - 1}) \tag{C.18}$$

where q is the number of rows or columns, *whichever is smaller*.

[††]We can demonstrate that using 120 degrees of freedom for the calculation will yield a value for N that is not much different from those that would be calculated using the other values. For instance, for $df_{res} = 60$, $\lambda = 11.5$, which would yield $N = 36.42$. For $df_{res} = 20$, $\lambda = 13.2$, which would yield $N = 41.8$. We can generally expect these sample sizes to vary by no more than 10 subjects. Cohen does provide a formula for obtaining a more exact value of N using an adjusted value for λ.[1]

[‡‡]Note that this value is identical to the phi coefficient, described in Chapters 23 and 25.

[§§]Note that this value is related to Cramer's V, described in Chapter 25.

Conventional Effect Sizes

Cohen offers values for conventional effect sizes: Small $w = .10$, medium $w = .30$, large $w = .50$. He suggests, however, that these values be used with caution, as the value of w will vary with the number of rows, columns, and degrees of freedom in a set of data, even when the true degree of association is the same.

Power and Sample Size Tables

Tables C.9.1 through C.9.4 provide power estimates for $\alpha = .05$ for degrees of freedom $= 1, 2, 3,$ and 4 associated with chi-square $[(R-1)(C-1)]$. To use the tables, we must specify the overall sample size (N) and the value of w. Table C.10 provides sample size estimates, based on a given α level and degrees of freedom. If the value for w is not given in the table, we can determine an exact N according to:

$$N = \frac{N_{.10}}{100w^2} \tag{C.19}$$

where $N_{.10}$ is the required sample size for $w = .10$ for the desired power and degrees of freedom.

Examples

2 × 2 Tables. To illustrate this application for a 2 × 2 contingency table, refer to the study described in Chapter 25, Table 25.5. This study examined the incidence of complications following open heart surgery in patients receiving breathing exercises or routine care (a 2 × 2 design). For these data, $\chi^2 = 2.49$ and $N = 40$. This study did not result in a significant chi-square test. We can apply these data to determine the probability of committing a Type II error using Equation C.17:

$$w = \sqrt{\frac{2.49}{40}} = \sqrt{.062} = .25$$

Using Table C.9.1, for 1 degree of freedom, this study achieves power between 24% and 47% (between $w = .20$ and .30). We can estimate power around 36%, with an associated probability of Type II error of 67%. We did not have enough subjects in this study.

To determine how many subjects we would need to achieve 80% power, we refer to Table C.10. For $w = .20$ (let's be conservative in our estimate), we need 196 subjects (substantially more than the original study used).

Larger Tables. Similarly, we can illustrate the calculation of w for larger tables, using the 2 × 4 study of hydrocortisone use shown in Table 25.4 (even though this study actually resulted in a significant value of chi-square, and we would not be concerned about power). For these data, $\chi^2 = 10.88$ with $N = 70$. With 4 rows and 2 columns, we will use $q = 2$ (the smaller number). According to Equation C.18,

$$w = \sqrt{\frac{10.88}{70(2-1)}} \sqrt{2-1} = .394$$

Using Table C.9.3, for 3 degrees of freedom, $N = 70$ and $w = .40$, we find that this study achieved 81% power.

REFERENCES

1. Cohen J. *Statistical Power Analysis for the Behavioral Sciences.* 2d ed. Hillsdale, NJ: Lawrence Erlbaum Associates, 1988.
2. Knapp TR. The overemphasis on power analysis. *Nurs Res* 1996;45:379–80.
3. Green SB, Salkind NJ, Akey TM. *Using SPSS for Windows: Analyzing and Understanding Data.* Upper Saddle River, NJ: Prentice-Hall, 1997.

TABLE C.1.1 POWER OF THE t-TEST FOR $\alpha_1 = .05$

n	.10	.20	.30	.40	.50	.60	.70	.80	1.00	1.20	1.40
8	07	10	13	19	25	31	38	46	61	74	85
9	07	11	15	20	27	34	41	50	66	79	88
10	08	11	16	22	29	36	45	53	70	83	91
11	08	12	17	23	31	39	48	57	74	86	94
12	08	12	18	25	33	41	51	60	77	89	96
13	08	13	18	26	34	44	54	63	80	91	97
14	08	13	19	27	36	46	57	66	83	93	98
15	08	13	20	28	38	48	59	69	85	94	98
16	09	14	21	30	40	51	62	72	87	95	99
17	09	14	22	31	42	53	64	74	89	96	99
18	09	15	22	32	43	55	66	76	90	97	99
19	09	15	23	33	45	57	68	78	92	98	
20	09	15	24	34	46	59	70	80	93	98	
30	10	19	31	46	61	74	85	92	99		
40	11	22	38	55	72	84	93	97			
50	12	26	44	63	80	91	97	99			
100	17	41	68	88	97						
200	26	64	91	99							

TABLE C.1.2 POWER OF THE t-TEST FOR $\alpha_2 = .05$

n	.10	.20	.30	.40	.50	.60	.70	.80	1.00	1.20	1.40
8	05	07	09	11	15	20	25	31	46	60	73
9	05	07	09	12	16	22	28	35	51	65	79
10	06	07	10	13	18	24	31	39	56	71	84
11	06	07	10	14	20	26	34	43	61	76	87
12	06	08	11	15	21	28	37	46	65	80	90
13	06	08	11	16	23	31	40	50	69	83	93
14	06	08	12	17	25	33	43	53	72	86	94
15	06	08	12	18	26	35	45	56	75	88	96
16	06	08	13	19	28	37	48	59	78	90	97
17	06	09	13	20	29	39	51	62	80	92	98
18	06	09	14	21	31	41	53	64	83	94	98
19	06	09	15	22	32	43	55	67	85	95	99
20	06	09	15	23	33	45	58	69	87	96	99
30	07	12	21	33	47	63	76	86	97		
40	07	14	26	42	60	75	87	94	99		
50	08	17	32	50	70	84	93	98			
100	11	29	56	80	94	99					
200	17	51	85	98							

Adapted from Tables 2.3.2 and 2.3.5 in Cohen J. *Statistical Power Analysis for the Behavioral Sciences,* ed 2. Hillsdale, NJ: Lawrence Erlbaum Associates, 1988. Used with permission of the publisher and author.

TABLE C.2 SAMPLE SIZES NEEDED FOR THE t-TEST

Power	.10	.20	.30	.40	.50	.60	.70	.80	1.00	1.20	1.40
$\alpha_1 = .05$											
.70	942	236	105	60	38	27	20	15	10	7	6
.80	1237	310	138	78	50	35	26	20	13	9	7
.90	1713	429	191	108	69	48	36	27	18	13	10
$\alpha_2 = .05$											
.70	1235	310	138	78	50	35	26	20	13	10	7
.80	1571	393	175	99	64	45	33	26	17	12	9
.90	2102	526	234	132	85	59	44	34	22	16	12

Adapted from Table 2.4.1 in Cohen J. *Statistical Power Analysis for the Behavioral Sciences,* ed 2. Hillsdale, NJ: Lawrence Erlbaum Associates, 1988. Used with permission of the publisher and author.

TABLE C.3.1   POWER OF THE F-TEST IN ANALYSIS OF VARIANCE FOR $\alpha = .05$ AND $df_b = 1$

n	.05	.10	.15	.20	.25	.30	.35	.40	.50	.60	.70	.80
5	05	06	07	08	11	13	16	20	38	29	50	61
6	05	06	07	09	12	15	20	34	35	47	60	71
7	05	06	08	10	14	18	23	28	41	55	68	79
8	05	06	08	11	15	20	26	32	47	62	75	85
9	05	07	09	12	17	22	29	36	52	68	80	89
10	05	07	09	13	18	25	32	40	57	73	85	93
11	05	07	10	14	20	27	35	44	62	77	88	95
12	05	07	10	15	22	29	38	47	66	81	91	97
13	05	07	11	16	23	32	41	51	70	84	93	98
14	05	08	11	17	25	34	44	54	73	87	95	98
15	06	08	12	18	26	36	47	57	76	89	96	99
16	06	08	12	19	28	38	49	60	79	91	97	99
17	06	08	13	20	30	40	52	63	82	93	98	
18	06	08	14	21	31	42	54	66	84	94	98	
19	06	09	14	22	33	44	57	68	86	95	99	
20	06	09	15	23	34	46	59	70	88	96	99	
30	06	11	21	34	49	64	77	87	97			
40	07	14	27	43	61	77	88	95	99			
50	07	16	32	52	71	85	94	98				
60	08	19	38	60	79	94	97	99				
80	09	24	48	72	89	97	99					
100	10	29	57	81	94	99						
120	11	34	65	88	94							
140	13	39	72	92	99							
160	14	44	77	95	99							
180	15	48	82	97								
200	16	52	86	98								

TABLE C.3.2   POWER OF THE F-TEST IN ANALYSIS OF VARIANCE FOR $\alpha = .05$ AND $df_b = 2$

n	.05	.10	.15	.20	.25	.30	.35	.40	.50	.60	.70	.80
5	05	06	07	09	11	14	17	22	32	44	56	69
6	05	06	07	10	13	16	21	26	39	53	67	79
7	05	06	08	11	14	19	25	31	46	62	76	87
8	05	06	08	12	16	22	28	36	53	69	83	92
9	05	07	09	13	18	24	32	40	59	75	88	95
10	05	07	10	14	20	27	35	45	64	81	91	97
11	05	07	10	15	21	30	39	49	69	85	94	98
12	06	07	11	16	23	32	42	53	74	88	96	99
13	06	08	11	17	25	35	46	57	77	91	97	99
14	06	08	12	18	27	38	49	61	81	93	98	
15	06	08	13	20	29	40	52	64	84	95	99	
16	06	08	13	21	31	43	55	94	86	96	99	
17	06	09	14	22	33	45	58	70	89	97	99	
18	06	09	14	23	34	48	61	73	90	98		
19	06	09	15	24	36	50	64	76	92	99		
20	06	09	16	26	38	52	66	78	93	99		
30	06	12	22	37	55	71	85	93	99			
40	07	15	29	48	68	84	94	98				
50	08	18	36	58	79	92	98	99				
60	08	21	42	67	86	96	99					
80	09	27	54	80	94	99						
100	11	32	64	88	98							
120	12	38	73	94	99							
140	14	44	79	97								
160	15	49	85	98								
180	16	54	89	99								
200	18	59	92									

TABLE C.3.3 POWER OF THE F-TEST IN ANALYSIS OF VARIANCE FOR $\alpha = .05$ AND $df_b = 3$

n	.05	.10	.15	.20	.25	.30	.35	.40	.50	.60	.70	.80
5	05	06	07	09	12	15	19	24	36	50	64	76
6	05	06	08	10	13	18	23	29	44	60	75	86
7	05	06	08	11	15	21	27	35	52	69	83	92
8	05	07	09	12	17	24	31	40	59	77	89	96
9	05	07	09	14	19	27	36	46	66	82	93	98
10	05	07	10	15	21	30	40	51	71	87	96	99
11	06	07	11	16	24	33	44	55	76	91	97	99
12	06	08	11	17	26	36	48	60	81	93	98	
13	06	08	12	19	28	39	52	64	84	95	99	
14	06	08	13	20	30	42	55	68	87	97	99	
15	06	08	13	21	32	45	59	71	90	98		
16	06	09	14	23	34	48	62	75	92	98		
17	06	09	15	24	37	51	65	78	94	99		
18	06	09	16	26	39	53	68	80	95	99		
19	06	09	16	27	41	56	71	83	96	99		
20	06	10	17	28	43	59	73	85	97			
30	07	13	25	42	61	79	90	96	99			
40	07	16	32	54	76	90	97	99				
50	08	19	40	65	85	96	99					
60	09	22	47	74	91	98						
80	10	29	61	86	97							
100	11	36	71	93	99							
120	13	43	80	97								
140	14	49	86	99								
160	16	55	94	99								
180	18	61	94									
200	19	66	96									

TABLE C.3.4 POWER OF THE F-TEST IN ANALYSIS OF VARIANCE FOR $\alpha = .05$ AND $df_b = 4$

n	.05	.10	.15	.20	.25	.30	.35	.40	.50	.60	.70	.80
5	05	06	07	09	12	16	21	26	40	55	70	83
6	05	06	08	10	14	19	25	32	49	66	81	91
7	05	06	09	12	16	22	30	39	58	79	88	96
8	05	07	09	13	19	26	35	45	65	83	93	98
9	05	07	10	14	21	29	40	51	72	88	96	99
10	06	07	10	16	23	33	44	56	78	92	98	
11	06	08	11	17	26	37	49	61	82	94	99	
12	06	08	12	19	28	40	53	66	86	96	99	
13	06	08	13	20	31	43	57	70	89	98		
14	06	08	13	22	33	47	61	74	92	98		
15	06	09	14	23	36	50	65	78	94	99		
16	06	09	15	25	38	53	68	81	95	99		
17	06	09	16	26	40	56	71	83	96			
18	06	09	17	28	43	59	74	86	97			
19	06	10	17	30	45	62	77	88	98			
20	06	10	18	31	47	65	79	90	99			
30	07	13	27	46	67	84	94	98				
40	07	17	36	60	81	94	99					
50	08	21	44	81	90	98						
60	09	24	52	80	95	99						
80	10	32	66	91	99							
100	12	40	77	96								
120	13	47	85	99								
140	15	54	91	99								
160	17	61	94									
180	18	67	97									
200	20	72	98									

Adapted from Tables 8.3.12 to 8.3.15 in Cohen, J. *Statistical Power Analysis for the Behavioral Sciences,* ed 2. Hillsdale, NJ: Lawrence Erlbaum Associates, 1988. Used with permission of the publisher and author.

TABLE C.4   SAMPLE SIZES NEEDED FOR THE ANALYSIS OF VARIANCE FOR $\alpha = .05$

Power	.05	.10	.15	.20	.25	.30	.35	.40	.50	.60	.70	.80
$df_b = 1$												
.70	1235	310	138	78	50	35	26	20	13	10	7	6
.80	1571	393	175	99	64	45	33	26	17	12	9	7
.90	2102	526	234	132	85	59	44	34	22	16	12	9
$df_b = 2$												
.70	1028	258	115	65	42	29	22	17	11	8	6	5
.80	1286	322	144	81	52	36	27	21	14	10	8	6
.90	1682	421	188	106	68	48	35	27	18	13	10	8
$df_b = 3$												
.70	881	221	99	56	36	25	19	15	10	7	6	5
.80	1096	274	123	69	45	31	23	18	12	9	7	5
.90	1415	354	158	89	58	40	30	23	15	11	8	7
$df_b = 4$												
.70	776	195	87	49	32	22	17	13	9	6	5	4
.80	956	240	107	61	39	27	20	16	10	8	6	5
.90	1231	309	138	78	50	35	26	20	13	10	7	6
$df_b = 5$												
.70	698	175	78	44	29	20	15	12	8	6	5	4
.80	856	215	96	54	35	25	18	14	9	7	5	4
.90	1098	275	123	69	45	31	23	18	12	9	7	5
$df_b = 6$												
.70	638	160	72	41	26	18	14	11	7	5	4	4
.80	780	195	87	50	32	22	17	13	9	6	5	4
.90	995	250	112	63	41	29	21	16	11	8	6	5
$df_b = 8$												
.70	548	138	61	35	23	16	12	9	6	5	4	3
.80	669	168	75	42	27	19	14	11	8	6	4	4
.90	848	213	95	54	35	24	18	14	9	7	5	4
$df_b = 10$												
.70	488	123	55	31	20	14	11	8	6	4	3	3
.80	591	148	66	38	24	17	13	10	7	5	4	3
.90	747	187	84	48	31	22	16	13	8	6	5	4

Adapted from Tables 8.4.4 and 8.4.5 in Cohen J. *Statistical Power Analysis for the Behavioral Sciences,* ed 2. Hillsdale, NJ: Lawrence Erlbaum Associates, 1988. Used with permission of the publisher and author.

TABLE C.5.1   POWER OF THE CORRELATION COEFFICIENT, r ($\alpha_1 = .05$)

					r				
n	.10	.20	.30	.40	.50	.60	.70	.80	.90
8	08	12	18	26	37	52	68	85	97
9	08	13	20	29	42	57	74	90	99
10	08	14	22	32	46	62	79	93	99
11	09	15	23	35	50	67	83	95	
12	09	15	25	38	54	71	87	97	
13	09	16	26	40	57	74	89	98	
14	10	17	28	43	60	78	91	98	
15	10	18	30	45	63	81	93	99	
20	11	22	37	56	75	90	98		
30	13	28	50	72	90	98			
40	15	35	60	83	96				
50	17	41	69	90	98				
60	19	45	76	94	99				
80	22	45	86	98					
100	26	64	82	99					
200	41	89							
500	72								
1000	94								

TABLE C.5.2   POWER OF THE CORRELATION COEFFICIENT, r ($\alpha_2 = .05$)

					r				
n	.10	.20	.30	.40	.50	.60	.70	.80	.90
8	06	07	11	16	25	37	54	75	94
9	06	08	12	19	29	43	62	82	97
10	06	08	13	21	33	49	68	87	98
11	06	09	14	23	36	54	73	91	99
12	06	09	16	26	40	58	78	93	99
13	06	10	17	28	44	63	82	95	
14	06	10	18	30	47	66	85	96	
15	06	11	19	32	50	70	88	98	
20	07	14	25	43	34	83	96		
30	08	19	37	61	83	95			
40	09	24	48	74	92	99			
50	11	29	57	83	97				
60	12	34	65	90	99				
80	14	43	78	96					
100	17	52	86	99					
200	29	81	99						
500	61	99							
1000	89								

Adapted from Tables 3.3.2 and 3.3.5 in Cohen, J. *Statistical Power Analysis for the Behavioral Sciences,* ed 2. Hillsdale, NJ: Lawrence Erlbaum Associates, 1988. Used with permission of the publisher and author.

TABLE C.6   SAMPLE SIZES NEEDED FOR THE CORRELATION COEFFICIENT, r

					r				
Power	.10	.20	.30	.40	.50	.60	.70	.80	.90
$\alpha_1 = .05$									
.70	470	117	52	28	18	12	8	6	4
.80	617	153	68	37	22	15	10	7	5
.90	854	211	92	50	31	20	13	9	6
$\alpha_2 = .05$									
.70	616	153	67	37	23	15	10	7	5
.80	783	194	85	46	28	18	12	9	6
.90	1047	259	113	62	37	24	16	11	7

Adapted from Table 3.4.1 in Cohen, J. *Statistical Power Analysis for the Behavioral Sciences,* ed 2. Hillsdale, NJ: Lawrence Erlbaum Associates, 1988. Used with permission of the publisher and author.

TABLE C.7   POWER OF THE F-TEST FOR REGRESSION ANALYSIS AT α = .05

λ

k	df_{res}	2	4	6	8	10	12	14	16	18	20	24	28	32	36	40
1	20	27	48	64	77	85	91	95	97	98	99					
	60	29	50	67	79	88	92	96	98	99	99					
	120	29	51	68	80	88	93	96	98	99	99					
	∞	29	52	69	81	89	93	96	98	99	99					
2	20	20	36	52	65	75	83	88	92	95	97	99				
	60	22	40	56	69	79	87	91	95	97	98					
	120	22	41	57	71	80	87	92	95	97	98					
	∞	23	42	58	72	82	88	93	96	97	99					
3	20	17	30	44	56	67	75	82	87	91	94	97	99			
	60	19	34	49	62	73	81	87	92	95	97	98				
	120	19	35	50	64	75	83	89	93	95	97	99				
	∞	19	36	52	65	76	84	90	93	96	98	99				
4	20	15	26	38	49	60	69	76	83	87	91	95	98	99		
	60	17	30	44	57	68	77	83	89	92	95	98	99			
	120	17	31	46	58	70	78	85	90	93	96	98	99			
	∞	17	32	47	60	72	80	87	91	94	96	99	99			
5	20	13	23	34	44	54	63	71	78	83	87	93	96	98	99	
	60	15	27	40	52	63	72	80	86	90	93	97	99			
	120	16	29	41	54	65	75	82	87	91	94	98	99			
	∞	16	29	43	56	68	77	84	89	93	95	98	99			
10	20	09	16	23	30	37	44	51	58	64	70	79	86	91	94	96
	60	10	20	30	39	48	56	65	72	78	83	90	95	97	99	99
	120	11	21	31	42	51	60	69	75	81	86	93	96	98	99	
	∞	12	21	32	43	54	64	72	79	85	89	94	98	99		
15	20	08	12	17	22	27	33	39	44	50	55	65	74	81	86	90
	60	09	15	22	30	38	46	54	61	67	73	83	89	94	96	98
	120	10	16	24	33	42	51	59	66	73	78	87	92	96	98	99
	∞	10	18	27	37	47	56	64	72	78	83	91	95	97	99	99
20	20	08	11	14	18	22	26	31	36	40	45	54	63	70	77	82
	60	08	13	19	25	31	38	45	52	58	64	75	83	89	93	96
	120	09	14	21	28	36	43	51	58	65	71	81	88	93	96	98
	∞	09	16	24	32	41	50	58	65	72	78	87	92	96	98	99

Adapted from Table 9.3.2 in Cohen, J. *Statistical Power Analysis for the Behavioral Sciences*, ed 2. Hillsdale, NJ: Lawrence Erlbaum Associates, 1988. Used with the permission of the publisher and author.

TABLE C.8 VALUES OF LAMBDA (λ) USED TO DETERMINE SAMPLE SIZE FOR THE *F*-TEST FOR REGRESSION ANALYSIS (α = .05)

k	df_{res}	.25	.50	.60	.67	.70	.75	.80	.85	.90	.95	.99
1	20	1.9	4.1	5.3	6.2	6.7	7.5	8.5	9.7	11.4	14.1	20.1
	60	1.7	3.9	4.9	5.8	6.2	7.0	7.9	9.1	10.6	13.2	18.7
	120	1.7	3.8	4.9	5.7	6.2	6.9	7.8	9.0	10.5	13.0	18.4
	∞	1.6	3.8	4.9	5.7	6.2	6.9	7.8	9.0	10.5	13.0	18.4
2	20	2.6	5.7	7.1	8.2	8.9	9.9	11.1	12.6	14.6	17.9	24.9
	60	2.3	5.1	6.4	7.4	8.0	8.9	10.0	11.3	13.2	16.1	22.4
	120	2.3	5.0	6.3	7.2	7.8	8.7	9.7	11.1	12.8	15.7	21.8
	∞	2.2	5.0	6.2	7.2	7.7	8.6	9.6	10.9	12.7	15.4	21.4
3	20	3.2	6.9	8.6	9.9	10.6	11.8	13.2	14.9	17.2	20.9	28.7
	60	2.8	6.0	7.5	8.6	9.3	10.3	11.5	13.0	15.0	18.3	25.1
	120	2.7	5.8	7.3	8.4	9.0	10.0	11.1	12.6	14.5	17.7	24.3
	∞	2.7	5.8	7.2	8.2	8.8	9.8	10.9	12.3	14.2	17.2	23.5
4	20	3.8	8.0	9.9	11.4	12.2	13.5	15.0	16.9	19.5	23.5	32.1
	60	3.3	6.8	8.5	9.7	10.4	11.5	12.8	14.4	16.6	20.1	27.4
	120	3.1	6.6	8.1	9.3	10.0	11.0	12.3	13.9	16.0	19.3	26.3
	∞	3.1	6.4	7.9	9.1	9.7	10.7	11.9	13.4	15.4	18.6	25.2
5	20	4.4	9.0	11.1	12.7	13.6	15.0	16.7	18.8	21.6	26.0	35.2
	60	3.7	7.5	9.3	10.6	11.3	12.6	14.0	15.7	18.0	21.7	29.4
	120	3.5	7.2	8.9	10.1	10.8	12.0	13.3	15.0	17.2	20.7	28.1
	∞	3.4	7.0	8.6	9.8	10.5	11.6	12.8	14.4	16.5	19.8	26.7
10	20	6.9	13.7	16.7	18.9	20.1	22.1	24.4	27.3	31.0	37.0	49.2
	60	5.3	10.5	12.8	14.5	15.4	17.0	18.7	20.9	23.8	28.3	37.7
	120	5.0	9.8	11.9	13.5	14.3	15.8	17.4	19.5	22.1	26.4	35.2
	∞	4.4	9.2	11.2	12.6	13.4	14.7	16.8	18.1	20.5	24.4	32.4
15	20	9.2	18.0	21.8	24.6	26.1	28.7	31.6	35.1	39.8	47.1	62.2
	60	6.7	13.1	15.8	17.8	18.9	20.7	22.8	25.3	28.7	33.9	44.7
	120	6.1	11.9	14.3	16.2	17.2	18.8	20.7	23.1	26.1	30.9	40.8
	∞	5.6	10.9	13.1	14.7	15.6	17.1	18.8	20.9	23.6	27.8	36.6
20	20	11.4	22.2	26.8	30.1	32.0	35.0	38.5	42.7	48.3	57.0	74.8
	60	8.1	15.4	18.5	20.8	22.1	24.1	26.5	29.4	33.2	39.1	51.2
	120	7.2	13.7	16.5	18.6	19.7	21.6	23.7	26.3	29.6	34.9	45.8
	∞	6.4	12.3	14.7	16.5	17.5	19.1	21.0	23.2	26.1	30.7	40.1

(Column group header: **Power**)

Adapted from Table 9.4.2 in Cohen, J. *Statistical Power Analysis for the Behavioral Sciences*, ed 2. Hillsdale, NJ: Lawrence Erlbaum Associates, 1988. Used with permission of the publisher and the author.

TABLE C.9.1   POWER OF THE χ^2 TEST AT α = .05 FOR *df* = 1

N	.10	.20	.30	.40	.50	.60	.70	.80	.90
25	08	17	32	52	70	85	94	98	99
30	08	19	38	59	78	91	97	99	
35	09	22	43	66	84	94	99		
40	10	24	47	71	89	97	99		
45	10	27	52	76	92	98			
50	11	29	56	81	94	99			
60	12	34	64	87	97				
70	13	39	71	92	99				
80	15	43	76	95	99				
90	16	47	81	97					
100	17	52	85	98					
120	19	59	91	99					
140	22	66	94						
160	24	71	97						
180	27	76	98						
200	29	81	99						
300	41	93							
500	61	99							
600	69								
700	75								
800	81								
900	85								
1000	89								

TABLE C.9.2   POWER OF THE χ^2 TEST AT α = .05 FOR *df* = 2

N	.10	.20	.30	.40	.50	.60	.70	.80	.90
25	07	13	25	42	60	77	89	96	99
30	07	15	29	49	69	85	94	98	
35	08	17	34	55	76	90	97	99	
40	08	19	38	61	82	93	98		
45	09	21	42	67	86	96	99		
50	09	23	46	72	90	97			
60	10	26	54	80	94	99			
70	11	30	61	86	97				
80	12	34	67	90	99				
90	12	38	72	93	99				
100	13	42	77	96					
120	15	49	85	98					
140	17	55	90	99					
160	19	61	93						
180	21	67	96						
200	23	72	97						
300	32	88							
500	50	99							
600	58								
700	66								
800	72								
900	77								
1000	82								

TABLE C.9.3 POWER OF THE χ^2 TEST AT $\alpha = .05$ FOR $df = 3$

N	.10	.20	.30	.40	.50	.60	.70	.80	.90
					w				
25	07	12	21	36	54	71	85	93	98
30	07	13	25	42	62	80	90	97	99
35	07	15	29	49	70	86	95	99	
40	07	16	32	55	76	90	97	99	
45	08	18	36	60	81	94	99		
50	08	19	40	65	86	96	99		
60	09	22	47	74	92	98			
70	09	26	54	81	95	99			
80	10	29	60	86	98				
90	11	32	66	90	99				
100	12	36	71	93	99				
120	13	42	80	97					
140	15	49	86	99					
160	16	55	90	99					
180	18	60	94						
200	19	65	96						
300	27	84							
500	44	98							
600	52	99							
700	59								
800	65								
900	71								
1000	76								

TABLE C.9.4 POWER OF THE χ^2 TEST AT $\alpha = .05$ FOR $df = 4$

N	.10	.20	.30	.40	.50	.60	.70	.80	.90
					w				
25	06	11	19	32	50	66	81	91	97
30	07	12	22	38	57	75	88	96	99
35	07	13	26	44	65	82	93	98	
40	07	14	29	50	72	88	96	99	
45	07	16	32	55	77	92	98		
50	08	17	36	60	82	94	99		
60	08	20	43	70	89	98			
70	09	23	49	77	94	99			
80	09	26	55	83	96				
90	10	29	61	88	98				
100	11	32	66	91	99				
120	12	38	75	96					
140	13	44	82	98					
160	14	50	88	99					
180	16	55	92						
200	17	60	94						
300	24	80	99						
500	40	96							
600	47	99							
700	54								
800	60								
900	66								
1000	72								

Adapted from Tables 7.3.15 to 7.3.18 in Cohen, J. *Statistical Power Analysis for the Behavioral Sciences,* ed 2. Hillsdale, NJ: Lawrence Erlbaum Associates, 1988. Used with permission of the publisher and author.

TABLE C.10 SAMPLE SIZES NEEDED FOR χ^2 FOR $\alpha = .05$

	w								
Power	*.10*	*.20*	*.30*	*.40*	*.50*	*.60*	*.70*	*.80*	*.90*
df = 1									
.70	617	154	69	39	25	17	13	10	8
.80	785	196	87	49	31	22	16	12	10
.90	1051	263	117	66	42	29	21	16	13
df = 2									
.70	770	193	86	48	31	21	16	12	10
.80	964	241	107	60	39	27	20	15	12
.90	1265	316	141	79	51	35	26	20	16
df = 3									
.70	879	220	98	55	35	24	18	14	11
.80	1090	273	121	68	44	30	22	17	13
.90	1417	354	157	89	57	39	29	22	17
df = 4									
.70	968	242	108	61	39	27	20	15	12
.80	1194	298	133	75	48	33	24	19	15
.90	1540	385	171	96	62	43	31	24	19
df = 6									
.70	1114	279	124	70	45	31	23	17	14
.80	1362	341	151	85	54	38	28	21	17
.90	1742	435	194	109	70	48	36	27	22
df = 8									
.70	1235	309	137	77	49	34	25	19	15
.80	1502	376	167	94	60	42	31	23	19
.90	1908	477	212	119	76	53	39	30	24
df = 9									
.70	1289	322	143	81	52	36	26	20	16
.80	1565	391	174	98	63	43	32	24	19
.90	1983	496	220	124	79	55	40	31	24
df = 12									
.70	1435	359	159	90	57	40	29	22	18
.80	1734	433	193	108	69	48	35	27	21
.90	2183	546	243	136	87	61	45	34	27

Adapted from Tables 7.4.6 to 7.4.9 in Cohen, J. *Statistical Power Analysis for the Behavioral Sciences,* ed 2. Hillsdale, NJ, Lawrence Erlbaum Associates, 1988. Used with the permission of the publisher and author.

APPENDIX

D

Transformation of Data

Many statistical procedures, like the *t*-test, analysis of variance, and linear regression, are based on assumptions about homogeneity of variance and normality that should be met to ensure the validity of the test. Although most parametric statistical procedures are considered robust to moderate violations of these assumptions, some modification to the analysis is usually necessary with striking departures. When this occurs, the researcher can choose one of two approaches to accommodate the analysis. The analytic procedure can be modified, by using nonparametric statistics or nonlinear regression, or the dependent variable, X, can be transformed to a new variable, X', which more closely satisfies the necessary assumptions. The new variable is created by changing the scale of measurement for X. In this appendix we introduce five approaches to *data transformation*.

The three most common reasons for using data transformation are to satisfy the assumption of homogeneity of variance, to conform data to a normal distribution, and to create a more linear distribution that will fit the linear regression model. Fortunately, the same transformation will often accomplish more than one of these goals.[1]

The most commonly used transformations are the square root transformation, the square transformation, the log transformation, the reciprocal transformation, and the arc sine transformation. The choice of which method to use will depend on characteristics of the data. Before we describe the guidelines for using each of these approaches, it may be helpful to illustrate the transformation process using the square root transformation.

The *square root transformation* ($X' = \sqrt{X}$) replaces each score in a distribution with its square root. This method is most appropriate when variances are roughly proportional to group means, that is, when $s^2/\overline{X}$ is similar for all samples. The square root transformation will typically have the effect of equalizing variances.

Suppose we were given two sample distributions shown on the left panel in Table D.1. These variances, $s_A^2 = 8.5$ and $s_B^2 = 26.5$, are obviously quite different from one another. We determine the applicability of the square root transformation by demonstrating that $s^2/\overline{X}$ is similar for both distributions: $s_A^2/\overline{X}_A = 2.15$ and $s_B^2/\overline{X}_B = 2.65$.

TABLE D.1.   EFFECT OF SQUARE ROOT TRANSFORMATION

	Original data (X)		Transformed data ($\sqrt{X}$)	
	A	B	A	B
	1	8	1.00	2.83
	3	7	1.73	2.65
	8	12	2.83	3.46
	6	5	2.45	2.24
	2	18	1.41	4.24
Σ	20	50	9.42	15.42
$\overline{X}$	4	10	1.88	3.08
s^2	8.5	26.5	.56	.61
$s^2/\overline{X}$	2.125	2.65		

Each score in both distributions is transformed to its square root on the right in Table D.1. As we can see, the effect of this transformation is a reduction in the discrepancy between the two variances; now $s_A^2 = .56$ and $s_B^2 = .61$. These transformed values can now be used in a statistical analysis.

When data contain many small numbers (equal or close to zero), the square root transformation is more valid using $X' = \sqrt{X} + .5$ as the converted score.

The *square transformation* $(X' = X^2)$ is used primarily in regression analysis when the relationship between X and Y is curvilinear downward; that is, slope steadily decreases as the value of the independent variable increases.[1] This transformation will cause the relationship to appear more linear. It will also have the effect of stabilizing variances and will normalize the dependent variable when the residuals are negatively skewed.

The *log transformation* $(X' = \log X)$ is most appropriately used when the standard deviations of the original data are proportional to the mean; that is, the ratio $s/\overline{X}$ (the coefficient of variation) will be roughly constant across distributions. In addition to equalizing variances, the log transformation is used most often to normalize a skewed distribution. In regression analyses, the log transformation can also be used to create a more linear relationship between X and Y when the regression model shows a consistently increasing slope.[1] When data are numerically small, the transformation should be made on the basis of $X' = \log X + 1$.[2] The effect of log transformation can be easily demonstrated by plotting scores on logarithmic or semilogarithmic graph paper.

The *reciprocal transformation* $(X' = 1/X)$ is used when the standard deviations of the original data are proportional to the square of the mean $s/\overline{X}^2$.[3] It is effective for attaining homogeneity of variance or normality. Use of this approach will minimize the skewing effect of large values of X, which will be close to zero in their reciprocal form. With numeric data close to zero, this transformation should be obtained by using $X' = 1/X + 1$.

The *arc sine transformation* $(X' = \arcsin \sqrt{X})$ is also called angular transformation. It is used when data are collected in the form of proportions or percentages, such as the proportion of successful responses in a given number of trials. The relationship $s^2 = \bar{X}$ $(1 - \bar{X})$ should be constant for all samples. This transformation is based on an angular scale, whereby each proportion, p, is replaced by the angle whose sine is $\sqrt{p}$. Angles are usually given in radians. Tables for arc sine transformations are provided in Fisher and Yates[4] and Snedecor and Cochran.[5]

CHOOSING THE BEST TRANSFORMATION

Selecting the best transformation may be a less than obvious task. Many researchers use trial and error to determine the transformation that is most successful at reorienting the data. Kirk has suggested a method that may be helpful in facilitating this decision.[3] He uses each transformation to convert the largest and smallest scores in each distribution. The difference between the largest and smallest score, or the range of the distribution, is calculated using the transformed values. The ratio of the larger to the smaller range is then calculated for each transformation. The transformation that produces the smallest ratio is selected. This process is illustrated in Table D.2.

Data are obtained from two treatment groups. For this example, the largest and smallest raw scores in each distribution are transformed using the square root, log, and reciprocal transformations. The differences between the transformed values of the smallest and largest scores is calculated. For example, the difference between the square roots of 18 and 10 (the largest and smallest scores in Distribution 1) is 1.08. The difference between the square roots of 40 and 20 (Distribution 2) is 1.85. For the square root transformation, the ratio of the larger to the smaller range is $1.85/1.08 = 1.71$. A similar ratio is calculated for each of the other transformations, as shown in Table D.2. The log transformation would be selected because it results in the smallest ratio.

When more than two distributions are compared, the ratio is calculated using the largest and smallest ranges for each transformation. For instance, suppose we added a third group to the data, and the differences between the square roots of the largest and smallest values were 1.08, 1.85, and 1.13. The ratio for this transformation would be formed using only 1.85 and 1.08, as these are the largest and smallest ranges for this transformation.

TABLE D.2.   TRANSFORMATION BASED ON LARGEST AND SMALLEST SCORES IN TWO DISTRIBUTIONS

	Treatment group		$\sqrt{X}$		log X		$1/X$	
	1	2	1	2	1	2	1	2
Largest	18	40	4.24	6.32	1.26	1.60	.06	.02
Smallest	10	20	3.16	4.47	1.00	1.30	.10	.05
Range	8	20	1.08	1.85	.26	.30	.04	.03
Ratio	$\dfrac{\text{range}_{\text{largest}}}{\text{range}_{\text{smallest}}}$		$\dfrac{1.85}{1.08} = 1.71$		$\dfrac{.30}{.26} = 1.15$		$\dfrac{.04}{.03} = 1.33$	

Once data are analyzed using transformed data, all further interpretations of data must be made using the transformed values. For example, epidemiologists have shown that the distribution of incubation periods of communicable diseases tends to be normally distributed on a logarithmic scale.[6] Therefore, further analyses of these data have used the log incubation period as the unit of measurement.[7]

There are situations where data will be of sufficient variability that no transformation will be successful at smoothing the data. When this occurs, the researcher may consider choosing a different response measure as the dependent variable, one that would be more evenly distributed. Alternatively, nonparametric statistics can be applied. These tests, discussed in Chapter 22, do not require normality or equal variances.

Tables are provided in many statistics texts to facilitate log, square, and square root transformations.[4,8] In addition, most computer programs provide a mechanism for data transformation prior to analysis.

REFERENCES

1. Kleinbaum DG, Kupper LL: *Applied Regression Analysis and Other Multivariable Techniques.* North Scituate, MA, Duxbury Press, 1978.
2. Winer BJ: *Statistical Principles in Experimental Design,* ed 2. New York, McGraw-Hill, 1971.
3. Kirk RE: *Experimental Design: Procedures for the Behavioral Sciences,* ed 2. Belmont, CA, Brooks/Cole, 1982.
4. Fisher RA, Yates F: *Statistical Tables for Biological, Agricultural and Medical Research,* ed 6. London, Longman, 1963.
5. Snedecor GW, Cochran WG: *Statistical Methods,* ed 6. Ames, Iowa University Press, 1967.
6. Sartwell PE: The distribution of incubation periods of infectious disease. *Am J Hyg* **51**:310, 1950.
7. Colton T: *Statistics in Medicine.* Boston, Little, Brown, 1974.
8. Dixon WJ, Massey FJ: *Introduction to Statistical Analysis,* ed 3. New York, McGraw-Hill, 1969.

E

Sample Informed Consent Form

UNIVERSITY HOSPITAL RESEARCH CONSENT FORM, PAGE 1

Title of Project: Treatment of the Painful, Stiff Shoulder
Principal Investigator: Jane Jones, MS, PT

PURPOSE OF RESEARCH

I have been informed that this study will test the effectiveness of two different physical therapy approaches to treating shoulder problems like mine. Both approaches are acceptable physical therapy interventions for this problem; neither involve my being hospitalized. This study will help physical therapists better understand the use of physical therapy services in the management of the painful, stiff shoulder.

PROCEDURE

I understand that I will be assigned by lot to receive either a conservative home-based therapy program or a more intensive clinic-based program of therapy. If I am assigned to the home-based program, I will be given a set of exercises to do everyday by myself at home, and will come to the clinic once a month where a physical therapist will review and adjust my exercise program. If I am assigned to the clinic-based program, I will be expected to attend physical therapy treatment sessions two to three times a week in addition to doing exercises at home.

I am aware that in addition to the ordinary care received, I will be examined and asked a series of questions by a research physical therapist. The physical therapist's examination consists of measuring range of motion, level of pain, and function of my shoulder. I have been asked to undergo these tests at the beginning of the study, at monthly intervals for six months, and at nine months after the start of the study. All tests will take place in the physical therapy department during regularly scheduled treatment sessions. I will not be asked to make a special trip to the clinic for these follow-up assessments.

RISKS AND DISCOMFORTS

I understand that I may experience some pain or discomfort during the examination or during my treatment. This is mainly the result of my condition, and the procedures of this study are not expected to exaggerate these feelings which are associated with the usual course of treatment.

BENEFITS

I understand that my participation in the study will have no direct benefit to me other than the potential benefit of the treatment which is planned to reduce my pain and increase my shoulder function. The major potential benefit is to find out which treatment program is more effective.

ALTERNATIVES

I understand that the two procedures being studied are standard ways of treating my problem, and I have been referred by my doctor to this clinic for a treatment program that ordinarily would be selected by the physical therapist. There are no other physical therapy alternatives offered in this clinic.

The following paragraphs contain the usual considerations involved in consenting to be a subject in a research study and are required by the Institutional Review Board of the University Hospital on all consent forms.

CONFIDENTIALITY

I understand that medical information produced by this study will become part of my hospital record and will be subject to the confidentiality and privacy regulations of the University Hospital. Information of a sensitive personal nature will not be part of the medical record, but will be stored in the investigator's research file and identified only by a code number. The code key connecting name to numbers will be kept in a separate secure location.

If the data are used for publication in the medical literature or for teaching purposes, no names will be used, and other identifiers, such as photographs and audio- or videotapes, will be used only with my special written permission. I understand I may see the photographs and videotapes and hear the audiotapes before giving this permission.

If an investigational drug or device is to be studied, then I understand that the Food and Drug Administration and the industrial sponsor are permitted to have access to my medical record and to the data produced by the study, for audit purposes. However, they are required to maintain confidentiality.

REQUEST FOR MORE INFORMATION

I understand that I may ask more questions about the study at any time. Jane Jones at 555-0000 is available to answer my questions or concerns. I understand that I will be informed of any significant new findings discovered during the course of this study which might influence my continued participation.

If during the study, or later, I wish to discuss my participation in or concerns regarding this study with a person not directly involved, I am aware that the Patient Care Representative (555-0001) is available to talk with me. A copy of this consent form will be given to me to keep for careful rereading.

REFUSAL OR WITHDRAWAL OF PARTICIPATION

I understand that my participation is voluntary and that I may refuse to participate or may withdraw consent and discontinue participation in the study at any time without prejudice to my present or future care at the University Hospital. I also understand that Jane Jones may terminate my participation in this study at any time after she has explained the reasons for doing so and has helped arrange for my continued care by my own physician or physical therapist, if this is appropriate.

INJURY STATEMENT

I understand that in the unlikely event of injury to me resulting directly from my participation in this study, if such injury were reported promptly, then medical treatment would be available to me, but no further compensation would be provided by the University Hospital. I understand that by my agreement to participate in this study I am not waiving any of my legal rights.

I have explained to _____ the purpose of the research, the procedures required, and the possible risks and benefits to the best of my ability.

_____   _____
Investigator   Date

I confirm that *Jane Jones* has explained to me the purpose of the research, the study procedures that I will undergo, and the possible risks and discomforts as well as benefits that I may experience. Alternatives to my participation in the study have also been discussed. I have read and I understand this consent form. Therefore, I agree to give my consent to participate as a subject in this research project.

_____   _____
Participant   Date

_____   _____
Witness to Signature   Date

Glossary of Terms

Numbers in parentheses indicate the chapter in which the term is introduced.

A–B design. A single-case design with two phases: A represents the baseline phase, and B represents the intervention phase. (12)

A–B–A design. A single-case withdrawal design in which a second baseline phase is introduced. (12)

abstract. A brief description of a research project, appearing at the beginning of a journal article or research proposal. (29,30)

accessible population. The actual population of subjects available to be chosen for a study. This group is usually a nonrandom subset of the target population. (8)

accidental sampling. (see *convenience sampling*)

active variable. An independent variable with levels that can be manipulated and assigned by the researcher. (7)

adherence. Compliance of subjects to a research protocol. (9)

adjusted means. Means that have been adjusted based on the value of a covariate in an analysis of covariance. (24)

adjusted odds ratio. Odds ratio, obtained from logistic regression, that is corrected for the influence of other variables in the equation. (27)

agreement. (see *percent agreement*)

alpha coefficient. (see *Cronbach's alpha*)

alpha level (a). Level of statistical significance, or risk of Type I error; maximum probability level that can be achieved in a statistical test to reject the null hypothesis. (18)

alphanumeric data. In data processing, the entry of values that contain symbols or letters. (28)

alternate forms reliability. Reliability of two equivalent forms of a measuring instrument. (5)

alternating treatment design. A single-case design in which two (or more) treatments are compared by alternating them within a session (or in alternate sessions). (12)

alternative hypothesis (H_1). Hypothesis stating the expected relationship between independent and dependent variables; considered the negation of the null hypothesis. The alternative hypothesis is accepted when the null hypothesis is rejected. (18)

analysis of covariance (ANCOVA). Statistical procedure used to compare two or more treatment groups while controlling for the effect of one or more extraneous variables (called covariates). (24)

analysis of variance (ANOVA). Statistical procedure appropriate for comparison of three or more treatment groups or conditions, or the simultaneous manipulation of two or more independent variables. (20)

analytic epidemiology. Epidemiologic approach for testing hypotheses about the relationship between specific exposures and disease outcomes. (15)

applied research. Research that is intended to address problems of practical interest. (1)

area probability sample.   A form of cluster sampling in which geographic areas serve as the units of analysis. (8)

ARIMA (autoregressive integrated moving average).   Statistical technique for analysis of data from time-series studies. (10)

array.   Arrangement of a distribution of data in which scores are sorted from lowest to highest values. (17)

assumptions.   Principles that are accepted as being true based on logic or theory, without proof or validation. (7)

attributable risk.   An estimate used to quantify the risk of disease in an exposed group that is attributable to the exposure, by removing the risk that would have occurred as a result of other causes (risk in the unexposed group). (15)

attribute variable.   An independent variable with levels that cannot be manipulated or assigned by the researcher, but that represent subject characteristics (such as age and sex). (7)

attrition (experimental mortality).   A threat to internal validity, referring to the differential loss of participants during the course of data collection, potentially introducing bias by changing the composition of the sample. (9)

audit trail.   Comprehensive process of documenting interpretation of qualitative data. (13)

autonomy.   The capacity of individuals to make decisions affecting their own lives and to act on those decisions. (3)

baseline phase.   In a single-case design, the initial phase (designated A) in which data are recorded before intervention is begun. (12)

basic research.   Research that contributes to basic knowledge, but that does not have immediate practical goals. (1)

beneficence.   Obligation to attend to the well-being of individuals engaged as research subjects. (3)

beta (b).   Probability of making a Type II error. (18)

between-groups variance.   That portion of the total variance in a set of scores that is attributed to the difference between groups. (19,20)

bimodal distribution.   A distribution having two modes. (17)

binomial variable.   (see *dichotomy*)

bivariate statistics.   Statistics involving the analysis of two variables for the purpose of determining the relationship between them, for example, correlation. (23)

blinding.   Techniques to reduce experimental bias by keeping the subjects and/or investigators ignorant of group assignments and research hypotheses. (9)

block.   Level of an attribute variable in which subjects are homogeneous on a particular characteristic. (9,10)

Bonferroni's correction.   A correction often used when multiple *t*-tests are performed, to reduce Type I error. The desired level of significance (a) is divided by the number of comparisons. The resulting value is then used as the level of signficance for each comparison to reject the null hypothesis. (21)

Boolean logic.   Use of the terms AND, OR and NOT for refining data base searches for professional literature. (7)

carryover effect.   A temporary or permanent change in behavior resulting from prior treatments. (10)

case–control study.   A design in analytic epidemiology in which the investigator selects subjects on the basis of their having or not having a particular disease and then determines their previous exposure. (15)

case study (report).   Type of descriptive research in which one individual or unit is studied in depth. (13,15)

celeration line.   In single-case research, a line that divides the data points within a phase into two equal halves, indicating the trend of the data within that phase. (12)

central tendency.   Descriptive statistics that represent "averages" or scores that are representative of a distribution; includes mean, median, and mode. (17)

centroid.   A point determined from the intersection of two means of two dependent variables (X, Y), used in multivariate analysis. (27)

changing criterion design.   In single-case research, a design for shaping behavior in which performance criteria for success change in each phase of the design. (12)

chi square test (c^2).   A nonparametric test applied to nominal data, comparing observed frequencies within categories to frequencies expected by chance. (25)

closed-ended question.   A question on a survey (interview or questionnaire) that offers a set of specific response choices that are mutually exclusive and exhaustive. (14)

cluster sampling.   A form of probability sampling in which large subgroups (clusters) are randomly selected first, and then smaller units from these clusters are successively chosen; also called multistage sampling. (8)

coding sheet.   Documentation used to record variable names and column locations for computer data processing. (28)

coding.   Setting numerical values for levels of categorical variables for use in data processing. (28)

coefficient alpha (Cronbach's alpha).   A reliability index used for estimating internal consistency in instruments composed of several items or questions. (5)

coefficient of determination (r^2).   Coefficient representing the amount of variance in one variable (Y) that can be explained (accounted for) by a second variable (X). (24)

coefficient of variation (CV).   A measure of relative variation, based on the size of the standard deviation relative to the mean, expressed as a percentage. (26)

cohort study.   A study design in which a specific group is followed over time. Subjects are classified according to their exposure status and followed to determine disease outcomes. (15)

completely randomized design.   An experimental design in which all groups have been randomly assigned. (10)

complex contrasts.   A multiple comparison strategy in which means from two or more groups are combined as a subset and compared with other individual means or subsets of means. (21)

concept.   An abstraction based on observation of behaviors or characteristics. (2)

concurrent validity.   A type of measurement validity; a form of criterion-related validity; the degree to which the outcomes of one test correlate with outcomes on a criterion test, when both tests are given at relatively the same time. (6)

confidence interval (CI).   The range of values within which a population parameter is estimated to fall, with a specific level of confidence. (18,19)

confounding.   The contaminating effect of extraneous variables on interpretation of the relationship between independent and dependent variables. (9)

consecutive sampling.   A form of non-probability sampling, where subjects are recruited as they become available. (8)

constant comparative method.   Inductive process in qualitative research that calls for continual testing of a theory as data are examined. (13)

construct.   An abstract concept that is invented to represent unobservable behaviors or ideas. (2)

construct validity.   A type of measurement validity; the degree to which a theoretical construct is measured by an instrument. (6)

content analysis.   A procedure for analyzing and coding narrative data in a systematic way. (13)

content validity.   A type of measurement validity; the degree to which the items in an instrument adequately reflect the content domain being measured. (6)

contingency table.   A two-dimensional table, with rows (R) and columns (C) representing categories of nominal or ordinal variables; also referred to as cross-tabulation. (25)

continuous variable.   A quantitative variable that can theoretically take on values along a continuum. (4)

contrast.   A comparison between two means, performed as part of a multiple comparison procedure. (21)

control group.   In an experiment, a group of subjects who resemble the experimental group, but who do not receive the experimental treatment, providing a baseline of comparison to interpret effects of treatment. (10)

convenience sampling.   A nonprobability sampling procedure, involving selection of the most available subjects for a study. (8)

convergent validity.   An approach in construct validation, assessing the degree to which two different instruments or methods are able to measure the same construct. (6)

correlation.   The tendency for variation in one variable to be related to variation in a second variable; those statistical procedures used to assess the degree of covariation between two variables. (23)

correlational research.   A descriptive research approach that explores the relationship among variables without active manipulation of variables by the researcher. (13)

counterbalancing.   Systematic alternation of the order of treatment conditions, to avoid order effects in a repeated measures design. (10)

covariate.   An extraneous variable that is statistically controlled in an analysis of covariance, so that the relationship between the independent and dependent variables is analyzed with the effect of the extraneous factor removed. (24)

criterion-related validity.   A type of measurement validity; the degree to which the outcomes of one test correlate with outcomes on a criterion test; can be assessed as concurrent validity or predictive validity. (6)

criterion-referencing.   Interpretation of a score based on its actual value. (6)

critical value.   The value of a statistic that separates the critical region; the value that defines a statistically significant result at the set alpha level. (18)

Cronbach's alpha.   Reliability index of internal consistency, on a scale of 0.00 to 1.00. (5, 26)

crossover design.   A repeated measures design used to control order effects when comparing two treatments, where half of the sample receives treatment A first followed by treatment B, and the other half receives treatment B first followed by treatment A. (10)

cross-sectional study.   A study based on observations of different age or developmental groups at one point in time, providing the basis for inferring trends over time. (13, 15)

cross-tabulation.   (see *contingency table*)

cross-validation.   The process of validating a test or statistical model by testing on a new group of subjects. (6)

cubic trend.   In trend analysis, a nonlinear function that takes two turns of direction. (21)

cumulative incidence (CI).   The number of new cases of a disease during a specified time period divided by the total number of people at risk; the proportion of new cases of a disease in a population. (15)

cut-off score.   Score used as the demarcation of a positive or negative test outcome. (6)

deductive reasoning.   The logical process of developing specific hypotheses based on general principles. (1)

default settings.   Settings in software programs that will occur automatically unless otherwise directed. (28)

degrees of freedom (*df*).   Statistical concept indicating the number of values within a distribution that are free to vary, given restrictions on the data set; usually N-1. (18)

Delphi survey.   Survey method whereby decisions on items are based on consensus of a panel. (14)

dependent variable.   A response variable that is assumed to depend on or be caused by another (independent) variable. (7)

descriptive epidemiology.   That area of epidemiology concerned with the distribution of disease in relation to person, place, and time. (15)

descriptive research. Research studies that are designed to describe the characteristics of individuals in specific populations. (13)

descriptive statistics. Statistics that are used to describe and summarize sample characteristics and their relationships. (17)

developmental research. A descriptive research approach designed to document how certain groups change over time on specific variables. (13)

deviation score $(X - X_-)$. The distance of a single data point from the mean of the distribution. The sum of the deviation scores for a given distribution will always equal zero. (17)

dichotomy (dichotomous variable). A nominal variable having only two categories, such as yes/no and male/female; a binomial variable. (7)

difference score (d). The difference between two scores taken on the same individual. (19)

directional hypothesis. A research hypothesis (or alternative hypothesis) that predicts the direction of a relationship between two variables. (7,18)

disablement model. Model of disability proposing a relationship among pathology, impairment, functional limitation and disability. (1)

discrete variable. A variable that can only be measured in separate units and that cannot be measured in intervals of less than 1. (4)

discriminant analysis. A multivariate statistical technique used to determine if a set of variables can predict group membership. (27)

discriminant validity. An approach in construct validation assessing the degree to which an instrument yields different results when measuring two different constructs; that is, the ability to discriminate between the constructs. (6)

dose-response relationship. The demonstration of a change over time that is proportional to the severity of a disease or the amount of exposure to a treatment. (15)

double-blind experiment. An experiment in which both the investigator and the subject are kept ignorant of group assignment. (9)

dummy variable. In regression procedures, the assignment of codes to a nominal variable, reflecting the presence or absence of certain traits. (27)

effect size. A statistical expression of the magnitude of the difference between two treatments or the magnitude of a relationship between two variables. (18, Appendix C)

effectiveness. Benefits of an intervention as tested under "real world" conditions, often using quasi-experimental methods. (10)

efficacy. Benefit of an intervention as tested under controlled experimental conditions, usually with a control group. (10)

eigenvalue. A measure of the proportion of the total variance accounted for by a factor in a discriminant analysis or factor analysis. (27)

empirical observation. The process of gathering information by direct observation. (1)

equivalence. (see *alternate forms reliability*)

error variance. That portion of the total variance in a data set that cannot be attributed to treatment effects, but that is due to differences between subjects. (19)

ethnography. An approach to qualitative research in which the experiences of a specific cultural group are studied. (13)

evaluation research. A research approach designed to determine the effectiveness of a program or policy. (16)

evidence-based practice. Concept whereby clinical practice and treatment choices are based on scientific evidence. (1)

exempt review. Exemption from review of a proposal by an Institutional Review Board for projects that do not involve direct contact with subjects, presenting no risk. (3)

expedited review. Accelerated review of a proposal by an Institutional Review Board, based on minimal risk. (3)

experiment.   A research study in which the investigator manipulates the independent variables and randomly assigns subjects to groups, and in which a control group or comparison group is used. (10)

experimental mortality.   (see *attrition*)

experimenter effects (experimenter bias).   Biases that are present in research data because of behaviors, expectations, or attitudes of those collecting the data. (9)

explained variance.   Between-groups variance; that portion of the total variance in a data set that can be attributed to the differences between groups or treatment conditions. (19)

exploratory research.   Research that has as its purpose the exploration of data to determine relationships among variables. (13)

ex post facto research.   Nonexperimental research that looks at relationships among variables, based on data that have already been collected or using all attribute variables. (9,13)

external validity.   The degree to which results of a study can be generalized to persons or settings outside the experimental situation. (9)

extraneous variable.   A variable that confounds the relationship between the independent and dependent variables. (9)

facets.   In generalizability theory, specific conditions under which reliability of a measurement can be generalized. (5,26)

face validity.   The assumption of validity of a measuring instrument based on its appearance as a reasonable measure of a given variable. (6)

factor.   1. A variable. (7) 2. A set of interrelated variables in a factor analysis. (27)

factor analysis.   An exploratory multivariate statistical technique used to examine the structure within a large set of variables and to determine the underlying dimensions that exist within that set of variables. (27)

factorial design.   An experimental design involving two or more independent variables, allowing for the interpretation of main effects and interaction effects. (10)

field.   An individual score or value entered into a data set, composed of one or more contiguous numerals or symbols. (28)

Fisher's Exact Test.   A nonparametric test, analogous to chi-square, used with extremely small samples. (25)

formative evaluation.   An assessment of a program or policy during developmental stages to determine how it should be implemented and the ongoing assessment of the operation of the program. (16)

Friedman two-way analysis of variance by ranks (c^2_r).   A nonparametric statistical procedure for repeated measures, comparing more than two treatment conditions of one independent variable; analogous to the one-way repeated measures analysis of variance. (22)

gamma.   Measure of association for categorical variables, based on Kendall's tau statistic. (25)

generalizability.   1. The quality of research that justifies inference of outcomes to groups or situations other than those directly involved in the investigation. (9) 2. The concept of reliability theory in which measurement error is viewed as multidimensional and must be interpreted under specific measurement conditions. (5)

gold standard.   An instrument that is considered a valid measure and that can be used as the standard for assessing validity of other instruments. (6)

goodness of fit test.   Use of chi square to determine if an observed distribution of categorical variables fits a given theoretical distribution. (25)

Greenhouse-Geisser correction.   A statistical correction for unequal variances with repeated measures analysis of variance. (20)

grounded theory.   An approach to collecting and analyzing data in qualitative research, with the goal of developing theories to explain observations and experience. (13)

Guttman scale. A cumulative scale designed so that agreement with higher-level responses assumes agreement with all lower-level responses. (14)

Hawthorne effect. The effect of subjects' knowledge that they are part of a study on their performance. (9)

histogram. A bar graph. (17)

historical controls. Use of subjects from previous research studies as controls for subjects in a current study. (10)

historical research. Research that seeks to examine relationships and facts based on documentation of past events. (16)

history effect. A threat to internal validity, referring to the occurrence of extraneous events prior to a posttest that can affect the dependent variable. (9)

homogeneity of variance. An underlying assumption in parametric statistics that variances of samples are not significantly different. (18,19)

Huynh-Feldt correction. A statistical correction for unequal variances with repeated measures analysis of variance. (20)

hypothesis. A statement of the expected relationship between variables. (7)

independent factor. An independent variable in which the levels represent independent groups of subjects. (7)

independent variable. The variable that is presumed to cause or determine a dependent variable; a variable that is manipulated or controlled by the researcher, who sets its "values" or levels. (7)

inductive reasoning. The logical process of developing generalizations based on specific observations or facts. (1)

inferential statistics. That branch of statistics concerned with testing hypotheses and using sample data to make generalizations concerning populations. (18)

informed consent. An ethical principle that requires obtaining the consent of the individual to participate in a study based on full prior disclosure of risks and benefits. (3)

institutional review board (IRB). That group in an institution that is responsible for reviewing research proposals that will involve human subjects to determine adherence to ethical principles. (3)

instrumentation effect. A threat to internal validity in which bias is introduced by an unreliable or inaccurate measurement system. (9)

intention-to-treat. Principle whereby data are analyzed according to group assignments, regardless of how subjects actually received treatment. (9)

interaction effect. The combined effect of two or more independent variables on a dependent variable. (10,20)

intercorrelations. A set of bivariate correlations for several variables within a sample. (23)

internal consistency. A form of reliability, assessing the degree to which a set of items in an instrument all measure the same trait. (5)

internal validity. The degree to which the relationship between the independent and dependent variables is free from the effects of extraneous factors. (9)

interquartile range. The difference between the first and third quartiles in a distribution. (17)

interrater reliability. The degree to which two or more raters can obtain the same ratings for a given variable. (5,26)

interrupted time-series design. A design involving a series of measurements over time, interrupted by one or more treatment occasions. (10)

interval scale. Level of measurement in which values have equal intervals, but no true zero point. (4)

intervening variable. (see *extraneous variable*)

intervention phase.   In single-case research, the phase in which intervention is introduced. (12)

intraclass correlation coefficient (ICC).   A reliability coefficient based on an analysis of variance; a generalizability coefficient. (26)

intrarater reliability.   The degree to which one rater can obtain the same rating on multiple occasions of measuring the same variable. (5,26)

item-to-total correlation.   Correlation of individual items in a scale with the total scale score; an indication of internal consistency. (5, 26)

justice.   Fairness in all aspects of the research process. (3)

kappa (k).   A correction factor for percent agreement measures of reliability, accounting for the potential effect of chance agreements. (26)

Kendall's tau (b and c).   Measure of association for ordinal variables. (25)

key words.   Words used to identify primary topics within an article for a literature search. (7)

known groups method.   A technique for construct validation, in which validity is determined by the degree to which an instrument can demonstrate different scores for groups known to vary on the variable being measured. (6)

Kruskal–Wallis one-way analysis of variance by ranks (H).   A nonparametric statistical procedure for comparing more than two independent groups representing levels of one independent variable; analogous to the one-way analysis of variance. (22)

lambda.   (*see Glossary of Statistical Symbols*)

Latin square.   A matrix of columns and rows used to assign sequences of treatments to control for order effects. (10)

Least squares method.   A method of fitting a regression line to a set of bivariate data so as to minimize the sum of the squared vertical deviations of Y values around that line. (24)

level.   1. The "value" or classification of an independent variable. (7) 2. In single-case research, the magnitude of the target behavior; changes in level are associated with differences in magnitude between the end of one phase and the beginning of the following phase. (12)

level of significance (a).   The probability that an observed effect could be attributed to chance; the standard for rejecting the null hypothesis; traditionally set at a = .05. (18)

Likert scale.   A summative scale based on responses to a set of statements for which respondents are asked to rate their degree of agreement or disagreement. (14)

limits of agreement.   Index of reliability between alternate forms of an instrument. (26)

line of best fit.   The regression line, representing the relationship between two variables, usually plotted on a scatter diagram. (24)

logical positivism.   A philosophy in which human experience is assumed to be limited to logical and controlled relationships between specific measured variables; providing a basis for quantitative research methods. (13)

logistic regression.   Multiple regression procedure where the dependent variable is a dichotomous outcome; predicts odds associated with presence or absence of the dependent variable based on the independent variables. (27)

logit.   A log odds ratio, used in logistic regression and Rasch analysis. (6, 27)

longitudinal study.   A study designed to collect data over time, usually for the purpose of describing developmental changes in a particular group. (13)

main effect.   The separate effect of one independent variable in a multifactor design. (10,20)

Mann–Whitney U test.   A nonparametric statistical test for comparing two independent groups; analogous to the unpaired t-test. (22)

matching.   Pairing of subjects on the basis of similarities on one or more variables. (9)

maturation effect.   A threat to internal validity, in which changes occur in the dependent variable as a result of the passing of time. (9)

Mauchly's test of sphericity.   (*see sphericity*).

maximum likelihood. A measure of probablity indicating the best odds of achieving accurate prediction of group membership with logistic regression. (27)

McNemar test. A nonparametric statistical test for nominal level measures, for correlated samples; a form of the chi square test. (25)

mean (X). A measure of central tendency, computed by summing the values of several observations and dividing by the number of observations. (17)

mean square (MS). In an analysis of variance, that value representing the variance; calculated by dividing the sum of squares for a particular effect by the degrees of freedom for that effect. (20)

measurement error. The difference between an observed value for a measurement and the theoretical true score; may be the result of systematic or random effects. (5)

median. A measure of central tendency representing the 50th percentile in a ranked distribution of scores; that is, that point at which 50% of the scores fall below and 50% fall above. (17)

MeSH headings. Medical Subject Headings. A system used by the National Library of Medicine to index resources. (7)

meta-analysis. Process of combining several studies of the same variables to determine overall outcome, based on effect size. (16)

method error. A form of reliability testing for assessing response stability based on the discrepancy between two sets of repeated scores. (26)

methodological research. Research designed to develop or refine procedures or instruments for measuring variables. (16)

mode. A measure of central tendency representing the most commonly occurring score. (17)

model. Symbolic representation of reality delineating concepts or variables and their relationships, often demonstrating the structural components of a theory or process. (2)

multicolinearity. The correlation between independent variables in a multiple regression equation, causing them to provide redundant information. (27)

multiple baseline design. In single-case research, a design for collecting data for more than one subject, behavior, or treatment condition. Baseline phases are staggered to provide control. (12)

multiple comparison test. A test of differences between individual means following analysis of variance, used to control for Type I error. (21)

multiple regression. A multivariate statistical technique for establishing the predictive relationship between one dependent variable (Y) and a set of independent variables $(X_1, X_2, \ldots)$. (27)

multistage sampling. (see *cluster sampling*)

multitrait-multimethod matrix. A process to demonstrate discriminant and convergent validity by examining intercorrelations for data derived from multiple methods on multiple characteristics. (6)

multivariate analysis. A set of statistical procedures designed to analyze the relationship among three or more variables; includes techniques such as multiple regression, discriminant analysis, and factor analysis. (27)

nominal scale. Level of measurement for classification variables; assignment of "values" based on mutually exclusive and exhaustive categories with no inherent rank order. (4)

nondirectional hypothesis. A research hypothesis (or alternative hypothesis) that does not indicate the expected direction of the relationship between variables. (7,18)

nonequivalent control group. A control group (or comparison group) that was not created by random assignment. (10)

nonparametric statistics. A set of statistical procedures that are not based on assumptions about population parameters, or the shape of the underlying population distribution; most often used when data are measured on the nominal or ordinal scales. (22)

nonprobability sample. A sample that was not selected using random selection. (8)

normal distribution.   A symmetrical bell-shaped theoretical distribution that has defined properties. (18)

normative research.   A descriptive research approach designed to determine normal values for specific variables within a population. (13)

norm referencing.   Interpretation of a score based on its value relative to a standard or "normal" score. (6)

null hypothesis (H_0).   A statement of no difference or no relationship between variables; the statistical hypothesis. (7,18)

observational research.   Research based on data collection through observation of subject characteristics, rather than experimental manipulation of variables; may include cohort, case-control or correlational studies. (15)

odds ratio (OR).   Estimate of relative risk in a case–control study. (15)

one-tailed test.   A statistical test based on a directional alternative hypothesis, in which critical values are obtained for only one tail of a distribution. (18)

open-ended question.   A question on a survey (interview or questionnaire) that does not restrict the respondent to specific choices, but allows for a free response. (14)

operational definition.   Definition of a variable based on how it will be used in a particular study; how a dependent variable will be measured, how an independent variable will be manipulated. (7)

order effects.   The sequential effect of one subject being exposed to several treatments in the same order; potentially manifested as carryover or practice effects. (10)

ordinal scale.   Level of measurement in which scores are ranks. (4)

outlier.   Numeric value that does not fall within the range of most scores in a distribution. (24)

paired *t*-test.   A parametric test for comparing two means for correlated samples or repeated measures; also called a correlated *t*-test. (19)

parameter.   A measured characteristic of a population. (17)

parametric statistics.   Statistical procedures for estimating population parameters and for testing hypotheses based on population parameters, with assumptions about the distribution of variables, and for use with interval or ratio measures. (18)

partial correlation.   A statistical technique for establishing the correlation between two variables, with the effect of a third variable removed; also called a first-order correlation. (27)

participant observation.   A method of data collection in qualitative research in which the researcher becomes a participant in the group that is being observed. (13)

Pearson product–moment coefficient of correlation (r).   A parametric statistical technique for determining the relationship between two variables. (23)

percentage agreement.   A reliability test for categorical variables, estimating the ability of researchers to agree on category ratings. (26)

percentile.   Data are divided into 99 equal ranks, or percentiles, with 1% of the scores in each rank. (17)

phenomenology.   An approach to qualitative research involving the study of complex human experience as it is actually lived. (13)

phi coefficient (r_f).   A nonparametric correlation statistic for estimating the relationship between two dichotomous variables. (23,25)

point biserial correlation (r_{pb}).   A correlation statistic for estimating the relationship between a dichotomy and a continuous variable on the interval or ratio scale. (24)

point estimate.   A single sample statistic that serves as an estimate of a population parameter. (18)

polynomial regression.   Regression procedure for nonlinear data. (24)

pooled variance estimate (s_p^2).   Estimate of population variance based on the weighted average of sample variances; used in the unpaired *t*-test when group variances are not significantly different (under conditions of homogeneity of variance). (19)

population. The entire set of individuals or units to which data will be generalized. (8)

posttest-only design. An experimental design in which only one measurement is taken following treatment. (10)

power (1-b). The ability of a statistical test to find a significant difference that really does exist; the probability that a test will lead to rejection of the null hypothesis. (18, Appendix C)

predictive validity. A form of measurement validity in which an instrument is used to predict some future performance. (6)

preference. In sequential clinical trials, the expression of which treatment is considered better within a sequential pair. (11)

prescriptive validity. Validity of a test as a basis for prescribing treatment. (6)

pretest-posttest design. An experimental design involving a pretest prior to intervention and a posttest following intervention. (10)

prevalence. The number of cases of a disease at a given point in time, expressed as a proportion of the total population at risk. (15)

probability sample. A sample chosen using randomized methods. (8)

prospective research. Research based on data that are collected in the present, following the progress of study subjects. (13)

purposive sample. A nonprobability sample in which subjects are specifically selected by the researcher on the basis of subjective judgment that they will be the most representative. (8)

quadratic trend. A nonlinear trend, with one turn in direction. (21,24)

quartile (Q). Three quartiles divide a distribution of ranked data into four equal groups, each containing 25% of the scores. (17)

quasi-experimental research. Comparative research approach in which subjects cannot be randomly assigned to groups or control groups are not used. (10)

quota sampling. Nonprobability sampling method in which stratification is used to obtain representative proportions of specific subgroups. (8)

random assignment. Assignment of subjects to groups using probability methods, where every subject has an equal chance of being assigned to each group. (9)

random error. A measurement error that is not constant, potentially increasing or decreasing the true score value to varying degrees. (5)

random sampling. Probability method of selecting subjects for a sample, where every subject in the population has an equal chance of being chosen. (8)

randomized block design. An experimental design in which one independent variable is an attribute variable, creating homogeneous blocks of subjects who are then randomly assigned to levels of the other independent variable. (10)

randomized clinical trial (RCT). An experimental study in which a clinical treatment is compared with a control condition, where subjects are randomly assigned to groups. (15)

range. A measure of dispersion equal to the difference between the largest and smallest scores in a distribution. (17)

rank biserial correlation (r_{rb}). A correlation procedure for estimating the degree of relationship between a dichotomy and an ordinal variable. (23)

rank sum test. A nonparametric statistical procedure, used to compare two independent samples; analogous to the unpaired t-test. (22)

Rasch analysis. Transformation of items on an ordinal scale to an interval scale, demonstrating the unidimensional nature of a scale. (14)

ratio scale. The highest level of measurement, in which there are equal intervals between score units and a true zero point. (4)

reactive measurement. A measurement that distorts the variable being measured, either by the subject's awareness of being measured or by influence of the measurement process. (9)

recall bias. The tendency for subjects to recall past events differentially depending on their current experiences or disease states. (14, 15)

receiver operating characteristic (ROC) curve. Curve that demonstrates the relationship between sensitivity and specificity at various cutoff points for a scale. (6)

regression analysis. A statistical procedure for examining the predictive relationship between a dependent (criterion) variable and an independent (predictor) variable. (24, 27)

regression coefficient. In a regression equation, the weight (*b*) assigned to the independent variable; the slope of the regression line. (24)

regression line. The straight line that is drawn on a scatter plot for bivariate data from the regression equation, summarizing the relationship between variables. (24)

regression toward the mean. A statistical phenomenon in which scores on a pretest are likely to move toward the group mean on a posttest because of inherent positive or negative measurement error; also called statistical regression. (5, 9)

relative risk (RR). Estimate of the magnitude of the association between an exposure and disease, indicating the likelihood that the exposed group will develop the disease relative to those who are not exposed. (15)

reliability. The degree of consistency with which an instrument or rater measures a variable. (5,26)

repeated measure (repeated factor). An independent variable for which subjects act as their own control; that is, all subjects are exposed to all levels of the variable. (7,10)

replication. The duplication of a research project for the purpose of determining if initial results can be repeated. (7)

research hypothesis. A statement of the researcher's expectations about the relationship between variables under study. (7)

residual ($Y - \hat{Y}$). In regression analysis, the difference between the value of the dependent variable predicted by the regression equation and the actual value. (24)

residualized gain score. A standardized value to reflect change, based on pretest scores, obtained through an analysis of covariance. (6)

response stability. Consistency with which a response is manifested over repeated trials. (5,26)

responsiveness. The ability of a test to demonstrate change. (6)

retrospective research. Research based on data that was collected in the past; may include data from medical records, surveys or data bases. (13)

risk. Any potential harmful physical or psychological effect from participation in research. (3)

risk–benefit ratio. An ethical principle that is an element of informed consent, in which the risks of a research study to the participant are evaluated in relation to the potential benefits of the study's outcomes. (3)

sample. Subset of a population chosen for study. (8)

sampling bias. Bias in a sample resulting from an overrepresentation or underrepresentation of specific attributes of the population. (8)

sampling distribution. A theoretical distribution of a statistic, based on the value of the statistic over an infinite number of samples. (18)

sampling error. The difference between an observed statistic from a sample and the population parameter. (18)

scatter plot. A graphic representation of the relationship between two variables. (24)

secondary analysis. An approach to research involving the use of data that were collected for another purpose, usually for the purpose of testing new hypotheses. (16)

selection bias. A threat to internal validity in which bias is introduced by initial differences between groups, when these differences are not random. (9)

semantic differential. A technique used to measure attitudes by asking respondents to rate concepts on a 7-point scale which represents a continuum across two extremes. (14)

sensitivity. A measure of validity of a screening procedure, based on the probability that someone with a disease will test positive. (6)

separate variance estimate.   Use of separate, rather than pooled, variance values when the assumption of homogeneity of variance is not met. (19)

serial dependency.   Correlation in a set of data collected over time, in which one observation can be predicted based on previous observations. (12)

sign test.   A nonparametric statistical procedure for comparing two correlated samples, based on comparison of positive or negative outcomes; analogous to the paired *t*-test. (22)

significance.   (see *statistical significance*)

significance level (a).   (see *alpha level*)

simple contrast.   In a multiple comparison, the contrast of two means to determine if they are significantly different from one another. (21)

single-factor design.   An experimental design involving one independent variable.

single-subject designs.   Research designs that provide an experimental model for the study of individuals over time. (12)

skewed distribution.   A distribution of scores that is asymmetrical, with more scores to one extreme. (17)

slope.   1. In regression analysis, the rate of change in values of Y for one unit of change in X. (24) 2. In single-case research, the rate of change in the magnitude of the target behavior over time. (12)

snowball sampling.   A nonprobability sampling method in which subjects are successively recruited by referrals from other subjects. (8)

social validation.   In single-case research, the process of demonstrating the acceptance of an intervention and behavior outcomes by the social community. (12)

Spearman–Brown formula.   The statistical procedure used to analyze split-half reliability; also called the Spearman–Brown prophecy formula. (5)

Spearman's rank correlation coefficient (r_s).   A nonparametric correlation procedure for ordinal data. (23)

specificity.   A measure of validity of a screening procedure, based on the probability that someone who does not have a disease will test negative. (6)

sphericity.   An assumption with repeated measures analysis of variance, wherein difference scores between pairs of conditions are assumed to have equal variances that are correlated with each other. (20)

split-half reliability.   A reliability measure of internal consistency based on dividing the items on an instrument into two halves and correlating the results. (5)

split middle line.   In single-case research, a line used to separate data points within one phase into two equal halves, reflecting the trend of the data within that phase (see *celeration line*). (12)

standard deviation (s).   A descriptive statistic reflecting the variability or dispersion of scores around the mean. (17)

standard error of measurement (SEM).   A reliability measure of response stability, estimating the standard error in a set of repeated scores. (26)

standard error of the estimate (SEE).   In regression analysis, an estimate of prediction accuracy; a measure of the spread of scores around the regression line. (24)

standard error of the mean (s_X).   The standard deviation of a distribution of sample means; an estimate of the population standard deviation. (18)

standardized residual.   In a chi square test, the contribution of each cell to the overall statistic. (25)

standardized response mean.   A measure of effect size, based on the ratio of mean change score divided by the standard deviation of the change scores. (6)

standardized score.   (see *z-score*)

statistic.   A measured characteristic of a sample. (12)

statistical conclusion validity.   The validity of conclusions drawn from statistical analyses, based on the proper application of statistical tests and principles. (9)

statistical hypothesis. (see *null hypothesis*)

statistical regression. (see *regression toward the mean*)

statistical significance. The term indicating that the results of an analysis are unlikely to be the result of chance at a specified probability level; rejection of the null hypothesis. (18)

stratification. The grouping of individuals in a population into homogeneous groups on some characteristic prior to sampling. (8)

summative evaluation. In evaluation research, the assessment of the effectiveness of a program or policy based on achievement of outcome goals. (16)

sum of squares (*SS*). A measure of variability in a set of data, equal to the sum of squared deviation scores for a distribution $(S(X - X)^2)$; the numerator in the formula for variance. Used in analysis of variance as the basis for partitioning between-groups and within-groups variance components. (17,20)

systematic error. A form of measurement error, where error is constant across trials. (5)

systematic sample. A probability sampling method where subjects are chosen from lists of population members using specified intervals, such as every 10th person. (8)

***t*-test.** A parametric test for comparing two means; also called Student's *t*-test (see paired *t*-test and unpaired *t*-test). (19)

target behavior. In single-case research, the behavior that is monitored over time. (12)

target population. The population to which results of a study will be generalized. (8)

test–retest reliability. The degree to which an instrument is stable, based on repeated administrations of the test to the same individuals over a specified time interval. (5)

theoretical sampling. A process of sampling in qualitative research, whereby subjects are recruited based on their match with the theory that has developed from prior work. (13)

theory. An abstract generalization that seeks to explain the relationship between observed phenomena. (2)

time-series design. A quasi-experimental design in which performance changes are assessed over time, prior to and following the administration of treatment. (10)

transformation. Mathematical conversion of a distribution to a different scale by a constant (such as square root or log) to change the shape or variance characteristics of the distribution. (Appendix D)

trend. 1. The shape of a distribution of scores taken over time, reflecting the distribution's linearity or lack of linearity. (21) 2. In single-case research, the direction of change in the target behavior within a phase or across phases. (12)

trend analysis. Part of an analysis of variance, used to assess trend within data taken over ordered intervals; can express data as linear, quadratic, cubic, and so on, reflecting the number of changes in direction in the data over time. (21)

triangulation. The use of multiple methods to document phenomena. (13)

two-standard deviation band method. A method of data analysis in single-subject research, to determine if there is a significant change across phases. (12)

two-tailed test. A statistical test based on a nondirectional alternative hypothesis, in which critical values represent both positive and negative tails of a distribution. (18)

Type I error. An incorrect decision to reject the null hypothesis, concluding that a relationship exists when in fact it does not. (18)

Type II error. An incorrect decision to accept the null hypothesis, concluding that no relationship exists when in fact it does. (18)

unexplained variance. (see *error variance*)

univariate analysis. Statistical procedures for analyzing one dependent variable. (27)

unpaired *t*-test. A parametric test for comparing two means for independent samples; also called an independent *t*-test. (19)

VAS. (see *visual analog scale*)

validity.   1. The degree to which an instrument measures what it is intended to measure. (6) 2. The degree to which a research design allows for reasonable interpretations from the data, based on controls (internal validity), appropriate definitions (construct validity), appropriate analysis procedures (statistical conclusion validity), and generalizability (external validity). (9)

variable.   A characteristic that can be manipulated or observed and that can take on different values, either quantitatively or qualitatively. (2,7)

variance (S^2).   A measure of variablity in a distribution, equal to the square of the standard deviation. (17)

visual analog scale.   A form of measurement utilizing a straight line, usually 10 cm in length, with anchors at either end representing the extremes of the characteristic being measured. (14)

washout period.   In a crossover design, that period of time between administration of the two treatments, allowing effects of the experimental treatment to dissipate. (10)

weighted kappa (k_w).   An estimate of percentage agreement, corrected for chance, based on weights reflecting levels of seriousness of disagreements. (26)

Wilcoxon signed-ranks test (T).   A nonparametric statistical procedure, comparing two correlated samples (repeated measures); analogous to the paired *t*-test. (22)

withdrawal design.   In single-case research, a design that involves withdrawal of the intervention. (12)

within-groups variance.   (see *error variance*)

Yates' correction for continuity.   In the chi square test, a correction factor applied when expected frequencies are too small, effectively reducing the chi square statistic. (25)

z-score.   The number of standard deviations that a given value is above or below the mean of the distribution; also called a standardized score. (17)

zero-order correlation.   A bivariate correlation. (27)

Glossary of Statistical Symbols and Abbreviations

Numbers in parentheses indicate the chapter in which the term is introduced.

Greek Letters

α	(alpha) Predetermined level of significance, usually set at .05; denotes risk of Type I error, or risk of falsely rejecting the null hypothesis (18)
α_1, α_2	One-tailed and two-tailed levels of significance, respectively (18)
α_{FW}	Familywise level of significance for a multiple comparison procedure; denotes risk of Type I error for a set (or family) of contrasts (21)
α_{PC}	Per comparison level of significance for a multiple comparison procedure; denotes risk of Type I error for each individual contrast (21)
β	(beta) Probability associated with Type II error, or risk of falsely accepting a null hypothesis (18)
ϵ	(epsilon) Statistic associated with repeated measures analysis of variance, used to adjust degrees of freedom to correct for unequal variances in the Greenhouse–Geisser and Huyhn–Feldt corrections (20)
θ	(theta) Effect size for proportions, used in sequential clinical trials (11)
κ	(kappa) Chance-corrected measure of agreement (26)
κ_W	Weighted kappa (26)
λ	(lambda) 1. A measure of association between categorical variables (25) 2. Index used to estimate power in multiple regression (App. C)
μ	(mu) Mean of a population (17)
ρ	(rho) Correlation coefficient for a population (23)
ϕ	(phi) Phi coefficient (23,25)
σ	(sigma) Standard deviation of a population (17)
σ^2	(sigma squared) Variance of population (17)
$\sigma_{\bar{X}}$	Standard error of the mean for a population (18)
Σ	(capital sigma) Read: "the sum of" (17)
χ^2	(chi square) Test of significance for nominal data; compares observed frequencies against a theoretical distribution (25)
χ^2_r	Test statistic for Friedman's two-way analysis of variance by ranks (22)

Abbreviations

a	Y-intercept (regression constant) in the equation for a straight line or regression equation (24)

ANOVA	Analysis of variance (20)
ANCOVA	Analysis of covariance (24)
AR	Attributable risk (15)
b	Regression coefficient in a regression equation; the slope of the regression line (24)
c	Number of comparisons within a multiple comparison procedure (21)
C	1. Contingency coefficient; measures degree of association in a contingency table. (25) 2. Number of columns in a contingency table (25)
CI	1. Confidence interval. (18,19) 2. Cumulative incidence (15)
CV	Coefficient of variation; expresses ratio of standard deviation to the mean, in percent (17,26)
d	1. Difference score. (19,22) 2. Effect size index for the t-test (Appendix C)
$\bar{d}$	Mean of a set of different scores (19)
D	Discriminant function score (27)
df	Degrees of freedom (18)
df_b	Degrees of freedom for the between-groups source of variance in analysis of variance (20)
df_e	Degrees of freedom for the error term (within-groups source of variance) in analysis of variance (20)
df_t	Total degrees of freedom (20)
f	1. Frequency. (17) 2. Effect size index for analysis of variance (Appendix C)
F	Test statistic for the analysis of variance (20)
H	Test statistic for the Kruskal–Wallis two-way analysis of variance by ranks (22)
H_0	Null hypothesis (18)
H_1	Alternative hypothesis (18)
HSD	Tukey's honestly significant difference multiple comparison test (21)
ICC	Intraclass correlation coefficient (26)
k	Number of independent groups (or means) in an analysis (20)
MANOVA	Multivariate analysis of variance (27)
ME	Method error (26)
MS	Mean square in an analysis of variance (20)
MS_b	Between-groups mean square (20)
MS_e	Error mean square, or within-groups mean square (20)
n	1. Number of subjects in a single sample (used in single-sample analyses) or in subgroups of a larger sample. (17) 2. Number of pairs in correlation or regression analyses (23)
N	Number of subjects in a population or total sample (17)
NK	Newman–Keuls multiple comparison test (21)
OR	Odds ratio (15)
p	1. Probability; represents the probability of Type I error associated with a specific test of significance. (18) 2. Number of means in a multiple comparison test. (21) 3. Number of independent variables in a multivariate analysis. (27) 4. Proportion of attribute X in a binomial distribution (23)

P	**1.** Percentile. (17) **2.** Prevalence (15)
q	**1.** Studentized range statistic, used in multiple comparison tests. (21)
Q	Quartile (17)
r	**1.** Pearson product–moment coefficient of correlation. (23) **2.** Range of ordered means in a multiple comparison test (21)
r^2	Coefficient of determination (correlation coefficient squared) (24)
r_S	Spearman rank correlation coefficient (23)
$r_{XY \cdot Z}$	First-order partial correlation of X and Y, with values of Z held constant (27)
r_{pb}	Point biserial correlation coefficient (23)
r_{rb}	Rank biserial correlation coefficient (23)
R	**1.** Multiple correlation coefficient, generated by a multiple regression analysis. (27) **2.** Number of rows in a contingency table. (25) **3.** Rank sum in nonparametric tests (22)
R^2	Multiple correlation coefficient squared; represents the proportion of variance in Y accounted for by several independent variables in a multiple regression analysis (27)
RR	Relative risk (15)
s	Standard deviation of a sample (17)
s^2	Variance of a sample (17)
s_d	Standard deviation of a set of difference scores (19)
$s_{\bar{d}}$	Standard error of a set of difference scores (19)
s_p^2	Pooled variance estimate (19)
$s_{\bar{X}}$	Standard error of the mean for a sample (18)
$s_{\bar{X}_1 - \bar{X}_2}$	Standard error of the difference between the means; used in calculation of the unpaired t-test and confidence intervals for differences between means (19)
SEE	Standard error of the estimate (24,27)
SEM	Standard error of measurement (26)
SS	Sum of squares (17,20)
SS$_b$	Between-groups sum of squares (20)
SS$_e$	Sum of squares for the error term, or within-groups sum of squares (20)
SS$_t$	Total sum of squares (20)
t	Test statistic for the comparison of two means (19)
$t(B)$	Test statistic for Bonferroni's multiple comparison (21)
T	**1.** Test statistic for the rank sum test. (22) **2.** Test statistic for the Wilcoxon signed-ranks test (22)
U	Test statistic for the Mann–Whitney U test (22)
V	Cramer's V coefficient, a measure of association for categorical variables (25)
$\bar{V}$	Mean vector in a multivariate analysis of variance (27)
x	Test statistic for the sign test, representing the number of scores with fewer signs (22)
X	**1.** A single score or datum. (17) **2.** An independent variable (7,24,27)
$\bar{X}$	Mean of a sample (17)

$\bar{X}_G$	Grand mean for a total sample composed of several subgroups; used in calculation of deviation scores for the analysis of variance (20)
Y	A dependent variable (7,24,27)
$\bar{Y}$	Mean for a sample of scores on variable Y (27)
$\hat{Y}$	Predicted value of the dependent variable in a regression equation (24,27)
z	Standardized score (17,18)

Symbols

$\approx$	Approximately equal to
$\neq$	Does not equal
$>, <$	Greater than, less than
$\geqslant, >=$	Greater than or equal to
$\leqslant, <=$	Less than or equal to
$\lvert X \rvert$	Absolute value of X without regard to sign

Index